Adult Emergency Medicine at a Glance

Thomas Hughes
Bt.MSC, MBA, MRCP, FRCS, FCEM
Consultant Emergency Physician
John Radcliffe Hospital, Oxford
Honorary Senior Lecturer in Emergency Medicine
University of Oxford

Jaycen Cruickshank
MCR, FACEM
Director of Emergency Medicine
Ballarat Health Services, Victoria, Australia
Senior Lecturer in Emergency Medicine
University of Melbourne, Victoria, Australia

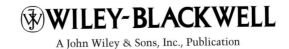
WILEY-BLACKWELL
A John Wiley & Sons, Inc., Publication

Library of Congress Cataloging-in-Publication Data
Hughes, Thomas, MSc.
Adult emergency medicine at a glance / Thomas Hughes, Jaycen Cruickshank.
p. ; cm.
Includes index.
ISBN 978-1-4051-8901-9
1. Emergency medicine--Handbooks, manuals, etc. I. Cruickshank, Jaycen. II. Title.
[DNLM: 1. Emergency Medicine--methods--Handbooks. 2. Adult. WB 105 H894a 2011]
RC86.8.H84 2011
616.02'5--dc22
2010024551

ISBN: 9781405189019

A catalogue record for this book is available from the British Library.

Set in 9 on 11.5 pt Times by Toppan Best-set Premedia Limited
Printed and bound in Malaysia by Vivar Printing Sdn Bhd

1 2011

Adult Emergency Medicine at a Glance

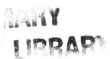

Contents

Preface

Emergency Medicine has undergone a quiet revolution over the past twenty years due to a variety of factors that have changed the way medicine is practiced.
- Increasing demand and expectations of medical care.
- Reduction of junior doctors' hours.
- An ageing population.
- Fragmentation of out of hours care.
- Reduced hospital bed-stay.
- Sub-specialisation of inpatient medical and surgical practice.
- Litigation.

These factors have pushed expert decision-making towards the front door of the hospital so that the correct diagnosis and treatment start as soon as possible in the patient's journey. As other specialties have moved away from the acute assessment and treatment of patients, Emergency Medicine has expanded to fill the vacuum left, and in doing so has increased its realm of practice substantially.

Emergency Medicine is exciting and confronting, intimidating and liberating – it is the chance to exercise and hone your diagnostic and practical skills in a well-supervised environment.

Clinical staff who work in the ED have all been through the inevitable feelings of fear, uncertainty and doubt that come with the territory, and want you to experience the enjoyment and satisfaction of working in an area of medicine that is never boring.

When trainees start Emergency Medicine, it is often the first time they have seen patients before any other staff. To use a traditional analogy, they have seen plenty of needles, and may be very good at recognising them, but now they are faced with haystacks, in which may be hidden a variety of sharp shiny objects.

Medical textbooks usually describe topics by *anatomy* or *pathology* (needles), e.g. heart failure, which tends to assume the diagnostic process. In this book we have tried to organise topics by *presentation* (haystacks), e.g. 'short of breath', and have tried to articulate the key features that help us find the needles.

We are both great fans of the 'At a Glance' series, and have enjoyed the challenge of combining the breadth of practice of adult Emergency Medicine with the concise nature of the 'At a Glance' format. We hope you enjoy this book and find it useful as you explore this most dynamic area of medicine.

Acknowledgements

We would like to thank Karen Moore and Laura Murphy at Wiley-Blackwell for their support and advice (and let's face it, patience) during the elephantine gestation of the book. Also Helen Harvey for understanding deadlines, and Jane Fallows for doing such a great job with the illustrations. We thank the students of Oxford and Melbourne Universities, whose inquiring minds keep us on our toes, and whose questions stimulated us to think of new ways to present the information we have used here. We are both lucky enough to have worked with an exceptional colleague, Philip Catterson, whose teamwork, leadership and hard work have helped us to achieve success in our jobs, and from whom we have learned the few interpersonal skills we have.

In addition TH would like to thank: Professor Christopher Bulstrode who has been an inspiration and mentor and without whose support the book would not have happened. My family, and particularly my wife Marina for her support. My work colleagues for continuing to tolerate me most of the time, and Jackie and Tracey, the ED secretaries who keep me in order. Nic Weir, Rob Janas and David Bowden for their help in sourcing images and the final preparation.

JC would like to thank: All the people who have taught me along the way, particularly Trevor Jackson and Steven Pincus. My parents Ron and Christine for making everything possible, and my wife Kerry and sons Jesse and Flynn for making everything worthwhile.

Thomas Hughes
Jaycen Cruickshank

List of abbreviations

AAA	abdominal aortic aneurysm		ED	Emergency Department
ABC	airway, breathing, circulation		EDTA	ethylene diamine tetraacetate
ABCD^2	acronym to assess stroke risk in a patient with TIA		ELISA	enzyme-linked immunosorbent assay
ABCDE	airway, breathing, circulation, disability, exposure		ENT	ear, nose and throat
ABG	arterial blood gases		EPL	extensor pollicis longus
ACE	angiotensin-converting enzyme		ESR	erythrocyte sedimentation rate
ACh	acetylcholine		ETT	endotracheal tube
ACJ	acromioclavicular joint		FAST	acronym for focused abdominal sonography in trauma; also face, arm, speech, time to call ambulance
ACL	anterior cruciate ligament of knee			
ACS	acute coronary syndrome		FB	foreign body
ACTH	adrenocorticotrophic hormone		FBC/FBE	full blood count/examination
AD	aortic dissection		FiO$_2$	fraction of inspired of oxygen (as %)
AF	atrial fibrillation		FFP	fresh frozen plasma
AIDS	acquired immunodeficiency syndrome		FOOSH	fall onto an outstretched hand
AMT4	four-point abbreviated mental test score		GA	general anaesthetic
AP	antero-posterior		GAβHS	group A β-haemolytic *Streptococcus*
APL	abductor pollicis longus		GCS	Glasgow Coma Scale/Score
AV	arteriovenous; also atrioventricular		GI	gastrointestinal
AVN	atrioventricular node		GP	general practitioner
AXR	abdominal X-ray		H1N1	swine flu virus
BDZ	benzodiazepine		H5N1	avian flu virus
BP	blood pressure		HbA$_{1c}$	glycated (glycosylated) haemoglobin
bpm	beats per minute		HCO$_3^-$	bicarbonate ion
CAGE	acronym for alcohol screening questions		hCG	human chorionic gonadotrophin
CAP	community-acquired pneumonia		HDU	high dependency unit
cAMP	cyclic adenonsine monophosphate		HHS	hyperosmolar hyperglycaemic state
CBRNE	chemical, biological, radiological, nuclear, explosive		HIV	human immunodeficiency virus
			HOCM	hypertrophic obstructive cardiomyopathy
CK	creatine kinase		HONK	hyperosmolar non-ketotic acidosis
CNS	central nervous system		HR	heart rate
CO	carbon monoxide		HVZ	herpes varicella zoster
COHb	carboxyhaemoglobin		IBS	irritable bowel syndrome
COPD	chronic obstructive pulmonary disease		ICP	intracranial pressure
CPAP	continuous positive airway pressure		ICU	intensive care unit
CPP	cerebral perfusion pressure		IgE	immunoglobulin E
CPR	cardiopulmonary resuscitation		IVDU	intravenous drug use
CRAO	central retinal artery occlusion		IVF	in vitro fertilisation
CRP	C-reactive protein		IVRA	intravenous regional anaesthesia
CRVO	central retinal vein occlusion		IVU	intravenous urogram
CT	computed tomography		JVP	jugular venous pressure
CTPA	CT pulmonary angiography		KUB	kidneys, ureters and bladder
CURB-65	confusion, urea, respiratory rate, blood pressure, age over 65 (acronym for pneumonia severity factors)		LA	local anaesthetic
			LCL	lateral collateral ligament of knee
			LFT	liver function test
			LMP	last menstrual period
CVP	central venous pressure		LNMP	last normal menstrual period
CXR	chest X-ray; also unit for X-ray dose, 1 CXR ≈ 3 days' background radiation		LOC	loss of consciousness
			LP	lumbar puncture
			LR	likelihood ratio
DIPJ	distal interphalangeal joint		LRTI	lower respiratory tract infection
DKA	diabetic ketoacidosis		MAOI	monoamine oxidase inhibitor
DM	diabetes mellitus		MAP	mean arterial pressure
DSH	deliberate self-harm		MCL	medial collateral ligament of knee
DUMBELS	diarrhoea, urination, miosis, bronchorrhoea/bronchospasm, emesis, lacrimation, salivation (acronym for clinical effects of organophosphate poisoning)		MCPJ	metacarpophalangeal joint
			MDI	metered dose inhaler
DVT	deep vein thrombosis			

MI	myocardial infarction		**RoSC**	return of spontaneous circulation
MR	magnetic resonance		**SAH**	subarachnoid haemorrhage
N₂O	nitrous oxide		**SAN**	sinoatrial node
NAC	*N*-acetylcysteine		**SARS**	severe acute respiratory syndrome
NICE	National Institute for Health and Clinical Excellence		**SDH**	subdural haematoma
NIV	non-invasive ventilation		**SoB**	short(ness) of breath
NNT	number needed to treat		**SOCRATES**	acronym for pain history
NNH	number needed to harm		**SOL**	space-occupying lesion
#NoF	fractured neck of femur		**SSRI**	selective serotonin reuptake inhibitor
NSAID	non-steroidal anti-inflammatory drug		**STD**	sexually transmitted disease
NSTEMI	non-ST segment elevation myocardial infarction		**STEMI**	ST segment elevation myocardial infarction
OD	overdose		**STI**	sexually transmitted infection
OP	organophosphate		**SVT**	supraventricular tachycardia
OPG	oral pantomogram		**TBSA**	total body surface area
ORIF	open reduction and internal fixation		**TCA**	tricyclic antidepressant
PA	postero-anterior		**TFT**	thyroid function test
PCL	posterior cruciate ligament of knee		**TIA**	transient ischaemic attack
PE	pulmonary embolism		**TIMI**	thrombolysis in myocardial infarction
PEA	pulseless electrical activity		**TMT**	tarsometatarsal
PEF	peak expiratory flow		**tPA**	tissue plasminogen activator
PEFR	peak expiratory flow rate		**U + E**	urea and electrolytes
PID	pelvic inflammatory disease		**UA**	unstable angina
PPCI	primary percutaneous coronary intervention		**URTI**	upper respiratory tract infection
PPI	proton pump inhibitor		**UTI**	urinary tract infection
PPM	permanent pacemaker		**VBG**	venous blood gases
PR	per rectum		**VF**	ventricular fibrillation
PT	prothrombin time		**V/Q**	ventilation/perfusion
PV	per vaginam		**VT**	ventricular tachycardia
RA	regional anaesthesia		**VVS**	vasovagal syncope
RBBB	right bundle branch block		**WCC**	white cell count

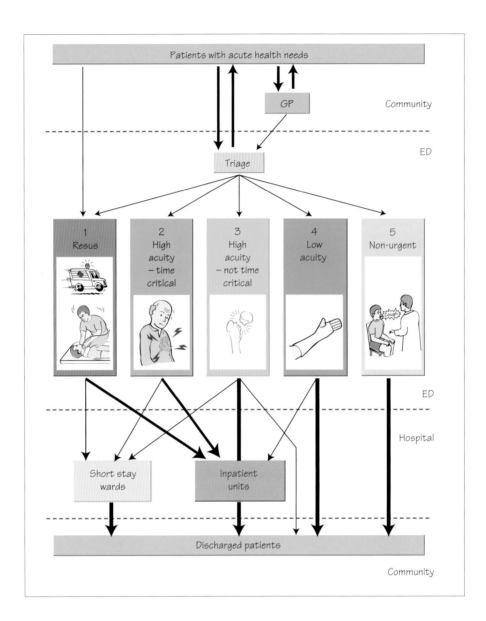

This chapter describes the way the Emergency Department operates, and some of the unwritten rules. The prevalence of Emergency Department-based drama generates plenty of misconceptions about what occurs in the Emergency Department. For instance, it is generally inadvisable to say 'stat' at the end of one's sentences, and neither of the authors has been mistaken for George Clooney!

What happens when a patient arrives at the Emergency Department?

Alert phone

Also known as the 'red phone' or sometimes 'the Bat-phone', this is the dedicated phone line that the ambulance service uses to pre-warn the Emergency Department of incoming patients likely to need resuscitation.

Triage

The concept of triage comes from military medicine – doing the most good for the most people. This ensures the most effective use of limited resources, and that the most unwell patients are seen first.

Nurses rather than doctors are usually used to perform the triage because doctors tend to start treating patients. Systems of rapid assessment and early treatment by senior medical staff can be effective, but risk diverting attention from the most ill patients.

Reception/registration
The reception staff are essential to the function of the Emergency Department: they register patients on the hospital computer system, source old notes and keep an eye on the waiting room. They have to deal with difficult and demanding patients, and are good at spotting the sick or deteriorating patient in the waiting room.

Waiting room
Adult and paediatric patients should have separate waiting rooms, and some sort of entertainment is a good idea. Aggression and dissatisfaction in waiting patients has been largely eliminated in the UK by the 4-hour standard of care: all patients must be seen and discharged from the Emergency Department within 4 hours.

Treatment areas in the Emergency Department
Resuscitation bays
Resuscitation bays are used for critically ill and unstable patients with potentially life-threatening illness. They have advanced monitoring facilities, and plenty of space around the patient for clinical staff to perform procedures. X-rays can be performed within this area.

High acuity area
This is the area where patients who are unwell or injured, but who do not need a resuscitation bay, are managed. Medical conditions and elderly patients with falls are common presentations in this area.

Low acuity area
The 'walking wounded' – patients with non-life-threatening wounds and limb injuries – are seen here. Patients with minor illness are discouraged from coming to the Emergency Department, but continue to do so for a variety of reasons.

There is a common misconception that patients in this area are similar to general practice or family medicine patients. Numerous studies have found that there is an admission rate of about 5% and an appreciable mortality in low acuity patients, whereas only about 1% of GP consultations result in immediate hospital admission.

Other areas
Imaging
Imaging, such as X-rays and ultrasound, are integral to Emergency Department function. Larger Emergency Departments have their own CT scanner.

Relatives' room
When dealing with the relatives of a critically ill patient and breaking bad news, doctors and relatives need a quiet area where information is communicated and digested. This room needs to be close to the resuscitation area.

Observation/short stay ward
This is a ward area close to the Emergency Department, run by Emergency Department staff. This unit treats patients who would otherwise need hospital admission for a short time, to enable them to be fully stabilised and assessed. The function of these units is described in Chapter 28.

Hospital in the home
Some hospitals run a 'hospital in the home' programme for patients who do not need to be in hospital but who need certain therapy, e.g. intravenous antibiotics, anticoagulation. The Emergency Department is the natural interface between home and hospital.

Culture of the Emergency Department
There is a much flatter (less hierarchical) organisational structure in the Emergency Department than most other areas in the hospital. This occurs because all levels of medical, nursing and other staff work together all the time, and the department cannot function without their cooperation. Ensuring good teamwork requires good leadership, an atmosphere of mutual respect and a bit of patience and understanding.

The resulting atmosphere can be one of the most enjoyable and satisfying places to work in a hospital. A feature of this less hierarchical culture that surprises junior doctors is that nurses will question their decisions; this is a sign of a healthy culture in which errors are less likely to occur, and is actively encouraged.

Emergency Department rules
Being a doctor in the Emergency Department is different from elsewhere in the hospital. There is nowhere to hide and, for the first time in most medical careers, you are responsible for making the decisions. On the positive side, there are plenty of people around to help you, who have all been through the same process.

Some basic advice:
- Write legible, timed, dated notes.
- Show respect for other professional groups and be prepared to learn from them.
- Do not be late for your shifts; do not call in sick less than 6 hours before a shift.
- Patients who re-present are high risk and need senior review.
- Take your breaks. You need them.
- Keep calm.
- If in doubt, ask.
- Do not pick up so many patients that you cannot keep track of them.
- Do not avoid work or avoid seeing difficult patients. We do notice.
- The nurse in charge is usually right.

With so many people working closely together in a stressful atmosphere, it is inevitable that conflicts will occur. Do not let them fester; some ground rules for resolving such conflicts are:
- Resolve it now.
- Do it in private.
- Do it face to face.
- Focus on facts.
- Criticise action, not person.
- Agree why it is important.
- Agree on a remedy.
- Finish on a positive.

A type of d-dimer test has a specificity of 50% and a sensitivity of 95%: this allows you to calculate the likelihood ratios to rule a condition in (+LR) or out (−LR)

$$+LR = \frac{Sn}{1-Sp} = \frac{0.95}{1-0.5} = 1.9 \qquad -LR = \frac{1-Sn}{Sn} = \frac{1-0.95}{0.5} = 0.1$$

A woman presents with a history suggestive of DVT, and her probability of having a DVT is low; about 5%, according to the Wells score (see Ch. 35).
The d-dimer test comes back negative.
What is the chance she has a DVT?

If the d-dimer test had come back positive, what is the chance she has a DVT?

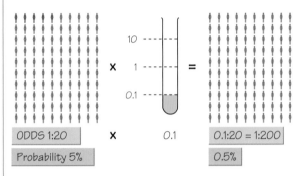

| ODDS 1:20 | × | 0.1 | 0.1:20 = 1:200 |
| Probability 5% | | | 0.5% |

The result (0.5%) is the risk of missing a DVT in **this patient**. Bearing in mind that no test is perfect, a result below 1% is generally taken as an acceptable level of risk

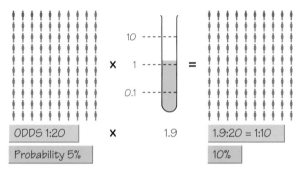

| ODDS 1:20 | × | 1.9 | 1.9:20 = 1:10 |
| Probability 5% | | | 10% |

Despite the positive d-dimer, this patient only has a **10%** chance of having a DVT

This shows that this d-dimer test is useful for excluding a DVT in a low-risk population, but that a positive test does not mean a DVT is present

A patient who has been immobile following a recent operation for cancer has pain in his lower leg. You assess his risk of DVT as about 50%, but the test comes back negative. What is the probability he has a DVT?

A young man with mild suprapubic pain, whom you estimate has a 1% chance of having a UTI, has a positive urine leucocyte test (+ LR = 5) on dipstick testing. What is the chance he has a UTI?

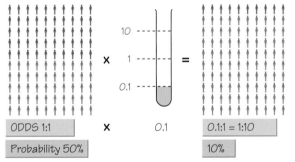

| ODDS 1:1 | × | 0.1 | 0.1:1 = 1:10 |
| Probability 50% | | | 10% |

Despite a negative d-dimer, he still has a 10% chance of having a DVT. D-dimer cannot 'rule out' DVT in a high risk patient

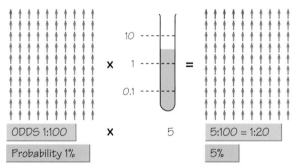

| ODDS 1:100 | × | 5 | 5:100 = 1:20 |
| Probability 1% | | | 5% |

Despite a positive test with a fairly high + LR he still only has a 5% chance of having a UTI because the condition was so unlikely in the first place

---

The Emergency Department is a diagnosis machine, taking people with a wide variety of symptoms, labelling them with a diagnosis, treating and then discharging them whenever safe to do so. There are plenty of opportunities for this process to go wrong, and it is important to understand how this can occur.

> 'If you listen carefully to the patient, they will tell you the diagnosis'. W Osler

Despite a couple of thousand years of medical education, we are still not really sure how the diagnostic process works.
- Some people work forward from history, examination and a shortlist of differential diagnoses.
- Others work backwards from a list of likely diagnoses to weight these according to symptoms and examination.
- Experts make their diagnoses by pattern recognition.

It may be that expertise occurs with the development of cognitive flexibility to use multiple diagnostic strategies to integrate and test the result.

Using tests

In the past, the Emergency Department used a few simple tests to inform decision-making. An X-ray of an injured limb has a binary outcome: broken/ not broken. As technology and the scope of Emergency Medicine has increased, the tests have become more numerous and less black and white, and there is a need to rationalise and manage the uncertainty generated.

The most common way of describing a test's performance is to use *sensitivity* and *specificity*.

Confusion matrix

Test result	Actual patient status (truth)	
	Disease present	Disease absent
Positive	True positive (A)	False positive (B)
Negative	False negative (C)	True negative (D)
Total no. patients	With disorder (A + C)	Without disorder (B + D)
	Sensitivity = A/(A + C) and	**Specificity = D/(B + D)**

For example, if a very *specific* test, e.g. Troponin I, is positive, we know that myocardial damage has occurred, because the number of false positives (B) is very low. Similarly, if a very *sensitive* test, e.g. CT scan for abdominal aortic aneurysm (AAA), comes back as negative, we know that it is very unlikely that the patient has an AAA as the number of false negatives (C) will be very low.

> **SpIN** – a very Specific test rules a condition **IN**.
> **SnOUT** – a very Sensitive test rules a condition **OUT**.

However, Emergency Departments use many tests that are not 100% sensitive or specific, and therefore a more powerful, but less intuitive, model is necessary to understand these tests: *likelihood ratios*, which are calculated from the specificity and sensitivity.

Treatment orders

Once the likely diagnosis has been made, a set of treatment orders needs to be decided and documented. A good acronym for this is DAVID, e.g., for an elderly patient with an open fracture of the tibia:
- **D**iet – nil by mouth
- **A**ctivities – elevate limb
- **V**ital signs monitoring – hourly limb observations
- **I**nvestigations – CXR, FBC, U+E
- **D**rugs/treatment – immediate i.v. antibiotics

Bayes' theorem

The chance of something being true or false depends not only on the quality of the test that one is performing, but *importantly*, how likely the event is in the first place.

Thomas Bayes, an eighteenth-century English priest, deduced the principles that underpin the way we use tests in medicine:

pre-test probability × likelihood ratio = post-test probability

To calculate this, we use odds (like horse racing odds) rather than probability, but the two are obviously very closely related.

The likelihood ratio is calculated from the test's sensitivity (Sn) and specificity (Sp) and is a much better measure of a test's clinical usefulness in ruling a disease in (positive LR) or out (negative LR).

$$+LR = \frac{Sn}{1-Sp} \qquad -LR = \frac{1-Sn}{Sp}$$

How do I define pre-test probability?

The triage process uses an expert nurse to assess clinical status and is an assessment of the probability of serious illness. The fact that a patient has arrived at the Emergency Department at all, rather than going to their own doctor, automatically means the probability of significant disease is relatively high.

Clinical decision rules are widespread in Emergency Medicine and help codify knowledge and explicitly define pre-test probability. However, unthinking application of such decision-support tools by clinicians without an appreciation of their flaws and limitations results in bad decisions and/or over-investigation.

A history and examination taken by an experienced clinician remains a very good predictor of pre-test probability of disease. As can be seen opposite, a test applied in an inappropriate population group, i.e. with a pre-test probability that is very high or very low, will give misleading results. Tests are best used in populations with an intermediate probability.

Using likelihood ratios in practice

It helps to think of the likelihood ratio as a multiplier that tells you how much more or less likely a disease is, once you have the result.

The particular advantage of likelihood ratios over other measures of a test's performance is that, as shown opposite, they can easily be applied to individual patients, not just populations.

A good test for ruling in a condition has a positive likelihood ratio of more than 10, meaning that if the patient has a positive test, it is 10 times more likely that they have the disease as a result of the positive test.

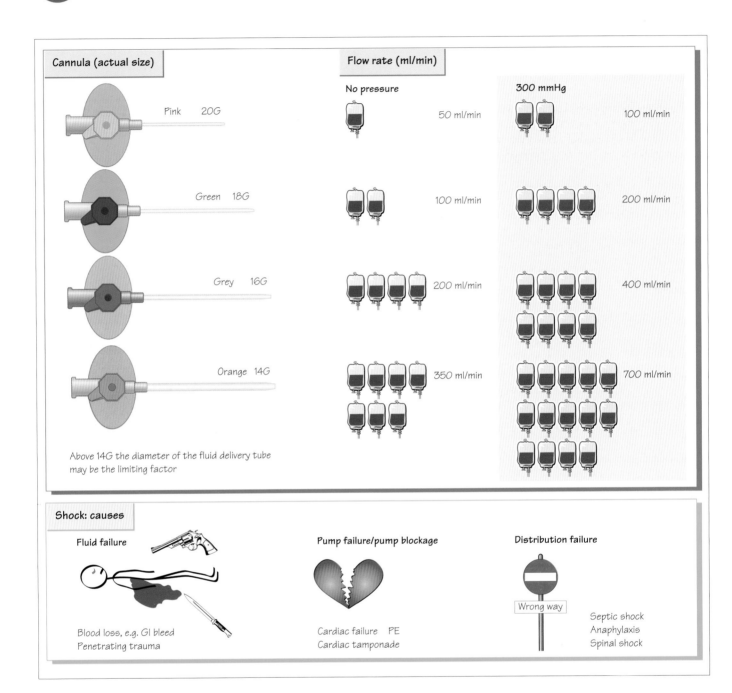

Cannula (actual size)

Pink   20G
Green   18G
Grey   16G
Orange 14G

Above 14G the diameter of the fluid delivery tube
may be the limiting factor

Flow rate (ml/min)

No pressure

50 ml/min
100 ml/min
200 ml/min
350 ml/min

300 mmHg

100 ml/min
200 ml/min
400 ml/min
700 ml/min

Shock: causes

Fluid failure

Blood loss, e.g. GI bleed
Penetrating trauma

Pump failure/pump blockage

Cardiac failure   PE
Cardiac tamponade

Distribution failure

Wrong way

Septic shock
Anaphylaxis
Spinal shock

Intravenous fluid therapy is a common medical treatment, but recently there has been a reassessment of the role of intravenous fluids as some of the hazards have become better understood.

Intravenous access

Poiseulle's Law governing fluid flow through a tube (assuming laminar flow):

$$Flow \propto \frac{Pr^4}{\eta L}$$

where P = pressure difference, r = radius, η = viscosity, L = length.

Therefore the ideal resuscitation fluid should be non-viscous, driven by pressure through a short, wide cannula. For resuscitation, or when giving blood (viscous), a 16 G or larger cannula is preferred. The large veins in the antecubital fossa and the femoral vein are good for resuscitation but are prone to infection and uncomfortable for patients in the long term. A pressure bag inflated to 300 mmHg doubles fluid flow.

Before cannulation the skin should be thoroughly cleaned using chlorhexidine in alcohol. A cannula in the forearm is (relatively) comfortable for the patient and less likely to become infected compared to other sites.

Special cases
• *Central lines* are very useful in very sick patients, patients with poor access or patients whose fluid balance is particularly difficult to regulate. Their length means that they are not ideal for delivering resuscitation fluids. Introducer sheaths offer a large bore central access.
• *Intraosseus needles* have to be drilled into adult bone to give fluid, but can be life-saving. Bone marrow aspirate may be used for blood cross-matching.
• *Venous cut-down* involves cutting the skin to be able to cannulate a vein under direct vision. The long saphenous vein 1 cm above and anterior to the medial malleolus, or the basilic vein in the antecubital fossa, are the most common sites for this.

Types of intravenous fluids
Crystalloids
Normal saline, Hartmann's solution and Ringer's lactate are solutions that match plasma osmolality. All can be used to resuscitate patients, and despite vigorous debate, no one variety has proven superior clinical outcomes.

Dextrose
50% dextrose is used to resuscitate hypoglycaemic patients. 10% dextrose is used to maintain a patient's blood sugar and prevent hypoglycaemia, and 5% is used to give 'free water' to avoid overloading with sodium or chloride.

Colloids
Colloids contain large molecules that help retain fluid within the intravascular space, which improves blood pressure in the short term. Unfortunately these molecules leak out of damaged capillaries, which may cause resistant oedema in the brain and lungs, which increases mortality in head-injured patients. Colloids may be helpful in sepsis, but should only be used by senior doctors.

Blood
A full cross-match takes 30 minutes but type-specific blood should be available within minutes. If blood is needed before the blood type is known, Group O Rhesus negative blood is used.

Whole blood as donated is the best substitute in trauma, but has a short shelf life (days). Separating blood cells into 'packed cells' extends storage time to 3 months, but deterioration may mean that the cells are not fully functional for 24 hours. The citrate used to stabilise blood binds calcium ions, which can cause problems in massive transfusions (>50% blood volume).

Fresh frozen plasma (FFP) or synthetic clotting factors can be used to correct clotting problems. Tranexamic acid, platelets and FFP are given as part of massive transfusion protocol.

Temperature
Evolution has given humans enzymes that function best at 37°C and pH ≈ 7.4. Blood clotting is impaired in a cold acidotic patient, e.g. trauma patient. Temperature <34°C and pH < 7.20 reduce clotting to 1% of normal. Laboratory measurements at 37°C will not accurately reflect the clinical picture. For this reason, clotting factors are given early in trauma resuscitation. Cold fluids (4°C) may be given after cardiac resuscitation as part of an active cooling strategy to preserve brain function.

Shock
Shock is defined as inadequate tissue perfusion, i.e. not meeting the metabolic demands of tissue. Pulse and blood pressure are bedside measures of tissue perfusion, but are insensitive. pH, PCO$_2$, lactate and mixed venous blood oxygen levels, measured from a central venous pressure (CVP) line, are better indicators.

Types of shock
The body pumps a limited amount of fluid around a series of closed loops. Problems occur when the fluid disappears, the pump fails or the fluid goes to the wrong loops.

Blood failure
Blood loss may be controlled or uncontrolled, internal or external. Severe dehydration may cause similar problems.

Pump failure
The heart may fail due to internal pump problems, e.g. myocardial infarction or heart failure, which impair the ability to pump. Alternatively the pump may fail because there is inflow obstruction (cardiac tamponade, tension pneumothorax) or outflow obstruction (pulmonary embolus, aortic dissection).

Distribution failure
Blood may be distributed to the wrong organs. Inappropriate vasodilation occurs in septic shock, anaphylaxis and spinal shock (due to loss of sympathetic tone below the injury) diverting blood away from vital organs.

Grades of shock
Compensated shock   BP → HR ↑
Young adults are able to compensate for loss of blood volume by vasoconstriction and increased cardiac output, maintaining a good BP and perfusion of vital organs.
Decompensated shock   BP ↓ HR ↑
The body's compensation mechanisms are overwhelmed, and the blood pressure falls rapidly.

Fluid resuscitation
Traditional teaching: 'Fill 'em up'
• Good blood pressure = good outcome.
• Poor blood pressure = poor outcome.
• Therefore give fluid/blood to achieve good blood pressure.
Unfortunately this is an oversimplification. Short-term poor perfusion is well tolerated and if blood loss has *not* been controlled:
• ↑ blood pressure = ↑ blood loss.
Increased blood loss is due to loss of vasospasm, dilution of clotting factors and dislodgement of clot.

Current teaching: 'minimal volume fluid resuscitation'
If there is *uncontrolled bleeding* (e.g. penetrating trauma, ruptured AAA), large-bore intravenous access is obtained. The minimum volume of fluid necessary to maintain cerebral perfusion or a systolic BP of 60–80 mmHg is used ('permissive hypotension'). The priority is urgent control of bleeding in the operating theatre.
Exception: if there is brain injury, the need to maintain cerebral perfusion pressure overrides hypotensive resuscitation.

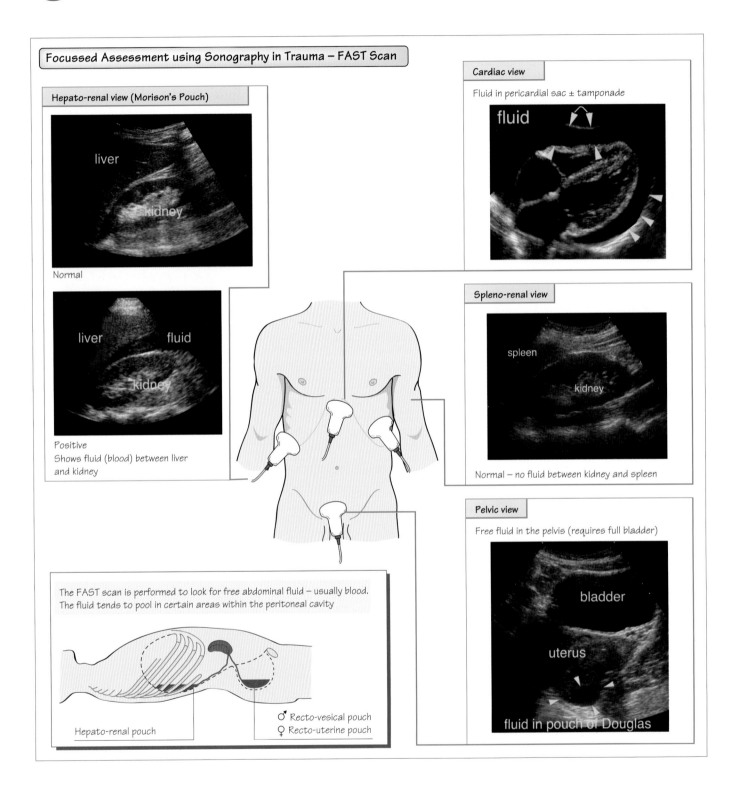

Focussed Assessment using Sonography in Trauma – FAST Scan

Hepato-renal view (Morison's Pouch)

liver

kidney

Normal

liver   fluid

kidney

Positive
Shows fluid (blood) between liver and kidney

Cardiac view

Fluid in pericardial sac ± tamponade

fluid

Spleno-renal view

spleen

kidney

Normal – no fluid between kidney and spleen

Pelvic view

Free fluid in the pelvis (requires full bladder)

bladder

uterus

fluid in pouch of Douglas

The FAST scan is performed to look for free abdominal fluid – usually blood. The fluid tends to pool in certain areas within the peritoneal cavity

Hepato-renal pouch

♂ Recto-vesical pouch
♀ Recto-uterine pouch

Imaging use in the Emergency Department has increased rapidly over the past few years due to technical advances and increasing pressure to move decision-making earlier in a patient's journey, and to prevent unnecessary hospital admissions. Ultrasound is now a core skill for senior Emergency Department doctors and new hospitals often have a CT scanner in the Emergency Department.

Plain radiography

Plain radiographs interpreted by the treating clinician are used for the majority of Emergency Department imaging. The advent of digital radiography has made real-time reporting by radiologists easier.

X-rays are ionising radiation and cause damage to tissues through which they pass. The energy released is proportional to the density of the tissue. Abdominal or thoracolumbar radiographs should not be performed in young people, especially females, without a very good reason, as the gonads are very radio-sensitive. In this book, X-ray doses are expressed in terms of chest radiographs (CXR). One CXR is approximately 3 days of background radiation.

X-rays are not therapeutic. If the result will not change management, radiographs should not be taken. Examples include uncomplicated rib fractures (when not worried about a pneumothorax), coccyx pain and stubbed toes other than the big toe. Soft tissues are poorly shown by plain films, making it an insensitive examination for joints that rely on these for stability, e.g. knee, shoulder.

Reading plain radiographs

1 Check the patient's name and the date of the film, particularly on digital radiography systems, which offer many opportunities for confusion.
2 There should be two good views of limbs: anterior-posterior and lateral.
3 If requesting imaging of more than one area, ask yourself if this is necessary. If not urgent, it may be better to re-examine the patient once they have had some analgesia, or obtain a senior opinion.
4 You will learn more from your radiology department if you engage with them and ask their advice rather than expecting a purely technical service.
5 Many Emergency Departments operate a system whereby the radiographer can flag an abnormality on the radiograph. You should not dismiss something that the radiographer has flagged as abnormal without obtaining a senior opinion.

Clinical ultrasound

Clinical (bedside) ultrasound use has increased exponentially with the availability of cheap robust ultrasound machines, and is now a core skill for Emergency Department doctors. Ultrasound has been described as the 'visual stethoscope' and is revolutionising the assessment and management of patients in the Emergency Department.

Ultrasound was initially used in the Emergency Department in the resuscitation room for:
• Detecting abdominal aortic aneurysms (AAA).
• Focused abdominal scanning in trauma (FAST) scans, searching for blood in the peritoneal cavity.
• Central venous line placement.

However, ultrasound use is now expanding to include:
• Shock assessment: cardiac function, vascular filling, signs of pulmonary embolus, together with the AAA and FAST scans.
• Basic echocardiography.
• Deep vein thrombosis (DVT) scanning.
• Early pregnancy scanning.
• Hepato-biliary scanning.

Disadvantages are that ultrasound is operator dependent, requires training and skill validation, and can divert attention from more important problems.

Computed tomography scan

As resolution and availability have increased and acquisition times have dropped, computed tomography (CT) has become an increasingly useful tool for the Emergency Department. CT is very good for bony injuries, and the trauma CT has proved to be more sensitive and specific than clinical examination in major trauma, but requires a very large radiation dose (1000 CXR).

Neck imaging in high-risk trauma is routinely done by CT (100 CXR), as plain films are insufficiently sensitive at detecting significant injury. Examples of high-risk injuries are a high-speed rollover road traffic collision, and also the elderly patient who falls forward, hitting their face ('fall on outstretched face'), who is at high risk of odontoid peg fracture, and in whom interpretation of plain radiographs is very difficult (see Chapter 11).

Modern CT scanners have enough resolution and speed to be able to resolve cardiac anatomy including the coronary arteries, pulmonary emboli and aortic dissection (400 CXR). CT brain scan (100 CXR) is an essential part of the assessment of stroke or the unconscious patient. CT KUB (kidneys, ureters and bladder; 400 CXRs) is the imaging of choice in renal colic.

Magnetic resonance scan

Magnetic resonance (MR) scanning is rarely used in the Emergency Department apart from possible cauda equina syndrome (acute central disc prolapse pressing on the cauda equina), giving bowel and bladder symptoms. MR scanning can be used to avoid the large radiation dose incurred by CT, e.g. investigating renal colic in young women.

Joints in which stability and function are mainly due to soft tissues, i.e. ligaments and cartilage such as the knee and shoulder, are well imaged by MR scanning, but it is generally difficult to access these directly from the Emergency Department.

Interventional imaging

Interventional imaging has an increasing role for a limited number of severe conditions. Interventional imaging is generally offered in larger hospitals, and together with trauma care, is one of the main drivers for centralisation of acute services into large hospitals.
• Primary percutaneous cardiac intervention with stenting has become the treatment of choice for patients with myocardial infarction.
• Endovascular treatments for patients with AAAs and aortic dissection are increasingly used. Neurosurgical bleeding from aneurysms is treatable by coils, as is otherwise uncontrollable bleeding in the pelvis, e.g. from pelvic fractures.

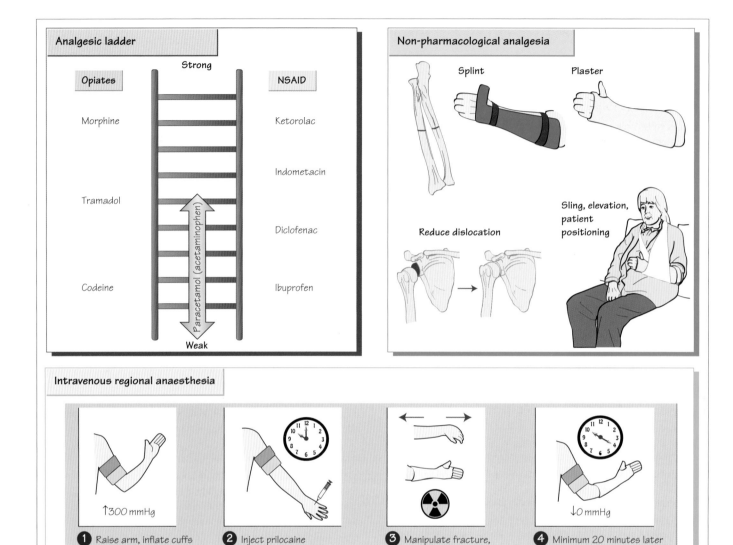

Analgesic ladder

Opiates — NSAID

Strong

Morphine — Ketorolac

Indometacin

Tramadol

Paracetamol (acetaminophen)

Diclofenac

Codeine — Ibuprofen

Weak

Non-pharmacological analgesia

Splint — Plaster

Reduce dislocation

Sling, elevation, patient positioning

Intravenous regional anaesthesia

1 Raise arm, inflate cuffs — ↑300 mmHg

2 Inject prilocaine

3 Manipulate fracture, plaster, X-ray

4 Minimum 20 minutes later — ↓0 mmHg

Patients often arrive at the Emergency Department in pain, and painkillers are often used before a definitive diagnosis is made. This is humane, and enables a thorough examination to be performed: there is no reason to withhold analgesia.

Patients are asked to rate the pain out of 10, with 0 being no pain, and 10 being the worst pain they can imagine. This procedure is repeated to gauge the effectiveness of the treatment and ensure the pain is controlled.

In general, a patient's reported pain is taken at face value: 'pain is what the patient feels' and is treated as such. Patients seeking opiates may fake pain, but this is rare.

Non-pharmacological analgesia

Splinting of fractures immobilises the bones, reducing pain. A patient's anxiety and pain makes them tense, which may make pain worse: a calm, supportive atmosphere and excellent nursing care help to keep the patient relaxed.

Nitrous oxide

Nitrous oxide (N_2O) combined with oxygen in a 1:1 mix in cylinders (Entonox®) is often used, particularly out of hospital. It is a short-term analgesic, effective only while the patient is breathing the gas, as it is rapidly cleared from the body. This 'laughing gas' is generally very safe, but should not be used in patients with a possible pneumothorax.

Paracetamol (acetaminophen) and compound analgesics

Paracetamol (acetaminophen) is effective and safe and can be given orally, rectally or intravenously. Compound analgesics consist of paracetamol combined with another analgesic, usually low-dose codeine. They come in different strengths, the weaker of which are sold without prescription. They are useful analgesics for patients to be able to take home on discharge, but prescribing the constituent drugs separately may allow more flexibility.

Moderate opiates

• *Codeine* is a common component of compound analgesics, and is effective but tends to cause constipation. *Oxycodone* and *dihydrocodeine* are more powerful variants of codeine, but offer little extra benefit, and have high abuse potential.
• *Tramadol* may be more effective than codeine. It has less abuse potential than other drugs of comparable potency but should be used with caution in the elderly.

Major opiates: morphine, fentanyl, pethidine (meperidine)

Opiates induce a feeling of well-being: patients, while still aware of the pain, are not distressed by it. Young patients with major fractures may require large doses of morphine, as will opiate addicts who need analgesia. Intravenous opiates are used because intramuscular absorption is unreliable and the intravenous route enables analgesia to be titrated to response.
• *Intravenous morphine* is the gold standard of Emergency Department analgesia. It is safe, predictable and effective. Morphine is not as lipid soluble as other opiates, so does not give a significant 'high'. Morphine often causes mild histamine release that should not be confused with an allergic reaction. The duration of action of morphine is approximately 3 hours.
• *Fentanyl* is a short-acting synthetic opiate that is particularly useful when performing short procedures, as it is cleared from the body within 30 minutes.
• *Pethidine* (meperidine) is quite lipid soluble and therefore sought after by opiate addicts as it crosses the blood–brain barrier, giving a 'high'. It offers no benefits over morphine and should not be used unless a patient has a definite allergy to morphine and there are no other alternatives.

Non-steroidal anti-inflammatory drugs

Injectable non-steroidal anti-inflammatory drugs (NSAIDs), e.g. *ketorolac*, are very effective in an Emergency Department setting. They are particularly useful in patients with broken bones, colicky pain (e.g. ureteric colic) and abdominal pain, but should be avoided in elderly patients or those with active bleeding. An equally effective alternative is a suppository (e.g. indometacin, diclofenac), which lasts for 16 hours.

Oral NSAIDs are useful as they can also be given to patients on discharge. *Ibuprofen* is the least powerful, but has a relatively benign side-effect profile.

Diclofenac and *indometacin* are more powerful NSAIDs but at a cost of increased risk of side-effects.

Local anaesthesia and nerve blocks

• *Lidocaine* 1% is the local anaesthetic (LA) most often used for wound management and is effective for 20–30 minutes without adrenaline, or for 40–60 minutes with adrenaline.
• *Adrenaline* mixed with lidocaine increases length of action and causes vasoconstriction giving a 'dry' wound that is much easier to assess, clean and close. Fear about using local anaesthetics with adrenaline in digits was related to high concentrations (1 : 10000); less than 1 : 100000 adrenaline is safe.
• *Bupivicaine* 0.25% is a long-acting local anaesthetic, lasting for 6–8 hours. Bupivicaine is highly protein bound: adrenaline does not increase duration of action.

A safe maximum dose of lidocaine for wound infiltration is 3 mg/kg, but with adrenaline is 6 mg/kg. For bupivicaine the maximum dose is 2 mg/kg. Local anaesthetic toxicity first causes perioral parasthesia, and then fits and arrhythmias, and is treated by lipid infusion.

Nerve blocks can offer very effective analgesia, e.g. digital and femoral nerve blocks. Bupivicaine and lidocaine can be mixed to provide a combination of rapid onset and long duration of action. Local anaesthetic can also be injected into joints, e.g. for shoulder dislocation.

A haematoma block can give good anaesthesia in minor fractures e.g. Colle's fractures (Chapter 15). The skin is carefully cleaned with alcohol and chlorhexidine and then up to 10 mL of local anaesthetic is injected into the fracture haematoma. After about 10 minutes reduction can be performed.

Intravenous regional anaesthesia (Bier's block)

Two intravenous cannulae are sited, one in the affected limb. A double cuff is placed on the affected limb (usually the arm), which is then lifted to exsanguinate it. The cuff is then inflated well above the systolic BP and local anaesthetic, e.g. prilocaine, injected. Bupivicaine should never be used for intravenous regional anaesthesia.

After waiting 5 minutes for the local anaesthetic to have maximal effect, the operation, e.g. fracture reduction, is performed. The cuff must not be deflated until *at least 20 minutes* have elapsed from injection of the local anaesthetic to avoid a bolus of undiluted local anaesthetic perfusing the heart, potentially causing asystole.

6 Airway management and sedation

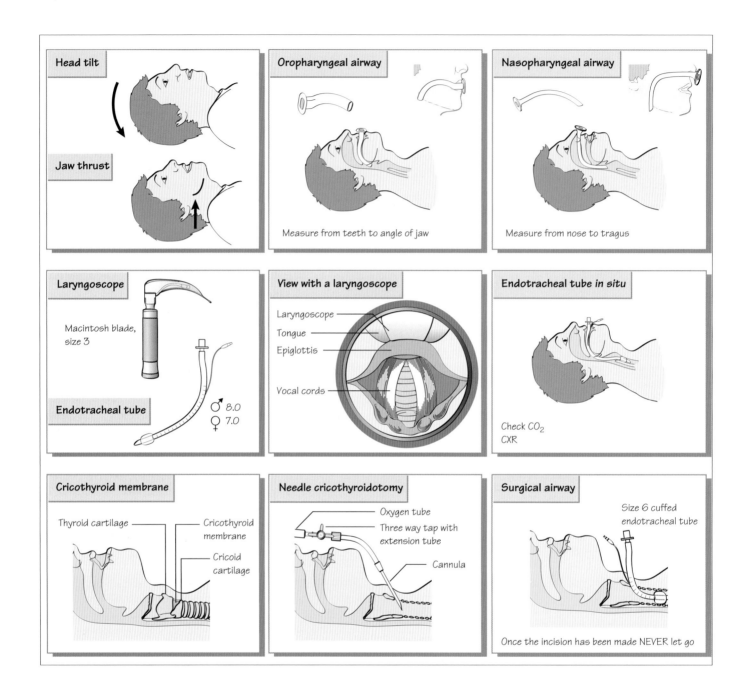

Head tilt

Jaw thrust

Oropharyngeal airway

Measure from teeth to angle of jaw

Nasopharyngeal airway

Measure from nose to tragus

Laryngoscope

Macintosh blade, size 3

Endotracheal tube

♂ 8.0
♀ 7.0

View with a laryngoscope

Laryngoscope
Tongue
Epiglottis
Vocal cords

Endotracheal tube in situ

Check CO_2
CXR

Cricothyroid membrane

Thyroid cartilage
Cricothyroid membrane
Cricoid cartilage

Needle cricothyroidotomy

Oxygen tube
Three way tap with extension tube
Cannula

Surgical airway

Size 6 cuffed endotracheal tube

Once the incision has been made NEVER let go

Airway management in the Emergency Department is more challenging than in the operating room as patients presenting to the Emergency Department must be assumed to be non-fasted, may be physiologically unstable, and may have head, neck or facial injuries.

Oxygenation and ventilation

Oxygenation is ensuring that the body has enough O_2; ventilation is ensuring that there is sufficient airflow to remove CO_2. Oxygen consumption is markedly increased in the acutely unwell patient, and giving high concentrations of oxygen supports the metabolic demands of the body in acute illness. However, high levels of oxygen may paradoxically make some ischaemic injury worse, e.g., brain/ heart due to vasoconstriction. A normal 'Hudson' O_2 mask can give inspired oxygen (FiO_2) concentrations of up to 60%. They should not be used with O_2 <4 L/min to prevent CO_2 build-up. A mask with a reservoir bag or a self-inflating bag-valve-mask can increase FiO_2 to about 90% with high flow (>10 L/min O_2). A

Venturi mask gives accurate low FiO_2 e.g. 28%. Nasal prongs give a variable amount of O_2 approx 25–30% but should only be used with low flow rates (2 L/min O_2).

Ventilatory failure

Under normal circumstances, an increased level of CO_2 is the main driver to breathe. Patients with chronic lung disease, usually COPD, become immune to this drive. For these 'blue bloater' patients, a low blood O_2 level drives breathing: their CO_2 level will be high.

If high FiO_2 is given to these patients, it reduces their respiratory drive, increasing their CO_2 levels further, making them sleepy, which further decreases their drive to breathe, etc. An oxygen saturation target of 91% in these patients balances the need for tissue oxygenation against that for ventilation.

WARNING

- O_2 should be prescribed, with a target saturation
- A patient with O_2 sat >96% probably does not need extra O2 unless high metabolic need, e.g., sepsis, trauma
- If FiO_2 has given a very high CO_2 level, reduce FiO_2 *slowly*
- If in doubt, give O_2 and obtain a senior review

Suction

A Yankauer suction catheter is used to suction blood, vomit or secretions in the oropharynx. To avoid causing the patient to vomit, do not suction the oropharynx if the patient is conscious, and 'only suck where you can see'.

Airway support

The jaw thrust, head tilt, oropharyngeal and nasopharangeal airways are illustrated opposite. The oropharyngeal airway is sized as the distance between the patient's teeth and the angle of the mandible. The nasopharyngeal airway should be the same length as the distance between the tip of the nose and the tragus of the ear.

Laryngeal mask airway

Emergency Department patients are not fasted and the laryngeal mask airway (LMA) does not prevent stomach contents being aspirated, nor can high ventilation pressures be achieved, as might be necessary in asthmatic patients. For these reasons the LMA is not a 'definitive' airway and is not normally used in the Emergency Department.

Endotracheal tube

The most common means to provide a definitive airway, the endotracheal tube (ETT), is a plastic tube that is inserted through the mouth (or rarely the nose) into the trachea. There is a cuff that is inflated to seal against the tracheal mucosa, and a radio-opaque line to indicate position on X-ray. The ETT should be secured, e.g. with tape, and the position checked by CO_2 monitoring and a chest X-ray.

Endotracheal tubes are sized by their internal diameter: 7.0 mm for an adult female, 8.0 mm for a male. There are markings indicating distance from the tip: this is to avoid the tube being pushed too far, e.g. down the right main bronchus, which is larger and straighter than the left.

The decision that the patient needs intubation is the responsibility of the doctor managing the airway. Factors indicating need for intubation include:

- Airway instability: bleeding into airways, airway burns.
- Coma: Glasgow Coma Scale (GCS) < 9, deteriorating level of consciousness, loss of protective laryngeal reflexes.
- Inadequate oxygenation: despite high inspired O_2 (FiO_2).
- Inadequate ventilation: patient tired/drowsy.
- Therapeutic reasons: control seizures, hypothermia.
- Pragmatic reasons: combative patient, need for transport.

A *laryngoscope* is needed to insert the ETT. In some countries, straight (Miller) blades are used; in others, curved (Macintosh) blades. These have a light to enable sight of the larynx.

McGill's forceps have a 'kink' in them to avoid the operator's hands obstructing the field of vision. They are useful for removing loose items in the oropharynx, and manipulating the ETT.

Surgical airway

Rarely, a situation occurs when it is not possible to intubate or ventilate a patient. In this situation, there are two options:

- A *needle cricothyroidotomy* will provide short-term oxygenation, but is not a definitive airway, and CO_2 levels will build up.
- A *surgical airway* through the cricoid membrane using a 6.0 mm cuffed ETT provides a definitive airway.

Procedural sedation

Procedural sedation is often performed in the Emergency Department to allow relocation of dislocations or for short painful procedures. *The person performing the sedation needs appropriate skills and experience to manage any potential situation, including the need for intubation.*

The procedure should be carried out in a resuscitation bay with full monitoring, oxygen and suction equipment. Two doctors should be present at all times to ensure that the doctor administering the sedation has their full attention on the patient's airway. The patient should be fasted for at least 4 hours, should give formal consent, and the doctor should stay with the patient until they are consistently responsive.

After sedation patients should not drive for a day and should be sent home in the care of a responsible adult with instructions to return if unwell.

- *Propofol* is a short-acting anaesthetic induction drug, but is used for sedation by giving as a series of small boluses, titrating for effect. Large doses of propofol abolish protective airway reflexes and may stop the patient breathing. Propofol has no analgesic properties so may need to be given with an analgesic, e.g. fentanyl.
- *Midazolam*, a short-acting benzodiazepine, may be used in combination with an opiate to provide sedation.
- *Ketamine* is a safe and predictable drug that is often used for paediatric sedation. It can be used for sedation and analgesia in adults, and may be combined with a short-acting benzodiazepine to minimise unpleasant emergence phenomena, e.g. hallucinations.

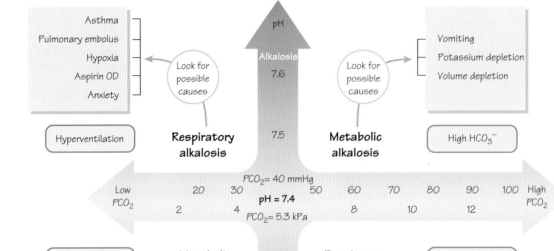

Asthma
Pulmonary embolus
Hypoxia
Aspirin OD
Anxiety

Look for possible causes

Vomiting
Potassium depletion
Volume depletion

Look for possible causes

Hyperventilation

Respiratory alkalosis

Metabolic alkalosis

High HCO_3^-

pH
Alkalosis
7.6
7.5

PCO_2 = 40 mmHg

| Low PCO_2 | | 20 | 30 | | 50 | 60 | 70 | 80 | 90 | 100 | High PCO_2 |

pH = 7.4

| 2 | | 4 | | 8 | 10 | 12 | |

PCO_2 = 5.3 kPa

Low HCO_3^-

Metabolic acidosis

7.3

Respiratory acidosis

Hypoventilation

Metabolic acidosis : Anion gap

Anion gap = $(Na^+ + K^+) - (HCO_3^- + Cl^-)$
normally about 8 mmol/l

A raised anion gap metabolic acidosis is caused by increased acid production or failure to excrete acid, e.g.
 – diabetic ketoacidosis
 – lactic acidosis
 – renal failure

A normal anion gap metabolic acidosis is generally caused by bicarbonate loss, e.g. gastrointestinal loss of alkaline fluid from diarrhoea or fistula

7.2
7.1
7.0
Acidosis
6.9
pH

The A-a gradient

In room air (21% oxygen) at sea level and with a pCO_2 of 40mmHg (5.3 kPa), the expected alveolar partial pressure of oxygen is:
P(Alveolar O_2) = P(inspired oxygen) − P(Alveolar H_2O) − P(Alveolar CO_2)

$$P_AO_2 = P_iO_2 - PH_2O - \frac{P_ACO_2}{R}$$ (1 kPa = 7.5 mmHg)

$$P_AO_2 = \frac{21}{100} \times (760 - 47) - \frac{40}{0.8} = 100 \text{ mmHg (13.3 kPa)}$$

This approximates to $P_AO_2 \approx 150 - \frac{5}{4} \times P_aCO_2$ mmHg

The A-a gradient is the difference between the expected (based on Alveolar oxygen) and the measured (the arterial) amount of oxygen in the blood

Normally this should be less than $\frac{Age}{4}$ + 4 mmHg

Warning

When the O_2 saturation is 88% (a drop of about 10%) the body's tissues are only receiving HALF the normal oxygen – the P_aO_2 is 50 mmHg (6.6 kPa)

Take home messages:

A very small difference in O_2 saturation equates to a very large difference in oxygen delivered to the tissues

Oxygen saturation monitoring is useful for trending, but if there are problems with oxygenation, only P_aO_2 from ABG can give the necessary information

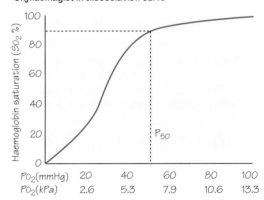

Oxyhaemaglobin dissociation curve

| PO_2(mmHg) | 20 | 40 | 60 | 80 | 100 |
| PO_2(kPa) | 2.6 | 5.3 | 7.9 | 10.6 | 13.3 |

Arterial blood gases

Arterial blood gas analysis provides information about oxygenation (O_2) and ventilation (CO_2), and metabolic disturbance. Some machines also provide electrolytes, lactate and carbon monoxide levels.

Indications for blood gas measurement

1 Diagnostic.
- Severe shortness of breath.
- Possible pulmonary embolus.

2 Assessment of severity of illness.
- Shock, severe sepsis.
- Diabetic ketoacidosis.
- Severe vomiting and diarrhoea.

3 Specific situations.
- Overdose of tricyclic antidepressants or aspirin.

Arterial puncture is painful and should only be performed if the result is going to change management. This is particularly important in young adults with chronic conditions. If just the pH is required, e.g. for a patient with diabetes, this may be obtained from venous blood.

The blood gas machine has three main sensors: pH, PaO_2 and $PaCO_2$. Other values such as bicarbonate and base excess are calculated from these values, not measured directly. Therefore you can deduce the problem using just these three values.

Oxygenation

Hypoxia occurs in two situations:

1 Not enough oxygen reaches the blood.
- High altitude: not enough oxygen in the air.
- Hypoventilation: neuromuscular disease, extreme fatigue
- Obstruction: asthma.

2 Not enough blood reaches the oxygen.
- Ventilation/perfusion (V/Q) mismatch: the lung tissue is intact but there is no blood passing through it, e.g. pulmonary embolus. If the arterial oxygen level fails to correct with 100% oxygen, this implies 'shunting', i.e. blood is bypassing the lung altogether.
- Alveolar dysfunction: the apparatus for gas exchange is not working, e.g. interstitial lung disease, pulmonary oedema.

The A-a gradient

If we know the fraction (%) of oxygen the patient is breathing in (=FiO_2) we can calculate the A-a gradient. The A-a gradient compares the *expected* amount of oxygen in the blood (= the amount of oxygen in the Alveolus), PAO_2, with the *actual* amount of arterial oxygen, PaO_2. Common causes of a large A-a gradient are:
- The blood not reaching the oxygen, e.g. pulmonary embolus.
- A barrier to effective gas exchange, e.g. pulmonary oedema.

Calculating the partial pressure of alveolar oxygen is shown opposite (R is the respiratory quotient and is related to diet).

Pulse oximetry

Pulse oximetry is very useful for monitoring patients, as it is non-invasive. The oxygen saturation is calculated by shining two beams of light through soft tissue, e.g. finger or earlobe, to estimate the fraction of haemoglobin carrying oxygen.

Unfortunately pulse oximetry has a significant flaw that can trip up the unwary. The blood value we want to measure is the PaO_2 = the amount of oxygen carried in arterial blood. Oxygen saturation is only a surrogate measure of the PaO_2: the graph (opposite) shows the relationship between the two.

Under normal circumstances, with an oxygen saturation of 100%, the PaO_2 is 13.3 kPa (100 mmHg).

WARNING

When the PaO_2 is *halved* to 6.6 kPa, the saturation is still 88%. Take-home message: O_2 saturation less than 97% is not good oxygenation.

Acid–base disturbance

Acidosis and alkalosis have a chicken/egg relationship with ventilation, (measured by $PaCO_2$) and respiratory effort: sometimes it is not always clear which came first. To analyse these problems, start with the acid–base disturbance, and then look at the $PaCO_2$.

Acidosis (pH < 7.35)

CO_2 low = metabolic acidosis

If the patient is acidotic and the $PaCO_2$ is low, it is likely the patient is breathing deeply to expel CO_2, to compensate for the metabolic acidosis by hyperventilation. This is often seen in diabetic ketoacidosis and is called Kussmaul breathing.

CO_2 high = respiratory acidosis

If the CO_2 is high, it is likely that this is at least partially responsible for the acidosis, although usually the acidosis is mixed (partly metabolic and partly respiratory).

The normal stimulus to breathe is increased blood CO_2 levels, so a high CO_2 level implies failure of adequate ventilation.

Some patients with lung disease (e.g. COPD) lose their sensitivity to increased blood CO_2 levels and therefore rely on low O_2 levels to drive their breathing. Giving these patients high concentrations of oxygen dangerously reduces their respiratory drive, resulting in a build-up of CO_2. The increase in CO_2 makes the patient sleepy, further reducing respiratory effort.

If faced with a patient who is on home oxygen or is known to have advanced COPD, the safest action is to give enough oxygen to ensure an oxygen saturation of about 91%. Any more than this may abolish the patient's drive to breathe.

Patients with chronically elevated CO_2 levels compensate for this by excreting acid (H^+) renally to rebalance the equation:

$$CO_2 + H_2O \Leftrightarrow HCO_3^- + H^+$$

Therefore these patients will have a chronically raised HCO_3^- (bicarbonate) level.

Alkalosis (pH > 7.45)

CO_2 low = respiratory alkalosis

Respiratory alkalosis is usually due to anxiety-related hyperventilation although marked hypoxia, e.g. from pulmonary embolus, may also cause this.

CO_2 high = metabolic alkalosis

Metabolic alkalosis is usually caused by loss of acid and/or dehydration, e.g. diarrhoea and vomiting.

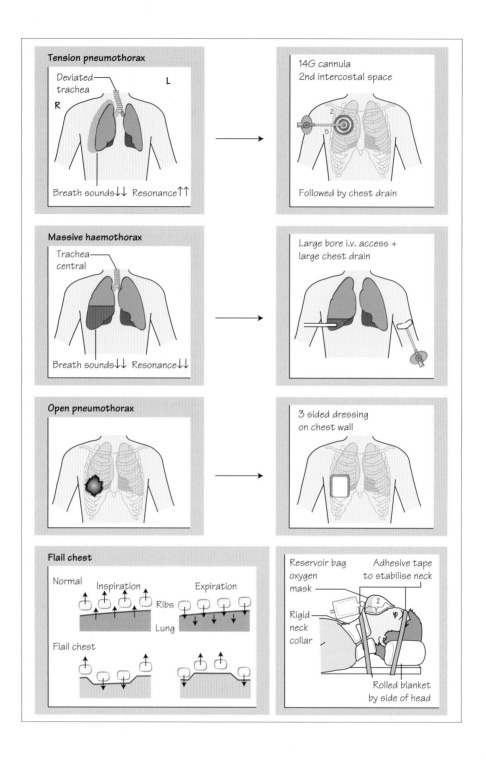

Trauma care has been much improved with systematic protocols that enable effective prioritisation of treatment. The first time one sees a trauma patient arriving in the Emergency Department can be confusing and intimidating as there are many things going on simultaneously.

Treatment priority

The *ABC* order of treatment reflects the relative importance of the different things that can go wrong. Under most circumstances, **A**irway problems will kill the patient before **B**reathing problems, before **C**irculation problems.

Problems are treated as they are found. If a problem is found and treated, or the patient deteriorates, one starts again with A and works through B and C.

Cervical spine protection is given highest priority to avoid catastrophic spinal injury.

> **WARNING**
>
> Head injuries are the cause of death in 70% of trauma deaths. It is critical to avoid *hypoxia* and *hypotension*, which cause secondary injury in head-injured patients.

Trauma team

Major trauma is managed by a trauma team of up to five doctors and nurses, led by a senior doctor. Team members perform specific roles, e.g. airway management, procedures. The role of the leader is to stand back and have an overview rather than perform procedures, but in a smaller Emergency Department this is not always possible.

Penetrating vs non-penetrating trauma

Penetrating trauma, caused by knives and guns, is relatively rare in Europe and Australia, where most trauma is 'blunt', e.g. motor vehicle crashes, falls, crush injuries. In penetrating trauma (and ruptured abdominal aortic aneurysm or ectopic pregnancy), blood may be lost faster than it can be replaced: it is *essential* for ongoing bleeding to be controlled immediately. This may require wound compression, tourniquets to stop bleeding, or immediate surgery.

Ambulance transfer and handover

Trauma patients are prepared for transfer by placing them onto a spinal board with their head and neck immobilised. When the ambulance arrives, the trauma team listens carefully to their structured handover: DeMIST.
- Demographics: age, sex, background.
- Mechanism of injury.
- Injuries sustained.
- Signs and symptoms.
- Treatment given.

The key points should be summarised back by the team leader to confirm understanding and prevent errors.

A: Airway and cervical spine protection

If a patient is not talking, check for stridor, or obstruction with blood/teeth/food, and normal chest wall movement with breathing. The tongue can fall back and cause an obstructed airway in a supine, unconscious patient.

Interventions
- Oxygen: 15 L/min using a mask with a reservoir bag.
- Inspect mouth and suction: only suck down side of mouth.
- Does the patient need a definitive airway? See Chapter 6.
- Cervical spine immobilisation (see opposite).

B: Breathing and ventilation

While there are many potential injuries to the chest, there are four breathing problems that are immediately life-threatening.

1 Tension pneumothorax

Tension pneumothorax occurs when a lung injury pumps air into the pleural space, building up pressure. Hypotension and respiratory difficulty are caused by high intrathoracic pressure and kinking of the great vessels. This causes distended neck veins, loss of breath sounds, and a trachea deviated *away from* the pneumothorax. *Tension pneumothorax is a clinical diagnosis, not a radiological one.*

Insert a large (16 or 14 G) intravenous cannula perpendicularly into the anterior chest wall in the second intercostal space in mid-clavicular line. A hiss of escaping air will be heard: leave in place and insert a chest drain as soon as possible.

2 Massive haemothorax

The patient may be in shock, and may have reduced air entry and dull percussion note, although this is often difficult to detect with the patient supine.

Ensure good intravenous access *before* placing a large bore (e.g. 32 Fr) chest drain, as draining the blood may precipitate bleeding, which may require resuscitation and immediate surgery.

3 Open pneumothorax

A large open chest wound gives a collapsed lung, loss of breath sounds and 'surgical emphysema' (air in the subcutaneous tissues that gives a crinkly feel).

Treat by applying an occlusive dressing over the wound that is secured on three sides only, thus acting as a one-way valve.

4 Flail chest

If multiple ribs are broken in more than one place, a segment of chest wall can move paradoxically, i.e. in the opposite direction to the rest of the chest during respirations. This markedly increases the work of breathing.

If a patient is becoming tired, intubation is necessary. If the flail segment is small, and respiratory function is good, analgesia can be achieved by an epidural or nerve blocks, but the patient should be closely monitored.

C: Circulation

Pulse and blood pressure are the key information – shock is described in Chapter 3.

Intravenous access should be a minimum of two 16 G cannulae. Blood should be sent to the laboratory for FBC (full blood count), U+E (urea and electrolytes), clotting, group and save, cross-matching, depending on clinical status of patient.

Stop the bleeding, warm the patient

Obvious bleeding sites should be compressed and dressed. Litres of blood can be lost into the pelvis or into femoral shaft fractures. A pelvic sling should be applied if there is a pelvic injury. Pelvic stability should never be assessed by compressing the pelvis. A traction splint, e.g., Thomas splint, stabilises and reduces pain and bleeding resulting from a femoral shaft fracture.

Pericardial tamponade

This produces similar signs to tension pneumothorax, with shock and distended neck veins, but *no tracheal deviation*. Heart sounds and ECG complex size may be reduced. Focused abdominal scanning in trauma (FAST) ultrasound scan should detect tamponade. Treatment depends on the nature of the trauma and clinical status of the patient, but is likely to require urgent thoracotomy.

Disability and neurological status

The Glasgow Coma Scale is described in Chapter 10.

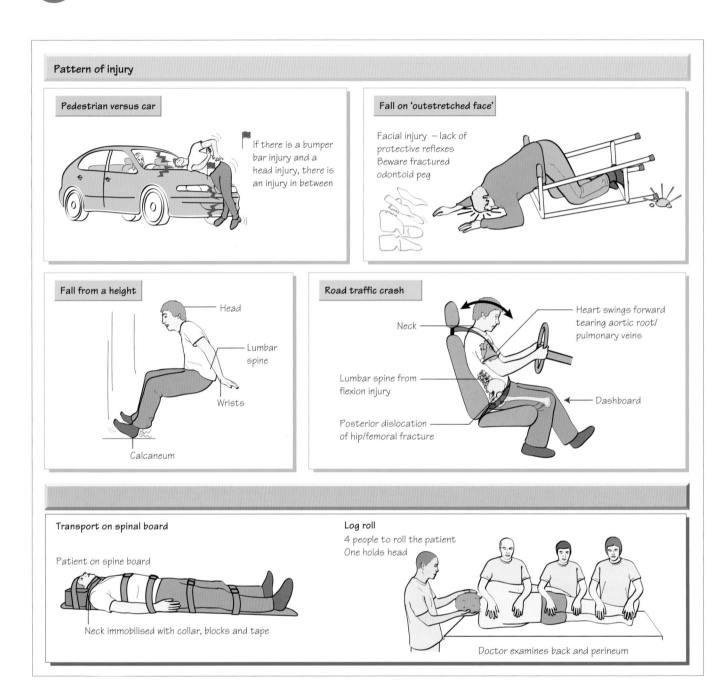

Pattern of injury

Pedestrian versus car

If there is a bumper bar injury and a head injury, there is an injury in between

Fall on 'outstretched face'

Facial injury – lack of protective reflexes
Beware fractured odontoid peg

Fall from a height

Head
Lumbar spine
Wrists
Calcaneum

Road traffic crash

Neck
Lumbar spine from flexion injury
Posterior dislocation of hip/femoral fracture
Heart swings forward tearing aortic root/pulmonary veins
Dashboard

Transport on spinal board

Patient on spine board
Neck immobilised with collar, blocks and tape

Log roll

4 people to roll the patient
One holds head
Doctor examines back and perineum

The secondary survey is a head-to-toe front and back, comprehensive review of the trauma patient to discover all injuries. This allows inpatient units to plan treatment. If an injury is missed at this stage it may not be picked up until it is too late to treat effectively, so thoroughness is essential. *This chapter will not cover limb injuries (Chapters 14–18), or head and neck injuries (Chapter 10).*

While the secondary survey proceeds, a number of other interventions take place:

- Analgesia, usually intravenous morphine, is humane, does not mask injuries and should be given early.
- Tetanus immunisation: give according to local protocol.
- Open fractures should be covered with a saline-soaked dressing and intravenous broad-spectrum antibiotics given immediately.
- A urinary catheter should be inserted if it is unlikely that the patient will be mobile within the next few hours. Urine should be dipstick tested, including βhCG in female patients.
- Arterial blood gases should be taken in severe trauma.

Log roll, perineal injury

The log roll is a technique to turn the patient while ensuring that the spine remains immobilised. It is used to examine the patient's back and perineum. A rectal examination is performed to look for blood, lack of tone/sensation or high-riding prostate which indicate bowel injury, spinal cord injury or urethral injury, respectively. Priapism occurs in spinal injury, while blood at the penile meatus implies urethral injury and the need for urological advice before catheterisation.

Patterns of injury

Knowledge about likely patterns of injury is helpful: discovery of one injury should prompt a search for related injuries.
• *Fall from a height*: the calcaneus is often broken, together with the wrists, and the lumbar spine from forced flexion.
• *Deceleration injury*: sudden flexion of the spine, as occurs in a motor vehicle collision, tends to cause injury at the junctions between the flexible parts of the spine (lumbar, cervical) and the more rigid thoracic spine. The vertebrae most often injured are C5/6 and T12/L1. Seatbelt injuries may cause injury to the small bowel or pancreas by squashing these against the vertebrae, particularly with lap-only seatbelts.
• *Abdominal trauma*: the spleen is immobile and sits just below the ribs, where it is vulnerable to damage. Splenic injury may initially be asymptomatic, followed by rupture days later, and so any left upper quadrant tenderness necessitates a CT. Liver lacerations may bleed extensively, as there are large vessels in the liver. The mobility of the bowel generally protects it from blunt injury, while the kidneys are quite well cushioned by soft tissue.
• *Spinal trauma*: if one spinal fracture is identified, there is a high probability that there is another fracture elsewhere, so the whole spinal column should be imaged with CT.
• *Penetrating injury*: for firearm injuries, aside from entry and exit wounds, the damage caused is proportional to the density of the tissue traversed and the energy (mass, velocity) of the projectile. This may be further complicated by cavitation, tumbling, internal deflection and secondary injury from fragments of bone.
• *Knife wounds* can be difficult to assess in the Emergency Department, particularly if the depth exceeds the width. Knowledge of the deep structures is essential to be able to recognise and predict complications, and this should be performed by someone with the necessary experience.

Imaging

Imaging is an integral part of the secondary survey, and occurs in parallel with the clinical examination and treatment.
• Bedside *ultrasound* scanning (Chapters 10 and 11) is used to identify causes of shock and patients who need urgent surgery rather than more examination/imaging.
• *Chest X-ray* concerns breathing and is therefore the most important plain X-ray film, and the first to be done.
• *Pelvis X-ray* relates to circulation: fractures of the pelvis may tear sacro-iliac veins, causing catastrophic bleeding. Pressure on the pelvis to 'test stability' may cause this bleeding, so must be avoided; however a pelvic X-ray is 60 CXRs, so should not be performed on patients who have minimal trauma.
• *Computed tomography* of head/neck/chest/abdomen and pelvis is now the 'gold standard' for severe trauma as it minimises the risk of missing injuries, and is quick to perform, at the cost of a substantial amount of radiation (1000 CXRs). The major contraindication to a CT scan is the unstable trauma patient, who needs urgent theatre to control bleeding, not a CT scan.
• *Cervical spine X-ray* is no longer routinely performed early in the assessment, providing the neck is immobilised. Plain X-ray of the cervical spine is not particularly sensitive at identifying injuries, and therefore any patient with a moderate or high chance of neck injury should have CT. This includes all patients requiring a CT scan of the brain, patients with a dangerous mechanism of injury (fall > 5 m, diving injury, rollover road traffic collision) or physiological abnormality (altered neurology).
• *Interventional radiology*: If there is sustained bleeding from poorly accessible sites (e.g. pelvis), embolisation of vessels may be life-saving.

Fluid resuscitation

Patients with significant injuries should have two large-bore intravenous cannulae inserted, but aggressive pursuit of 'normal' measures of pulse and blood pressure may be counterproductive (Chapter 3). For patients with head injury see Chapters 10 and 11.

As described in Chapter 3, hypothermia (<35°C) or severe acidosis (pH < 7.20) will reduce in-vivo clotting function to a fraction of normal, and together they are a lethal combination. An important intervention in the resuscitation stage is to keep the patient warm, using a warm air blanket, warmed intravenous fluids and warmed humidified oxygen.

There is debate over the optimum transfusion strategy, but recent military experience suggests early use of blood and blood products produces better outcomes.

Surgical resuscitation

In cases where there is ongoing bleeding that cannot be controlled, the abdomen and/or chest are opened and the bleeding areas packed in 'damage control surgery'. Major fractures are immobilised with external fixators. The patient is then transferred to the intensive care unit (ICU) for stabilisation prior to further surgery at a later time.

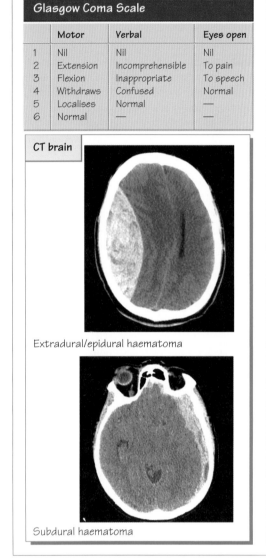

Glasgow Coma Scale

	Motor	Verbal	Eyes open
1	Nil	Nil	Nil
2	Extension	Incomprehensible	To pain
3	Flexion	Inappropriate	To speech
4	Withdraws	Confused	Normal
5	Localises	Normal	—
6	Normal	—	—

CT brain

Extradural/epidural haematoma

Subdural haematoma

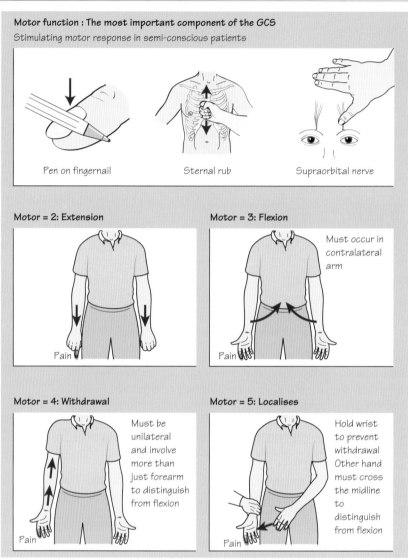

Motor function : The most important component of the GCS

Stimulating motor response in semi-conscious patients

Pen on fingernail   Sternal rub   Supraorbital nerve

Motor = 2: Extension

Pain

Motor = 3: Flexion

Must occur in contralateral arm

Pain

Motor = 4: Withdrawal

Must be unilateral and involve more than just forearm to distinguish from flexion

Pain

Motor = 5: Localises

Hold wrist to prevent withdrawal Other hand must cross the midline to distinguish from flexion

Pain

This chapter covers patients who have suffered a significant head (Glasgow Coma Scale; GCS < 13) and/or neck injury, often as part of multi-system trauma (Chapters 8 and 9). Of trauma-related deaths, 70% are from head injury, and many of these deaths are preventable.

• *Primary brain injury* occurs at the moment of trauma. Prevention is the only way to minimise primary injury, which is why collection of injury data is an integral part of Emergency Medicine. Seatbelts, helmets, car and road design all prevent primary brain injury, as does road safety enforcement (speeding, drink driving).

• *Secondary brain injury* occurs after trauma, and may be preventable by expert medical care. The most common preventable conditions that cause secondary brain injury are *hypoxia* and *hypotension*.

• *Cervical spine injury*: in the context of a major head injury, a cervical spine injury is assumed until proved otherwise. All patients should arrive at the Emergency Department immobilised on a spinal board with a cervical collar and supports.

Aside from an AMPLE history (Chapter 9), information from witnesses may be available from the ambulance crew. Periods of loss of consciousness and amnesia before or after the event are helpful to assess neurological damage.

Airway, breathing and cervical spine

The patient is immobilised on a spinal board, with a rigid cervical collar, together with blocks and tape. Immobilisation is painful after about 20 minutes, and pressure sores can develop in patients with reduced sensation and/or mobility. The patient should be safely removed from the board as soon as possible, usually as part of the log roll in the secondary survey.

If a patient does need to be intubated and ventilated (Chapter 6), it is very important to establish objective neurological status (see Disability, below) *before intubation*, as it is impossible afterwards due to the muscle paralysis necessary for ventilation.

Circulation

Having established that the blood will be oxygenated, the next challenge is to ensure that enough blood is perfusing the brain. This is dictated by:

cerebral perfusion pressure (CPP) =
mean arterial pressure (MAP) – intracranial pressure (ICP)

The brain's normal self-regulation of CPP is impaired in brain injury: it is critical that MAP does not fall below 80 mmHg. CPP can be maintained by increasing MAP or reducing ICP. MAP can be increased by giving intravenous fluids and inotropes (e.g. adrenaline) according to the CVP and MAP. ICP can be reduced by reducing venous pressure: avoid excessive intravenous fluid and elevate the head of the bed by 30°.

Disability

This refers to the brief structured assessment of functional neurological impairment as a result of the head injury.

Glasgow Coma Scale

The Glasgow Coma Scale (GCS) was devised in the 1970s before the advent of CT to predict the need for neurosurgical intervention. The motor component is the most important, but also the most difficult to assess. If the GCS is not assessed using optimal stimulation, poor-quality information will be collected, resulting in poor decisions. Pressing on a fingernail with a pen, and firm sternal pressure, are commonly used; if a spinal injury is possible, pressure on the supraorbital nerve in the supraorbital notch is effective.

Pupil size and reactivity

The pupils' size and reactions give useful information about the patient's neurological status, assuming that no drugs that influence the pupil size (e.g. atropine, adrenaline) have been given.
• If the pupils are of normal diameter (3–5 mm) and reactive, this suggests underlying normal function, and is associated with a good outcome.
• If one pupil is fixed and dilated, this may indicate that the brain on the same side is under increased pressure, stretching the IIIrd nerve.
• If both pupils are small, this suggests either opiate overdose or brainstem injury.
• Having both pupils fixed and dilated is associated with a poor outcome, unless caused by drugs (e.g. atropine, adrenaline) or local eye injury.

Focal limb movement deficit

If limb movement differs from one side to the other (excluding direct reasons e.g. broken arm) consider whether there may be a spinal or brain injury.

Investigations

Any necessary investigations are integrated into the primary and secondary trauma survey as described in Chapters 8 and 9.

Bedside investigations

• Blood glucose monitoring must be early and then regularly repeated in all cases of neurological impairment in the Emergency Department.

Laboratory investigations

• An alcohol level is only useful if negative. If positive it does not rule out the need for imaging. Some countries have mandatory blood testing for all road trauma patients.
• FBC/U + E/clotting profile/blood group and hold.
• ABGs/lactate ensure accurate assessment of oxygenation, ventilation and shock.

Imaging

• CT brain and neck.
• MRI is not indicated in the initial assessment, but may be useful to assess spinal cord injury.

Management

After stabilisation and CT scan, a decision needs to be made about what further care is necessary. The process to achieve this depends on local policy, but there are essentially four groups of patients:

Urgent neurosurgery

This small but important group comprises patients with extradural (epidural), intracerebral or posterior fossa bleeding. Some subdural bleeds, e.g. those resulting in marked midline shift, may also require surgery.

Intensive care

These patients need a period of ventilation in an ICU, which has facilities for ICP monitoring using a bolt drilled through the skull, and that offers ready access to neurosurgery, should this become necessary.

Ward care

Ward care is for patients who need close neurological monitoring on a normal ward with the ability to have an urgent medical review should their condition deteriorate. The Emergency Department observation ward is sometimes used for this group of patients. Post-injury care including follow-up is advisable, as even patients with apparent normal function after head injury can have significant problems (e.g. poor concentration, emotional lability) that are helped by psychological support.

Catastrophic head injury

If the CT shows no chance of survival, this must be explained to the patient's relatives in sympathetic but unambiguous terms. Organ donation should be sought by a member of staff experienced at explaining this, as the opportunity to donate organs is usually very much appreciated in the long term.

11 Minor head and neck injury

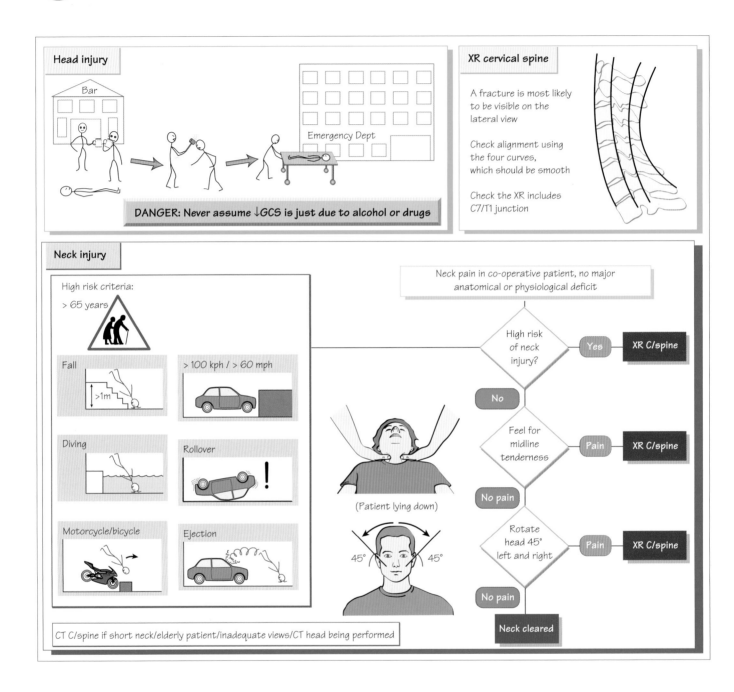

Head injury

Bar

Emergency Dept

DANGER: Never assume ↓GCS is just due to alcohol or drugs

XR cervical spine

A fracture is most likely to be visible on the lateral view

Check alignment using the four curves, which should be smooth

Check the XR includes C7/T1 junction

Neck injury

High risk criteria:

> 65 years

Fall

>1m

> 100 kph / > 60 mph

Diving

Rollover

!

Motorcycle/bicycle

Ejection

(Patient lying down)

45°   45°

CT C/spine if short neck/elderly patient/inadequate views/CT head being performed

Neck pain in co-operative patient, no major anatomical or physiological deficit

High risk of neck injury? — Yes → XR C/spine

No

Feel for midline tenderness — Pain → XR C/spine

No pain

Rotate head 45° left and right — Pain → XR C/spine

No pain

Neck cleared

Minor head and neck injuries are extremely common reasons to attend the Emergency Department. Within this group of patients there is a very small number who have sustained serious damage: the challenge is to accurately and efficiently identify these. This task is complicated by the fact that alcohol is involved in more than half of these cases. Minor head injury is defined as Glasgow Coma Scale (GCS) 13 or above, and may be associated with a period of loss of consciousness (LOC), and/or amnesia.

Guidelines use clinical features to identify low-risk patients who can safely be discharged and high-risk patients who need further investigation.

Imaging
• Skull radiography (5 CXR) is not helpful as it cannot exclude significant brain injury: only CT brain (100 CXR) can do this.
• Radiography of cervical spine (5 CXR) is appropriate in patients with a low to moderate probability of injury. X-ray

of cervical spine comprises three views: AP, lateral and (odontoid) peg.
• In patients with a high likelihood of neck injury *or* when the X-ray of cervical spine is not of adequate diagnostic quality *or* if a CT brain scan is indicated as well, then a CT cervical spine scan (100 CXR) is preferable.

Head injury: clinical assessment

This should include details about mechanism of injury, previous medical history, loss of consciousness and symptoms since. The key points to establish are:
• Mechanism of injury: pedestrian or cyclist vs vehicle, or ejected from vehicle, or fall >1 metre.
• Age ≥65 years.
• Vomiting >1 episode.
• Pre-traumatic amnesia >30 minutes.
• Seizure.
• Warfarin or coagulopathy.
• GCS < 15 after 2 hours in Emergency Department.
• Suspected skull fracture (open or depressed or skull base).
• Focal neurological deficit.
If any of the above factors is present, it is likely that the patient will need a CT brain scan (100 CXR).

Neck injury: clinical assessment

History: high-risk factors
• GCS <15, unstable physiologically.
• Age >65 years.
• Prior neck problems, neurology.
• Fall >1 metre.
• Axial load to head, e.g. diving, rollover crash.
• Motor vehicle crash involving high speed, ejection from vehicle, bicycle, motorcycle or recreational vehicle.
If a patient has neck pain and any of these features, arrange imaging.

Examination
Look Look for fixed flexion deformity of the neck.
Feel While a clinician stabilises the head, take the collar off and feel for midline tenderness over the spinous processes.

Tenderness over the trapezius muscles is common but does not necessitate imaging. If either Look or Feel is abnormal, arrange imaging, otherwise test movement:

Move Ask the patient to rotate their head 45° left and right.

If this is possible without pain and the above tests have been performed by a doctor with the appropriate training and experience, the neck is 'cleared'.
If any of the findings are abnormal, arrange imaging.

Other investigations
• Investigations indicated as per Chapters 8 and 9.
• Blood glucose.
• Alcohol testing, whether breath or blood, is only useful if it is negative. If positive, it is dangerous to assume that all symptoms are due to the alcohol.

Common diagnoses

Concussion: mild traumatic brain injury
After ruling out significant brain injury, the patient may be discharged to the care of another adult with written head injury instructions. These should express clearly the reasons to return to the Emergency Department, e.g. vomiting or drowsiness.

The patient should be warned about common symptoms following a mild head injury (e.g. poor concentration, labile mood): psychological follow-up may be helpful.

Acute neck sprain
Patients should be warned that pain and stiffness is likely to be worse the following day and that it is important to use sufficient analgesia, e.g. NSAID ± codeine, to keep the neck mobile. The term 'whiplash' is best avoided as it has medicolegal implications. It is interesting that in countries without a compensation culture, acute neck sprains do not cause long-term disability.

Soft foam collars discourage neck movement, preventing recovery and encouraging psychological dependence, so should not be used. Semi-rigid collars (e.g. Philadelphia) are sometimes used for patients with a stable neck injury on expert advice.

Diagnoses not to miss

Reason for fall or injury
Elderly patients who present with a fall may have been on the floor for a prolonged period: look for hypothermia, pressure sores, rhabdomyolysis (Chapter 29). Think about possible causes (e.g. urinary tract infection, postural hypotension or arrhythmia), and keep an open mind about possible elder abuse or domestic violence.

Occult cervical spine fracture
Elderly patients with facial injuries may have fallen so fast they have not been able to protect their face, and therefore are at high risk of cervical spine fractures, especially of the odontoid peg. Have a low threshold for requesting CT, as plain radiographs are usually uninterpretable.

Extradural (epidural) haematoma
A fracture of the temporal bone overlying the middle meningeal artery may cause a large bleed. The classical presentation is of deterioration following a lucid interval; if diagnosis and surgery are rapid, a good outcome is common.

Subdural haematoma
Patients at high risk of subdural haematoma (SDH) include the elderly with recurrent falls, alcoholics and those on anticoagulants. SDH may present following an acute injury, or as a chronic deterioration, and often has a poor prognosis whether surgery is performed or not, due to the underlying conditions.

Cervical spine fracture
C2 and C5/6 injuries are most common. Document and monitor neurological and respiratory function carefully. Insertion of a catheter, pressure area care, and correction of spinal shock using intravenous fluids are essential basic treatments.

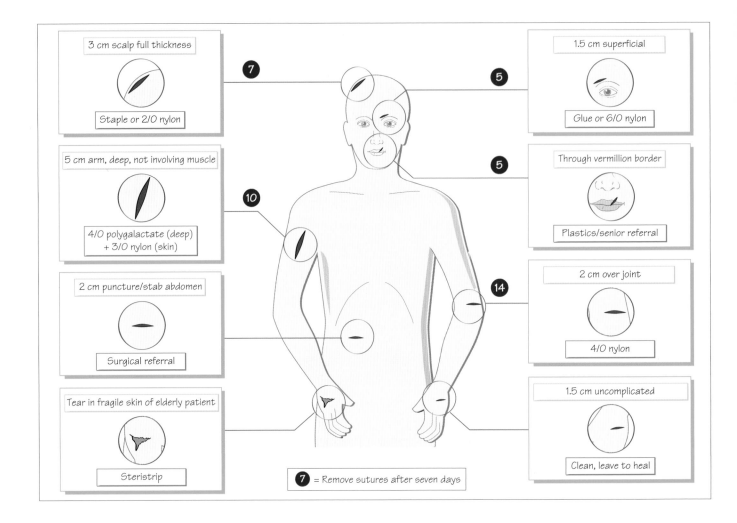

3 cm scalp full thickness

Staple or 2/0 nylon

5 cm arm, deep, not involving muscle

4/0 polygalactate (deep)
+ 3/0 nylon (skin)

2 cm puncture/stab abdomen

Surgical referral

Tear in fragile skin of elderly patient

Steristrip

1.5 cm superficial

Glue or 6/0 nylon

Through vermillion border

Plastics/senior referral

2 cm over joint

4/0 nylon

1.5 cm uncomplicated

Clean, leave to heal

7 = Remove sutures after seven days

Wounds often involve visible areas, the face and upper limb, where cosmetic as well as functional outcome is important. Wounds are generally *incised* – caused by sharp objects, or *lacerated* – caused by blunt force. An *abrasion* is a wound where the upper layers of the skin are removed, but there is no surface break. A wound where the depth exceeds the width or length is described as a *puncture* wound.

Resuscitation
Bleeding should be stopped using direct pressure or tourniquets: blind clamping should be avoided. Bleeding from scalp wounds can be controlled by full-thickness sutures using 2/0 nylon.

Any wound near a fracture is assumed to communicate with it, and should be covered by a clean saline-soaked dressing and antibiotics administered *immediately*.

Toxic bites (e.g. from snakes, spiders) should be treated according to local protocols. Snake bites can be painless, and venom may cause paralysis or catastrophic anticoagulation. Antivenom derived from animal serum is quite toxic in itself, so should not be given unless toxicity is certain.

History
Medical notes from the Emergency Department are used to write legal reports: avoid words like 'cut' or 'stab wound' unless you are an expert. Unless you witnessed the injury, use 'alleged' and quote the patient's own words wherever possible, e.g. 'Alleged assault – patient says was "hit with bottle outside a nightclub".' Accurate descriptions with *measurements*, diagrams and photographs are very helpful. Occupation/hobbies, hand dominance, allergies and tetanus status should be recorded.

Examination
Look Assess skin loss and viability, contamination, cut muscle or crush injury.

Feel Test motor and sensation (before local anaesthetic infiltration).

Move Test muscle and tendon and muscle function while observing the wound. If the wound is very painful, this is best done after infiltration of local anaesthetic.

Foreign body

Examination cannot reliably exclude foreign bodies (FBs), which are common in motor vehicle accidents, puncture wounds and clenched fist injuries. Imaging is not necessary for most wounds; X-ray if the FB is radio-opaque, i.e. metal or most glass. Ultrasound is useful, but is operator dependent.

Management

Assess the wound

Is the wound complex or dirty?
• Complex: the wound is large, involves crushed tissue, FBs, injection under pressure or extends into deep structures like muscles, tendons or joints. These wounds have a high risk of infection or compartment syndrome (Chapter 15).
• Dirty: if there is obvious contamination or the wounds is >6 hours old. Patients with reduced immune function (e.g. diabetes, steroids) are at increased risk of infection.

Consider the reason for the wound (e.g. fall, domestic violence), and any other potential injuries.

Is it safe to close the wound in the Emergency Department?

All complex or obviously contaminated wounds should be referred for exploration and closure in an operating theatre.

The options for wound closure are:
• Primary closure – close the wound immediately. This gives the neatest scar, but risks infection by trapping bacteria within the wound.
• Delayed primary closure – clean, give antibiotics for 48 hours, then close. This reduces the risk of infection in dirty wounds.
• Secondary healing – allow the wound to heal on its own. It heals more slowly, and there is more risk of scarring.

Analgesia

Local anaesthetic (LA) is injected around wounds to allow thorough cleaning and suturing (Chapter 5). Lidocaine 1% ± adrenaline (epinephrine) 1 : 100 000 is the most commonly used LA. Pain on LA injection is reduced by using a small needle, warming the LA and injecting slowly through wound edges. For wounds to be glued, use *topical* lidocaine with adrenaline applied onto a piece of gauze, cover and leave for 20 minutes.

Clean the wound

A tourniquet can be used to ensure a bloodless field. Hair near a wound may need to be cut or shaved, but not eyebrows or eyelashes. Use a syringe and 19 G needle and drinking-quality water to irrigate the wound under pressure: guard against splashback by wearing a mask and eyewear. Remove non-viable tissue and ensure embedded grit is removed to prevent tattooing.

Close the wound

Sutures

Interrupted non-absorbable nylon sutures allow drainage and minimise tissue tension and ischaemia. If there are potential spaces within the wound where a haematoma could form, or there would be tension on the skin sutures, deep absorbable sutures (e.g. polygalactin/polyglycolic acid) are used.

Timing of suture removal is a balance between scarring (shorter time better) and wound strength (longer time better). For facial wounds, 5 days is best; for wounds over extensor surfaces of joints, 14 days.

Glue, adhesive strips, staples, dressings

Tissue glue (similar to domestic Superglue®) or adhesive strips are effective for simple wounds, providing the wound edges are easily opposed without tension. The effectiveness of adhesive strips is increased by pre-coating the skin with Friar's Balsam. Staples are a fast way of closing linear wounds that do not need a perfect cosmetic result, especially scalp, limb or self-harm wounds.

If the wound is dry, a clear vapour permeable dressing allows inspection. If there are exudates, a dressing that is absorbent yet non-adherent is preferable.

Tetanus, antibiotic prophylaxis

Wounds that are dirty or complex are prone to tetanus. If a patient has had full tetanus immunisation, further boosters are not necessary unless the wound is heavily contaminated, e.g. with soil), in which case tetanus immunoglobulin is given.

Antibiotics are not a substitute for adequate wound cleaning. Antibiotics are indicated in wounds at high risk of infection or with established infection: flucloxacillin covers *Staphylococcus* and *Streptococcus*.

Special situations

Bites

Bite wounds from humans or animals are prone to infection due to the combination of crushed tissue and inoculation with saliva. Wounds should be cleaned and 5 days of broad-spectrum antibiotics (e.g. co-amoxiclav) prescribed.

Needlestick

Wounds that risk hepatitis or HIV transmission should be thoroughly cleaned. Blood should be taken and local policies consulted about follow-up.

Pre-tibial lacerations

Elderly patients can tear the thin skin over the anterior tibia. The skin should be stretched to cover as large an area as possible and early plastic surgery review arranged.

Facial wounds

Facial wounds are closed up to 24 hours after injury as cosmesis is important, and the excellent blood supply provides some protection against infection. Antibiotic ointment can be used instead of systemic antibiotics.

13 Burns

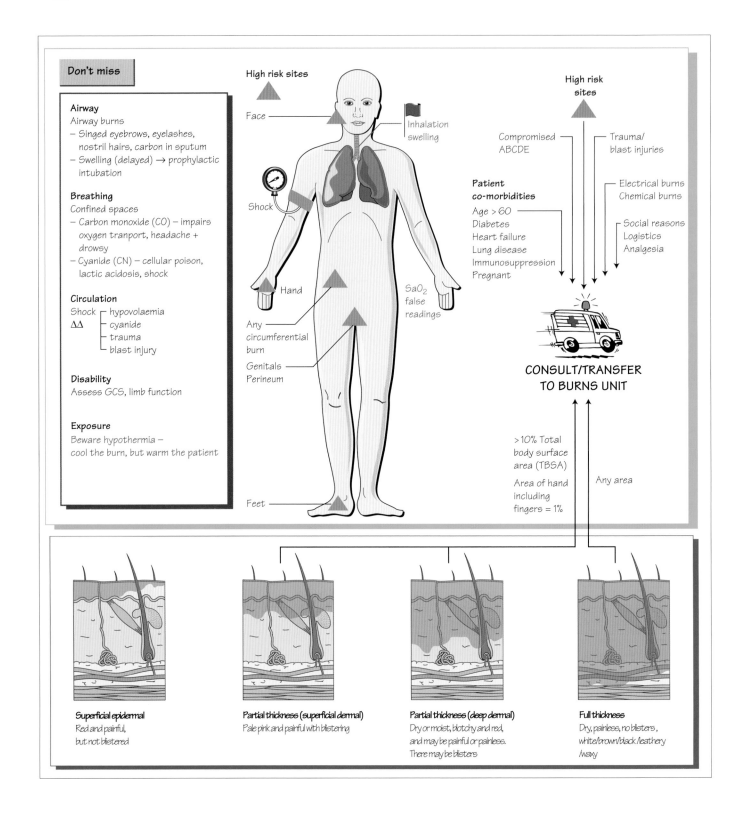

Don't miss

Airway
Airway burns
– Singed eyebrows, eyelashes, nostril hairs, carbon in sputum
– Swelling (delayed) → prophylactic intubation

Breathing
Confined spaces
– Carbon monoxide (CO) – impairs oxygen tranport, headache + drowsy
– Cyanide (CN) – cellular poison, lactic acidosis, shock

Circulation
Shock ┌ hypovolaemia
ΔΔ   ├ cyanide
       ├ trauma
       └ blast injury

Disability
Assess GCS, limb function

Exposure
Beware hypothermia –
cool the burn, but warm the patient

High risk sites

Face

Inhalation swelling

Shock

Hand

Any circumferential burn

Genitals
Perineum

SaO_2 false readings

Feet

High risk sites

Compromised ABCDE

Trauma/ blast injuries

Electrical burns
Chemical burns

Patient co-morbidities

Age > 60
Diabetes
Heart failure
Lung disease
Immunosuppression
Pregnant

Social reasons
Logistics
Analgesia

CONSULT/TRANSFER TO BURNS UNIT

>10% Total body surface area (TBSA)

Area of hand including fingers = 1%

Any area

Superficial epidermal
Red and painful, but not blistered

Partial thickness (superficial dermal)
Pale pink and painful with blistering

Partial thickness (deep dermal)
Dry or moist, blotchy and red, and may be painful or painless. There may be blisters

Full thickness
Dry, painless, no blisters, white/brown/black/leathery /waxy

Burns are a common problem, but the vast majority are relatively minor. Serious burns undergo initial assessment and resuscitation as per any trauma (Chapter 8).

History

Eye-witness accounts from ambulance personnel or witnesses are helpful in assessing the risk of associated problems such as trauma (jumping from buildings) or blast injuries. Patients trapped in confined spaces may have inhalation injuries or exposure to toxic gases such as carbon monoxide and cyanide.

AMPLE history (Chapter 9) and tetanus immunisation status are important.

Resuscitation

The patient

- *Airway:* look for signs of inhalation injury: carbon/soot in nostrils or mouth, singed eyebrows/eyelashes/nostril hairs, facial burns, and any orophayryngeal redness or swelling, change in voice or stridor.

Upper airway burns require urgent prophylactic intubation with an armoured (crushproof) endotracheal tube, as the face and oropharynx swell massively within a few hours.

- *Breathing:* oxygen via a reservoir mask for all patients.
- *Circulation:* two large-bore intravenous cannulae, through burned skin if necessary. Take blood for FBC, U+E, LFTs (liver function tests), CK (creatine kinase), group and save, clotting.

The burn

- *Stop the burning:* remove clothes, chemicals, initial cool water.
- *Treat the pain:* large doses of morphine are required for large burns. Pain is caused by air movement over the burn: clingfilm can help analgesia.
- *Secondary survey:* look for signs of other injuries, e.g. jumping from a height, blast injuries. Look for burned areas needing escharotomy (incision of the burn to prevent constriction of underlying tissues), e.g. limbs with circumferential burns, thorax.
- *Measurement of the burn:* size of patient's hand including fingers ≈1% TBSA (total body surface area).
- *Intravenous fluids:* see below.
- *Tetanus:* tetanus immunoglobulin should be given according to local protocol.
- *No antibiotics:* antibiotics should not be given routinely.
- *Investigations:* bedside urinalysis, ECG; blood tests as above, chest X-ray.
- *Transfer:* consider the need to contact a burns unit.
- *Keep warm:* although initial cooling may be helpful, burns patients are at risk of hypothermia. Wrap burned areas in clingfilm and place patient in dry, sterile sheets. Use warm air heating blanket and warmed humidified oxygen to minimise heat loss.

Complicated or non-thermal burns such as those from bitumen, chemicals, and electrical injuries require expert assessment, as the injury may be more extensive than is immediately apparent.

Intravenous fluids

Widespread capillary damage results in massive loss of intravascular fluid and protein. Give warmed crystalloids using the Parkland formula and monitor urine output.

Parkland formula for intravenous fluids in burns

2–4 mL × (% burn) × (bodyweight in kg) over 24 hours; half given in first 8 hours, the rest over 16 hours.

Minor burns

These can be dressed in many ways according to local practice including:

- Dry non-adherent dressings.
- Gel-based hydrocolloid dressings.
- Adhesive woven dressing direct to skin.
- Silver sulphasalazine cream (never on face).
  Discharged patients need:
- A clear management plan including analgesia, community support and medical and nursing follow-up.
- In elderly patients consider an Occupational Therapy assessment to identify risks of further injury.

Carbon monoxide and cyanide poisoning

Carbon monoxide poisoning occurs in fires, but is also a mode of suicide; it is most commonly caused by inadequately ventilated heating. Symptoms are often non-specific, e.g. headache, nausea and vomiting that resolves when out of the house.

Carbon monoxide has a much higher (200×) affinity for haemoglobin than oxygen. Oxygen saturation monitors cannot differentiate between carboxyhaemoglobin (COHb) and oxyhaemoglobin, so give falsely normal readings. COHb is measured in blood gas analysers: venous blood may be used. Smokers and city dwellers may have COHb levels of up to 10%.

Treatment of COHb levels above 10% is by 100% oxygen, which reduces the half-life of COHb from 240 to 75 minutes. Hyperbaric oxygen has not been shown to give additional benefit.

Cyanides are formed by furniture burning in enclosed spaces. Diagnosis and treatment is described in Chapter 47.

Electrical burns (including lightning)

Electricity follows the path of least resistance, which tends to be nerves, blood vessels and, to a lesser extent, muscle. Skin burns – entry and exit points – may appear relatively minor, and the full extent of electrical burns may not be apparent immediately.

High-voltage (>600 V) injuries produce heat injury in underlying tissues and can cause cardiac damage and compartment syndrome. If a patient hit by lightning makes it to hospital, their chances of survival are good. Admit all patients with high-voltage burns, but patients exposed to domestic electricity (110–220 V AC) may be discharged if they have a normal ECG and no evidence of burns or systemic injury.

Chemical burns

Seek early expert advice with chemical burns. Both alkaline and acid substances can burn the skin: alkalis such as drain cleaner and cement are generally worse as acids tend to precipitate proteins, preventing deep burns. Water is used until pain resolves and pH is neutral.

Hydrofluoric acid burns deeply and painfully, binding calcium ions, causing local and systemic hypocalcaemia. Treatment is by local or systemic calcium gluconate, which can be given as a gel, injection into the wound, intravenously (like IVRA) or intra-arterially.

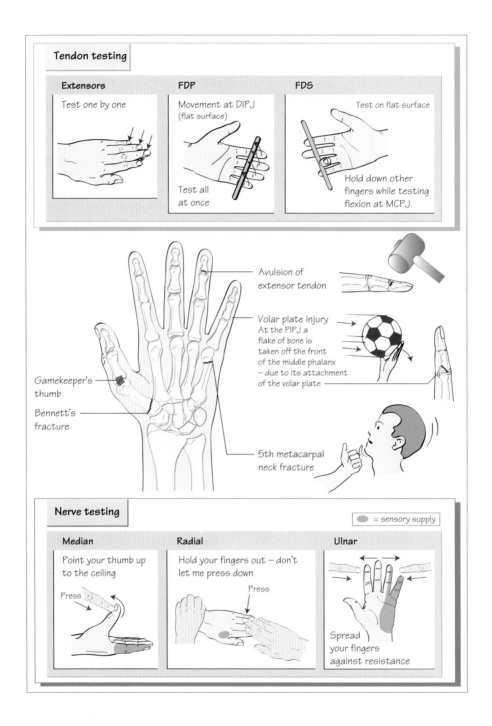

Hand injuries are a common presentation to the Emergency Department, and the importance of good hand function in day-to-day life requires excellent results. The spectacular range of hand function relies on complex interplay between muscles, tendons, bones and ligaments, all of which may be damaged.

History and examination
Hand dominance, job and hobbies are essential parts of the history. The mechanism of injury may suggest a likely pattern of injury, e.g. a fifth metacarpal fracture following a fight. If there is no history of injury, consider infection (e.g. septic arthritis) or inflammation (e.g. rheumatoid arthritis).

It can be confusing to describe lesions in relation to the anatomical position, so the terms volar or palmar, and dorsal are used, rather than anterior and posterior. Similarly, radial and ulnar are used rather than medial or lateral. Names of digits (thumb/index/middle/ring/little) should be used, rather than numbers.

Look Look for swelling/bruising and compare hands. Check the skin over the knuckles for wounds: human 'bites' need treatment (Chapter 12).

Feel Feel the carpal and metacarpal bones and joints and the 'anatomical snuff box' (Chapter 15).

Move Ask the patient to make a fist: check the fingers are in line, pointing to the scaphoid.
• Check sensory and motor function. Two-point discrimination testing can reveal subtle sensory loss.
• Check the extensor and flexor tendon function.
• Test the thumb ligaments.
• Ask the patient to grip your index and middle fingers 'as tight as they can'.

Management
Immobilise and elevate
Neighbour/buddy strapping involves strapping an injured finger to an adjacent finger, providing protection against hyperextension while still allowing good function.

Volar slab: a strip of plaster on the palmar/volar side of the hand with the wrist in extension and the metacarpophalangeal joints (MCPJs) in flexion provides support and prevents contraction of tendons or muscles.

Multiple layers of elastic or plaster strapping around the thumb is called a thumb 'spica', and provides protection against abduction or hyperextension.

The compartments of the hand have little room to accommodate soft tissue swelling, so elevation in a sling is used to keep the hand above the heart. Rings should be removed.

The majority of hand injuries can be managed as outpatients or by GPs; however, open fractures, or those listed below under 'Do not miss', should be reviewed by the inpatient team.

Common injuries
Metacarpal neck fractures
Little or ring finger metacarpal neck fractures caused by punch injuries are quite stable. Angulation <30° gives a good functional outcome. If more angulated, the fracture may be reduced by flexing the MCPJ to 90° and pushing dorsally.

Fractures and dislocations of the phalanges
Dislocations and fractures with marked deformity should be reduced in the Emergency Department using N_2O/O_2 or a ring block. Mid-shaft or spiral fractures may be unstable due to fracture pattern or muscle action, and require operative fixation, particularly if there is any rotational deformity.

Hammer/mallet finger
Forced flexion of the extended distal phalanx pulls a flake of bone off the distal phalanx. Treat with a mallet splint to ensure the patient does not flex their distal phalanx at all for 6 weeks.

Thenar eminence sprain
The powerful muscles of the thenar eminence can be torn by forced abduction of the thumb – a common injury when falling on a slippery surface, e.g. skiing or skating. More serious injuries, e.g. Bennett's/scaphoid fractures must be excluded.

Nail and fingertip injuries
Injuries to the fingertip are common, and require X-ray to exclude bone injury, but rarely need operative treatment. If the nail is displaced, remove under ring block, trim, and use as a dressing for the nailbed. Nailbed injuries rarely need treatment.

Lacerations
Uncomplicated lacerations (that do not involve underlying structures) on the hand and digits less than 2cm long do not require suturing, providing the wounds are not at high risk of infection (Chapter 12). Clean, dress and consider topical antibiotic ointment. Above this size, sutures are usually used. Ensure that distal neurovascular function is documented.

Fish-hook injury
Fish-hooks have a barb to prevent fish (or humans) from pulling the hook out. After anaesthetising the area, it may be necessary to advance the hook through the skin to cut off the barb and allow removal.

Diagnoses not to miss
Bennett's fracture
This is a fracture of the base of the thumb or first metacarpal bone, caused by thumb hyperextension. It is unstable and needs operative fixation.

Gamekeeper's thumb
Gamekeeper's thumb is a tear of the ulnar collateral ligament of the thumb at MCPJ level by forced abduction. Complete tears do not heal without surgery.

Tendon injuries
Tendon injuries are easy to miss unless the tendons are individually tested. Tendon lacerations can occur when an extensor, or less commonly, a flexor tendon hits a sharp object, particularly when the is running over a bony prominence. Complete tendon division requires operative repair.

Tendon sheath infection
Tendons run in fibrous sheaths that protect and lubricate the tendon. If infection penetrates the sheath, it may track down the finger and into the hand. Such infections need urgent drainage, washout and antibiotic treatment.

Amputations
All amputations involving bone loss should be referred and reimplantation considered, especially for thumb and index fingers. The amputated part should be wrapped in clean cloth, and then put in a plastic bag inside an ice bath. The amputated part should not touch ice. Successful reimplantation of digits severed distal to the distal interphalangeal joint (DIPJ) is unlikely as the nerves, arteries and veins are too small.

15 Wrist and forearm injuries

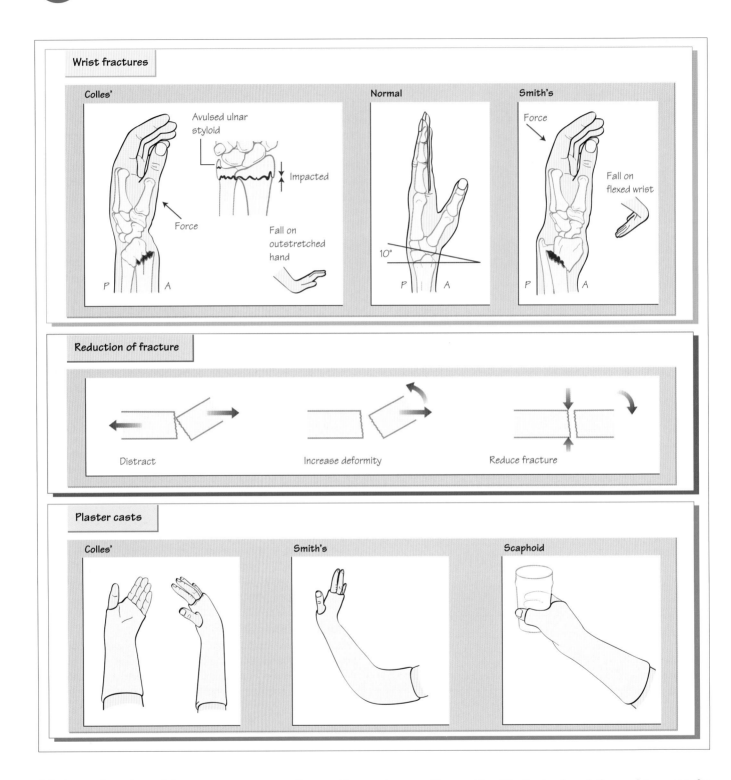

Injuries to the wrist and forearm are common, often resulting from a fall onto an outstretched hand (FOOSH). It can be difficult to distinguish subtle fractures from soft tissue injury on clinical history and examination alone, so X-ray is usually necessary.

Fractures of normal bones imply *high-energy* injuries, whereas a fracture occurring as a result of a *low-energy* injury implies poor bone quality – a *'fragility fracture'*, and the need to screen for osteoporosis.

In any injury affecting the upper limb, dominance (handedness) and occupation and hobbies must be recorded. If the injury is the result of a fall, consider further investigations (Chapter 30).

 Adult Emergency Medicine at a Glance, 1st edition. © Thomas Hughes and Jaycen Cruickshank. Published 2011 by Blackwell Publishing Ltd.

Examination: look, feel, move

Compare with opposite side, and look for swelling/bruising. A full range of elbow flexion, pronation and supination makes significant injury unlikely. The radial, median and ulnar nerve function in the hand should be checked (Chapter 14).

Management of fractures: principles

Pain should be controlled by splintage and analgesic drugs before imaging. Elevation of the arm in a sling reduces soft tissue swelling and pain. *If there is any evidence of neurovascular deficit or tenting of the skin by fractures, urgent reduction will be necessary.*

If there is a skin wound over a fracture, this makes it an *open fracture*. Antibiotics ± anti-tetanus treatment must be given *immediately*. The wound should be covered with a saline-soaked dressing, and the patient should go to theatre for debridement as soon as possible.

Plaster of Paris casts are used to hold the fracture in position while it heals. Rings should be removed before plaster is applied, as the digits will swell.

Compartment syndrome results from swelling of muscle within fascia compartments, e.g. of the forearm, leg or foot. If untreated, the muscle dies, resulting in untreatable ischaemic contracture. Patients should be warned about the symptoms: numbness, pain and cold digits. If a patient has pain on passive stretching of a muscle, compartment syndrome is likely; a palpable pulse *does not exclude* compartment syndrome. If elevation does not solve the problem, the plaster *must* be released, and a surgeon *must* review.

Common diagnoses
Colles' fracture

This is a fracture of the distal radius occurring in *osteoporotic* bone resulting from *low-energy* impact, e.g. FOOSH. The fracture may be impacted and the tip of the ulna is often avulsed. Dorsal angulation gives the wrist a 'dinner fork' appearance.

The fracture should be reduced in the Emergency Department using haematoma block and nitrous oxide, or intravenous regional anaesthesia (Chapter 5). Good wrist function depends on restoration of the length of the radius, and avoidance of steps in the articular surface. On the lateral X-ray view, the articular surface of the radius is normally 10° angulated towards the palm. This is often difficult to achieve by reduction, but a neutral (0°) position is satisfactory.

High-energy distal radius fracture

This injury occurs in *normal* bones as a result of *high-energy* impact, e.g. falling off a bicycle. In comparison to a Colles' fracture, there is more likely to be comminution (multiple bone fragments), more soft tissue damage and more pain: intravenous opiates are necessary.

To achieve good function, these fractures need excellent ('anatomical') reduction and may ultimately require operative fixation with plates or wires. A good reduction in the Emergency Department using intravenous regional analgesia or procedural sedation (Chapter 6) minimises soft tissue swelling and may avoid the need for further intervention.

Smith's fracture

A Smith's fracture is sometimes called a reverse Colles' fracture: it is a distal radius fracture, but instead of dorsal angulation, there is volar (palmar) angulation. However, Smith's fractures often occur in *normal* bone, when they are *high-energy* injuries. The structures on the volar (palmar) side of the wrist are at risk of injury, particularly the median nerve.

A Smith's fracture is inherently unstable, and almost always needs open reduction and internal fixation (ORIF) (e.g. with a plate and screws), although a good reduction in the Emergency Department is usually the first step in the management.

Diagnoses not to miss
Scaphoid fractures

The difficulty in diagnosis and the consequences of failure to diagnose make this fracture a frequent source of litigation. The history is usually FOOSH, and clinical signs are pain:

- In the 'anatomical snuffbox' between extensor pollicis longus (EPL) and abductor pollicis longus (APL).
- On axial thumb compression.
- On pressing over the scaphoid tubercle.

A patient with clinical signs of scaphoid injury requires a 'scaphoid view' X-ray. If this demonstrates a fracture, the joint should be immobilised as shown opposite.

Even if the X-ray does *not* show a fracture, the patient should still be immobilised in a splint or plaster cast, and sent home to have a definitive investigation, e.g. repeat X-ray, in 1 week, or CT or MR scan, to prove or refute the diagnosis of scaphoid fracture.

The reason for this approach is that 20% of patients have fractures of the scaphoid that are *not visible* on plain X-ray until at least 1 week after injury. If the scaphoid fracture is missed, avascular necrosis and non-union can result in early osteoarthritis and disabling stiffness of the wrist.

If you perform an X-ray of the scaphoid, it is illogical and therefore medicolegally indefensible not to follow up with a definitive investigation.

Fractures of shaft of radius and ulna

The X-ray must include the joint above and below to ensure that there is no dislocation. These fractures need ORIF.

- *Nightstick fracture*: a mid-shaft transverse fracture of the ulna, usually a 'defence injury' when the forearm is raised to protect the head ('nightstick' is the US term for a police truncheon). Consider possible causes, e.g. domestic violence.
- *Monteggia fracture*: fracture of *proximal* third of ulna and dislocation of the head of the radius at the elbow.
- *Galeazzi fracture*: fracture of *distal* third of radius with associated dislocation of distal radio-ulnar joint; rare.

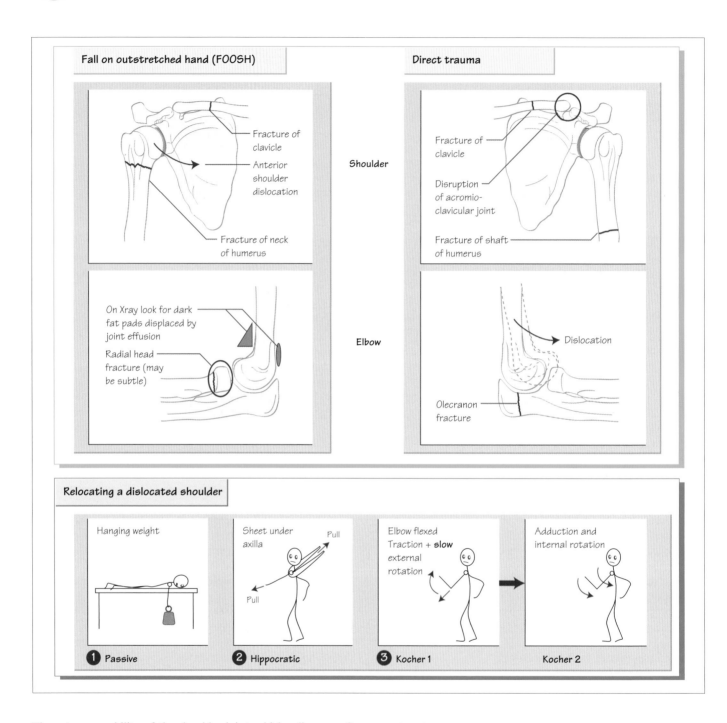

The extreme mobility of the shoulder joint, which relies on soft tissues – muscles, ligaments and cartilage – for stability, comes at a price. The shoulder is relatively unstable, and prone to stiffness if not used. There is a wide range of injury patterns, which change according to the age of the patient.

History

In any injury affecting the upper limb, dominance (handedness) and occupation and hobbies must be recorded. Shoulder pain can also be referred, e.g. cardiac, diaphragmatic, respiratory.

Injury is usually caused by either a fall onto outstretched hand (FOOSH) or direct trauma.

Examination

Look Compare with the other side.

Feel Start at the medial end of the clavicle and work laterally, feeling for tenderness of clavicle, coracoid process, acromioclavicular (AC) joint, humeral head and greater tuberosity.

Feel the olecranon, epicondyles and radial head. An elbow effusion may be felt below the radial head.

Move Limited or painful shoulder movement warrants an X-ray; very little movement will be possible with a dislocated shoulder or fracture. A full range of elbow extension makes fracture unlikely.

Neurovascular examination
Specific injuries and their corresponding neurovascular deficits are:
- Shoulder dislocation and fracture neck of humerus: test the axillary nerve – loss of sensation over lower deltoid area.
- Humeral shaft fractures – radial nerve.
- Medial epicondyle fracture – ulna nerve injury.
- Elbow dislocations – brachial artery and median nerve.

Imaging
Plain X-rays are indicated in most patients presenting with shoulder pain and reduced range of movement after trauma. Elbow fractures are very unlikely if there is full elbow extension. Fractures are difficult to see and radiographs should be examined carefully for evidence of an effusion: the dark shadows caused by the anterior and posterior fat pads.

Management
Analgesia is achieved by immobilisation (e.g. sling), and oral analgesics before imaging. Patients with severe pain and deformity require intravenous opiates and early assessment. Early active movement of the shoulder is important to avoid stiffness in the elderly.

Ensure urgent orthopaedic referral for:
- Any fracture with neurovascular compromise.
- Open fractures, which require urgent antibiotics.

Common diagnoses
Fractured clavicle
This injury most commonly occurs at the junction between the middle and outer third. Most heal with good function by providing rest in a sling and analgesia.

Acromio-clavicular joint injuries
Acromio-clavicular joint (ACJ) injuries are caused by fall onto tip of shoulder, causing disruption to the ACJ and ligaments. With complete disruption, the clavicle will 'float' above the acromion. ACJ injuries are treated with analgesia, rest in a sling and physiotherapy in the first instance, but the more severe grades of disruption may need fixation later.

Dislocated shoulder
The shoulder usually dislocates anteriorly (95%) from a fall with the arm in the 'hailing a taxi' position – the humerus is externally rotated and abducted. The humeral head may be palpable and the patient will support the arm, holding it by their side.

There are many different reduction techniques, each with their own proponents. It is generally best to start with a passive technique that requires only nitrous oxide/oxygen analgesia and can be conducted by nursing staff. The active techniques require intravenous analgesia ± sedation (Chapter 6).
- **Passive: hanging weight technique.** The patient lies prone on a couch with the arm hanging down with a 2–5 kg weight suspended from their wrist.

- **Active: Hippocratic technique.** Traction of the patient's arm, together with mild rotation. The traditional method of counter-traction involved the doctor's 'stockinged foot' in the patient's axilla. The modern version uses a sheet under the axilla so an assistant at the head of the bed can provide counter-traction.
- **Active: modified Kocher's technique.** This technique must not be rushed and requires good analgesia and sedation.
  1 Flex elbow, continuous gentle traction.
  2 Using the forearm as a lever, the humerus is externally rotated to almost 90° *very slowly* to overcome pectoral spasm.
  3 The arm is brought across the body and the humerus internally rotated to achieve reduction.

Reduction should be confirmed on X-ray, which may show any damage to the humeral head. Patients with a first dislocated shoulder should have the shoulder immobilised for 6 weeks to allow the capsule to heal. Patients with multiple dislocations need surgery to stabilise the shoulder.

Fractured neck of humerus
This injury is common in the elderly, due to FOOSH; underlying causes for falls should be sought (Chapter 30). Early mobilisation with appropriate analgesia is necessary to avoid long-term stiffness ('frozen shoulder') that may be far more disabling than the original injury. Displaced fractures may require reduction ± fixation.

Dislocated elbow
Hyperextension of the elbow forces the humerus anteriorly over the coronoid process of the ulna. Neurovascular status should be checked, and this should be reduced by traction under sedation.

Fractured head of radius
This is the most common elbow fracture, which can be difficult to see on plain X-ray, although the elbow effusion 'fat pad sign' will be visible. Diagnosis can be confirmed by tenderness over the radial head, and reduced pronation/supination. Most fractures make a good recovery with analgesia and early mobilisation.

Fractured shaft of humerus
Twisting injuries produce spiral fractures, bending injuries transverse fractures. Radial nerve injury can occur in fractures of the middle third of the humerus.

Diagnoses not to miss
Posterior dislocation of shoulder
This injury is most common after epileptic fits or electrical injury forcing contraction of the strong latissimus dorsi muscles. Posterior dislocation is difficult to spot on X-ray: there is reduced glenohumeral overlap and the greater tuberosity is not visible, creating the 'lightbulb sign': the humeral head appears symmetrical. If in doubt, ask for an axillary view X-ray.

Scapular fracture
Scapular fractures can be difficult to see on X-ray, but are usually very painful due to distension of the tight capsule and may need admission for analgesia. Significant energy is necessary to fracture a scapula, and other injuries should be sought.

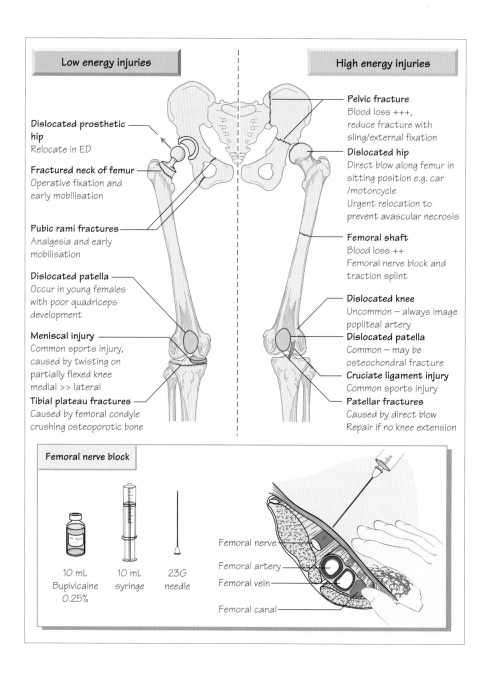

Low energy injuries

Dislocated prosthetic hip
Relocate in ED

Fractured neck of femur
Operative fixation and early mobilisation

Pubic rami fractures
Analgesia and early mobilisation

Dislocated patella
Occur in young females with poor quadriceps development

Meniscal injury
Common sports injury, caused by twisting on partially flexed knee medial >> lateral

Tibial plateau fractures
Caused by femoral condyle crushing osteoporotic bone

High energy injuries

Pelvic fracture
Blood loss +++, reduce fracture with sling/external fixation

Dislocated hip
Direct blow along femur in sitting position e.g. car /motorcycle
Urgent relocation to prevent avascular necrosis

Femoral shaft
Blood loss ++
Femoral nerve block and traction splint

Dislocated knee
Uncommon – always image popliteal artery

Dislocated patella
Common – may be osteochondral fracture

Cruciate ligament injury
Common sports injury

Patellar fractures
Caused by direct blow
Repair if no knee extension

Femoral nerve block

10 mL
Bupivicaine
0.25%

10 mL
syringe

23G
needle

Femoral nerve
Femoral artery
Femoral vein
Femoral canal

Back pain

Lumbar back pain is a common presentation to the Emergency Department, and can be very challenging to manage. Patients may arrive at the Emergency Department with an agenda that includes hospital admission for analgesia and rehabilitation. This is not practical or desirable: after exclusion of significant pathology, early mobilisation is the most effective treatment. Back pain may also be caused by hip disease and retroperitoneal organs, e.g. aorta, pancreas.

Red flags

There are four conditions that must not be missed.
1 Abdominal aortic aneurysm (Chapter 19).

2 Malignancy.
3 Epidural abscess or haematoma.
4 Large prolapsed disc causing neurological deficit or cauda equina syndrome.

Therefore any history and examination must document the following.
- Age, back pain history, history of malignancy.
- Pain at rest, pain wakes at night.
- History of trauma, fever, intravenous drug use, anticoagulation.
- Straight leg raising, angle, crossed leg raise.
- Power at each joint (flexion, extension).
- Reflexes: knee, ankle, plantar.

• Incontinence, perineal anaesthesia, reduced anal tone (implies possible cauda equina syndrome).

Crossed straight leg raising: lifting the *unaffected* leg reproduces pain in the other leg. This is a very sensitive indicator of nerve root irritation, e.g. from a prolapsed disc.

If there are no abnormalities and the patient is otherwise well, the diagnosis is likely to be mechanical back pain.

Investigations

Investigations are rarely necessary if no red flag symptoms. MRI is the gold standard for investigating spinal neurological problems. Urgent MRI scanning is indicated if cauda equina is suspected. Lumbar spine X-ray (70 CXR) is only indicated with a history of trauma or if malignancy is suspected.

Management

A positive but firm attitude to encourage mobilisation may be necessary: Emergency Department nursing staff are particularly skilled at this.

The combination of an NSAID (e.g. ketorolac) and paracetamol/codeine-based analgesia is a good starting point. Diazepam acts as a muscle relaxant if there is significant spasm, but should only be given for a couple of days.

Hip and knee injury

The hip is an inherently stable joint, which requires substantial energy to disrupt. The knee's stability depends on muscles, tendons, ligaments and cartilage, all of which are vulnerable to injury. Osteoporotic bone is vulnerable to low-energy injuries, i.e. 'fragility fractures' such as fractured neck of femur (#NoF).

Examination

Look Assess gait and inspect for joint swelling or asymmetry. Look for shortening and external rotation (#NoF) or flexion and internal rotation (dislocation of hip). Swelling of the knee joint may be due to a joint effusion. Acute traumatic effusion occurs as a result of bleeding from bony or ligamentous injury.

Feel Areas of tenderness may indicate fracture, e.g. patella, head of fibula. Knee effusion is detected by pushing the patella down so it makes contact with the anterior surface of the femoral condyle – 'patellar tap'.

Move Assess all hip movements. Internal/external rotation at the hip is a sensitive test for fractures. Assess range of movement of knee, specifically for pain or instability (ligament injury) or locking/unlocking (meniscus tear/loose body).
• Knee ligamentous stability: ACL, PCL, LCL, MCL (anterior and posterior cruciate, lateral and medial collateral ligaments).
• Knee meniscal stability: Apley's test.
• Patellar stability: apprehension test.

Neurovascular examination

Knee dislocation damages the popliteal artery, which *always* needs expert vascular assessment. The common peroneal nerve is at risk in lateral knee injuries: test for dorsiflexion of foot and sensation over dorsum of foot.

Investigations
Bedside investigations
• Blood glucose, urine dipstick, ECG in patients with falls.

Laboratory investigations
• FBC and group and save indicated in all patients with pelvic or femur fractures, as bleeding is often underestimated.

Imaging
• In frail elderly patients, even low amounts of energy can cause fractures. All possible hip fractures should have an X-ray of the pelvis and lateral hip. The pelvis and pubic rami are brittle ring structures, and like a 'Polo' ® mint, they can never be broken in one place only.
• The Ottawa knee rules prevent unnecessary knee X-rays.
• CT is useful for pelvic and tibial plateau fractures.
• MRI is the gold standard for the diagnosis of knee injuries and occult hip fractures.

Treatment

Lower limb fractures are painful. Intravenous opiates are often necessary. A femoral nerve block gives effective analgesia for femoral fractures at/below the trochanter. Femoral shaft fracture requires a traction splint.

Knee

A tense, painful knee haemoarthosis should be aspirated. This also allows examination of cruciate function, reduces intra-articular adhesions, or confirms haemarthrosis vs. blood-stained effusion. By putting the aspirate into a bowl, fat globules floating on the surface will be seen if there is a fracture.

Most patients with isolated knee injuries will be able to go home in a knee brace or a Robert Jones bandage (a wool and crepe bandage built up to support the extended knee) with outpatient clinic follow-up.

Hip and femur

Fractured neck of femur is common in the elderly and requires operative fixation. Consider possible causes for falling (Chapter 29).

A patient who has a clinically suspected fractured neck of femur but normal X-rays needs admission and further investigation. These patients often have fractured pubic rami, or impacted fractures seen on further imaging, e.g. MR.

The Ottawa knee rules

X-ray if:
>55 years
Tender at head of fibula
Tender patella
Inability to flex to 90°
Inability to weight bear (4 steps, limping allowed) both immediately and in the Emergency Department.

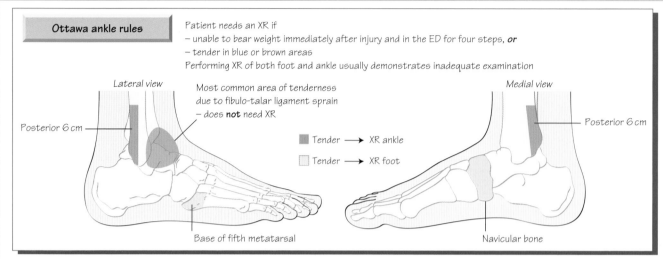

Ottawa ankle rules

Patient needs an XR if
– unable to bear weight immediately after injury and in the ED for four steps, **or**
– tender in blue or brown areas
Performing XR of both foot and ankle usually demonstrates inadequate examination

Lateral view

Most common area of tenderness due to fibulo-talar ligament sprain
– does **not** need XR

Posterior 6 cm

⬛ Tender ⟶ XR ankle
⬜ Tender ⟶ XR foot

Base of fifth metatarsal

Medial view

Posterior 6 cm

Navicular bone

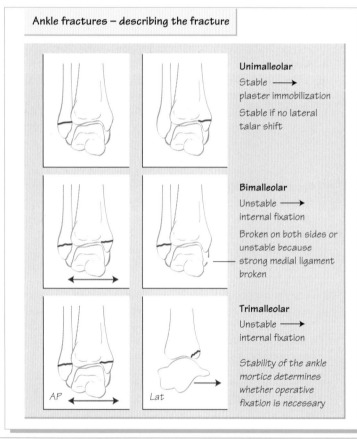

Ankle fractures – describing the fracture

Unimalleolar
Stable ⟶ plaster immobilization
Stable if no lateral talar shift

Bimalleolar
Unstable ⟶ internal fixation
Broken on both sides or unstable because strong medial ligament broken

Trimalleolar
Unstable ⟶ internal fixation
Stability of the ankle mortice determines whether operative fixation is necessary

AP   Lat

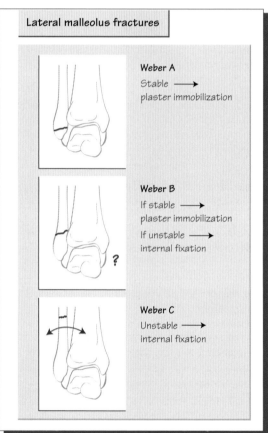

Lateral malleolus fractures

Weber A
Stable ⟶ plaster immobilization

Weber B
If stable ⟶ plaster immobilization
If unstable ⟶ internal fixation

Weber C
Unstable ⟶ internal fixation

History
Mechanism of injury
High-energy injuries commonly result from axial loading, direct blows or crush injuries, e.g. falls or jumps, motor vehicle accidents. Tibial shaft injuries are severe, and risk neurovascular injury and compartment syndrome.

Low-energy injuries tend to occur from twisting at the ankle joint, particularly ankle inversion. The medial tibiotalar ligament is strong, unlike the weaker fibulotalar and fibulocalcaneal ligaments on the lateral side. Hence most ankle sprains are on the lateral side, caused by inversion of the foot.

Examination

Look A dislocated ankle will look deformed. Bruising and swelling around ankle and foot is not specific for fracture, although bruising over the calcaneus is likely to indicate a fracture.

Feel Widespread mild soft tissue tenderness is common in ankle injuries and needs to be differentiated from specific areas of bony tenderness. Examination must never be rough, but if poor-quality information is collected from the clinical examination, poor-quality decisions will be made. Check neurovascular status.

Move The function of the foot and ankle is critically dependent on the subtalar joint. Support the calcaneus in your non-dominant hand and use your dominant hand to:
- Flex and extend at the ankle.
- Invert and evert at the subtalar joint.
- Twist the forefoot while holding the calcaneum tight.

Imaging
- A dislocated ankle should be reduced before taking X-rays.
- Use the Ottawa rules (opposite).
- Ordering both foot and ankle radiographs together implies inadequate examination.
- CT is useful in injuries to the mid and hindfoot.
- Radiographs of toes other than the big toe are unlikely to change management, and should not generally be performed.

Management
Patients with an open fracture must have intravenous antibiotics urgently; the injury should be photographed and then covered in a saline-soaked dressing pending urgent theatre. Taking a picture of the wound is useful for the surgeon as it will be covered by dressing and plaster.

Analgesia includes splintage and reduction of fractures. Elevation will reduce pain and tissue oedema, which facilitates surgery, and reduces the risk of compartment syndrome. Neurovascular status must be recorded, particularly before and after fracture/dislocation reduction.

Disposal: who can go home?
Admit patients with the following.
- Open fractures.
- Dislocated ankles.
- Failed closed reduction/unstable fracture.
- Fractured talus or calcaneus.
- Tarsometatarsal dislocation: Lisfranc injury.

Patients with stable fracture pattern injuries, who are unlikely to need surgery and who have no evidence of complications, can usually go home. The initial cast should be either a backslab or a split cast; this is because swelling will occur over the first 24 hours after injury. Casts should ensure that the foot is at 90° to the leg to maintain soft tissue length, except for Achilles tendon plasters, which are plantarflexed.

Patients should receive written instructions covering monitoring for signs of neurovascular compromise/compartment syndrome, (Chapter 15) cast care, advice to elevate the limb and follow-up arrangements. If crutches are necessary, patients should be shown how to use them.

Common diagnoses
Ankle sprain
If a fracture is ruled out using a decision rule or radiograph, the likely diagnosis is a 'sprained ankle' – partial rupture of the lateral ligament complex, e.g. fibulo-talar and fibular-calcaneal.

In addition to short-term rest, ice and elevation, patients may benefit from physiotherapy. Compression bandages do not help, but for more severe sprains, immobilisation in a backslab for one week, together with crutches, is advisable.

Ankle fractures
The mortice joint of the ankle is responsible for its structural integrity. If the mortice is intact on one side, the fracture will be stable, and may be managed in plaster. If both sides are unstable, internal fixation will be necessary.

Gastrocnemius tear
The calf muscle may tear in a sudden contraction, common in tennis. Treatment is rest, analgesia and physiotherapy.

Achilles tendon rupture
Occurs when jumping (basketball, racquet sports) – or due to quinolone antibiotics. Squeezing the calf muscles normally causes foot plantarflexion – this does not occur with a complete rupture, which can be confirmed by ultrasound. Complete rupture is repaired, but partial rupture is managed in plaster.

Metatarsal fracture
The second and third metatarsals are most affected by stress fractures. The tendon of peroneus brevis attaches at the base of the fifth metatarsal. Inversion injuries may cause avulsion of this tendon with a flake of bone.

Avulsion fractures
These are easily missed in the 'sprained foot'. Look specifically at the navicular, talus, cuboid and the inferior border of the malleoli for a flake of bone that has been avulsed by a ligament.

Diagnoses not to miss
Talar fracture
Falls on an inverted foot, or forced foot dorsiflexion ('aviator's fracture') may cause a talar fracture. The talus has a central role in both ankle flexion/extension and inversion/eversion. Fractures of the talus often have poor outcomes due to a circuitous blood supply, with high rates of avascular necrosis.

Tarsometatarsal (Lisfranc) dislocation
These injuries are rare, complex and often missed. The history may be of a crush type injury. Typical signs and symptoms include pain, swelling over midfoot (TMT joints) and the inability to bear weight. X-ray findings are subtle and may appear normal. Consider this diagnosis if pain is very high despite no apparent deformity.

Calcaneal fracture
Calcaneal fractures are generally caused by a fall from a height. Fractures are usually comminuted and are associated with fractures of the lumbar spine and wrists, which should be examined carefully.

19 Abdominal pain

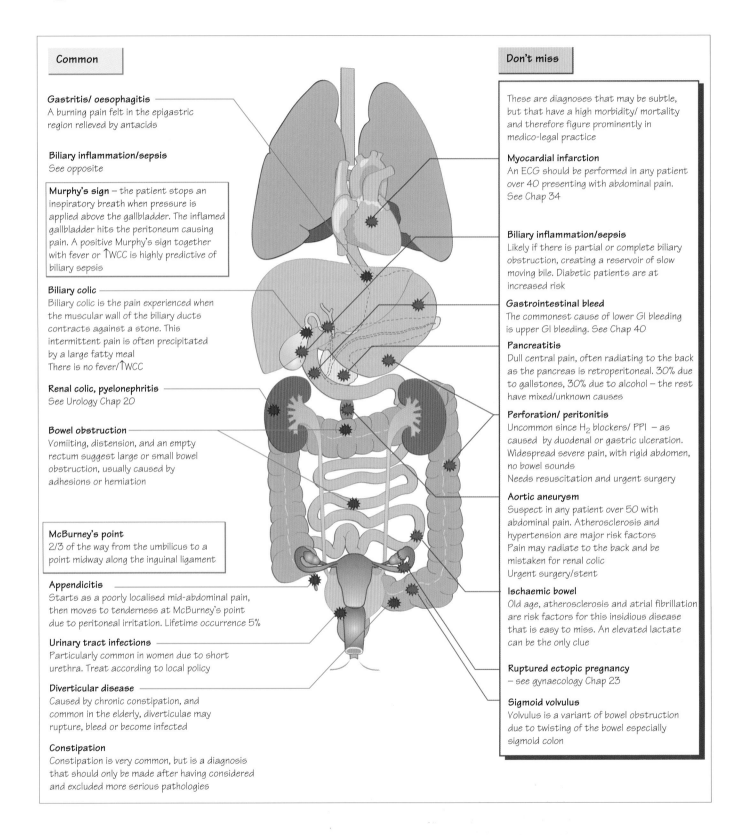

The abdominal cavity contains the organs that digest food, filter blood and enable reproduction, any of which may give rise to abdominal pain. As with chest pain, patients presenting with a 'textbook' collection of symptoms are the exception rather than the rule.

History

A focused history should be taken, concentrating on the nature and timing of the pain and its associations. Most abdominal space relates to food processing, therefore the relationship of pain to food intake/excretion is important, e.g. pain related to large or fatty meals suggests gallstones. Date of last menstrual period (LMP) is essential information to obtain from any woman of childbearing age.

Nature of the pain

There are three common sorts of abdominal pain.
• *Colicky pain:* pain that comes and goes in spasms, and is usually the result of peristalsis failing to move a solid mass, e.g. the ureter attempting to move a stone to the bladder. The patient may move about, seeking a comfortable position.
• *Peritonism:* the sharp, well-localised pain resulting from inflammation of the parietal (outer) peritoneal surface – peritonitis. The patient lies still to avoid moving the inflamed surfaces.
• *Distension pain* results from an organ or bowel being stretched. The pain is poorly localised and may be felt as central abdominal pain. When the bowel is distended by gas, it may be tympanic: the abdomen sounds 'hollow' when percussed.

Less common types of pain are:
• *Mucosal pain:* burning pain due to inflammation of the mucosa, e.g. reflux of gastric acid into the oesophagus, urinary tract infection (UTI), sexually transmitted infection (STI).
• *Ischaemic pain:* poorly localised gnawing/cramping pain caused by inflammation progressing to ischaemic necrosis, e.g. menstruation, ischaemic bowel.
• *Referred pain:* pain occurring in a different area, e.g. cardiac ischaemia may be perceived as abdominal pain. Conversely, pain from within the abdomen may be perceived elsewhere, e.g. shoulder tip pain from diaphragmatic irritation, penile pain from renal colic, and back pain from retroperitoneal structures.

To make things more complicated, a single pathophysiological process may cause different types of pain simultaneously.

Examination
Inspection

From the end of the bed: is the patient well/ill/critically ill? Immunosuppressed patients may appear deceptively well despite significant disease. Also beware patients with neuropathy, e.g. diabetics who may not experience 'normal' pain. Patients who cannot get comfortable or who are constantly moving are likely to have colicky pain. Patients who lie very still are likely to have peritonitis.

Palpation, percussion and auscultation

Poorly localised general pain is usually felt around the umbilicus, but specific point tenderness suggests peritonitis. Increased bowel sounds are caused by obstruction; absent bowel sounds indicate peritonitis. Rectal examination is an important part of the examination, and stool should be tested for blood.

Investigations
Bedside investigations
• Blood glucose.
• Urine dipstick.
• Urinary βhCG in any woman of childbearing age.
• Ultrasound is used by emergency physicians to rule out abdominal aortic aneurysm or to look for intra-abdominal fluid. If the expertise is available, it may be useful in patients with other diseases, e.g. gallstones.

Laboratory investigations
• FBC, U+E, LFTs and amylase/lipase in all patients.
• Arterial blood gases including lactate in sick patients.
• Group and save/cross-match blood if patient likely to go to theatre.

Imaging
• An erect chest X-ray detects free air from a perforated bowel.
• A supine abdominal X-ray (60 CXR) will demonstrate obstruction but is otherwise unlikely to be helpful.
• Ultrasound is good for biliary, urinary and gynaecological causes of pain.
• CT (300 CXR) is very good at demonstrating most abdominal pathology but is a high dose of radiation.
• MRI is good for imaging abdominal organs, but is not widely available.

Management
• *Resuscitation* and urgent surgical opinion if clinically unwell. Oxygen for all unwell patients together with observation and monitoring in a suitable clinical area.
• *Intravenous fluids* are an important part of resuscitation, but also replace ongoing fluid losses (Chapter 3). A nasogastric tube keeps the stomach empty, e.g. if there is bowel obstruction.
• *Analgesia:* intravenous morphine with anti-emetic is humane, safe and does not impede diagnosis. Intravenous or rectal NSAID, e.g. ketorolac, is good for peritoneal pain and relaxes smooth muscle so is good for colicky pain, although should be avoided in the elderly.

Disposal: who can go home?

Any patient who has abdominal pain requiring ongoing morphine needs to be admitted. Patients who appear well, in whom serious pathology has been excluded, and whose pain has not recurred after analgesia has worn off, are usually safe to discharge. Other patients should be reviewed by the relevant surgical team.

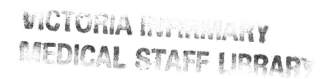

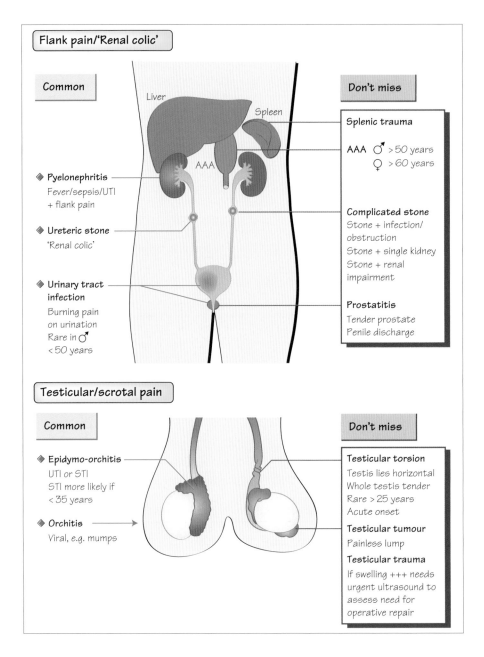

Flank pain/'Renal colic'

Common

- ◆ Pyelonephritis
  Fever/sepsis/UTI + flank pain
- ◆ Ureteric stone
  'Renal colic'
- ◆ Urinary tract infection
  Burning pain on urination
  Rare in ♂ < 50 years

Liver
Spleen
AAA

Don't miss

Splenic trauma

AAA ♂ > 50 years
♀ > 60 years

Complicated stone
Stone + infection/ obstruction
Stone + single kidney
Stone + renal impairment

Prostatitis
Tender prostate
Penile discharge

Testicular/scrotal pain

Common

- ◆ Epidymo-orchitis
  UTI or STI
  STI more likely if < 35 years
- ◆ Orchitis
  Viral, e.g. mumps

Don't miss

Testicular torsion
Testis lies horizontal
Whole testis tender
Rare > 25 years
Acute onset

Testicular tumour
Painless lump

Testicular trauma
If swelling +++ needs urgent ultrasound to assess need for operative repair

The urinary tract includes the kidneys, ureters, bladder, (prostate), urethra, and external genitalia. Symptoms perceived by patients reflect the embryological origin as well as the current anatomy of these organs.

History

Any previous history of urogenital problems, and a specific focus on:
- *Colicky pain:* intense pain that comes and goes suggests intermittent contraction of a hollow organ, e.g. ureter. Patients with ureteric colic cannot find a comfortable position. Pain may be referred to the genitals.
- *Back pain:* the kidneys are retroperitoneal.

- Ask about urinary frequency, flow, blood or clots.
- *Fever:* with chills and rigors (shaking) suggests sepsis (Chapter 38).
- *Dysuria:* burning pain when passing urine implies urethral inflammation. Abnormal discharge from the genitals suggests STI.
- *Sexual history:* if other symptoms suggest it is likely to be relevant.

Examination

A patient with active renal colic will move around, trying in vain to find a comfortable position; other causes of intra-abdominal pain are usually alleviated by lying still. The abdomen should be palpated for alternative causes of pain (e.g. abdominal aortic aneurysm (AAA), cholecystitis) and the kidneys should be examined for tenderness.

In a patient unable to void urine, a palpable tender bladder that is dull to percussion suggests urinary retention. The external genitalia should be examined if symptomatic, including rectal examination if prostatitis is suspected.

Investigations
Bedside investigations
- Ultrasound: can rule out AAA.
- Blood glucose.
- Swabs from urethra/cervix if appropriate.
- Urine dipstick testing is a rule-out test: if leucocytes, nitrites, blood and protein are all negative, the urine does not need to be sent for culture, unless the patient is immunosuppressed. If nitrites and leucocytes are negative, infection is unlikely (-LR = 0.16), but if the patient's symptoms are very suggestive of UTI, the urine may be sent for culture.
- βhCG
- Urine microscopy – red cell casts imply glomerular bleeding, rather than bleeding elsewhere in the urinary tract.

Laboratory investigations
- FBC, U+E
- LFTs, amylase if abdominal pain.

Imaging
- Ultrasound is operator and body mass index dependent, can detect bladder size, ureteric and renal pelvis dilatation resulting from obstruction but cannot reliably detect stones.
- CT KUB (kidney, ureters, bladder) detects stones and other intra-abdominal pathology, but involves significant radiation (300 CXR). MRI is an alternative that avoids irradiation.
- Contrast radiography: intravenous urogram (IVU; 250 CXR) has been superseded by CT, but X-ray KUB (75 CXR) can track radio-opaque stones.

Common diagnoses
Urinary tract infection/pyelonephritis
Females are more prone to UTIs due to the short urethra. Drinking large quantities of water may help flush out mild infection, but more serious infection needs treatment for 3 days with antibiotics: trimethoprim or nitrofurantoin are common recommendations. Men with UTIs and women with recurrent UTIs need antibiotics for 7 days and should be reviewed in an outpatient clinic.

Pyelonephritis occurs when a UTI ascends to the kidney(s). The patient is systemically unwell with fever, loin/back pain, rigors, headache, nausea and vomiting. The kidney(s) are tender on palpation. Emergency Department treatment includes antibiotics (e.g. gentamicin), analgesia and intravenous fluids. Patients who respond to this may be discharged with oral antibiotics (e.g. co-amoxycillin) and GP follow-up.

Urinary tract stones
Some patients, usually for unknown reasons, form stones in their renal pelvis. If the stones pass into the ureter, they cause intense colicky pain, 'renal colic' and microscopic haematuria (90%).

> **WARNING**
>
> 'Renal colic' in a male over 50 years old is AAA until proven otherwise.

NSAIDs, e.g. ketorolac i.v. or diclofenac p.r., are rapidly effective at relaxing ureteric smooth muscle. Morphine is useful for ongoing pain; pethidine (meperidine) should be avoided – opiate-seeking should be suspected if it is requested.

CT confirms the diagnosis, and informs treatment decisions. If there is a stone of less than 5 mm and the pain has resolved, discharge patient on regular NSAID or tamsulosin (an alpha blocking drug that also helps stones pass) with outpatient clinic review.

Patients who are discharged should be warned to return if they develop fever or further significant pain. Otherwise, or if there is evidence of infection, urinary obstruction, renal failure or single kidney, discuss with urology team.

Urinary retention
Urinary retention may occur due to mechanical obstruction or neurological impairment, causing acute or chronic retention that may cause renal damage. Ultrasound can confirm a large residual volume of urine in the bladder after voiding.

Catheterisation should be performed urgently to relieve obstruction and pain. If dipstick testing indicates that the patient's urine is likely to be infected, then catheterisation should be covered by a single shot of gentamicin. If there are blood clots in the bladder, a large irrigation catheter may be needed to flush out the bladder.

If urinary retention occurs in a patient with back pain, consider cauda equina compression (Chapter 17). Constipation, e.g. from opiate analgesics, can cause urinary retention: treating the constipation resolves the retention.

Sexually transmitted disease
Dysuria and/or discharge makes STI more likely than torsion, but if there is any doubt, an ultrasound can confirm normal testicular perfusion. Swabs should be taken and the patient should be followed up in an STI clinic for contact tracing.

Diagnoses not to miss
Testicular torsion
Common in early adulthood, the spermatic cord twists, causing testicular ischaemia. Torsion is diagnosed clinically by a tender, high-riding testis: ultrasound may confirm the diagnosis, but must not delay surgical exploration.

Infected obstructed kidney
The combination of urinary obstruction and infection can rapidly destroy a kidney. Evidence of possible infection should be sought in patients who have obstruction, e.g. stones, in their urinary tract.

Prostatitis
UTIs are uncommon in men, and prostatitis should be considered. The diagnosis is confirmed by a tender prostate on rectal examination, after which urine is taken for culture. Prolonged antibiotic treatment is necessary, e.g. ciprofloxacin for 3 weeks.

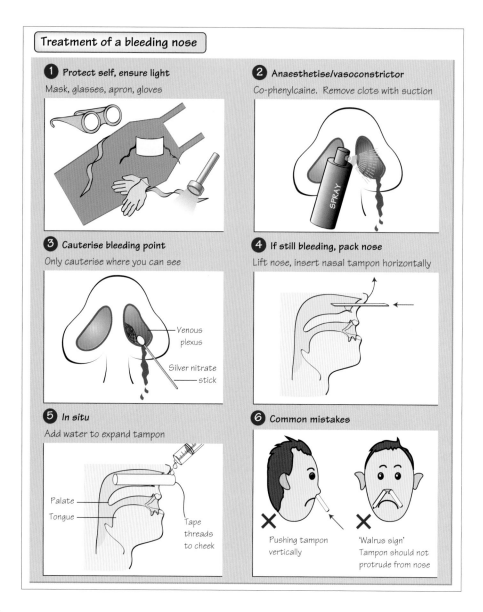

Treatment of a bleeding nose

① Protect self, ensure light
Mask, glasses, apron, gloves

② Anaesthetise/vasoconstrictor
Co-phenylcaine. Remove clots with suction

SPRAY

③ Cauterise bleeding point
Only cauterise where you can see

Venous plexus

Silver nitrate stick

④ If still bleeding, pack nose
Lift nose, insert nasal tampon horizontally

⑤ In situ
Add water to expand tampon

Palate
Tongue
Tape threads to cheek

⑥ Common mistakes

Pushing tampon vertically

'Walrus sign' Tampon should not protrude from nose

Ear, nose and throat (ENT) examination needs patience and practice to master. Patients may cough or sneeze, showering you with their body fluids, so protect yourself with gloves, apron, mask and eye protection. Adequate light and topical anaesthesia makes examination easier and your patient more comfortable.

Ear
Common diagnoses
Otitis media/sinusitis
Ear pain is usually caused by infection in the middle ear – otitis media. The eardrum appears dull with prominent blood vessels. Sinusitis presents as headache and a feeling of pressure in the face. These are self-limiting conditions caused by a viral upper respiratory tract infection, blocking drainage from airspaces within the head. Analgesics and decongestant drugs are helpful; antibiotics are not.

Otitis externa
Otitis externa or 'swimmer's ear' is a localised infection of the ear canal, which becomes congested with discharge and debris. Otitis externa is treated with topical antibiotics and steroids, applied using a wick of cotton wool.

Ruptured ear drum
Commonly caused by trauma, barotrauma or infection, a ruptured ear drum normally heals within 2 months. Patients should avoid immersing the ear in water.

Vertigo
Vertigo causes a sensation of *spinning*; it is not just 'feeling faint/light-headed'. Vertigo is caused by conflicting sensory information from ears, eyes and joints. The problem is usually due to peripheral (sensory) problems rather than central (brain) ones.

- A *peripheral* cause is likely if the patient has hearing loss, tinnitus, ear infection, headache, nausea and vomiting.
- A *central* cause is likely if the patient has motor symptoms or cardiovascular risk factors, e.g. atrial fibrillation.

Use the Dix-Hallpike test to differentiate central from peripheral causes. If there are central signs, check blood glucose and ECG – consider transient ischaemic attack (TIA)/stroke or other neurological cause (Chapter 42).

If the patient has no hearing loss, the most common cause of vertigo is vestibular neuronitis, usually caused by a (viral) upper respiratory tract infection. Prochlorperazine (an anti-emetic) +/− intravenous fluids is particularly effective. Antihistamines are structurally similar drugs and can also be used. Vestibular labyrinthitis is similar, but patients may have hearing loss and tinnitus.

Nose and face
Common presentations
Nosebleed
Most patients bleed from venous plexi in the anterior part of the nose – Little's area. Some (usually elderly) patients may have bleeding from the posterior part of their nasal cavity. Ask about warfarin and antiplatelet drugs such as aspirin and clopidogrel. Check FBC/clotting in older patients. Pack the nose and admit according to local protocols.

Facial fractures
Assess stability of upper teeth and mandible, and sensation over the face. If there is a fracture of the orbital floor, examine the eye movements (Chapter 22). Radiographic facial views are necessary, but are difficult to interpret – look for asymmetry. If there is mandibular injury, request XR OPG (oral pantomogram): fractures of the neck of the mandible can be difficult to spot.

Fractured nose
A patient with a painful swollen nose following trauma is likely to have broken their nose. X-rays do not change management. The patient should be discharged and reviewed in 5–7 days in an Ear, Nose and Throat clinic.

Do not miss
Septal haematoma
Septal haematoma – a swelling from the medial side of a fractured nose, usually in a young adult. This requires urgent drainage to prevent avascular necrosis of the cartilage.

Throat
Common presentations
Tonsillitis/pharyngitis
Pharyngitis and tonsilitis can be caused by bacteria or viruses. Viral pharyngitis is more likely if the patient has runny nose/conjunctivitis/diarrhoea. Group A β-haemolytic *Streptococcus* (GAβHS) is responsible for 10% of pharyngitis, and is treated by penicillin/erythromycin if three or more of the following criteria are present.
- Fever.
- Exudate on the tonsils.
- Tender anterior neck lymph nodes.
- Lack of cough.

If two or more criteria are present, rapid antigen tests can be used to identify those patients with GAβHS. Complications of untreated GAβHS are uncommon, and over-treatment with antibiotics is self-reinforcing. Patients who are systemically unwell with extensive bacterial pharyngitis need admission for intravenous penicillin and fluids.

Foreign body in throat/oesophagus
The site of pain suggests location of the foreign body.
- Unilateral pain – foreign body above cricopharyngeus.
- Pain in submandibular region – foreign body in tonsillar fossa.
- Pain around larynx – foreign body in posterior tongue.

If there is pain on every swallow, the foreign body is probably still there; if there is just vague discomfort, the foreign body has probably gone. Radiography is useful for bones, but fishbones, a common cause, are not very radio-opaque.

If there is no danger of the foreign body causing obstruction were it to be pushed into the trachea, it may be removed under direct vision using forceps or suction. Otherwise it is likely the foreign body will need to be removed under general anaesthesia.

Foreign bodies stuck in the oesophagus will often move with a combination of glucagon (which relaxes the lower oesophageal sphincter) and fizzy drink. Failure necessitates endoscopy.

Diagnoses not to miss
Quinsy (peritonsillar abscess)
Quinsy causes a painful, asymmetrically swollen throat with difficulty opening the mouth or swallowing and a 'plummy' voice. Treated by aspiration or drainage in theatre, together with antibiotics.

Epiglottitis, retropharyngeal abscess, Ludwig's angina
These rare but dangerous infections can cause upper airway obstruction, giving stridor, a whistling sound worse on inspiration. Patients are unwell with high fever, sitting forward, with a stiff neck, drooling saliva they are unable to swallow. Treatment is urgent anaesthetic and ENT airway assessment and antibiotics.

Postoperative bleeding
Postoperative bleeding is often a result of infection: these patients should always be reviewed by the Ear, Nose and Throat team.

Dental
Dental pain is usually caused by dental caries leading to local infection (pulpitis) and abscesses. Affected teeth are tender to percussion and temperature. Treatment is analgesia and advice to see a dental practitioner. Antibiotics are not normally indicated.

Wounds inside the mouth rarely need treatment as they heal very rapidly, and saliva has a natural antibacterial action. Exceptions are 'through and through' lacerations (through oral mucosa, muscle and facial skin) or lacerations involving the tip of the tongue.

An avulsed tooth should be replaced in the socket immediately if it is to survive. If this is not possible, the patient should carry the tooth between cheek and teeth. A dentist can place a splint to keep the tooth in place.

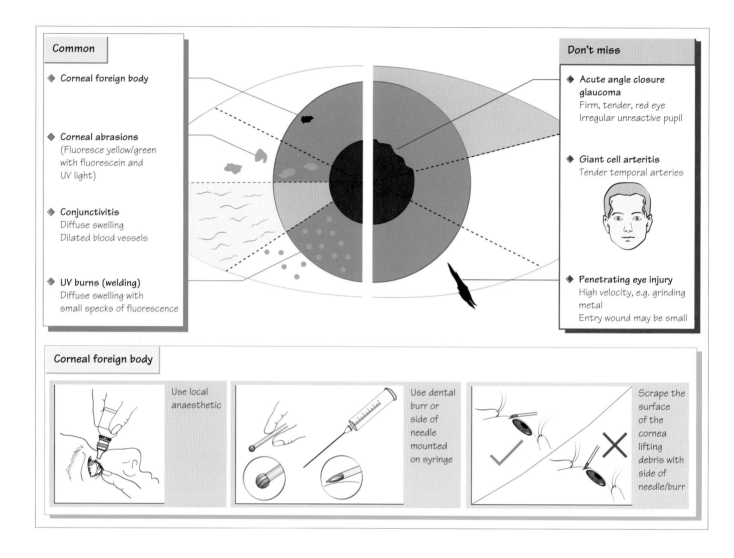

52 *Adult Emergency Medicine at a Glance,* 1st edition. © Thomas Hughes and Jaycen Cruickshank. Published 2011 by Blackwell Publishing Ltd.

Eye problems seen in the Emergency Department are usually the result of trauma affecting the anterior part of the eye, but can also be manifestations of systemic, CNS or vascular disorders.

A brief general history should include details of diabetes, stroke, hypertension, neurological or cardiac problems and drug treatment. Ask about trauma and the use of hand or power tools prior to the symptoms, as shards of metal or ceramic material are common foreign bodies.

Ask about previous eye problems including treatment, and corrective lenses if worn. If vision is impaired, was the deterioration sudden or gradual?

Examination

Topical anaesthetic drops are necessary if the eye is painful. Check the label carefully as different eye drops are often stored together. Any eye that has had topical anaesthesia must be padded until painful again, to protect the eye while normal protective reflexes are lost. Never give the patient anaesthetic drops to take home.

- *Visual acuity must be recorded for every patient (use glasses if worn, pinhole if glasses not available).*
- *Examine* the skin around the eye and evert the eyelids to check for foreign bodies.
- *Visual fields* are particularly important when retinal or cerebrovascular disease is suspected.
- *Eye movements* should be tested and feelings of double vision sought. Nystagmus and conjugate eye movements are indicative of cerebellar and brainstem function.
- *Pupils* should be examined for size, symmetry and reaction to light.
- *Ophthalmoscopy* is necessary if there is loss of visual acuity.

Slit lamp examination

The slit lamp illuminates and magnifies the cornea and the anterior chamber of the eye. Fluorescein dye makes corneal abnormalities fluoresce yellow-green in ultraviolet light. Intraocular pressure measurement is essential if there is any possibility of glaucoma.

Common diagnoses

Corneal abrasion or foreign body

Foreign bodies embedded in the cornea are usually caused by use of power tools without eye protection. The patient presents with a red, painful, watering eye, and the foreign body is usually easily visible. Use fluorescein to show corneal damage.

Use topical anaesthesia and remove the foreign body and any rust ring scraping with a dental burr or the side of a needle bevel (mount the needle on a syringe barrel to aid manipulation). Treat with antibiotic ointment, which lubricates and protects the healing cornea, and arrange review in 36–48 hours, to assess healing and check for missed foreign body or residual rust.

Welder's arc/flashburn

Electrical arc welding generates intense ultraviolet light. If a dark glass shield is not used, severe bilateral pain and redness develops several hours later. Fluorescein reveals corneal inflammation with tiny dots of fluorescence. Treatment is systemic analgesia and protection/padding of the eyes for the 2–3 days it takes to resolve.

Conjunctivitis

The patient presents with red eyes with watery discharge, usually *bilateral*, and associated with *normal visual acuity.* The cause may be one of the following.
• *Viral:* most common, sometimes after an upper respiratory tract infection, very transmissible; advise the patient to wash hands and avoid sharing towels, but no treatment is necessary.
• *Allergic:* advise the patient to use topical and systemic antihistamines available from pharmacies.
• *Bacterial:* rapid onset, purulent – consider *Gonococcus* or *Chlamydia.*

Conjunctivitis should improve within 10 days; if not, an ophthalmology review is necessary.

Subconjunctival haemorrhage

This dramatic appearance is caused by rupture of a subconjunctival vein and spread of blood below the conjunctiva. No treatment is necessary unless it occurs in the context of head injury, when it indicates a skull base fracture.

Diagnoses not to miss

Globe rupture

If globe rupture is suspected, a ring bandage is placed around the eye to prevent any pressure on the globe. Intravenous antibiotics, analgesics and anti-emetics are given: urgent CT and refer.

Intra-ocular foreign body

Suspect if there is the feeling of a foreign body and the possibility of high-energy material, yet little or no corneal damage. Urgent CT and refer.

Acute angle closure glaucoma

Rare below 60 years of age, this presents with pain, headache, blurred vision with haloes around lights, and nausea. The eye is red, feels firm, and there is a mid-sized irregular unreactive pupil.

High intraocular pressure confirms the diagnosis: treatment is intravenous acetazolamide and urgent referral.

Giant cell arteritis

Occurring in the elderly, rapid visual loss is associated with headache, jaw claudication (pain on chewing), tender temporal arteries and a pale and swollen optic disc on fundoscopy. An erythrocyte sedimentation rate (ESR) >50 is likely, but the gold standard for diagnosis is temporal artery biopsy. Commence high-dose steroids immediately and refer.

Dendritic ulcer

These branching ulcers, caused by herpes simplex virus (HSV) infection are best seen with fluorescein, but can be mistaken for abrasions. Treat with topical antivirals and refer.

Orbital floor (blowout) fracture

Patients with a facial fracture should be checked for an upward gaze palsy by holding the patient's head still and moving a finger upwards 50 cm from the face. Diplopia suggests tethering of the inferior rectus muscle/soft tissue, preventing upward gaze, and need for referral.

Central retinal artery/vein occlusion

Central retinal artery occlusion (CRAO) causes *sudden* painless loss of vision, with a pale fundus except for a red macular spot, and is caused by emboli, atherosclerosis or giant cell arteritis. Central retinal vein occlusion (CRVO) is similar, but of slower onset, and is associated with diabetes and hypertension, giving swollen oedematous retinal vessels. Immediate referral is necessary for both.

Transient ischaemic attack

Patients with a transient ischaemic attack (TIA) affecting their visual cortex describe 'a curtain coming down' on their vision – sometimes known as amaurosis fugax (Chapter 42).

Retinal detachment

Retinal detachment presents with gradual visual deterioration, floaters, flashes or field defects in middle-aged or myopic patients or in patients with diabetes. Opthalmoscopy in the Emergency Department cannot detect all cases of retinal detachment, so consider ultrasound and refer.

Ophthalmic varicella zoster virus

Shingles affecting the trigeminal nerve can manifest with pain or sensory symptoms, which precede the vesicular rash. Treat with oral acyclovir and refer.

Orbital cellulitis/endophthalmitis

Any suspicion of infection in the orbit needs antibiotics, CT and referral. Pain on eye movement indicates deep infection.

Acute inflammatory eye conditions

A number of conditions can present with painful visual disturbance, and red eyes. These differ from conjunctivitis in that visual acuity is *not* normal, and referral is necessary.

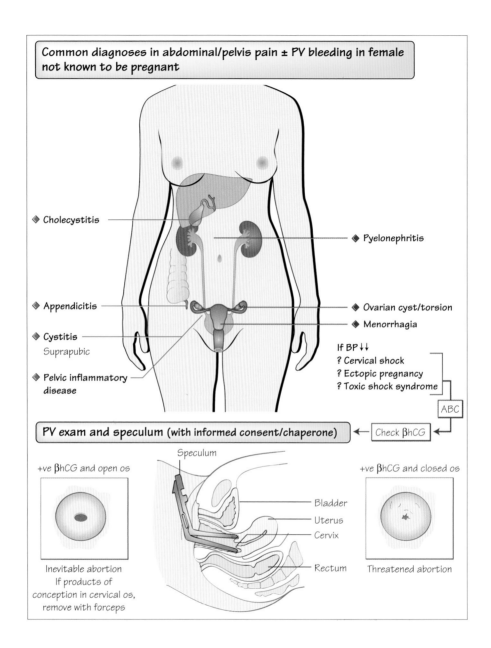

Common diagnoses in abdominal/pelvis pain ± PV bleeding in female not known to be pregnant

◆ Cholecystitis
◆ Pyelonephritis
◆ Appendicitis
◆ Ovarian cyst/torsion
◆ Menorrhagia
◆ Cystitis
Suprapubic
◆ Pelvic inflammatory disease

If BP↓↓
? Cervical shock
? Ectopic pregnancy
? Toxic shock syndrome

ABC

PV exam and speculum (with informed consent/chaperone) ← Check βhCG ←

Speculum

+ve βhCG and open os

Inevitable abortion
If products of conception in cervical os, remove with forceps

Bladder
Uterus
Cervix
Rectum

+ve βhCG and closed os

Threatened abortion

Assume that any woman of childbearing age is pregnant until proven otherwise. Pregnancy up to the time of foetal viability (approx 23/40 weeks) is managed by gynaecology, after that by obstetrics.

Resuscitation

PV bleed + abdo pain + shock = ruptured ectopic pregnancy

A ruptured ectopic pregnancy can bleed faster than blood can be replaced. Immediate surgery is necessary: ensure large bore intravenous access, with minimal volume resuscitation (Chapter 3). Speculum examination allows exclusion of possible alternatives: 'cervical shock' (see below) or toxic shock syndrome (Chapter 38).

History

Enquire about:
• Possible pregnancy, menstrual cycle including last normal menstrual period (LNMP);
• Previous pregnancies/miscarriages and Rhesus status, if known;
• Pain – site/nature and associations/radiation – shoulder tip suggests peritoneal irritation/onset – rapid/slow;
• Bleeding/discharge – volume/nature;
• Sexual history including sexually transmitted infections (STIs);
• General symptoms, and those that might indicate other causes for abdominal pain, e.g. fever, bowel and urinary symptoms (Chapters 19 and 20).

Examination

Lower abdominal tenderness suggests a gynaecological cause for pain, but also consider other causes of abdominal pain, particularly appendicitis (Chapter 19) or bowel obstruction. Estimate fundal height in pregnancy.

Speculum and internal examination

A chaperone must always be present when performing internal examination. With speculum examination, take swabs first if necessary. In bleeding in early pregnancy, if the os is open, this indicates an 'inevitable abortion'. If closed, it suggests a 'threatened abortion' or ectopic pregnancy. Manual examination allows assessment of pain on cervical movement – 'cervical excitation', which occurs in pelvic inflammatory disease (PID).

Investigations
Bedside investigations
- Urinalysis, βhCG, STI swabs, ultrasound.

Laboratory investigations
- FBC.
- Blood group if pregnancy possible.
- Quantitative βhCG according to local protocol.

Imaging
- Ultrasound is sensitive for detecting the intrauterine gestational sac and is now an essential component of assessment of problems in early pregnancy. If there is no intrauterine sac and the quantitative βhCG is >1500 units it is assumed that there is an ectopic pregnancy. There is a small risk (↑with IVF) of *heterotopic* pregnancy – simultaneous ectopic *and* intrauterine pregnancy.
- A full bladder is essential for transabdominal ultrasound, providing a 'window' through which the pelvic organs are seen. Transvaginal ultrasound can detect a gestational sac at about 4–5 weeks, 1 week before it would be visible on abdominal ultrasound.

Common diagnoses
Bleeding in early pregnancy

Significant vaginal bleeding occurs in 20% of pregnancies, and of these, half will abort. Ultrasound is essential in the assessment of these patients. Possible diagnoses include the following.
- *Ectopic pregnancy:* Presents with abdominal pain and bleeding. A positive βhCG (quantitative >1500 units) and an empty uterus confirms the diagnosis. While *ruptured* ectopic pregnancy requires resuscitation and immediate surgery as described above, many patients with stable ectopic pregnancy are treated medically, preserving the fallopian tubes.
- *Threatened abortion:* mild pain, bleeding, closed cervical os: if intrauterine gestational sac seen, reassure as most settle.
- *Inevitable abortion:* ongoing pain and bleeding, open cervical os: refer.
- *Missed abortion:* the fetus dies but is not expelled: refer.
- *Incomplete abortion:* ongoing pain/bleeding but no sac: refer.
- *Complete abortion:* closed os, no sac on ultrasound, no ongoing symptoms: no further treatment necessary.

If diagnosis is uncertain and the quantitative βhCG is below 1500 units, the quantitative βhCG should be repeated 48 hours later – in normal pregnancy, levels should double within this time.

In all cases, consider anti-D immunoglobulin, provide information about support groups, and arrange outpatient follow-up.

Vomiting in mid pregnancy

Vomiting is common between weeks 6/40 and 16/40. Exclude alternative causes, treat symptomatically with intravenous fluids and metoclopramide, and discharge with follow-up if otherwise well.

Menorrhagia

After ruling out pregnancy, this common symptom is treated with tranexamic acid and mefenamic acid, with GP review.

Pelvic inflammatory disease

Vaginal discharge, fever and pelvic pain, with cervical excitation on examination. Consider STIs – take swabs and arrange follow-up for contact tracing according to local protocol.

Mid-cycle pain

This sharp pain, localised to one side of the lower abdomen, results from rupture of the ovarian follicle during ovulation. After excluding pregnancy and more serious pathology (e.g. appendicitis), reassure and advise simple analgesia: paracetamol/NSAIDs.

Diagnoses not to miss
Cervical shock

Products of conception in the cervical canal can provoke a very intense parasympathetic response, resulting in extreme bradycardia and shock. Removal of the tissue results in rapid resolution of the symptoms.

Ovarian pathology

Many ovarian cysts are incidental findings on ultrasound and cause no symptoms. Ovarian torsion is rare, and may present with non-specific low/mid abdominal pain.

Pre-eclampsia/eclampsia

The triad of hypertension, proteinurea and oedema can occur from week 12/40 to the immediate postpartum period, but is most common in the third trimester. If untreated, this can progress to full eclampsia with seizures.

Magnesium is used to increase the seizure threshold, benzodiazepines being relatively ineffective. The foetus should be monitored, and delivered at the earliest safe opportunity.

Rhesus auto-immunisation

Auto-immunisation occurs if a significant amount of rhesus-positive foetal blood mixes with rhesus-negative maternal blood, causing foetal haemolysis in future pregnancies. Consider in abortion or trauma affecting a pregnant woman. A Kleihauer test detects foetal blood, but may miss small amounts. Anti-D immunoglobulin should be given according to local guidelines.

Bleeding in late pregnancy

Large amounts of blood may be lost, so large-bore cannulae are necessary. Urgent obstetric review is necessary.
- *Placental abruption:* bleeding occurs between the placenta and the uterine wall, jeopardising the foetus.
- *Placenta praevia:* the placenta extends over the cervical os, and bleeding may occur as the uterus enlarges.

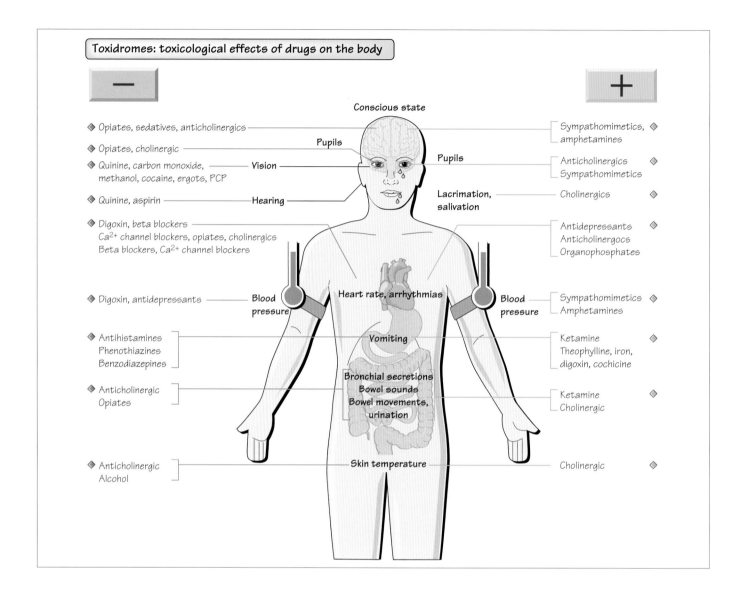

Toxidromes: toxicological effects of drugs on the body

Conscious state

− side:
- Opiates, sedatives, anticholinergics
- Opiates, cholinergic — Pupils
- Quinine, carbon monoxide, methanol, cocaine, ergots, PCP — Vision
- Quinine, aspirin — Hearing
- Digoxin, beta blockers
  Ca^{2+} channel blockers, opiates, cholinergics
  Beta blockers, Ca^{2+} channel blockers
- Digoxin, antidepressants — Blood pressure
- Antihistamines
  Phenothiazines
  Benzodiazepines
- Anticholinergic
  Opiates
- Anticholinergic
  Alcohol

Central labels:
- Pupils
- Lacrimation, salivation
- Heart rate, arrhythmias
- Blood pressure
- Vomiting
- Bronchial secretions
  Bowel sounds
  Bowel movements, urination
- Skin temperature

+ side:
- Sympathomimetics, amphetamines
- Anticholinergics
  Sympathomimetics
- Cholinergics
- Antidepressants
  Anticholinergocs
  Organophosphates
- Sympathomimetics
  Amphetamines
- Ketamine
  Theophylline, iron, digoxin, cochicine
- Ketamine
  Cholinergic
- Cholinergic

Self-poisoning is the most common toxicological problem: serious adverse effects are rare with good basic supportive management. The difficulty of performing human toxicological research means that the evidence base is very limited. Expert advice on the management of poisoning is available through a system of national poisons information centres.

National Poisons Information	
Australia	13 11 26
Canada	911/local Poison Control Centre
Ireland	01 809 2566
New Zealand	0800 764 766
UK	0870 600 6266
USA	1 800 222 1222

History

A straightforward, non-judgemental tone can help establish rapport. The details of the ingestion (e.g. drugs, alcohol, suicide note, social factors and precipitants) should be documented.

Resuscitation: ABCDE

Airway Ensure the airway is open and protected, give oxygen if unwell.

Breathing Ensure adequate respiratory rate and oxygenation saturation.

Circulation Look for signs of shock, obtain intravenous access and bloods.

Shock responds to intravenous fluid in most cases.

Arrhythmias may need antidotes before usual treatments are effective (Chapter 25).

Disability Pupils and Glasgow Coma Scale, seizures, agitation.

Exclude hypoxia and hypoglycaemia.

Toxidromes are groups of physical findings suggesting certain drug ingestions (see opposite).

Agitation can be a medical emergency, putting staff and patients at risk. A combination of physical restraint and chemical sedation may be required (Chapter 27).

Many toxic seizures are self-limiting. Benzodiazepines are first-line treatment; barbiturates are second-line. Phenytoin should *not* be used in seizures related to toxic ingestions as its mechanism of action (Na^+ channel blockade) is the same as the cause of many such fits.

Exposure Check temperature, check for trauma or evidence of intravenous drug use (IVDU).

Examination

Any patient who is comatose or has major ABC derangement needs resuscitation first. Poisoning can be difficult to detect clinically: patients may be asymptomatic despite having taken a lethal dose.

It is easy to assume that all signs and symptoms are attributed to poisoning. Impaired consciousness may be due to a head injury.

Management

Supportive care is the mainstay of management: ensuring the patient does not come to harm while the drugs are eliminated. Supportive care is a continuation of the principles of resuscitation above. The patient should be nursed in an environment close to a critical care area where close monitoring is possible. The observation unit of an Emergency Department is ideal.

Risk assessment

Patients should be assessed early for their risk of coming to harm:
- Risk of deterioration: patients who have taken particularly toxic drugs that may have delayed presentation, e.g. tricyclic antidepressants, beta blockers, digoxin. These patients should be observed in a high acuity area until the danger is passed.
- Risk of absconding: patients who try to leave may be intoxicated, confused, attention-seeking, psychotic, seriously depressed and intent on finishing the job, or sometimes just bored. An assessment of their mental capacity is essential (Chapter 26), to allow detention of the patient against their wishes if necessary.

Minimising systemic toxicity

Systemic effects of drugs are minimised by:
- *Decontamination* – minimisation of drug absorption.
- *Elimination* – maximising drug removal.
  Specific poisons and their treatments are discussed in Chapter 25.

Decontamination
Activated charcoal

Charcoal is 'activated' by superheating, increasing its surface area to volume ratio to $900m^2/g$, i.e. the area of a tennis court per gram. Activated charcoal *ad*sorbs drugs, minimising gut *ab*sorption. Charcoal also adsorbs drugs excreted in the bile, some of which would normally be reabsorbed by the body: the enterohepatic circulation.

Charcoal appears helpful if given soon after ingestion, ideally within one hour. It should be given only if:
- the patient is alert, and drinks it voluntarily OR
- the patient is intubated.

Charcoal is not helpful in poisoning due to alcohols (ethanol, methanol, ethylene glycol), hydrocarbons, alkalis, acids or metals.

Gastric washout, Ipecac

Gastric washout is rarely performed, as it is unlikely to offer benefit over charcoal, and carries the risk of aspiration. Washout is appropriate in a patient presenting within a few hours of ingestion of a highly toxic overdose who has already been intubated. Charcoal can be instilled after the washout. Ipecac is a plant extract that causes vomiting; it is rarely used, as it can cause serious GI side effects.

Whole bowel irrigation

Whole bowel irrigation is performed by infusing a clear inert solution (polyethylene glycol) orally until no drug residue is passed. It is useful for slow-release preparations not adsorbed by charcoal, e.g. iron, lithium. It requires close nursing supervision and is messy and so is usually performed in the intensive care unit (ICU).

Elimination
Repeated charcoal

Repeat doses of activated charcoal prevent reabsorption (and therefore enhance elimination) in drugs that undergo enterohepatic recirculation, e.g. theophylline, anti-epileptic drugs and digoxin.

Diuresis

Urinary alkalinisation enhances excretion of weak acids such as aspirin. Forced diuresis with large fluid volumes is dangerous as circulatory overload can occur.

Haemodialysis

Haemodialysis is used in severe poisoning by drugs that cannot be removed by other means, e.g. aspirin, lithium.

Investigations in poisoning

Bedside investigations
Blood glucose
ECG

Laboratory investigations
Paracetamol level at least 4 hours after ingestion
Salicylate level if history of aspirin ingestion or acidosis
Other drug levels rarely helpful in the Emergency Department
FBC, U+E
ABG, lactate in sick patients
CK if patient has been unconscious for lengthy period

Imaging
Chest X-ray if possible aspiration
Abdominal X-ray rarely necessary, but shows radio-opaque tablets such as iron, lithium
CT of head: the clinical presentation of many poisonings often overlaps with conditions that may cause intracranial bleeding/ swelling. An urgent CT scan should be obtained if there is a possibility of traumatic injury or any doubt about the diagnosis

---

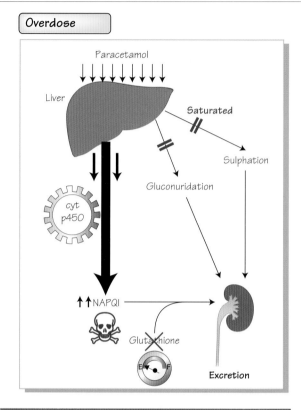

Normal paracetamol dose

Paracetamol
Liver
45% Sulphation
45%
Gluconuridation
10%
cyt p450
NAPQI → Excretion
Glutathione
E F
Excretion

Overdose

Paracetamol
Liver
Saturated
Sulphation
Gluconuridation
cyt p450
↑↑NAPQI → Excretion
Glutathione
E F
Excretion

Paracetamol toxicity

Plasma paracetamol level →
Toxic
Not toxic
4 hours   Time →

Antidotes	
Poison	**Antidote/treatment**
Benzodiazepines	Supportive care
Beta blockers	Glucagon, inotropes, pacemaker
Calcium channel blockers	Calcium, inotropes, glucagon
Carbon monoxide	Oxygen
Digoxin	Digibind (Fab fragments)
Ethylene glycol	Ethanol, fomepizole
Hydrofluric acid	Calcium gluconate
Insulin, hypoglycaemics	Glucose/dextrose >10%, glucogon
Iron	Desferoximine
Methanol	Ethanol, fomepizole
Opiates	Naloxone
Organophosphates	Atropine, pralidoxime
Paracetamol	n-acetyl-cysteine, methionine
Tricyclic antidepressants	Sodium bicarbonate
Warfarin	Clotting factors/vitamin K

Paracetamol (acetaminophen)

Paracetamol overdose (OD) is the most common toxicological emergency and the most common cause of liver transplant and death due to poisoning. Patients who start N-acetylcysteine (NAC) within 12 hours of ingestion are very likely to survive.

Mechanism of action

In overdose, normal pathways of paracetamol metabolism become saturated, forcing paracetamol down an alternate pathway: the first stage is performed by a cytochrome p450 enzyme, forming a hepatotoxic compound called NAPQI. Under normal circumstances, the NAPQI is quickly cleared from the liver by conjugation with glutathione.

After about 10 hours, the liver's supply of glutathione is exhausted, and NAPQI accumulates, damaging cells. Intravenous N-acetylcysteine prevents hepatic damage from NAPQI by substituting for glutathione; methionine is an oral alternative, given over several days.

Patients at increased risk of toxicity

Drugs that induce p450, such as anti-epileptics, and chronic alcohol consumption, increase the rate of formation of NAPQI. Patients with low hepatic glutathione stores, such as those with HIV, anorexia or cystic fibrosis, may also be at increased risk of hepatotoxicity.

Management

Measurement of paracetamol levels before 4 hours after ingestion is unhelpful, except to exclude paracetamol ingestion. The graph opposite predicts the need for NAC in patients above the line. NAC is given as a front-loaded infusion. Patients presenting more than 24 hours after ingestion may still benefit from NAC.

Patients who present more than 8 hours after ingestion and who have ingested >150 mg/kg paracetamol should have paracetamol levels measured and NAC commenced on arrival. Other patients should wait until the paracetamol level is known.

The prothrombin time (PT) is the single best indicator of hepatic function. Patients whose PT is rising 24 hours after ingestion should continue NAC; a PT level >36 sec at 36 hours suggests serious damage. Hepatic and renal function is monitored using PT, LFTs and U+Es.

Antidepressants

Tricyclic anti-depressants (TCAs) such as amitriptyline, imipramine and doxepin are highly toxic in overdose, and are the second most common cause of overdose deaths. By comparison, the SSRI antidepressants are much safer in overdose.

The toxic effects of tricyclic antidepressants are mainly a result of blockade of fast sodium channels, resulting in membrane-stabilising effects on cardiac and neurological cells. They also have an anticholinergic action. CNS effects include seizures, agitation and coma, while cardiotoxicity causes hypotension and ventricular arrhythmias.

Supportive management with close monitoring is essential. Acidosis and progressive lengthening of the QT_c may occur. A QRS >120 msec predicts toxicity; >160 msec indicates imminent seizures and/or ventricular fibrillation (VF).

Sodium bicarbonate is an effective antidote. The alkali reduces the free drug and the large sodium load helps overcome the blockade. Phenytoin should not be used for seizures as it also blocks sodium channels.

Opiates

Opiate overdose causes coma, hypoventilation and small pupils. Patients who are apnoeic or in whom the cause for coma is in doubt, e.g. possible trauma, should be given naloxone, a short-acting antagonist.

In patients who are breathing, it is best to just give oxygen and wait, as there are hazards in giving naloxone.
• Danger to staff from needles around intravenous drug users.
• Naloxone causes acute opiate withdrawal symptoms, which may dissuade drug users from calling for help in the future.
• Naloxone is short-acting, so there is a danger that a patient may wake, run away and collapse when the naloxone wears off. Therefore if naloxone is indicated, it should be a large dose, e.g. 1.6 mg i.m.

In patients who have (iatrogenic) opiate-induced hypoventilation where one does not want to reverse the analgesic effect – just the hypoventilation, this may be reversed by very small doses of i.v. naloxone e.g. 40–80 µg. Naloxone infusion may be necessary with long-acting opiates.

Benzodiazepines

Benzodiazepines (BDZ) are often taken as part of a mixed overdose. Benzodiazepines have a very good safety record in overdose and may protect against seizures e.g. when taken with tricyclic antidepressants.

Flumazenil is a short-acting benzodiazepine antagonist that can precipitate acute benzodiazepine withdrawal and intractable seizures, so should not be used in the Emergency Department.

Alcohol

Ethanol is often taken with overdoses. Paradoxically this may provide a degree of protection from the toxic effects of some overdoses by competing for metabolic pathways.

Toxic alcohols such as methanol and ethylene glycol (antifreeze) are metabolised by alcohol dehydrogenase to toxic compounds. Toxicity can be prevented by either blocking alcohol dehydogenase using fomepizole, or giving ethanol, which is preferentially metabolised. The toxic alcohol can be removed by haemodialysis.

Salicylates

Aspirin overdose, while relatively common, rarely needs treatment. Most patients with significant overdose complain of tinnitus. Direct stimulation of the respiratory centre gives initial hyperventilation and respiratory alkalosis, progressing later to a metabolic acidosis. High levels of salicylates indicate the need for alkaline diuresis (dilute sodium bicarbonate i.v.) or haemodialysis.

Digoxin

Digoxin overdose may be acute or chronic. Chronic digoxin overdosage will give bradycardia, and patients complain of yellow/green vision – xanthopsia. Acute digoxin overdose may cause coma, brady- or tachyarrhythmias. Digoxin has a specific antidote – digoxin antibody fragments.

Iron

Iron overdose is uncommon, but serious. Abdominal X-radiography can identify number and progress of tablets, and serum iron concentrations predict toxicity. Gastrointestinal absorption of iron is normally tightly regulated. In overdose, damage to the gut mucosa allows unregulated iron absorption, exacerbating toxicity. Bowel decontamination with whole bowel irrigation and chelation using intravenous deferoxamine may be necessary.

Stuffers and packers

Body *stuffers* are usually street-level drug dealers who are caught and decide to swallow the evidence. Body *packers* are people who seek to smuggle drugs by concealing them within the body. Pyrexia >38°C or pulse >120 indicate significant toxicity – benzodiazepines are useful for agitation.

Stuffers are more likely to suffer toxic effects as the drugs are not packaged to withstand gastrointestinal transit, although the drugs are relatively impure, compared to those ingested by packers. Abdominal radiography and ultrasound can diagnose packers, who need charcoal and whole bowel irrigation.

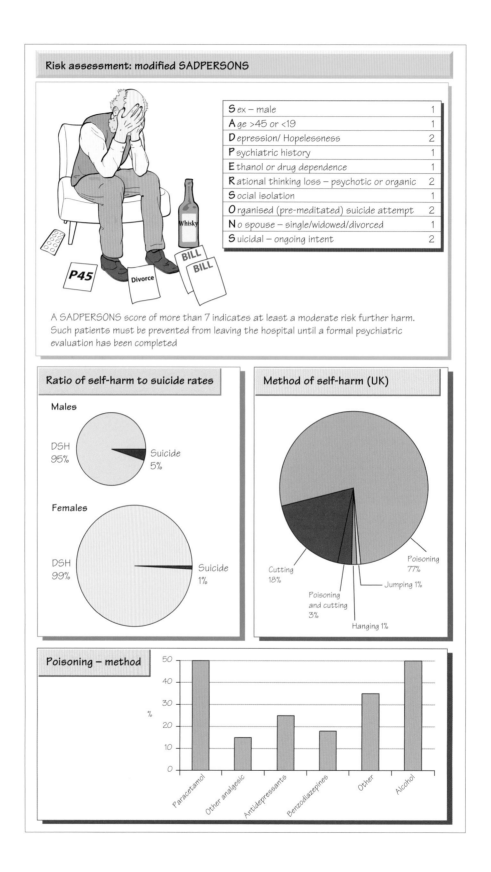

Risk assessment: modified SADPERSONS

S ex – male	1
A ge >45 or <19	1
D epression/ Hopelessness	2
P sychiatric history	1
E thanol or drug dependence	1
R ational thinking loss – psychotic or organic	2
S ocial isolation	1
O rganised (pre-meditated) suicide attempt	2
N o spouse – single/widowed/divorced	1
S uicidal – ongoing intent	2

A SADPERSONS score of more than 7 indicates at least a moderate risk further harm. Such patients must be prevented from leaving the hospital until a formal psychiatric evaluation has been completed

Ratio of self-harm to suicide rates

Males

DSH 95%   Suicide 5%

Females

DSH 99%   Suicide 1%

Method of self-harm (UK)

Poisoning 77%
Cutting 18%
Poisoning and cutting 3%
Jumping 1%
Hanging 1%

Poisoning – method

(Bar chart with y-axis % from 0 to 50; categories: Paracetamol, Other analgesic, Antidepressants, Benzodiazepines, Other, Alcohol)

Deliberate self-harm

Most of the patients who self-harm (e.g. overdose or cut themselves) do so as a response to a stress in their life. Common precipitants are problems with relationships or finances.

The majority of deliberate self-harm (DSH) patients seen in the Emergency Department do not have ongoing suicidal intent; of those presenting with an overdose, only a very small fraction go on to commit suicide. Therefore the challenge is to identify patients with a high ongoing risk of suicide.

The modified SADPERSONS scoring system can identify patients at high risk of subsequently committing suicide. The SADPERSONS score should not be viewed in isolation; other indicators that a suicide attempt is associated with a high level of intent are:
- *A violent method*, e.g. hanging, falls, weapons.
- *Avoidance of discovery* where the person has attempted to avoid being found.
- *Premeditation*: most suicide attempts are impulsive, and often related to alcohol consumption. Evidence of having 'put one's affairs in order', e.g. making or changing a will, suggests a high degree of planning. 'Suicide notes' are common, but a carefully considered letter is a more worrying indicator than a scrawled note.

DSH patients need medical treatment if necessary and, if assessed as low risk, may be discharged with appropriate community-based follow-up. If at moderate or high risk, these patients should have a psychiatric assessment before discharge.

Personality disorders

Within the group of DSH patients there are many more patients with personality disorders than with mental illnesses such as depression or schizophrenia. A personality disorder is *not* a mental illness per se, but a pattern of behaviour that is consistently outside social norms. Patients with personality disorders are orientated, do not have hallucinations, delusions or thought disorders; they have normal senses and memory.

Patients with a personality disorder may present in a very similar way to a patient with mental illness. Both may harm themselves, and students are often surprised to find that doctors and nurses appear unconcerned by these patients. This is because patients with personality disorders may be manipulative and attention-seeking, and indifference to their behaviour is less likely to reinforce it.

There are three distinct subgroups of personality disorders:

A Suspicious/odd behaviour
B Impulsive/antisocial/emotionally manipulative behaviour
C Anxious/dependent behaviour.

The patients seen in the Emergency Department with self-harm tend to be from group B, who are more likely to be emotionally labile and form fragile relationships. The label 'borderline personality disorder' stems from the outdated notion that these patients were 'on the border' between psychosis and neurosis. Patients with group B personality disorders may also have drug and alcohol problems and chaotic lives.

Patients with personality disorders are not generally helped by treatments used for serious mental illness: psychiatrists try to avoid admitting them to hospital as this can make the situation worse.

Capacity, consent and ethics

Sometimes a patient may refuse treatment for a potentially life-threatening overdose, or may want to leave the Emergency Department before their treatment is complete. The doctor must then assess whether the patient's autonomy should be overridden to allow treatment.

Ethics

The ethical principles that guide medical treatment are:
- *Beneficence* – doing good.
- *Non-maleficence* – not doing harm.
- *Autonomy* – respecting a patient's decisions.
- *Justice* – fairness.

In some countries, this situation is covered by mental health legislation, in others by legislation covering consent. In England and Wales, the Mental Capacity Act (2005) formalised a framework to assess patients whose mental capacity to consent to treatment is in doubt.

Mental capacity

Assesment of mental capacity is person, time and decision specific: can *this* person make *this* decision at *this* time?

To establish mental capacity to a patient must be able to:
- *Understand* the choices being presented to them
- *Retain* the information about the choices for enough time to be able to
- *Weigh* the relative merits of the choices, then be able to
- *Communicate* the decision to others.

If a patient fails the test for mental capacity (most commonly on the ability to weigh information rationally) then this decision and the reasons for it must be recorded in the notes. Treatment that is necessary to preserve the patient's life may then proceed against the patient's wishes. This may include sedation necessary to safely permit life-saving interventions.

Mental capacity can be difficult to assess in patients with pre-existent disabilities or communication difficulties, and these points may help guide assessment.
- Everything possible should be done to maximise a patient's capacity.
- An unwise decision by the patient does not automatically prove lack of capacity.
- Capacity should be presumed until evidence to the contrary.
- Decisions should act in the best interests of the patient.
- If a decision has to be made, it should be the least restrictive option that meets the patient's needs.

Advance Directives

Advance Directives, sometimes (confusingly) known as 'living wills', are a legally binding method to specify treatment decisions in the event that a patient does not have capacity to make those judgements. Not all countries have similar legislation, and such documents must be signed and witnessed, preferably by a medical witness who can verify that the patient had capacity to make that decision at that time.

The advance directive should include a statement that the treatment should be withheld *even if the patient's life is put at risk*.

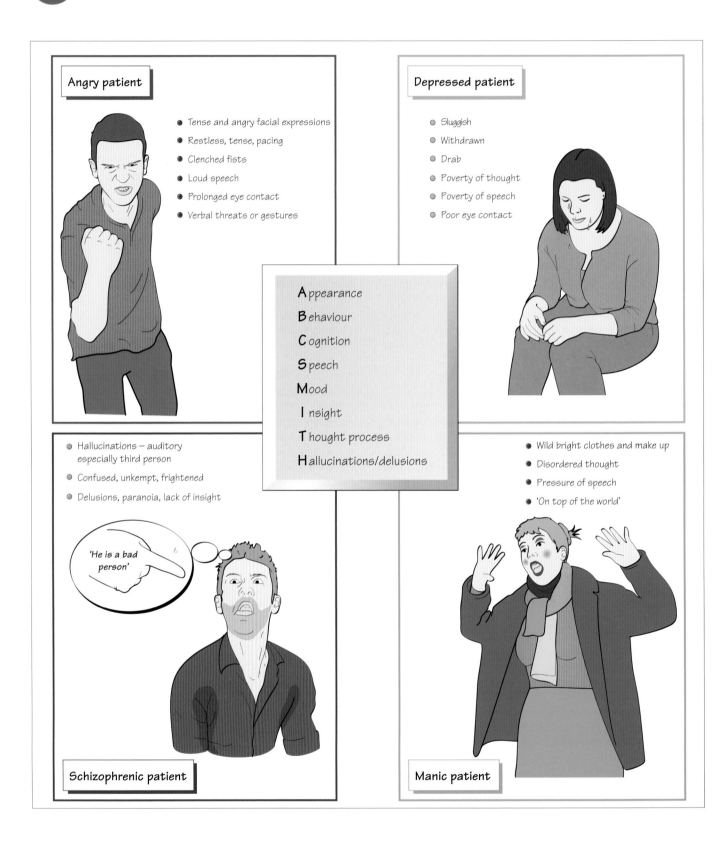

Angry patient

- Tense and angry facial expressions
- Restless, tense, pacing
- Clenched fists
- Loud speech
- Prolonged eye contact
- Verbal threats or gestures

Depressed patient

- Sluggish
- Withdrawn
- Drab
- Poverty of thought
- Poverty of speech
- Poor eye contact

Appearance
Behaviour
Cognition
Speech
Mood
Insight
Thought process
Hallucinations/delusions

- Hallucinations – auditory especially third person
- Confused, unkempt, frightened
- Delusions, paranoia, lack of insight

'He is a bad person'

Schizophrenic patient

- Wild bright clothes and make up
- Disordered thought
- Pressure of speech
- 'On top of the world'

Manic patient

Mental state examination: ABCSMITH

The mental state examination is a structured way of collecting and presenting information about patients with psychiatric symptoms.

Appearance grooming/hygiene/dress/eye contact
Behaviour agitation/withdrawn/gestures/co-operation
Cognition inattention/orientation/reasoning
Speech speed/fluency/pressure/volume
Mood sad/happy/angry/flat/labile/apathetic
Insight presence/degree
Thought process content/possession/speed/flow
Hallucinations/delusions presence/organisation/system

The acutely disturbed patient

The majority of incidents of agitation and aggression in the Emergency Department are related to drug and alcohol use. Often it is not possible to immediately identify the underlying cause, e.g. drug or alcohol use or withdrawal, personality disorder, acute mental illness or delirium brought on by an organic disease process. Therefore any treatment system must be robust enough to deal with all these possibilities.

Principles
Prediction and prevention
Patients with a risk or history of violence should be searched by hospital security before being seen by clinical staff. Observation of patients may pick up warning signs. Patients should be interviewed in a quiet room that has outward-opening doors and an alarm system. Adequate numbers of staff should be nearby.

De-escalation and observation
De-escalation is the verbal and non-verbal behaviour that is used to calm a potentially confrontational situation. Seclusion is an option if a suitable room is available, together with a staff member for observation.

Disturbed patients respond positively to honesty and respect and can be presented with options. Limited negotiation may be attempted, e.g. to persuade the patient to take an oral benzodiazepine, but both sides must understand that failure to comply will result in restraint. Such negotiation is more likely to be effective when backed with a credible 'show of force'.

Restraint
If de-escalation has not worked, then restraint is necessary to protect the patient, other patients, the public and members of staff.

If physical restraint is to be used, a minimum of six trained staff are necessary to minimise the risk of injury to staff or the patient. Restraint is initially physical, followed by pharmaceutical sedation. Whenever a patient is restrained or sedated, close clinical and physiological monitoring is essential to ensure patient safety.

Review
When a patient has been restrained or sedated, they should be examined thoroughly for signs of organic disease. Psychiatric wards have limited medical facilities and it is prudent to perform any screening tests in the Emergency Department. This should include bedside tests – urine/glucose, bloods if indicated, e.g. FBC, U+E, LFTs, Ca^{2+}, TFTs (thyroid function tests). Chest X-ray, CT brain and lumbar puncture may be necessary depending on the history, e.g. head trauma.

Sedation
- *Benzodiazepines*, e.g. lorazepam, midazolam, diazepam. These drugs are generally safe and predictable. Routine users of benzodiazepines develop tolerance to these drugs, which will therefore have minimal effect.
- *Neuroleptics*, e.g. haloperidol, chlorpromazine, droperidol. These 'major tranquillisers' offer prolonged sedation and are the first choice for patients with psychotic features.

Benzodiazepines and neuroleptics can be usefully combined for the most agitated patients. Current UK recommendations favour lorazepam and/or haloperidol. If a patient is co-operative, these may be administered orally, otherwise intramuscular injection is effective.

Delerium (organic) or psychiatric symptoms

It can be difficult to distinguish organic from psychiatric disease. Delirium is the cognitive and consciousness impairment that may result from organic disease, e.g. sepsis, drugs, metabolic disorders.

Organic disease is suggested by:
- rapid onset
- fever
- non-sensory neurological abnormalities
- disorientation and confusion
- visual hallucinations.

Psychiatric disease is suggested by:
- chronic symptoms, previous psychiatric problems
- delusional beliefs, paranoia, disorganised thought processes
- auditory hallucinations – especially third person.

Patients with psychiatric illness may also have organic disease. Alcohol and drug use and/or withdrawal may cloud the picture and may need to resolve or be treated before a definitive decision can be made.

Factitious disorders

The Emergency Department sees a small number of particularly challenging patients with symptoms that have no organic basis: factitious disorders or Munchausen's syndrome. The Internet ensures that such patients are well informed about what symptoms they might have. It is very easy for doctors to become part of the problem, by continuing to search for disease despite absence of objective evidence of any disease process.

The symptoms may be very dramatic, yet the patient may appear unconcerned. The patient may appear to be in great distress, yet their pulse and blood pressure will be normal. Pseudocoma, pseudoseizures, dramatic and non-anatomical patterns of paralysis may occur. True factitious illness should be differentiated from malingering or drug-seeking where there is an obvious secondary gain.

Patients with a history of factitious illness may also develop organic illness. Safe diagnosis of factitious diseases using the minimum investigations necessary can be difficult, and early involvement of a senior doctor is advisable. When challenged, these patients usually leave rapidly and have no interest in engagement with psychiatric services.

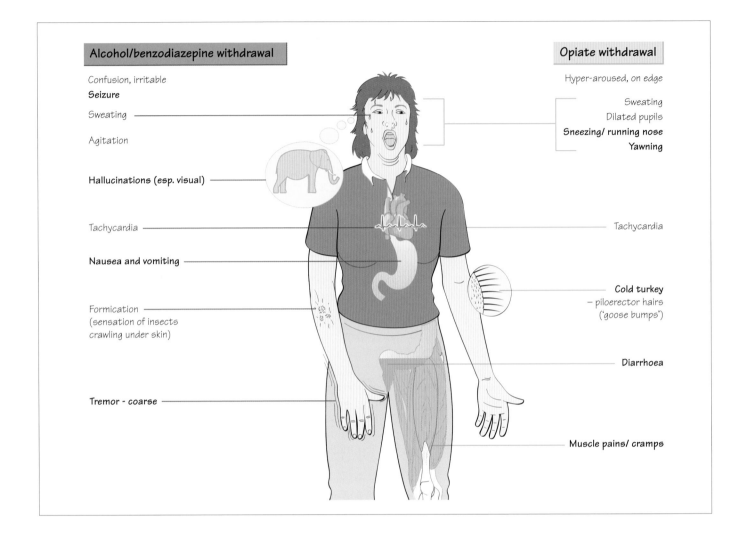

Alcohol/benzodiazepine withdrawal

Confusion, irritable
Seizure
Sweating
Agitation
Hallucinations (esp. visual)
Tachycardia
Nausea and vomiting
Formication
(sensation of insects
crawling under skin)
Tremor - coarse

Opiate withdrawal

Hyper-aroused, on edge
Sweating
Dilated pupils
Sneezing/ running nose
Yawning
Tachycardia
Cold turkey
– piloerector hairs
('goose bumps')
Diarrhoea
Muscle pains/ cramps

Observational medicine units are an expansion of traditional Emergency Department activity. Patients who are likely to be fit for discharge within 24 hours are held in a unit managed by the Emergency Department.

The reason for the rise of observational medicine is the pressure to better use hospital beds in the main part of the hospital, together with a better appreciation of the risks of hospitalisation. Emergency physicians are less inclined to hold onto patients than other specialties and are motivated to ensure rapid discharge wherever possible.

Features that differentiate an observational medicine ward from other wards in the hospital are:
• Frequent consultant-led ward rounds, e.g. three times a day, to ensure rapid progress and decision making.
• A discharge plan is necessary for entry to the unit.
• Ready availability of other health professionals, e.g. physiotherapists, occupational therapists, social workers.

The observation unit should not be used as an alternative to making a decision. There should be rapid turnover of patients: bed occupancy is often 200–300% per day.

Minor injury in elderly patient

A relatively minor injury in an older patient may have a disproportionate effect on their ability to cope safely at home. Common injuries, often the result of a fall, that may incapacitate patients include fracture of the neck of the humerus, Colles' fracture and fractured pubic rami. There are a vast number of potential causes for elderly patients to fall, but common medical causes that can be diagnosed and treated within the Emergency Department include:
• Arrhythmias: ECG.
• Postural hypotension: lying and standing blood pressure.
• Infections: urine dipstick, chest X-ray.
• Medication: polypharmacy increases the risk of drug interactions and adverse effects.

Review in the observation unit by a multidisciplinary team, which includes occupational therapy, physiotherapy and social workers as well as medical and nursing staff, can ensure a rapid, safe discharge from hospital.

Homelessness

The Emergency Department is sometimes the only medical contact that homeless people have. Appropriate emergency medical care is given but it is not the job of the Emergency Department to resolve the multiple chronic and social problems these patients often have. Mental illness and drug and alcohol dependence are common in this group, but there is a limited amount that the Emergency Department can do unless there is ongoing community support.

'Frequent flyers'

There is a small group of patients who come to the Emergency Department very often. This is usually due to a combination of factors, which may include personality disorders, drug and alcohol problems, self-harm, loneliness, homelessness and mental illness. These are difficult patients to manage as they are often very experienced at manipulating healthcare staff. It is best if they are looked after by the most senior staff available, to avoid one group of health professionals being played off against another.

Domestic violence and elder abuse

An Emergency Department visit is an opportunity for intervention: staff need to be alert to the possibility of non-accidental injury in vulnerable people. Drug and alcohol problems often coexist with domestic violence. Emergency Department staff cannot force someone to seek help, but can provide contact details and a quiet area with a telephone. Elder abuse may be particularly difficult to diagnose due to the high rate of natural falls and bruising, together with poor memory.

Drugs and alcohol

Although drug and alcohol dependence are often managed by psychiatrically trained doctors, they are *not* mental illnesses per se. However, drug and alcohol use often coexists with mental illness; this could be viewed as the patient's self-medicating.

Patients sometimes present to the Emergency Department seeking 'a detox'. A detoxification is a (usually temporary) drug-free period. The Emergency Department is not the place for elective management of withdrawal of drugs or alcohol: this can be safely managed in the community.

Patients who are dependent on drugs or alcohol often end up in the Emergency Department as a result of falls, fights, and so on. These patients may experience withdrawal in the Emergency Department, and this must be identified and managed, otherwise they may have seizures or the patient will leave, compromising their medical care. Withdrawal symptoms do not respect class or educational attainment, and one must be alert to symptoms in unexpected patients.

If alcohol problems are suspected, use the CAGE questionnaire (Chapter 29) and, if positive, expect to have to manage withdrawal, and ensure the patient is aware of community support on discharge.

Alcohol and benzodiazepine withdrawal

Withdrawal from alcohol and benzodiazepines is potentially dangerous, as fits may occur. *Thiamine*, usually combined with other B and C vitamins, is given to prevent Wernicke's encephalopathy (characterised by confusion, ataxia, ophthalmoplegia and nystagmus) and Korsakoff's psychosis, the disastrous irreversible consequences of chronic thiamine deficiency common in alcoholics.

Alcohol withdrawal is generally best managed using front-loaded oral *diazepam*, which has active metabolites with a long half-life (2–4 days). Large doses of diazepam, e.g. 20 mg every one to two hours, are given according to symptoms; multiple doses are often required.

Once the patient's symptoms have been controlled, the patient does not have to stay in hospital, and does not need diazepam on discharge, as its pharmacokinetics will ensure a tapering dose of benzodiazepines.

Opiate withdrawal

Opiate withdrawal is unpleasant, but not dangerous. Musculoskeletal symptoms respond to NSAIDs; high-dose diazepam helps with agitation and nausea. Clonidine, an alpha antagonist with mild opiate agonist properties, can also be used.

Other patient groups

Other patient groups who often end up in the observation ward include:
- Overdose (Chapters 24 and 25).
- First fit (Chapter 43).
- Minor head injury (Chapter 11).
- Post-sedation (Chapter 6).

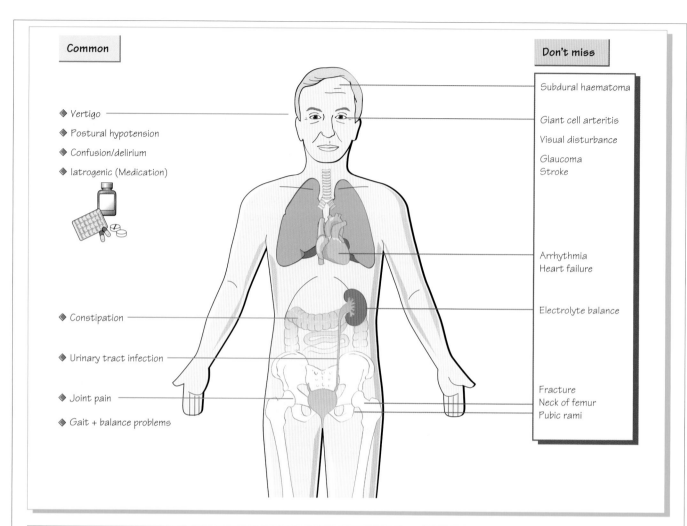

Common

- Vertigo
- Postural hypotension
- Confusion/delirium
- Iatrogenic (Medication)
- Constipation
- Urinary tract infection
- Joint pain
- Gait + balance problems

Don't miss

Subdural haematoma

Giant cell arteritis
Visual disturbance
Glaucoma
Stroke

Arrhythmia
Heart failure

Electrolyte balance

Fracture
Neck of femur
Pubic rami

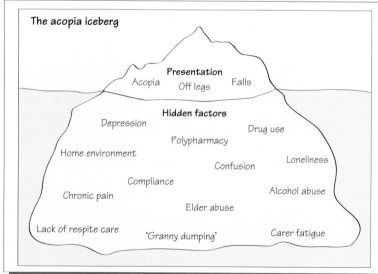

The acopia iceberg

Presentation
Acopia   Off legs   Falls

Hidden factors

Depression
Drug use
Polypharmacy
Home environment
Loneliness
Confusion
Compliance
Alcohol abuse
Chronic pain
Elder abuse
Lack of respite care
'Granny dumping'
Carer fatigue

CAGE screening for alcohol problems

| Have you tried to **C**ut down your drinking? |
| Do you get **A**nnoyed when people criticise your drinking? |
| Do feel **G**uilty about your drinking? |
| Do you sometimes have an **E**ye-opener in the morning? |

A score of 2 suggests alcohol problems;
3 or 4 is diagnostic
[The +LR for a score of 1,2,3,4 are 1.5, 4.5, 13,
100 respectively, and the −LR for a score of 0 is 0.14]

Abbreviated mental test (AMT4)

| Age |
| Year |
| Date of Birth |
| Prime Minister/President |
| A score of less than 4 indicates mental impairment |

Caring for patients with multiple long-term conditions, frailty, and functional or cognitive impairment is an increasing challenge for families and health and social services. These patients often present to the Emergency Department with a relatively minor functional decline, but one that renders the patient 'off their legs', 'bedbound' or 'acopic' (unable to cope).

The Emergency Department can offer a rapid, thorough, medical and social assessment, with the aim of making an early decision as to whether the patient should be:
- Discharged home ± increased nursing/social support.
- Transferred to a rehabilitation bed.
- Admitted to a medical bed.

Such decisions require the range of skills of many different health professionals to be integrated, but can provide safe and effective care and avoid unnecessary acute hospital admissions.

History

An early part of the history and examination of these patients should be their Abbreviated Mental Test (AMT4) score. If this suggests impairment (score less than 4), the rest of the history may need cautious interpretation. It is always useful to corroborate the history from at least one other source (carer, relative).

Key questions are:
- Why is the patient here now?
- Is there a (reversible) reason for a loss of function?

Presenting complaints
- *Precipitants*: ask in detail about any recent symptoms, specifically adequacy of oral intake, loss of weight, bowel or urinary symptoms, and symptoms of infection.
- *Falls*: falls are common and a careful history is necessary to work out the aetiology. Ask about the frequency and pattern of falls, possible precipitants such as problems with gait and balance, and syncope/pre-syncope.
- *Medications*: an accurate list of medications and doses, including recent changes, provides insight into the current medical conditions being managed and possible drug interactions and side-effects, both of which are common in the elderly. Assess likely compliance with medication.
- *Cognition*: what is the current level of function, cognitive and mental status, vs the usual level? Ask about alcohol consumption and mood disturbance. Many patients successfully conceal high alcohol consumption: use the CAGE questions.

Ask about family and social supports, and if external services are currently in place to support the patient with their Activities of Daily Living (ADLs) at their home.

Examination
General examination
Look for evidence of infection, chest and urine being the most common. Minor trauma may cause occult hip and pelvic fractures in an osteoporotic patient.

Cardiorespiratory examination
Look for valvular disease and heart failure. Postural hypotension is common and should be excluded in every patient.

Neurological examination
Assess speech, gait and cerebellar function. Look for weakness or changes in reflexes that would indicate stroke. Full sensory examination of limbs is not practical in the Emergency Department, but pinprick and vibration should be performed to search for evidence of peripheral neuropathy (diabetes, vitamin B_{12}/folate/thiamine deficiency).

The rare but treatable condition of normal pressure hydrocephalus occurs in elderly patients and presents as ataxia, incontinence and confusion. CT confirms the diagnosis.

Investigations
Bedside investigations
- Blood glucose.
- ECG.
- Urine dipstick.
- Lying and standing blood pressure.

Laboratory investigations
- FBC and U+E.
- Creatine kinase for any patient 'found on floor'.

Imaging
- Chest X-ray.
- CT head if risk of subdural haematoma, or if stroke is suspected.

Management
Identify medically reversible reasons for a loss of function. This might include treatment of urinary tract infection, constipation, or stopping a recently commenced medication. Beware occult fractures of neck of femur and neck. CT or MRI may be necessary in cases where there is pain but an equivocal plain X-ray examination.

Patients may require new equipment (e.g. a walking aid), a home hazards assessment, or additional home or community services. These may be combined with a rehabilitation programme involving exercise and physical therapy.

Disposal: who can go home?
Patients at risk of falls require a formal falls risk assessment before discharge, and either admission or early referral to a falls clinic. Reversible medical conditions identified and treated within the Emergency Department (e.g. UTI, mild hyponatraemia, polypharmacy) do not necessitate hospital admission.

Discharge patients who appear well, in whom serious pathology has been excluded and who are safe to return to their normal home environment after screening by the multidisciplinary team.

30 Syncope, collapse and falls

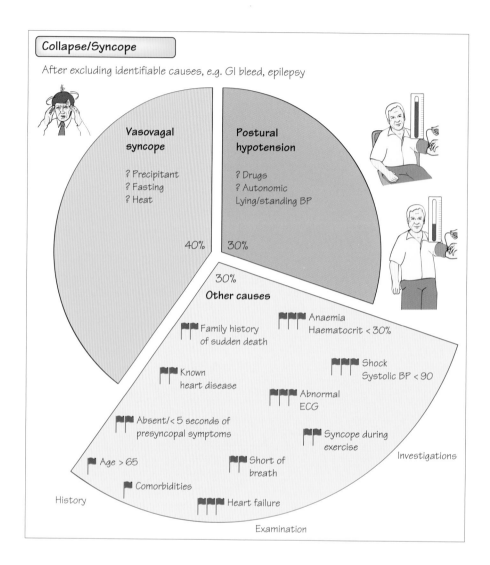

Collapse/Syncope

After excluding identifiable causes, e.g. GI bleed, epilepsy

Vasovagal syncope
? Precipitant
? Fasting
? Heat

Postural hypotension
? Drugs
? Autonomic
Lying/standing BP

40%

30%

30%
Other causes

Family history of sudden death

Anaemia Haematocrit < 30%

Known heart disease

Shock Systolic BP < 90

Abnormal ECG

Absent/< 5 seconds of presyncopal symptoms

Syncope during exercise

Age > 65

Short of breath

Comorbidities

Heart failure

Investigations

History

Examination

Syncope is a brief loss of consciousness that resolves spontaneously and completely. It is distinct from vertigo, seizures, coma and states of altered consciousness. Syncope accounts for 1–2% of Emergency Department visits but 6% of hospital admissions.

History

A detailed history taken as soon as possible after the event offers the best chance to achieve an accurate diagnosis. Patients are by definition asymptomatic by the time they have reached the Emergency Department and may not remember the event. An eyewitness account is therefore particularly valuable in corroborating what happened during the episode, particularly in estimating duration of loss of consciousness and any possible seizure activity.

Single most important question: 'Do you remember falling?'

Nature of the episode: first episode, or recurrent?
Environment
• Lying down/seated, with absent or brief prodromal symptoms (? cardiac).
• Within 2 minutes of standing (? postural hypotension).
• Stressor (pain or emotional upset) with longer prodromes and associated pallor, sweating, nausea or vomiting (? vasovagal/arrhythmia).
• Head rotation or movement (? carotid sinus sensitivity); visit to the toilet (? micturition or defecation syncope); or coughing (? cough syncope).
• Exertion (? cardiac arrhythmia, HOCM), hot/cold?

Prodromal symptoms Prodomal symptoms might be things like 'feeling faint', 'feeling like I was going to pass out', 'feeling the

 Adult Emergency Medicine at a Glance, 1st edition. © Thomas Hughes and Jaycen Cruickshank. Published 2011 by Blackwell Publishing Ltd.

room spin around me'. Prodromal symptoms that last a few seconds suggest an arrhythmia, those lasting a few minutes suggest vasovagal syncope.

What happened during the syncope? Witnesses may report falls or trauma during the episode. A few seconds of mild tonic-clonic activity may be caused by syncope 'anoxic jerks', and do not necessarily signify epilepsy. Absence seizures mimic syncope.

What happened after the syncope? A long period of confusion occurs after generalised seizures. Neurological deficits, e.g. hemiparesis, may occur after a seizure ('Todd's palsy') or may represent a TIA/stroke (Chapter 42).

Medical and drug history
Polypharmacy, drug interactions and compliance are a particular problem in the elderly. Antihypertensive agents and vasodilators, e.g. for angina or cardiac failure, cause postural hypotension, and many psychoactive drugs prolong the QT interval.

Examination
Examination focuses on the cardiac and neurological systems. Examine specifically for carotid bruits, valvular disease, outflow obstruction or evidence of heart failure. All patients should have postural blood pressure measured.

Abdominal pain may indicate bleeding or abdominal aortic aneurysm (AAA). Rectal examination should be performed, with testing for blood using a faecal occult blood testing kit.

Tongue biting (lateral margins) or incontinence suggests a seizure, but absence does not rule it out. Neurological examination should include a Glasgow Coma Scale (Chapter 10), cranial nerves, limb tone, power and reflexes.

Investigations
Bedside investigations
- Glucose and ECG in all patients. ECG monitoring may capture intermittent (paroxysmal) arrhythmias.
- Urine for UTI and βhCG if pregnancy possible.
- Ultrasound to rule out AAA.

Laboratory investigations
- FBE, U+E, troponin if cardiac disease a possibility.

Imaging
- CT is indicated if there is suspicion of a seizure, or new/focal neurological findings.

Treatment: identify or stratify
Identify
After resuscitation if necessary, patients with an identifiable cause of their syncope should be managed according to the cause.
- Syncope + shortness of breath = shortness of breath (Chapter 36).
- Syncope + chest pain = chest pain (Chapters 34 and 35).
- Syncope + headache = headache (Chapter 41).
- Syncope + gastrointestinal bleed = gastrointestinal bleed (Chapter 40).

Also identifiable from the history and examination will be patients with the two most common causes for syncope:

Vasovagal (neurocardiogenic) syncope
Vasovagal syncope (VVS) causes about 40% of syncopal episodes, and may be precipitated by a stressful event, or lack of food or drink. VVS is usually preceded by pallor, sweating, nausea and dizziness, but in the elderly, these prodromal symptoms may be short or non-existent.

Vagal parasympathetic outflow causes bradycardia; when cardiac output falls, the sympathetic-driven tachycardia and vasoconstriction fails to remedy the situation in time, and there is transient loss of cerebral perfusion. When the patient collapses, venous return increases and cardiac output is restored.

As VVS is a 'benign' diagnosis, there is a significant danger that junior Emergency Department doctors attribute a patient's syncope to VVS too easily: all such patients should be reviewed by a senior doctor.

Postural hypotension
Under normal circumstances, moving from lying or sitting to standing causes a reflex rise in heart rate and blood pressure, to maintain cerebral perfusion. Drugs (vasodilators) and autonomic dysfunction (diabetes, Parkinson's disease) may interfere with this response, which causes about 30% of syncope episodes.

To test for postural hypotension, the BP should be measured repeatedly after moving to vertical, until the BP rises. Treatment is by treating the underlying cause, with appropriate follow-up by GP or outpatient clinic.

Stratify
One is then left with approximately 30% of patients with no clear cause for the syncope, and the aim shifts to risk stratification. Clinical guidelines have not proved robust, but key criteria predicting need for admission are shown opposite. Of these criteria, cardiac failure seems a particularly important predictor of sudden death, probably due to ventricular arrhythmias.

Diagnoses not to miss
Conditions predisposing to tachyarrhythmia
- *Long QT syndromes (>460 msec)* may be congenital or acquired. Correct electrolyte abnormalities, and avoid medications that prolong QT (e.g. phenothiazines, benzodiazepines, antidepressants).
- *Short PR interval (<120 msec)* together with a slurred upstroke of QRS complex (delta wave) suggest an accessory pathway between the atria and ventricles, e.g. Wolff-Parkinson-White syndrome.
- *Brugada syndrome (RBBB with ST elevation V1–3) and short QT interval (<300 msec)* are congenital conditions that predispose to ventricular arrhythmias.

Conditions predisposing to bradyarrthmia
Sinus node dysfunction, heart block and vagal hypersensitivity – see Chapter 31.

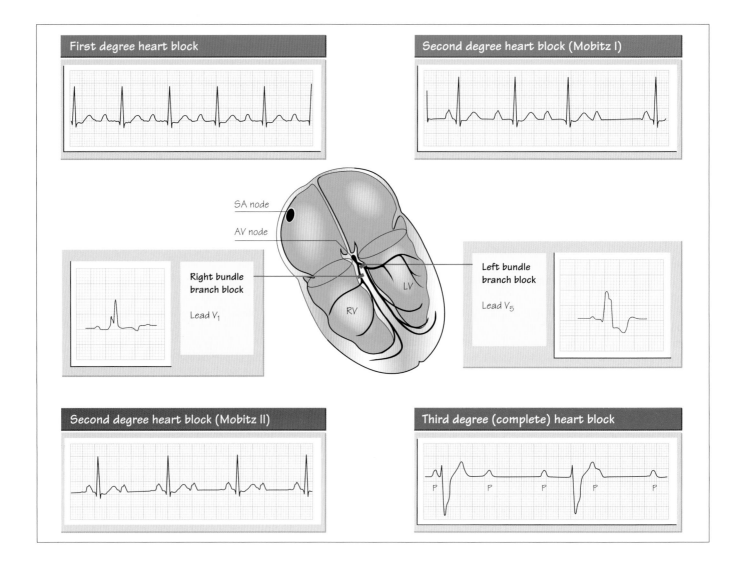

Bradycardia is a heart rate below 60 beats per minute (bpm). Bradyarrhythmia is rhythm disturbance with a ventricular rate below 60 bpm. Bradyarrhythmias usually result from a defect in the heart's intrinsic conduction system or drugs affecting these areas.

The different parts of the conduction system have different intrinsic rates of depolarisation.
- 60 bpm: sinoatrial node (SAN).
- 50 bpm: atrioventricular node (AVN).
- 40–50 bpm: bundle of His leading to right and left (anterior and posterior) bundles of specialised conductive myocardial cells that conduct from AVN down the interventricular septum.
- 30–40 bpm: ventricular myocardium – the Purkinje fibres that distribute depolarisation around the myocardium.

Therefore, under normal circumstances, the SAN is the pacemaker, as it has the fastest intrinsic rate. If the SAN fails, the AVN takes over as the pacemaker but with a slower rate. If the AVN fails, the ventricles will beat on their own, but at a very slow rate.

Investigations
Bedside investigations
- Blood glucose.
- ECG.
- Cardiac device interrogation. If the patient has an implanted device, e.g. pacemaker, this may have recorded what occurred.

Laboratory investigations
- U+E, LFTs. Ensuring $K^+ > 4$ mmol/L, minimises the risk of arrhythmias.
- Thyroid function tests (TFTs).
- Troponin I.
- Ca^{2+}, Mg^{2+}.

Imaging
- Chest X-ray.
- Echocardiogram.

Common diagnoses
Right bundle branch block
Blockage of the single right bundle does not cause bradycardia, is relatively common and not necessarily pathological: it can be a normal variant. On ECG there is a broad RSR wave (i.e. M-shaped, ≥ 0.12 sec = 3 small squares wide) in the leads looking at the right side of the heart, V1 and V2.

Left bundle branch block
Blockage of both the left bundles, anterior and posterior, is always pathological, and may be a feature of acute coronary syndrome (ACS). Left bundle branch block (LBBB) implies significant damage to the interventricular septum and, although it does not cause bradycardia, it slows conduction of the wave of depolarisation, impairing contraction of the ventricle. The ECG shows a broad RSR wave (i.e. M-shaped, ≥ 0.12 sec = 3 small squares wide) in the leads looking at the anterolateral side of the heart II, aV_L and V_{3-6}. The abnormal depolarisation and repolarisation of the left ventricle means that ST abnormalities normally associated with ACS cannot be interpreted.

First-degree heart block
In first-degree heart block, *all 'P' (atrial) waves are conducted, but slowly*. The delay occurs in transmission through the AVN, resulting in a P-R interval of more than 0.20 sec = 5 small squares = 1 big square. On its own, first-degree heart block does not need treatment.

Second-degree heart block: Mobitz type I
In second-degree heart block, *some 'P' (atrial) waves are not conducted*. Mobitz type I (Wenkebach) results in a progressive delay in conduction of P waves through the AVN until a P wave is not conducted. This is a relatively benign phenomenon, and can occur in inferior myocardial infarction (MI) as the right coronary usually (70%) supplies the AVN, but rarely needs pacing.

Diagnoses not to miss
Second-degree heart block: Mobitz type II
In second-degree heart block, *some 'P' (atrial) waves are not conducted*. Intermittent conduction of P waves in a fixed ratio, i.e. 1:2, 1:3 is termed Mobitz type II. Mobitz type II heart block implies significantly more damage to the conducting system than Mobitz type I, particularly in the context of an anterior myocardial infarction, when pacing is necessary.

Third-degree (complete) heart block
Third-degree heart block occurs when *no 'P' (atrial) waves are conducted*. The atria beat regularly, as do the ventricles, but there is no association between the two. An artificial pacemaker is usually necessary to preserve cardiac output, and to avoid long pauses which may precede asystolic cardiac arrest.

Extreme bradycardia, pauses
Pauses between ventricular beats of over 2 seconds and heart rates below 50 bpm are likely to be significant, especially if the patient is symptomatic. Possible causes include:
- *Sinus node dysfunction* (sick sinus syndrome, brady/tachy syndrome) may cause both bradycardia and tachycardia at different times, and occurs in older patients due to fibrosis of the sinus node. Inpatient assessment for permanent pacemaker (PPM) ± antiarrhythmics is usually necessary.
- *Vagal hypersensitivity*: e.g. micturition syncope, carotid sinus hypersensitivity – abnormal sensitivity of the heart to normal vagal stimulation can result in bradycardia and pauses. Treatment is by avoidance (sitting down, avoiding pressure on neck) and cardiology review for consideration of further measures (drugs, PPM).
- *Iatrogenic*: Excessive beta blocker, digoxin or rate-controlling calcium channel blocker.
- *Normal finding*: Athletes may have heart rates in the 40s and occasionally in the 30s. This may be accentuated by the normal physiological 'sinus arrhythmia' resulting from changes in venous return due to variation of intrathoracic pressure.

Electrolytes and the patient's thyroid function should be checked, as subclinical hypothyroidism is common in the elderly. Treatment is by treating the underlying cause, but in the acute setting, *atropine* 500 micrograms i.v. blocks the vagal tone, and can be repeated to a maximum of 3 mg.

If further stimulation is required, a low-dose adrenaline infusion or a temporary pacemaker may be necessary. Some defibrillators can perform transthoracic pacing by delivering small electric currents between the pads on the chest to stimulate the heart to beat.

Bifascicular and trifascicular block
The combination of right bundle branch block and left axis deviation, which signifies partial left bundle branch block, is known as bifascicular block. The combination of bifascicular block and first-degree heart block is known as trifascicular block, which is not a good descriptor.

It is particularly important to identify these blocks in patients presenting with falls, or who will need surgery. Trifascicular block may intermittently become complete heart block, particularly during anaesthesia.

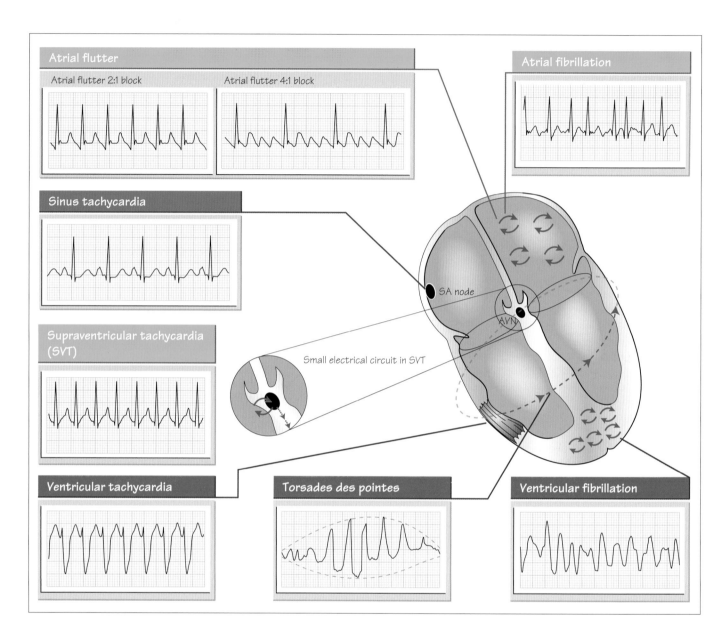

Tachycardia vs tachyarrhythmia

Tachycardia is a heart rate above 100 beats per minute (bpm). Tachyarrhythmia is a rhythm disturbance with a ventricular rate of more than 100 bpm.

Narrow vs broad complex

Tachyarrhythmias usually occur because the heart's intrinsic rate regulation system described in the previous chapter is overridden. The QRS complexes are caused by ventricular depolarisation. If the ventricle's normal (fast) electrical distribution system, the Bundle of His and left and right bundles, are still used by the arrhythmia, then the QRS complexes will be *narrow*, as usual.

However, if the impulse bypasses this network, and instead relies on (slow) conduction between normal cardiac muscle cells, the ECG complexes will be *broad*.

Regular vs irregular

Regular complexes imply a degree of stability in the underlying electrical circuits, whereas irregular complexes are caused by chaotic electrical activity.

Paroxysmal

Arrhythmias that are not consistent, i.e. come and go, are termed 'paroxysmal'.

Clinical assessment

A rapid assessment needs to be performed to assess whether the patient is significantly unwell; this is usually fairly clear. It can be more difficult is to establish whether the tachyarrhythmia is the cause of the patient being unwell, or a response to an underlying cause. If it is a simple tachycardia, then often there is an underlying cause. Further assessment and treatment depends on the arrhythmia found.

Investigations

Bedside investigations
- Blood glucose.
- ECG.
- Cardiac device interrogation. If the patient has an implanted device, e.g. pacemaker, this may have recorded what occurred.

Laboratory investigations
- U+E, LFTs. Ensuring $K^+ > 4$ mmol/L, minimises the risk of arrhythmias.
- Thyroid function tests (TFTs).
- Troponin I.
- Ca^{2+}, Mg^{2+}.

Imaging
- Chest X-ray.
- Echocardiogram.

Common diagnoses: atrial

Sinus tachycardia
Sinus tachycardia occurs when the heart is driven faster than usual. Causes include:
- Response to illness, e.g. shock, sepsis.
- Drugs – β_2 agonists such as salbutamol.
- Thyrotoxicosis.
- Anxiety – if other causes excluded.
  Treatment is correction of the underlying cause.

Atrial flutter/fibrillation
The chaotic micro-circuits of *atrial fibrillation* (AF) are seen as an *irregular baseline* of the ECG, whereas the larger, more consistent, *atrial flutter* waves are seen as a *sawtooth* pattern at 300 bpm. Of these flutter impulses, only some are conducted through the AVN to the ventricles: a simple ratio governs this, e.g. 2:1 giving 150 bpm, 3:1 giving 100 bpm or 4:1 giving 75 bpm.

In atrial *fibrillation*, conduction is not consistent, resulting in a heartbeat that is irregular in *time* but also in *volume*, as there is no atrial contraction to fill the ventricles consistently.

Treatment depends on patient stability, myocardial status and duration of arrhythmia.
- A patient who is unwell with a low blood pressure due to atrial fibrillation needs urgent electrical cardioversion, with sedation.
- Patients who are stable may be cardioverted with drugs, or, if the arrhythmia is likely to be chronic (older patients), the ventricular rate may be controlled using beta blockers or digoxin.
- If the patient is stable and the arrhythmia has been present for more than 48 hours, they should be fully anticoagulated before cardioversion to prevent embolism of intracardiac blood clots that may have formed.

- Drugs commonly used for cardioversion include flecainide (only if the heart is structurally normal), amiodarone or sotalol.
- Anticoagulation should be considered in patients who have long-term or paroxysmal atrial fibrillation, as this reduces the risk of stroke.
- If the patient has heart failure and atrial fibrillation, both need to be treated.

Supraventricular tachycardia

Commonly causing a ventricular rate of 160–180 bpm, supraventricular tachycardia (SVT) is caused by an abnormal electrical circuit in or near the AVN. Every time an impulse goes round the circuit, it also sends an impulse down the Bundle of His.

Treatment aims to break the electrical circuit by reducing transmission in the AVN. This can be achieved by:
- Increasing the vagal drive to the AVN, e.g. Valsalva manoeuvre (ask patient to blow plunger out of a 10 mL syringe) or carotid sinus massage.
- Pharmacologically blocking the AVN using adenosine, which temporarily upsets the adenosine/cAMP balance, preventing transmission for a few seconds.

If a patient has SVT but has a ventricular conduction problem, e.g. left bundle branch block, this may look like VT. If SVT is treated as VT, no harm will come to the patient, but if VT is treated as SVT, great harm may occur. A simple yet robust rule of thumb is:

Broad Complex Tachycardia + Ischaemic Heart Disease
= Ventricular Tachycardia

Diagnoses not to miss: ventricular
See also Chapter 33.

Ventricular tachycardia
Ventricular tachycardia usually results from a single focus of abnormal electrical activity within the ventricles that produces rapid ventricular activation at about 180–220 bpm. Patients who are unstable with VT, e.g. low blood pressure or chest pain, require immediate electrical cardioversion. Patients who are stable may be cardioverted with drugs, e.g. amiodarone.

Torsades des pointes
Meaning 'twisting of points', this rare arrhythmia is caused by the focus of VT moving around the myocardium. Because the ECG sees this three-dimensional activity in one plane, the amplitude of the VT appears to vary like a sine wave. Treatment is as for VT, together with intravenous magnesium.

Ventricular fibrillation
Chaotic electrical activity in the ventricles – ventricular fibrillation (VF) – means there are no organised cardiac contractions, and therefore no cardiac output. Without electrical cardioversion to restore normal rhythm, or cardiopulmonary resuscitation (while awaiting cardioversion), there will be no blood perfusing the brain, which is irreversibly damaged within 5 minutes.

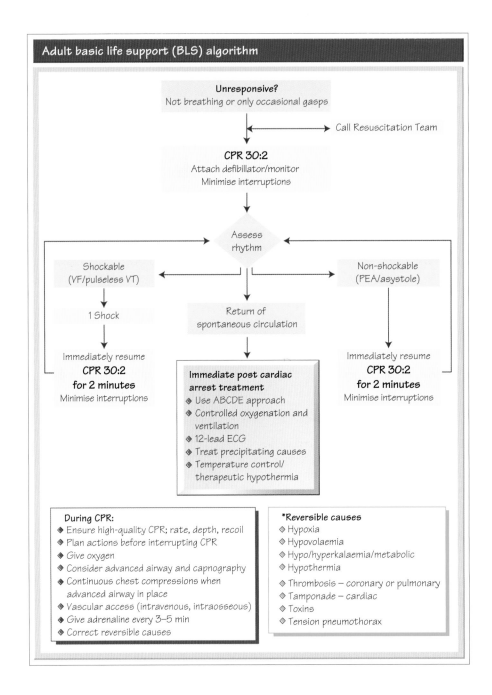

Adult basic life support (BLS) algorithm

Unresponsive?
Not breathing or only occasional gasps

→ Call Resuscitation Team

CPR 30:2
Attach defibrillator/monitor
Minimise interruptions

Assess rhythm

Shockable
(VF/pulseless VT)

1 Shock

Immediately resume
CPR 30:2
for 2 minutes
Minimise interruptions

Return of spontaneous circulation

Non-shockable
(PEA/asystole)

Immediately resume
CPR 30:2
for 2 minutes
Minimise interruptions

Immediate post cardiac arrest treatment
◆ Use ABCDE approach
◆ Controlled oxygenation and ventilation
◆ 12-lead ECG
◆ Treat precipitating causes
◆ Temperature control/ therapeutic hypothermia

During CPR:
◆ Ensure high-quality CPR; rate, depth, recoil
◆ Plan actions before interrupting CPR
◆ Give oxygen
◆ Consider advanced airway and capnography
◆ Continuous chest compressions when advanced airway in place
◆ Vascular access (intravenous, intraosseous)
◆ Give adrenaline every 3–5 min
◆ Correct reversible causes

*Reversible causes
◇ Hypoxia
◇ Hypovolaemia
◇ Hypo/hyperkalaemia/metabolic
◇ Hypothermia
◇ Thrombosis – coronary or pulmonary
◇ Tamponade – cardiac
◇ Toxins
◇ Tension pneumothorax

Ischaemic heart disease is common, and arrhythmias are a common mode of death in otherwise normal 'hearts too good to die'. These arrhythmias are treatable with cardiopulmonary resuscitation (CPR) and defibrillation, which has been one of the success stories of pre-hospital medicine.

Research into causes and treatment of cardiac arrest using human subjects is ethically challenging, which explains the lack of high-level evidence in this area, and why international guidelines can change radically. Ventricular fibrillation and tachycardia are described in Chapter 32.

Asystole

Asystole is the complete absence of electrical activity and is the final pathway for all untreated cardiac arrests, and therefore may indicate that the heart is functionally dead. However there are reversible causes of asystole: see the '4Hs and 4Ts' opposite.

Pulseless electrical activity

Pulseless electrical activity (PEA) occurs when the ECG trace looks normal(ish), i.e. one would expect the rhythm to result in cardiac output, but there is no pulse. This suggests that the heart is beating, but there is some mechanical reason for its lack of output:

- Tension pneumothorax increases hemithoracic pressure, and also causes mediastinal shift, which kinks the great vessels (aorta and vena cavae).
- Hypovolaemia: there is no blood to pump.
- Tamponade: fluid in the pericardiac sac under pressure prevents venous inflow in diastole.
- Thrombosis: thrombus obstructing right ventricular outflow (pulmonary embolus) or coronary arteries (myocardial infarction).

These and other potentially reversible causes of arrest are listed opposite – the '4 Hs and 4Ts'.

Cardiopulmonary resuscitation

Chest compressions

Chest compressions provide a (reduced) cardiac output by squeezing the heart between the sternum and the spine. Chest compressions need to be of adequate force, depth (one-third of chest wall diameter) and rate – 100/minute to be effective. Even short gaps in compressions significantly reduce the effective coronary perfusion, so must be avoided wherever possible.

Ventilation

The role of ventilation compared to chest compression has been progressively downgraded. Performing ventilation is a barrier to members of the public starting CPR, and chest compressions alone give a similar outcome in most adult situations. This is not the case in children, where hypoxia is the commonest cause of cardiac arrest.

Care must be taken with intubated asthma/ COPD patients: over-ventilation results in hyperexpanded lungs and increased intrathoracic pressure. This in turn reduces venous return to the heart, causing PEA cardiac arrest. Sustained pressure over the anterior chest wall decompresses the chest, restoring venous return.

Drugs

Adrenaline/vasopressin

Adrenaline/epinephrine reduces blood flow to muscle and the gut, preserving blood flow to vital organs: the myocardium, the brain and the kidneys. It is given once every 4 minutes. Anoxic damage to the brain and the kidney predict a poor outcome from an ICU admission. Vasopressin (ADH) is given once only and has a similar action to adrenaline; however, it is more expensive and no survival advantage has been demonstrated.

Amiodarone

Amiodarone is an anti-arrhythmic drug given for persistent ventricular fibrillation or broad complex tachycardia. All anti-

arrhythmic drugs reduce heart contractility (negatively inotropic), which is undesirable in cardiac arrest, but amiodarone seems the 'least bad' in this respect.

Defibrillation

Defibrillation is indicated in ventricular arrhythmias (VT/VF) with no pulse. Defibrillators use a DC (monophasic) or AC (biphasic) pulse of electric current to depolarise the entire heart simultaneously. Biphasic defibrillators are smaller, lighter, and as effective as the older monophasic machines.

The success of defibrillation depends on the time to defibrillation. If *no CPR is performed*, this is a linear relationship, with 90% success at 1 minute, to 0% at 10 minutes. If CPR is performed, the rate of deterioration is much slower, and brain and kidney will remain perfused.

When giving defibrillation, every 5 seconds between stopping chest compressions and defibrillation halves the chance of successful defibrillation.

Automatic defibrillators that help the rescuer with a series of voice prompts have been successfully used by non-experts, and *no training is necessary to use them*. They are widely available in public areas such as transport hubs and large entertainment venues.

Return of spontaneous circulation

In the case of return of spontaneous circulation (ROSC), there are a number of things to remember in addition to 'Airway/Breathing/ Circulation'.

A Arterial blood gas/audit
B Blood pressure
C CXR, cool patient, consider PPCI + stent
D Draw blood for U+E, troponin
E Electrocardiogram (ECG)
F Family – speak to the family
G Gratitude – thank resuscitation team
H Handover to inpatient medical team and
I Intensive care

When to stop resuscitation?

This can be a difficult decision and should be made by the most senior person present. Futility of further treatment is judged on the patient's pre-arrest functional state (particularly their exercise tolerance), length of time of resuscitation and response to treatment.

Patients who have potentially treatable causes, e.g. drug overdose, or who have been cooled prior to their arrest may make a full normal recovery after hours of CPR. However, if there is no reversible cause and no ventricular activity 30 minutes after the start of resuscitation, there is little point in continuing.

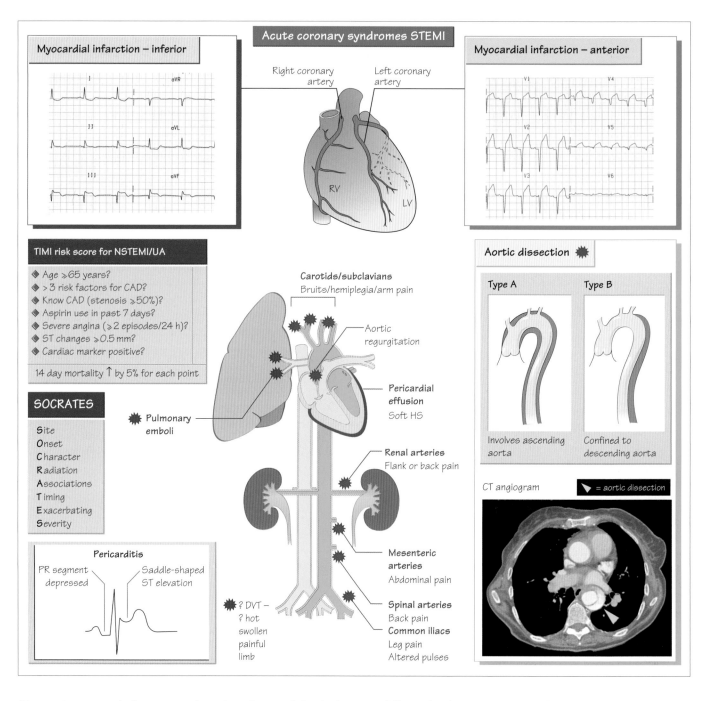

Acute coronary syndromes STEMI

Myocardial infarction – inferior

Myocardial infarction – anterior

Right coronary artery

Left coronary artery

TIMI risk score for NSTEMI/UA

◆ Age ≥65 years?
◆ > 3 risk factors for CAD?
◆ Know CAD (stenosis ≥50%)?
◆ Aspirin use in past 7 days?
◆ Severe angina (≥2 episodes/24 h)?
◆ ST changes ≥0.5 mm?
◆ Cardiac marker positive?

14 day mortality ↑ by 5% for each point

Carotids/subclavians
Bruits/hemiplegia/arm pain

Aortic regurgitation

SOCRATES

Site
Onset
Character
Radiation
Associations
Timing
Exacerbating
Severity

Pulmonary emboli

Pericardial effusion
Soft HS

Renal arteries
Flank or back pain

Mesenteric arteries
Abdominal pain

Spinal arteries
Back pain
Common iliacs
Leg pain
Altered pulses

? DVT –
? hot
swollen
painful
limb

Pericarditis

PR segment depressed

Saddle-shaped ST elevation

Aortic dissection

Type A

Type B

Involves ascending aorta

Confined to descending aorta

CT angiogram

▼ = aortic dissection

Chest pain can result from many thoracic and even abdominal organs. This chapter, together with Chapter 35 concentrates on the 'big three' – acute coronary syndrome (ACS), aortic dissection (AD) and pulmonary embolus (PE) and their differential diagnoses. These diagnoses are often difficult to make, and are a common area for medico-legal action.

History

Patients presenting with a 'textbook' collection of symptoms are the exception rather than the rule, and therefore the history must carefully probe the exact natures of the pain; use the acronym SOCRATES (see above).

• *Dull pain*: retrosternal or left-sided pain that is tight, crushing or heavy in nature, and may radiate to the left arm, shoulder or jaw, suggests acute coronary syndrome. Cardiac ischaemia is exacerbated by exercise or stress, relieved by rest, nitrates or oxygen. Autonomic phenomena such as nausea, anxiety or sweating are particularly associated with myocardial ischaemia, as is radiation of pain to both arms or the use of the clenched fist on the chest wall to demonstrate the pain.

- *Sharp pain*: sharp, well-localised pain, exacerbated by breathing and coughing, suggests pleuritic irritation: consider pulmonary embolism and other causes (Chapter 35).
- *Sudden-onset tearing or ripping pain radiating to back/intrascapular region* suggests aortic dissection.
- *Breathlessness* is a common feature of pulmonary embolism and acute coronary syndrome, and may be the only symptom in elderly or diabetic patients. Breathlessness as the main complaint is covered in Chapter 36.

Previous medical history should include risk factors for atherosclerosis – family history, smoking, hypertension, diabetes and hyperlipidaemia. A history of cocaine use should be sought, particularly in young patients with chest pain.

Investigations
Bedside investigations
- ECG: reviewed by doctor within 5 minutes of arrival, interpretation written and initialled.
- Glucose: tight glucose control is important in ACS.

Laboratory investigations
- FBC, U+E.
- Troponin I: baseline and 8–12 hours from onset of pain.
- D-dimer: only if low-risk patient (Chapters 2 and 35).

Imaging
- Erect chest X-ray, preferably PA; AP magnifies the mediastinum.
- CT (300 CXR) with contrast can detect PE, AD and MI. Perfusion (Q) scan (70 CXR) can be used to detect PE in patients with normal chest X-ray.
- Ultrasound confirming DVT supports a diagnosis of PE.

Treatment
Patients should be triaged to an area with full monitoring and nursing care.

MONA is a useful acronym.

Oxygen should be given to keep the saturation above 96%, together with *Aspirin* to chew in all patients who might have ACS.

Oxygen and *Nitrates* may relieve the pain associated with ACS, but if not, intravenous *Morphine* should be given, titrated to pain.

Acute coronary syndromes
ACS is a useful umbrella term reflecting the common symptoms resulting from coronary artery occlusion due to atherosclerotic plaque.

ST elevation myocardial infarction (STEMI)
This term covers the 'traditional' MI: patients with chest pain of more than 20 minutes and *ST elevation >1 mm in two or more contiguous leads*, EXCEPT chest leads V_2 and V_3 where ST elevation must be >1.5 mm (female) or >2 mm (male). Contiguous in this sense means from the same angle e.g. II, III and aV_F or V_4, V_5, aV_L.

Aspirin gives a similar level of benefit to thrombolysis with a fraction of the risk or cost. If nothing else, give aspirin to chew. Other drugs that may be used in ACS include glycoprotein IIb/IIIa blockers, low molecular weight heparin, beta blockers, statins and ACE inhibitors.

Primary percutaneous coronary intervention (PPCI) Opening the coronary artery using a balloon, then holding it open using a stent is the optimum treatment for STEMI treatment if it can be performed within 2 hours of patient presentation.

Thrombolysis Dissolves blood clot using drugs. It is used in situations where PPCI is not immediately available. There is a 1% risk of catastrophic, e.g. cerebral bleeding.

Non-STEMI/unstable angina (UA)
Some patients have myocardial infarction without ST elevation (non-STEMI) or UA, ischaemic chest pain at rest with ST depression. These patients must be distinguished from those who have had a recent MI, as the troponin remains raised for up to 14 days. Immediate PPCI/thrombolysis do not give the same benefit in NSTEMI/UA as in STEMI, therefore treatment is to stabilise and investigate.

The TIMI score (opposite) assists with risk stratification of these patients according to local protocol, e.g.
- Patients with TIMI >2 should be admitted and have an exercise test or other investigation if the troponin 9–12 hours after pain is negative.
- Patients with TIMI ≤2 can be observed in the ED and sent home if the troponin is negative at 6–9 hours with outpatient clinic follow-up.

The GRACE score is a more complicated alternative to TIMI scoring, but does not appear to be significantly superior in the Emergency Department setting.

Pericarditis
Pericarditis is inflammation of the pericardium, usually caused by a viral infection, renal failure or post-MI/cardiac surgery. Pericarditis typically causes a sharp pain over the left chest, worse when lying flat, but relieved when sitting forward.

A high-pitched scratchy 'sandpaper' rub can often be heard on examination. The ECG may show saddle-shaped ST elevation, which must be differentiated from STEMI.

Pericarditis usually responds well to NSAIDs, but in cases where there is doubt, or evidence of complication, e.g. pericardial effusion or high jugular venous pressure (JVP), an echocardiogram should be performed.

Aortic dissection
A defect in the elastic middle layer of the aortic wall allows blood to flow in, progressively stripping apart the layers. Old age, hypertension and connective tissue disorders such as Marfan's syndrome predispose to dissection. Dissection may involve branches off the aorta, presenting as stroke or MI (usually inferior) and with a diverse range symptoms (see opposite).

Most (90%) patients describe a severe 'tearing' pain radiating to the back between the scapulae. The blood pressure may differ between arms and legs. The chest X-ray may show a wide mediastinum, but a normal chest X-ray does not rule out dissection, nor can a transthoracic echocardiogram. The definitive investigation is CT with contrast.

Careful control of blood pressure prevents extension: labetalol ± vasodilators are used to achieve a systolic BP <120 mmHg. Type A dissection needs surgery or endovascular stenting; type B is usually managed with blood pressure control only.

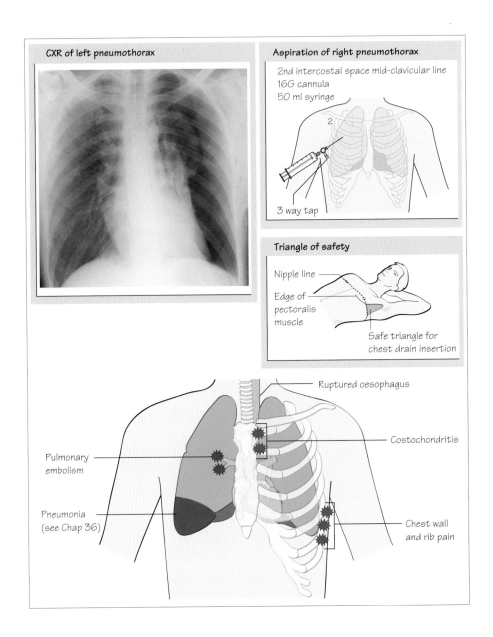

CXR of left pneumothorax

Aspiration of right pneumothorax

2nd intercostal space mid-clavicular line
16G cannula
50 ml syringe

3 way tap

Triangle of safety

Nipple line

Edge of pectoralis muscle

Safe triangle for chest drain insertion

Ruptured oesophagus

Costochondritis

Pulmonary embolism

Pneumonia (see Chap 36)

Chest wall and rib pain

This chapter concentrates on non-cardiovascular causes of chest pain, but there is inevitable overlap with the previous and subsequent chapters, particularly in the history and examination.

History

Non-cardiovascular chest pain is usually caused by inflammation of the soft tissues, which give a sharp or stabbing pain, often described as 'pleuritic' pain. A SOCRATES (Chapter 34) pain history may give pointers to possible causes.

• Pulmonary embolism: shock, syncope, sudden-onset SOB, previous deep vein thrombosis/pulmonary embolism (DVT/PE), malignancy, immobility, haemoptysis.
• Pneumothorax: past history of same or asthma/ chronic obstructive pulmonary disease (COPD), breathlessness.
• Chest infections: cough, sputum, breathlessness and fever (Chapter 36).

• Pericarditis: central sharp pain, recent viral infection, pain worse supine and relieved by sitting or leaning forward (Chapter 34).
• Costochondritis: following viral upper respiratory tract infection.
• Cracked rib: if trauma.
• Vomiting: ruptured oesophagus.

Examination

Tenderness over the chest wall, and reproduction of the *same pain* on palpation, suggests costochondritis or a fractured rib, but does not rule out any of the other, more serious causes of chest pain.

The legs should be checked for calf pain, oedema, swelling and prominent veins that may indicate a deep vein thrombosis. The abdomen should be palpated to look for conditions that could cause pain in the chest, e.g. epigastric pain, liver or gall bladder disease.

Investigations

Bedside investigations
- ECG.

Laboratory investigations
- FBC, U+E.
- D-dimer only if PE suspected *and* low risk.

Imaging
- Chest X-ray (erect, PA).

Common conditions

Pulmonary embolus and deep vein thrombosis

Pulmonary embolism is a notoriously difficult diagnosis due to a wide spectrum of presentations, from the moribund patient with a large 'saddle' embolus occluding their pulmonary arteries to the COPD patient with mild pain and breathlessness. The same is true with DVT: physical signs are inconsistent and overlap with normal findings.

Investigations for PE/DVT are similarly ambiguous; there is no simple, cheap test capable of accurately ruling out PE or DVT in *any* patient. The use of a d-dimer test is discussed in Chapter 2, but *should only be used in low-probability patients.* To complicate things further, there are different d-dimer tests, ELISA (enzyme-linked immunosorbent assay) being the most sensitive.

Wells score for PE	
Clinical signs of DVT	3
PE most likely diagnosis	3
Heart rate >100 bpm	1.5
Immobilisation or surgery <4/52	1.5
Previous definite PE/DVT	1.5
Haemoptysis	1
Active cancer	1
Score <2 = 3% chance of PE (low)	
Score 2–6 = 20% chance of PE (mod)	
Score >6 = 50% chance of PE (high)	
Alternative cutoff	
Score ≤4 = PE unlikely	
Score >4 = PE likely	

Wells score for DVT	
Active cancer	1
Paralysis, paresis or plaster	1
Immobilisation or surgery <4/52	1
Tenderness over deep veins	1
Entire leg swollen	1
Calf swelling >3 cm difference	1
Pitting oedema	1
Collateral superficial veins	1
DVT not most likely diagnosis	−2
Score ≤0 = 3% chance of DVT (low)	
Score 1–2 = 25% chance of DVT (mod)	
Score >2 = 75% chance of DVT (high)	

In the case of a patient with a moderate to high pre-test probability, definitive imaging needs to be performed to prove or disprove the diagnosis. In the case of PE this is CTPA (300 CXR) or Q (perfusion) scan (70 CXR) ± ventilation scan (70 CXR). For DVT an ultrasound is the usual choice. The main value of the CXR is in excluding other causes of chest pain/SOB.

Features that are positive in PE	%
Respiratory rate >16 breaths/minute	92
↑ A-a gradient (Chapter 7)	90
Breathlessness	85
Tachycardia >100/minute	80
Sharp chest pain	75
Fever >37.8°C	45
Haemoptysis	30
Dull chest pain	15
$S_I Q_{III} T_{III}$	10

Treatment of DVT/PE is by anticoagulation; thrombolysis is sometimes used in severe cases but is controversial. If there is high probability of PE/DVT or significant delay before investigation, anticoagulation should be started before investigation. Many patients with uncomplicated DVT/PE are now investigated and treated as outpatients.

Pneumothorax (spontaneous)

Pneumothorax is air in the pleural space, between the lung and the chest wall. Primary pneumothorax occurs in individuals without other chest pathology: risk factors are smoking, being thin and male. Secondary pneumothorax may occur due to trauma (e.g. rib fractures) or lung pathology (e.g. bullae, COPD). Breathlessness and chest pain are common symptoms.

Treatment is guided by the type, size and symptoms of the pneumothorax seen on chest X-ray. Patients with uncomplicated pneumothorax <2 cm (≈50% hemithorax volume) can be discharged with outpatient review, and instructions to return if ↑SOB. Patients with a larger pneumothorax should have a maximum of two attempts at aspiration through the second intercostal space in the mid clavicular line.

In secondary pneumothorax, symptomatic patients, patients >50 years and those with a complete pneumothorax are likely to need a chest drain. Small-diameter chest drains (10–14 Fr) are used for pneumothorax, as they are less traumatic, using Seldinger technique.

Costochondritis, chest wall pain and fractured rib

Inflammation of the costochondral cartilages at the edge of the sternum produces sharp pain when the ribs move with breathing. This inflammation often occurs after a viral upper respiratory tract infection. A similar sharp pain may be caused by a rib fracture. If there is no evidence of any more significant problem, treat with NSAIDs.

Diagnosis not to miss

Ruptured oesophagus

This is a rare consequence of severe vomiting or straining. Pain is a consistent finding and there may be dysphagia, haematemesis, subcutaneous emphysema and pneumothorax. Diagnosis is by a combination of chest X-ray, contrast swallow and CT. Management includes resuscitation, antibiotics and urgent surgical review.

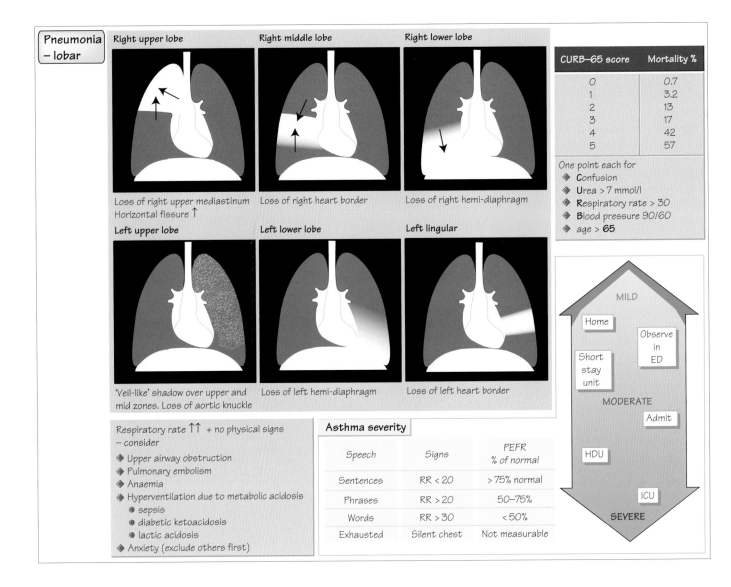

Pneumonia – lobar			

Right upper lobe
Loss of right upper mediastinum
Horizontal fissure ↑

Right middle lobe
Loss of right heart border

Right lower lobe
Loss of right hemi-diaphragm

Left upper lobe
'Veil-like' shadow over upper and mid zones. Loss of aortic knuckle

Left lower lobe
Loss of left hemi-diaphragm

Left lingular
Loss of left heart border

CURB–65 score	Mortality %
0	0.7
1	3.2
2	13
3	17
4	42
5	57

One point each for
- Confusion
- Urea > 7 mmol/l
- Respiratory rate > 30
- Blood pressure 90/60
- age > 65

MILD — Home — Observe in ED — Short stay unit — MODERATE — Admit — HDU — ICU — SEVERE

Respiratory rate ↑↑ + no physical signs – consider
- Upper airway obstruction
- Pulmonary embolism
- Anaemia
- Hyperventilation due to metabolic acidosis
  - sepsis
  - diabetic ketoacidosis
  - lactic acidosis
- Anxiety (exclude others first)

Asthma severity

Speech	Signs	PEFR % of normal
Sentences	RR < 20	> 75% normal
Phrases	RR > 20	50–75%
Words	RR > 30	< 50%
Exhausted	Silent chest	Not measurable

History

Feeling 'short of breath' (SoB) generally indicates a problem with the lungs; however, it can also be a feature of cardiac disease, metabolic disturbance, anaemia and anxiety. Exacerbating or relieving factors such as exercise/position or timing (at night/early morning) are helpful.

Abrupt onset of SoB associated with sharp chest pain suggests pneumothorax, or pulmonary embolism (PE; Chapter 35). Dull chest pain and SoB implies a cardiac cause (Chapter 34).

Examination

Assess 'work of breathing', and vital signs: temperature, BP, heart rate, respiratory rate and accessory muscle use. Inability to talk, exhaustion, cyanosis and bradycardia are preterminal signs. Specific findings that should be sought include:

- *Wheeze*: a musical noise usually heard *in expiration*, due to partial obstruction of small airways. This may be caused by bronchospasm (asthma), loss of lung elasticity causing collapse (chronic obstructive pulmonary disease; COPD) or obstruction by mucus or fluid. Fluid in the terminal bronchioles (pulmonary oedema) may cause 'cardiac asthma', due to left-sided heart failure. Wheeze audible only over one part of the lung suggests bronchial obstruction, e.g. foreign body or compression – malignancy.
- *Crackles*: crackles are caused by airway opening, so are generally *inspiratory*. Coarse crackles ⇒ fluid (pulmonary oedema), or infection in small airways. Fine crackles are heard in chronic lung diseases.
- *Stridor*: a whistling noise worse *on inspiration*, due to partial upper airway obstruction.
- *Sputum*: increased production of sputum and green colour suggest infectious illness. Pink, frothy sputum occurs in pulmo-

nary oedema. Blood-stained sputum (haemoptysis) is usually due to infections (80%), but may also occur in lung cancer or PE.

- *Reduced air entry* and chest wall movement with:
  - percussion note dull, ↑ breath sounds ⇒ consolidation;
  - percussion note dull, no breath sounds ⇒ pleural effusion;
  - percussion note hyperresonant, ↓ breath sounds ⇒ pneumothorax.

Investigations

Investigations are determined by symptoms – mild asthma exacerbations do not require investigations other than peak expiratory flow (PEF). Arterial blood gases (ABGs) are painful and should be limited to patients in whom they are likely to influence management, e.g. O_2 saturation <92%.

Bedside investigations

- Peak expiratory flow meter for all patients with asthma/COPD (pre- and post-bronchodilator).
- Urine for *Legionella* or streptococcal urinary antigen.
- Blood glucose, ECG.

Laboratory investigations

- FBC, U+E.
- ABGs (Chapter 7).
- Blood cultures and atypical pneumonia serology indicated only in patients with severe pneumonia.

Imaging

- Chest X-ray – rarely needed in straightforward asthma.
- CT is very good for imaging lungs and CT pulmonary angiography (CTPA) (300 CXR) is the imaging of choice for possible PE, although a Q (perfusion) scan (70 CXR) can be used in patients without lung pathology who have a normal chest X-ray.

Management

Check airway, give oxygen. If the patient has type II respiratory failure (e.g. from COPD) and is on long-term oxygen, give oxygen to achieve a saturation of approximately 91%.

Pneumonia

A patient with fever, cough and pleuritic chest pain has pneumonia until proven otherwise. In community-acquired pneumonia (CAP), the clinical or X-ray features do not accurately predict the organism responsible.

The CURB-65 scoring tool is helpful to predict the need for admission/intensive treatment, but must be moderated by the patient's social circumstances and general condition. For a stable patient with CAP and a CURB-65 score of 0 who does not need to be admitted, amoxicillin is usually the first-choice antibiotic. For more serious or complex infections such hospital-acquired pneumonia, immunosuppression, cancer, HIV, and high-risk groups (travellers, intravenous drug users), consult local antibiotic guidelines that reflect local patterns of disease and organism sensitivity.

Asthma and chronic obstructive pulmonary disease

Asthma can be unpredictable: ensure early senior assessment in ill patients. The main danger for both asthma and COPD patients is *tiredness*, which results in a vicious cycle of raised PCO_2, exhaustion and hypoventilation. In addition a few asthmatics may have extreme *tightness*, where tight bronchoconstriction makes it very difficult to move any air in and out of the alveoli – the 'silent chest'.

Treatment is guided by regular PEF measurements: the mainstay is *oxygen* and β_2 *agonist bronchodilators* (e.g. salbutamol, 5 mg) delivered by oxygen-driven nebuliser or metered dose inhaler (MDI) and spacer. In severe cases, the nebulisers are given continuously. Intravenous β_2 agonists are rarely necessary as adequate drug delivery is usually possible with nebulisers.

- *Steroids* are given to reduce inflammation in the small airways. Intravenous hydrocortisone 100 mg should be used in unwell patients, but milder cases may have oral prednisolone 50 mg. Antibiotics are not indicated unless there is evidence of infection.
- *Anticholinergics* (e.g. nebulised ipratropium bromide) are used in more severe cases of asthma and all cases of COPD, but only need to be given once every 4 hours.
- *Magnesium sulphate* and *aminophylline* are second-line drugs used for severe asthma, but use is controversial.
- *Non-invasive ventilation* (NIV) is used in both COPD and asthma to reduce the work of breathing, and to try to avoid intubation. *Intubation and ventilation* is sometimes necessary if the patient is tired and their PCO_2 is rising.

Most COPD patients who arrive at the Emergency Department will require admission to hospital. Asthmatics who revert to a PEF >75% normal after having three nebulisers over an hour and a dose of steroids over 1 hour, can usually be discharged. Patients being discharged from the Emergency Department should have:

- A written asthma plan.
- 3–5 days of oral prednisolone 30–50 mg.
- An agreed review, e.g. GP or outpatient clinic.
- Inhaler technique check.

Acute pulmonary oedema

These patients often present in the early morning with extreme SoB, crackles and sometimes wheeze – 'cardiac asthma'. The underlying problem is acute left ventricular failure, usually due to myocardial ischaemia/infarction which pushes the patient to the 'wrong' side of the Frank-Starling curve. Treatment is oxygen, aspirin and reducing cardiac preload using nitrates, continuous positive airway pressure (CPAP) and angiotensin-converting enzyme (ACE) inhibitors in the short term and loop diuretics, e.g. furosemide, in the medium term.

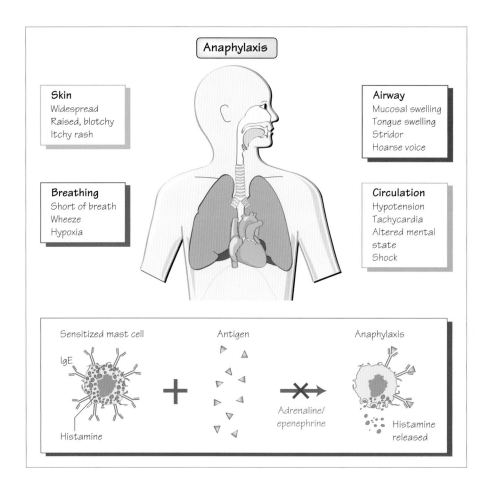

Anaphylaxis is a severe, life-threatening systemic IgE-mediated hypersensitivity reaction. Anaphylaxis causes compromise of airway, breathing and circulation, together with a characteristic itchy skin rash. Deaths occur because of late treatment or under-treatment. Adrenaline as an intramuscular injection is very safe as the localised vasoconstriction it provokes effectively makes it slow release.

The short time course of anaphylaxis means the stimulus is usually known. Ask about a history of atopy, and specific triggers (e.g. stings, nuts, food) and medications (e.g. antibiotics, anaesthetic agents, NSAIDs and angiotensin-converting enzyme (ACE) inhibitors) and contrast media.

WARNING

Don't be afraid of adrenaline/epinephrine

Airway

Visible swelling of upper airway (tongue and throat), stridor and hoarseness are very worrying signs.

In upper airway obstruction, oxygen saturations are meaningless – do not be reassured by a normal saturation.

Give adrenaline 500 micrograms i.m. immediately and get senior help urgently.

Give high-flow oxygen via a reservoir mask.

Breathing

Shortness of breath, wheeze, respiratory rate, use of accessory muscles of breathing may progresses to fatigue, hypoxia/cyanosis and respiratory arrest.

Give adrenaline 500 micrograms i.m. immediately (if not already done) and get senior help.

Circulation

Massive vasodilatation leads to anaphylactic shock and circulatory collapse.

Give adrenaline 500 micrograms i.m. immediately (if not already done) and get senior help.

Disability

Shock may result in altered conscious state.

Exposure

Remove the antigen if possible, e.g. wasp sting.

There is usually a widespread red rash, which is itchy (urticaria), and there may be angioeodema (deep tissue swelling).

Why give adrenaline?

Anaphylaxis is caused by mast cells releasing histamine in response to IgE-mediated stimulus. Adrenaline stabilises the mast cells, preventing further histamine release. It also has other beneficial effects:
- Beta-2 agonist in lungs, counteracting bronchospasm.
- Counteracts vasodilation.

By giving the injection intramuscularly, the local vasoconstriction it provokes means the adrenaline is released slowly, avoiding tachycardia and hypertension. If ongoing symptoms persist after 5 minutes, repeat the dose of intramuscular adrenaline.

If symptoms persist despite the repeat dose of adrenaline, or the patient is very unwell with incipient airway obstruction, a senior doctor may consider using bolus doses of 50–100 μg of adrenaline (= 0.5–1 mL of the 1:10000 premixed resuscitation syringes) with a flush. This may make the patient feel unwell and have a tachycardia, but usually rapidly resolves the symptoms.

Secondary drugs for anaphylaxis

Corticosteroids

Systemic corticosteroids take at least 30 minutes to have an effect, even when given intravenously, but they may be helpful in preventing recurrence of reaction – a biphasic reaction.
- Hydrocortisone, 100 mg i.v.
- Prednisolone, 50 mg oral.

Antihistamines (H$_1$ antagonists)

These are second-line agents and *should not be used before adrenaline* to treat anaphylaxis, but may be suitable for treating mild allergy, particularly the itchy urticarial rash. The sedating antihistamines seem more effective in the acute phase:
- Diphenhydramine, 25–50 mg i.v.
- Chlorphenamine, 10–20 mg i.v.

The role of H$_2$ antagonists, such as ranitidine, is controversial; they may have a role as an additional treatment to H$_1$ antagonists in severe anaphylaxis.

Anaphylaxis mimics

ACE inhibitors are responsible for anaphylactoid facial swelling, which occurs without any obvious precipitant, but is differentiated from anaphylaxis by absence of rash. It is probably caused by bradykinin build-up as swapping to an angiotensin II blocker (-sartan) prevents further episodes.

Scrombotoxin poisoning is seen when people eat fish, particularly tuna, that is past its prime. The scrombotoxin has a histamine-like effect, giving a red itchy rash, but no systemic upset. Notify public health officials. Treatment is supportive.

Morphine causes direct histamine release but without systemic upset, and this does not represent allergy.

Other diagnoses that can be confused with anaphylaxis include vasovagal syncope, syndromes associated with flushing (e.g. carcinoid), panic attacks, angioedema and other causes of shock.

Investigations

Investigations should not delay the resuscitation.

Bedside investigations
- Blood glucose, ECG

Laboratory invstigations
- FBC, U+E, ABGs if indicated
- Mast cell tryptase levels
  - useful if the diagnosis is in doubt;
  - one initial sample (minimum) with optional samples at 2 and 24 hours.

Management

Patients with an anaphylactic reaction should be observed for 4–6 hours as there is a risk of recurrence of symptoms – 'rebound' phenomenon. Review by a senior clinician determines need for further treatment or a longer period of observation, e.g.
- Patients with a previous history of biphasic reactions or reactions with the possibility of continuing absorption of allergen;
- Severe reactions with no apparent cause;
- Reactions in patients with severe asthma;
- Patients presenting in the evening or at night, or those who may not be able to respond to any deterioration.

Disposal: who can go home?

Discharge a patient who has anaphylactic reaction only once the patient is stable and:
- has been reviewed by a senior clinician;
- has been given education and clear written instructions to avoid allergen, and return to hospital if symptoms return;
- has been given 3 days of antihistamines and oral steroids
- has been considered for an adrenaline auto-injector (Epi-pen®);
- has a plan for follow-up, including referral to allergy specialist, and contact with the patient's GP;
- alert has been noted in patient's medical record (written/electronic).

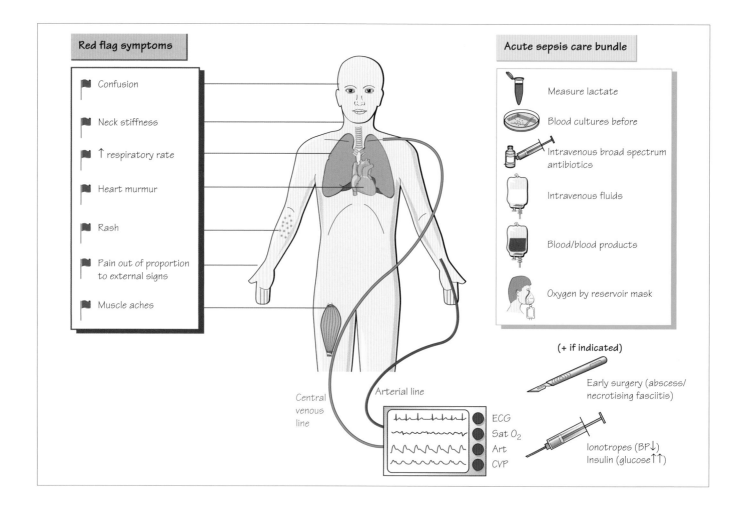

Red flag symptoms

- ⚑ Confusion
- ⚑ Neck stiffness
- ⚑ ↑ respiratory rate
- ⚑ Heart murmur
- ⚑ Rash
- ⚑ Pain out of proportion to external signs
- ⚑ Muscle aches

Acute sepsis care bundle

- Measure lactate
- Blood cultures before
- Intravenous broad spectrum antibiotics
- Intravenous fluids
- Blood/blood products
- Oxygen by reservoir mask

(+ if indicated)

- Early surgery (abscess/necrotising fasciitis)
- Ionotropes (BP↓)
  Insulin (glucose↑↑)

Central venous line   Arterial line

ECG
Sat O₂
Art
CVP

Patients with fever and infections are a very common problem in the Emergency Department. Amongst the many straightforward cases of viral or bacterial infection are small numbers of patients with life-threatening sepsis: this chapter concentrates on the more severe end of the spectrum.

There is very good evidence of the importance of early diagnosis and aggressive resuscitation of patients with severe sepsis. Intensive resuscitation with invasive monitoring and vasoactive drug support must start in the Emergency Department if the patient is to have the best chance of survival.

Uncomplicated sepsis
Infection with no evidence of systemic effects

Severe sepsis (mortality 30%)
Infection + sepsis-induced hypoperfusion/organ failure

Septic shock (mortality 50%)
Infection + systolic blood pressure <90 mmHg despite adequate fluid resuscitation

---

History

There are many non-specific features such as fever, vomiting, muscle aches and pains, headache and malaise that are present in both viral infections and systemic sepsis.

Specific features are localising symptoms that suggest a focus for the infection, e.g. dysuria, cough and production of green sputum. Rigors (like shivering) and high fever >38°C make bacteraemia more likely.

Ask about immunisation, comorbidities, e.g. diabetes, heart/liver/renal failure, medications esp. immunosuppressants, drug use and contact with sick people or travel in the last 6 months.

Examination

From the end of the bed:
- Is the patient well/ill/critically ill?
- Is the patient in an appropriately monitored area?
- Does the patient have oxygen?

Localising signs
- Upper respiratory tract infection (URTI): pharyngitis, tonsillitis, otitis media, sinusitis (Chapter 21).

- Lower respiratory tract infection (LRTI/pneumonia): the commonest cause of septic shock (Chapter 36).
- UTI/pyelonephritis: Gram-negative septicaemia a common cause of septic shock (Chapter 20).
- Gastroenteritis (Chapter 40).
- Meningitis: the classic signs are reduced state of consciousness, neck stiffness, headache, vomiting, photophobia together with a high fever. The non-blanching, re/dark purple vasculitic rash is only caused by meningococcal sepsis/meningitis. Neck stiffness may be absent in 30% of cases.

Investigations
Bedside investigations
- Blood glucose, urine test, βhCG.

Laboratory investigations
- FBC, U+E, LFTs, arterial blood gas (ABG).
- Lactate level: lactate results from anaerobic metabolism, and is a useful marker of the severity of tissue hypoperfusion.
- C-reactive protein (CRP), according to local protocol.
- Clotting screen/Group and Save.
- Blood cultures if severe sepsis/septic shock/neutropenic/immunosuppressed or suspected endocarditis.
- Urine culture, pneumococcal and *Legionella* antigen.
- Lumbar puncture/meningococcus PCR if indicated.

Imaging
- Chest X-ray.
- CT head: if meningitis suspected, treat first.

Management
Oxygen, broad-spectrum antibiotics and intravenous fluids are the mainstays of treatment. Time to antibiotics is crucial – they should never be delayed, e.g. waiting for CT or LP. The notion of a 'bundle' of care is often used, which is a set of goals to achieve within that point of the patient pathway (opposite). For severe or transmissible infectious diseases such as meningitis, the diagnosing doctor has a duty to notify the health authorities to trace contacts and ensure prevention of further cases.

Disposal: who can go home?
Patients who appear well, in whom serious infection has been excluded, and who can tolerate oral fluids and medication are usually safe to discharge. Patients need a letter to their GP, with specific mention of tests that need follow-up, e.g. cultures.

Common diagnoses
Cellulitis
Cellulitis is a bacterial infection (usually *Staphylococcus* and/or *Streptococcus*) of the skin and subcutaneous tissues resulting in pain, erythema, swelling and warmth. Patients with underlying diseases such as venous stasis, peripheral vascular disease or diabetes are particularly vulnerable. Minor skin wounds or intravenous cannula sites allow organisms to enter the skin.

Mild cellulitis is treated with oral flucloxacillin or a first-generation cephalosporin. Monitoring is helped by drawing a line around the red area, so it is obvious if the cellulitis is increasing. Admission and intravenous treatment is necessary for more severe cases and those with underlying diseases.

Diagnoses not to miss
Severe sepsis and meningitis
In uncomplicated sepsis and meningitis, there is narrow window of opportunity to catch the disease *before* the patient becomes critically unwell with severe sepsis. Rapid disease progression means that antibiotics (e.g. ceftriaxone 2 g i.v.) must be given as soon as the disease is suspected, together with the other parts of the 'care bundle'.

> rash + unwell = meningococcal septicaemia
> meningococcal septicaemia + meningitis =
>   meningococcal meningitis

If there is meningitis without rash, give dexamethasone with the first dose of antibiotics and also consider encephalitis.

Public health officials should be notified.

Immunocompromised patients
Sepsis occurring in an immunocompromised patient is life-threatening. Neutropenia (<1/mm^3) usually occurs approximately 10 days after chemotherapy. Other immunocompromised patients include: haematological malignancy, HIV/AIDS, and those on immunosuppressive medication, e.g. tacrolimus, methotrexate, ciclosporin, prednisolone.

These patients need urgent high-dose broad-spectrum antibiotics and admission. Patients on steroids cannot produce extra endogenous steroids as part of the stress response; therefore extra exogenous steroids must be given.

Travellers
Consider malaria, typhoid fever, dengue fever, hepatitis and sexually transmitted diseases such as HIV or gonorrhoea. Patterns of disease change faster than books are written, so consult an infectious disease physician.

Toxic shock syndrome
A widespread red rash together with features of septic shock, caused by an exotoxin from staphylococcal/streptococcal infection in a (forgotten) vaginal tampon.

Infective endocarditis
Presenting with an insidious combination of fever, malaise, night sweats, heart murmur and embolic phenomena, there is usually a history of valvular heart disease or intravenous drug use.

Necrotising fasciitis and gas gangrene
These severe soft tissue infections should be considered if there is fever together with pain ± gas in soft tissues that is out of all proportion to the clinical appearance. Early antibiotics, together with rapid aggressive surgical debridement, are necessary.

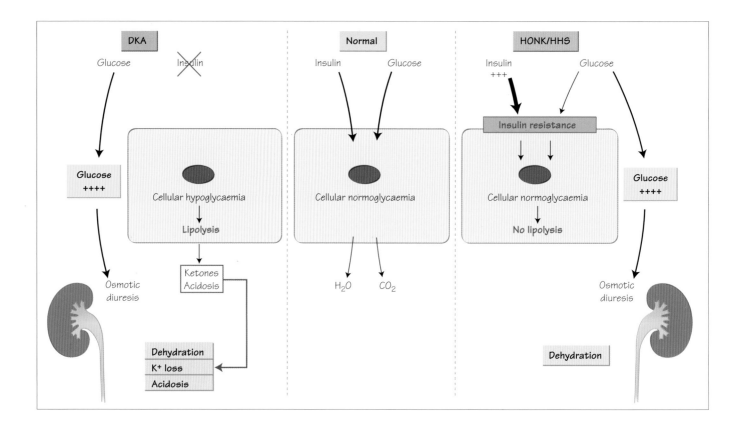

Diabetes

Diabetic emergencies result from either lack of (diabetes mellitus (DM) type 1) or resistance to (DM type 2) insulin and the treatments for these conditions. Young adults with diabetes often go through a period of suboptimal control: treatment of acute problems of this difficult chronic disease should be sympathetic and collaborative.

What sort of diabetes/control does this patient have?

As patients with DM(2) are sometimes treated with insulin, confusion can occur; these rules of thumb may help.
• If the patient has a high body mass index, they probably have DM(2).
• A patient with DM(1) and good diabetic control will have four or more injections of insulin per day, will know their HbA_{1c} (which will be low), and will be prone to hypoglycaemia.
• A patient with DM(1) and poor diabetic control will have one or two injections of insulin per day, may not know their HbA_{1c} and will be prone to diabetic ketoacidosis (DKA).

History

The history should cover the type of diabetes, its history and complications, i.e. atherosclerotic (MI/CVA), neurological (peripheral neuropathy/retinopathy), renal.

Why has the patient attended now? What are the stressors/factors that have caused the disease to decompensate? For example, infections/illness/psychological.

Examination

Look for diseases that may have triggered a loss of diabetic control, e.g. UTI, pneumonia.

In people with long-standing diabetes, absence of pain does not mean absence of disease: neuropathy can mask significant disease. Myocardial infarction or abdominal conditions such as infection or pancreatitis may be painless. The feet are particularly vulnerable – look at the soles for evidence of neuropathy, ulceration or infection, and consider osteomyelitis.

Investigations
Bedside investigations

• Blood glucose: treat hypoglycaemia as below. Hyperglycaemia readings above 20 mmol/L are inaccurate, and not useful in guiding treatment.
• ECG: myocardial infarction (MI) may occur in patients less than 30 years old with poorly controlled diabetes.
• Urine or blood should be checked for ketones.
• pH measurement: a venous pH is adequate in all but the most sick patients and avoids painful arterial puncture.

Laboratory investigations
- FBC, U+E, BG/VBG, clotting.
- Pseudo-hyponatraemia may occur in patients with very high levels of glucose, due to the method of measurement.
- Serum osmolality if hyperosmolar non-ketotic acidosis/hyperosmolar hyperglycaemic state (HONK/HHS) suspected.

Imaging
- Chest X-ray in all HONK/HHS or severe DKA.

Common diagnoses

Hypoglycaemia (glucose < 3 mmol/L)
Hypoglycaemia occurs as a result of too much insulin, too much exercise, too little carbohydrate or a combination of these. Most patients recognise the symptoms of hypoglycaemia, and self-treat with oral glucose, followed by complex carbohydrates. Untreated, they become confused and eventually comatose. A bedside blood glucose check is essential for all such patients, whether they are known to have diabetes or not.

Treatment
Treatment of hypoglycaemia in the Emergency Department is 50 mL of glucose 50% if i.v. access is available, 1 mg glucagon i.m. if not. If there is recurrent hypoglycaemia, an infusion of glucose 10% is necessary. Patients with hypoglycaemia due to long-acting preparations of insulin or oral hypoglycaemics should be admitted.

Diabetic ketoacidosis
The majority of DKA episodes occurs in patients with known diabetes, but new diagnoses are made on the history of polyuria, polydipsia, weight loss and dehydration. The rapid sighing deep 'Kussmaul' breathing serves to remove CO_2 – respiratory compensation for the metabolic acidosis.

To diagnose DKA requires diabetes, ketones and acidosis.
- Blood glucose >11 mmol/L
- Ketones in urine or blood
- pH <7.30 (venous blood)

The pH correlates the severity of DKA – the most severe being pH <7.10. In addition to diagnosing DKA, it is important to search for a cause, which is often omission of insulin or illness.

Treatment principles
DKA occurs because glucose cannot enter cells without insulin. Without glucose, cells switch to metabolising fat, producing organic acids. High blood glucose forces osmotic diuresis, resulting in electrolyte loss and dehydration. Treatment aims to replace the massive fluid and electrolyte loss, and allow the body to normalise the pH. Treatment protocols vary but common features are:

- *Resuscitation phase*: 30 mL/kg, i.e. about 2 litres of i.v. normal saline, given over 1 hour. Soluble insulin is started at 6 units/hour using an infusion pump.
- *Rehydration phase*: gradual rehydration avoids rapid intracellular osmotic/sodium shifts that may cause (fatal) CNS oedema or demyelination. As the insulin takes effect, potassium enters the cells with insulin and glucose, and serum potassium drops sharply. Normal saline is continued at a reduced rate, e.g. 250 mL/hour, but with potassium, e.g. 40 mmol/L initially. Regular U+E measurement should take place to monitor the potassium.

Insulin infusion (0.1 units/kg/hour) is continued at a fixed rate until blood ketones are cleared, using an infusion of 10% glucose to prevent hypoglycaemia. If blood ketone measurement is not available, insulin may be given on a sliding scale according to the glucose level. Education about the importance of regular insulin may help prevent further episodes.

Rare diagnoses

Hyperosmolar non-ketotic or hyperosmolar hyperglycaemic state
HONK/HHS occurs in DM(2) patients: insulin resistance allows small amounts of glucose to enter cells. This is enough to prevent lipolysis, so hyperglycaemia occurs, but acidosis does not. Hyperglycaemia results in osmotic diuresis and a hyperosmolar state that develops more slowly than DKA – over days rather than hours, which eventually results in coma.

A patient with HONK/HHS is therefore markedly hyperosmolar (>320 mOsm/kg) and hyperglycaemic (>40 mmol/L), but not acidotic. Rehydration to correct these deficits should be slow, spread over several days, to avoid (fatal) CNS oedema or demyelination. Anticoagulation is necessary to prevent the hyperviscous blood forming clots, and underlying causes (e.g. UTI, pneumonia) should be sought. ICU/HDU care should be considered as mortality is high.

Hypoadrenalism
The most common cause of adrenal suppression is exogenous – pharmacological steroids given for more than 5 days suppress endogenous steroid production. Extra stress (e.g. infection, trauma) will require extra steroid (e.g. hydrocortisone) for the body to respond effectively.

Endogenous hypoadrenalism – Addison's disease – is fortunately very rare, as the features of the classic presentation of slim, hyperpigmented female with hypotension, hyponatraemia, hyperkalaemia and abdominal pain are very inconsistent and easy to overlook in the Emergency Department. Diagnosis is confirmed by the lack of endogenous steroid production when synthetic adrenocorticotrophic hormone (ACTH) is given (short synacthen test).

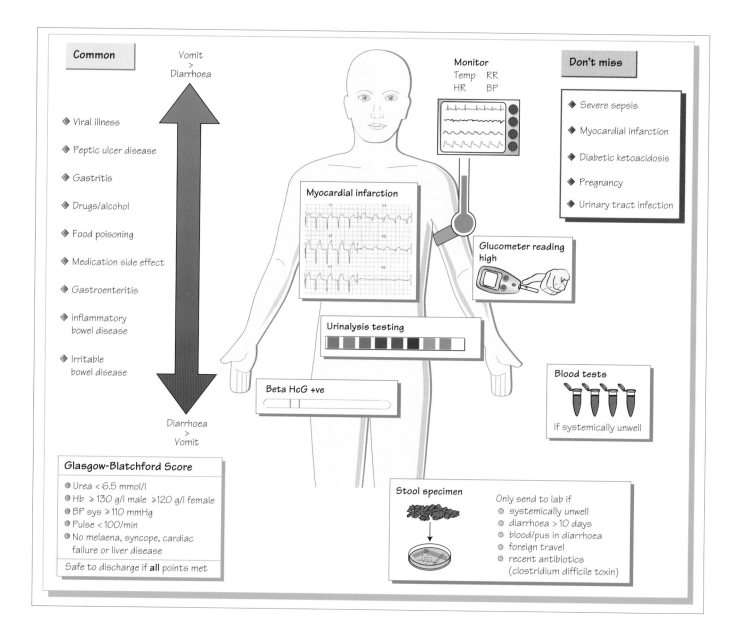

Common

Vomit > Diarrhoea

- Viral illness
- Peptic ulcer disease
- Gastritis
- Drugs/alcohol
- Food poisoning
- Medication side effect
- Gastroenteritis
- inflammatory bowel disease
- Irritable bowel disease

Diarrhoea > Vomit

Monitor

Temp RR
HR   BP

Don't miss

- Severe sepsis
- Myocardial infarction
- Diabetic ketoacidosis
- Pregnancy
- Urinary tract infection

Myocardial infarction

Glucometer reading high

Urinalysis testing

Beta HcG +ve

Blood tests

If systemically unwell

Glasgow-Blatchford Score

- Urea < 6.5 mmol/l
- Hb ⩾ 130 g/l male ⩾120 g/l female
- BP sys ⩾110 mmHg
- Pulse < 100/min
- No melaena, syncope, cardiac failure or liver disease

Safe to discharge if **all** points met

Stool specimen

Only send to lab if
- systemically unwell
- diarrhoea >10 days
- blood/pus in diarrhoea
- foreign travel
- recent antibiotics (clostridium difficile toxin)

History

Vomiting

The amount, frequency and nature of the vomit should be recorded. Heavily bile-stained or faecal vomit implies obstruction. A few streaks of blood in the vomit after repeated vomiting suggests a small ('Mallory-Weiss') tear at the gastro-oesophageal junction, but large amounts of fresh blood in the vomit may indicate bleeding from the oesophagus or stomach. Dark-brown changed blood ('coffee grounds') vomit occurs with stomach or duodenal pathology, e.g. ulcer or gastritis.

Diarrhoea

The amount, frequency and nature of diarrhoea are important. Bleeding from the distal large bowel and anorectal area will be

bright red. More proximal bleeding makes the stools black and shiny with a distinctive smell – melaena, but iron therapy also causes black stools.

Lower gastrointestinal tract bleeding can be caused by some infections, but should always raise suspicion of inflammatory bowel disease or malignancy. Upper gastrointestinal bleeding is a common cause of lower gastrointestinal bleeding.

Other history

Food, travel and medication (including recent antibiotic use) history should be taken. A history of rigors, muscle aches and headache suggests sepsis (Chapter 38). A history of contact with viral gastroenteritis is helpful but does not rule out other causes. Alcohol history is important, particularly when liver disease is suspected – use the CAGE score (Chapter 29). Abdominal pain may be a feature of infectious diarrhoea and inflammatory bowel disease, but if pain is the predominant symptom see Chapter 19.

Examination

Inspection
Look for shock: tachycardia, hypotension, cool peripheries – assess level of dehydration. Document presence of jaundice, anaemia (pale conjunctivae) or oedema (low protein state or heart failure)

Palpation and percussion
Look for surgical causes such as peritonitis, appendicitis (Chapter 19). A rectal examination is an essential part of the assessment – stools should be checked for blood using faecal occult blood testing kit. Constipation ± overflow diarrhoea is a common problem in the elderly.

Investigations

Bedside investigations
- Digital rectal examination with testing for faecal blood.
- Blood glucose, urinalysis and ECG.

Laboratory investigations
- FBC, U+E, Group and Save.
- LFTs, amylase.

Imaging
- Abdominal X-ray (60CXR) is rarely helpful unless bowel obstruction is suspected.
- Chest X-ray (erect) will demonstrate gas under the diaphragm if there is a perforation of the bowel.

Management
Resuscitation/oxygen if unwell, observation and monitoring. If bleeding and shock, obtain large-bore intravenous access, notify blood bank and the gastroenterology/surgical team.

Vomiting is treated by treating underlying causes. Metoclopramide or prochlorperazine are first-line treatments. Persistent vomiting may require $5HT_3$ antagonist such as ondansetron.

Treat dehydration with intravenous crystalloid solutions. Potassium replacement is necessary in persistent vomiting, as the kidneys lose K^+ to retain H^+ ions, causing hypokalaemia.

Common diagnoses

Gastritis/oesophagitis/peptic ulcers
Symptoms are 'heartburn', or burning epigastric pain. Risk factors include smoking, alcohol, aspirin and NSAIDs. Treated by antacids/H_2 blockers/proton pump inhibitors (PPI). Follow-up should be arranged to detect *H. pylori*, which can be treated with antibiotics. For ruptured peptic ulcer see Chapter 19.

Mallory-Weiss tear
A small tear at the gastro-oesophageal junction resulting from vomiting, producing blood streaks in the vomit. If the Glasgow-Blatchford Score is 0, the patient may be discharged with no follow-up, otherwise admit and observe.

Gastroenteritis
The majority of gastroenteritis is viral in origin, and treatment is supportive only. If the patient is unwell, consider toxin-mediated (e.g. staphylococcal) or invasive disease due to food poisoning (e.g. *E. coli*, *Campylobacter*), travel-related illness (e.g. *Salmonella*, *Shigella*) or inflammatory bowel disease. *Clostridium difficile* infection occurs after broad-spectrum antibiotic use, and produces a toxin detectable in stools.

Patients who are not dehydrated, in whom serious pathology has been excluded, are usually safe to discharge. Educate patients about oral rehydration using small sips of diluted fruit juice or sugar-containing fruit drinks diluted 1:5 with water to make oral rehydration fluid. The elderly and those with heart failure may need admission, but most patients can be safely discharged.

Rectal bleeding (haematochezia)
Localised bleeding in or near the anal canal is commonly caused by anal fissures or haemorrhoids. If the patient is well, they can be reassured in the ED, but patients should have follow-up to exclude more serious causes. Inflammatory bowel disease, diverticulitis and lower GI carcinoma should be considered in patients who are unwell.

Anorectal abscess
More common in patients with inflammatory bowel disease and diabetes, these large abscesses cause poorly localised pain. Keep nil by mouth and refer for surgical drainage.

Constipation, irritable bowel syndrome
Patients who are well but have intermittent abdominal pain, bloating and diarrhoea, often have a diagnosis of irritable bowel syndrome (IBS) or constipation with overflow, but these can only be safely diagnosed once serious pathology has been excluded.

Diagnoses not to miss

Inflammatory bowel disease
Exacerbation of inflammatory bowel disease (ulcerative colitis, Crohn's disease) commonly presents with intermittent bloody diarrhoea and abdominal pain. Weight loss and systemic manifestations such as mouth ulcers, rashes, joint and eye problems may be present. The gastroenterology team must be informed about any patient with inflammatory bowel disease presenting with gastrointestinal symptoms, even if the patient needs surgical care.

Oesophageal varices
Oesophageal varices are caused by portal hypertension, usually secondary to cirrhotic liver disease. Catastrophic bleeding can result, exacerbated by coagulopathy due to lack of (hepatically manufactured) clotting factors and platelet dysfunction. Treatment is by resuscitation and urgent endoscopy.

Lower gastrointestinal tract cancer
Cancer should always be considered in lower gastrointestinal bleeding. While the patient may not need admission, it is important to make sure that these symptoms are followed up.

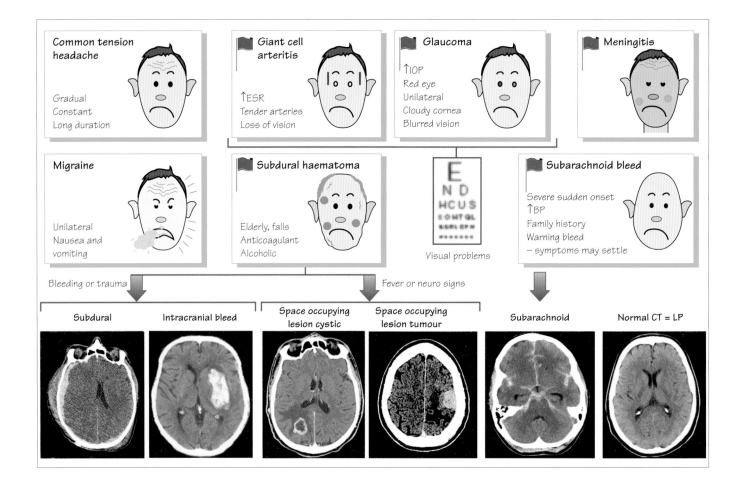

History

Many conditions cause headache – local, systemic and non-organic. As there are usually no clinical findings, the history is everything.

• Is this the first episode, or a recurrent headache? Longstanding headaches are unlikely to be life-threatening.

A unilateral headache is typical of migraine, cluster headaches, or giant cell arteritis. Descriptions such as pressure, tightness, throbbing, are not specific for particular diagnoses. Other associated symptoms that should be sought:

• Focal neurological symptom (migraines, space-occupying lesion).
• Nausea and vomiting (migraine, infections, ↑intracranial pressure; ICP).
• Alcoholism, anticoagulant medication (subdural haematoma).
• History of recent trauma (concussion, subdural haematoma).
• Worse on waking, or on straining/bending over/coughing (↑ICP).
• Fever, photophobia, neck stiffness (meningitis).
• Visual disturbance, (migraine, glaucoma, giant cell arteritis).
• Pain/tenderness on the side of head, jaw claudication (pain on chewing), visual disturbance (giant cell arteritis).

Reduced consciousness, confusion, seizures or focal neurological symptoms suggests a significant problem.

> **WARNING**
>
> Sudden-onset headache = subarachnoid haemorrhage until proven otherwise

The headache of subarachnoid haemorrhage may be described as 'like being hit over the back of the head' and may occur with peaks of blood pressure, e.g. exercise or sexual intercourse.

Examination
Inspection

From the end of the bed – is there evidence of recent trauma, excessive bruising, rash, photophobia, altered state of consciousness or irritability? Assess consciousness state using the Glasgow coma scale (Chapter 10).

Neurological examination

There may be no neurological signs in subarachnoid haemorrhage (SAH). Intracranial space-occupying lesions may result in focal signs; look for upper motor neuron signs – focal weakness with increased tone, reflexes, upgoing plantar reflex.

General examination findings on the basis of the history:
- Fever, look for focus of infection, e.g. ENT.
- Cranial nerve examination.
- Meningism implies inflammation of the meningeal layers covering the brain and spinal cord. Movement of the neck or straight leg raising may cause pain.
- In patients over 50 years, check temporal artery tenderness and intraocular pressure.

Investigations

Bedside investigation
- Blood glucose.

Laboratory investigations
- FBC/CRP/blood cultures if infectious cause.
- INR/clotting if on warfarin or suspected coagulopathy.
- ESR if suspected giant cell arteritis.

Lumbar puncture

Lumbar puncture (LP) must not be performed in drowsy or unconscious patients, due to risk of death from coning ($\uparrow$ICP forces the brain through the foramen magnum, compressing the brainstem). LP must not delay treatment if there is suspicion of meningitis. In possible SAH, LP should be performed at least 12 hours after the onset of headache to allow xanthochromia time to develop. Xanthochromia is the yellow coloration of CSF that occurs when bilirubin leaks from red blood cells, and should be measured quantitatively in the laboratory.

Imaging
- High resolution CT (100 CXR) is sensitive at detecting SAH within 12 hours of onset of pain. MR is good for detecting late-presenting SAH.

Management

Treatment of patients with specific symptoms is discussed below. NSAIDs should not be given to patients with possible intracranial bleeding. Mild dehydration often exacerbates headache: a combination of the following treatments is usually effective.
- *Fluids*: two litres of normal saline.
- *Analgesia*: paracetamol, NSAID, codeine.
- *Anti-emetic*: metoclopramide, prochlorperazine, chlorpromazine.

The combination of chlorpromazine and i.v. fluids seems particularly effective for migraine. Opiate analgesia should be avoided, as there is a high risk of dependence, especially with pethidine (meperidine).

Disposal: who can go home?

Any patient who has severe headache not responding to standard treatments requires admission (10% of patients). Patients who have responded well to treatment, in whom serious pathology has been excluded, are safe to discharge.

Common diagnoses

Tension headache

Very common, multiple possible triggers including psychosocial stressors. Gradual onset of a bilateral/generalised headache, with relatively constant nature over time.

Migraine

Migraines are common, female > male, often with a family history. Many patients will recognise their typical symptoms: unilateral, preceded by nausea and/or visual disturbance ± temporary unilateral numbness. Migrainous neuralgia/cluster headaches are rare, and present with brief (< 30 minutes) episodes of eye, facial or head pain or autonomic symptoms clustered in time.

Diagnoses not to miss

Subarachnoid haemorrhage

Subarachnoid haemorrhage (SAH) may be caused by cerebral aneurysms, arteriovenous (AV) malformations, hypertension or head trauma. SAH may occur at any age but is most common between 40 and 60 years. A large SAH typically presents with acute headache, progressing to coma, and is not difficult to diagnose, but the outlook is often poor.

A small bleed with subtle symptoms is difficult to diagnose, as the history may be the only guide that this may be a warning bleed. Identification and intervention in this group of patients may prevent a catastrophic bleed. If the history is good for a SAH and CT is normal, LP is necessary: MRI or CT angiography can resolve equivocal results.

Meningitis and encephalitis

It can be difficult to distinguish between a viral infection from meningitis or encephalitis, as they may present with a similar picture of fever, headache and neck stiffness (Chapter 38). Immediate empirical antibiotic ± antiviral treatment is vital, followed by lumbar puncture if appropriate.

Subdural haematoma

Elderly and/or alcoholic patients who tend to fall are at risk of chronic subdural haematoma (SDH), especially if there is an increased bleeding risk, e.g. warfarin. Physical examination cannot exclude a subdural haematoma: low threshold for CT is required.

Space-occupying lesion

Patients presenting with a headache and new neurological symptoms need a CT to exclude intracranial pathology, e.g. bleeding, space-occupying lesions (SOL).

Giant cell arteritis

Must be considered in patients >50 years with unilateral headache ± visual disturbance, jaw claudication, tenderness over temporal artery. If ESR$\uparrow$, commence on steroids and refer for temporal artery biopsy.

Glaucoma

Acute glaucoma can present with a unilateral headache, and visual disturbance (Chapter 22).

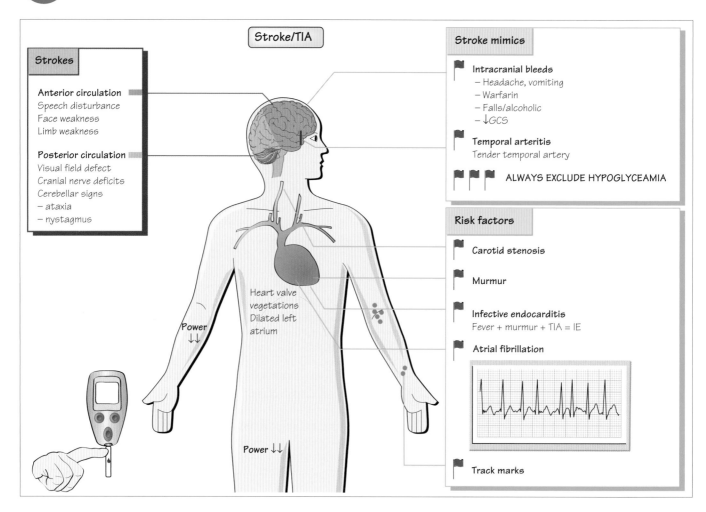

Stroke is a major cause of mortality and chronic disability. The advent of thrombolysis for stroke has prompted campaigns to increase public awareness of stroke symptoms e.g. 'FAST – face, arm, speech, time to call ambulance'. Stroke thrombolysis in carefully selected patients reduces disability in survivors. Strokes can be prevented by identification, investigation and treatment of transient ischaemic attack (TIA) patients at high risk of stroke.

Clinical assessment

The time of onset, type and duration of symptoms is critical to decision-making. Many patients have an indistinct onset of stroke symptoms, e.g. have woken with symptoms, and are therefore ineligible for thrombolysis. History and examination should cover:
• Time of onset.
• Risk factors for atherosclerosis (diabetes, smoking, hypertension, ↑cholesterol, family history).
• Risk factors for embolism, e.g. atrial fibrillation (AF), valvular disease, coagulopathy.
• Contraindications to thrombolysis.
• A brief but thorough neurological examination.
• Consider stroke mimics (see below).

Investigations
Bedside investigations
• Blood glucose.
• ECG.

Laboratory investigations
• FBC, U + E, clotting.

Imaging
• Immediate CT/MR to exclude haemorrhage if inside thrombolysis window. Unconscious patients may need intubation to perform CT safely.
• Chest X-ray.

Stroke

A stroke is defined as a 'focal neurological deficit of cerebrovascular cause that persists beyond 24 hours'.

Stroke subtypes: clinical syndromes
• *Anterior circulation infarction* (40%): limb weakness combined with visual field loss and/or cortical dysfunction (e.g. aphasia/apraxia) suggests a partial (20%) or complete (20%) cortical infarc-

tion. If the dominant hemisphere is affected, aphasia and apraxia are common, whereas involvement of the non-dominant hemisphere gives contralateral hemi-neglect.

• *Lacunar infarction* (30%) of the internal capsule results in motor/sensory loss affecting two or more of face, arm and leg *without* visual or speech disturbance.

• *Posterior circulation infarction* (15%): visual problems and/or cerebellar symptoms (ataxia, nausea/vomiting) and cranial nerve deficits are the hallmark of a posterior infarction, although weakness and sensory deficits may also occur.

• *Haemorrhage* (15%) intracerebral (10%), subarachnoid (5%). Warfarin therapy, early vomiting, severe headache, drowsiness and hypertension are common in these patients.

Stroke mimics

• *Hypoglycaemia* must be excluded on arrival. Hypoglycaemia can give a strikingly similar clinical picture to stroke, is easy to diagnose and treat, and if untreated will result in significant neurological damage.

• *Seizures* may give a transient hemiplegia, 'Todd's palsy'.

• Recent trauma or falls suggest *subdural* haematoma.

• Fever suggests *infection*, e.g. sepsis, meningitis, encephalitis, brain abscess, septic emboli.

• A history of cancer warrants exclusion of brain *metastases* using CT with contrast.

• *Migraine* can give a transient hemiparesis, visual, speech or sensory symptoms.

• *Giant cell arteritis*: suspect if visual disturbance in patients over 50 years old. Check for tender temporal artery, raised ESR (Chapter 22).

• Isolated lower motor neurone facial weakness could be due to *Bell's palsy*. Symmetrical normal forehead movement ('raise your eyebrows') implies an upper rather than a lower motor neurone deficit. Inflammation affecting the facial nerve gives unilateral facial muscle weakness. Although most cases will resolve over a few weeks, prednisolone for 10 days improves recovery if started within 3 days of onset. Inability to close the eye needs ophthalmology review.

• *Functional* (psychological/psychiatric) disorders may present as stroke, e.g. somatisation.

ROSIER score

This simple scoring system is better at *excluding* stroke than diagnosing it (+LR = 6.5; −LR=0.09) using a cutoff of 1, i.e. ROSIER ≥1 = stroke more likely, ROSIER <1 = stroke less likely.

ROSIER score for stroke	
Clinical sign	Score
LOC or syncope	−1
Seizure	−1
Asymmetric face weakness	+1
Asymmetric arm weakness	+1
Asymmetric leg weakness	+1
Speech disturbance	+1
Visual field defect	+1

If total ≥1 stroke more likely (+LR = 6.5)
If total <1 stroke unlikely (−LR = 0.09)

Treatment

Ischaemic stroke

Patients with ischaemic stroke, confirmed by clinical symptoms and absence of bleeding on CT, *and* who are less than 3 hours from symptom onset are eligible for thrombolysis. After establishing absence of contraindications and obtaining informed consent, thrombolysis is performed with tissue plasminogen activator (tPA).

While some patients benefit greatly from thrombolysis, at a population level the picture is more complicated. Within 3 hours of onset, NNT ≈10, i.e. ten patients have to be treated to save one life or prevent one dependent patient, at the cost of intracranial bleeding (often fatal) in about 5% of patients (NNH ≈20). Beyond 3 hours, the risk/benefit ratio is less favourable.

If the patient has an ischaemic stroke but is not eligible for thrombolysis, aspirin should be started immediately. To prevent aspiration, patients should have a swallowing assessment before being given food or drink. Pressure area care and adequate hydration are essential in immobile patients.

Haemorrhagic stroke

Intracranial bleeding in patients on anticoagulants has a poor prognosis, and must be rapidly halted using fresh frozen plasma or prothrombin complex concentrate (expensive) and vitamin K. Surgical treatment should be considered.

Transient ischaemic attack

A transient ischaemic attack is a focal CNS disturbance caused by transient brain ischaemia from emboli or thrombosis with *complete resolution* within 24 hours. This can make differentiation from stroke difficult; patients with a neurological deficit that is resolving spontaneously should not receive thrombolysis.

The ABCD² score estimates the short-term risk of stroke. Patients with high scores must be investigated and treated urgently to prevent a stroke, e.g.

• Carotid stenosis: endarterectomy
• Atrial fibrillation, cardiac failure: anticoagulation
Antiplatelet therapy, e.g. aspirin, should be started immediately if TIA suspected and no contraindications.

Antiplatelet therapy, e.g. aspirin, should be started immediately if TIA suspected and no contraindications.

ABCD² score for TIA	
Clinical detail	Score
Age >60 years	1
Blood pressure > 140/90	1
Clinical features:	
Unilateral weakness	2
Speech disturbance without weakness	1
Duration	
>60 mins	2
10–60 mins	1
Diabetes	1

Total >4 = high risk – need urgent investigation
Total >5 = 8% risk of stroke in next 48 hours

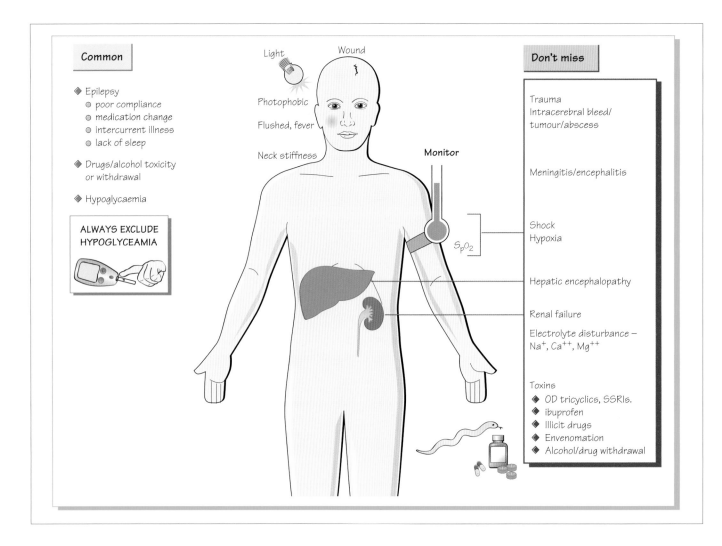

Seizures are the result of electrical 'storms' in the brain. Most seizures occur in people with known epilepsy: these patients often do not come to hospital unless the seizure is different from their normal pattern, or occurs in public. Most seizures last less than 5 minutes, so will have finished by the time the patient reaches the Emergency Department.

In a *generalised* or *tonic-clonic* seizure, the patient loses consciousness, their body tenses (*tonic* phase) and then undergoes a series of rhythmic contractions affecting all their muscles (*clonic* phase). *Partial* seizures exhibit a wide spectrum of patterns of motor activity and sensory disturbance according to the area of brain affected.

Primary seizures occur in patients with no underlying pathological cause. Secondary seizures occur as a result of some pathophysiological process.

Stop the seizure

The ABC rules apply, but with caveats. Never try to splint or force the mouth open. Patients may be cyanosed during the active phases of seizures, but if there is upper airway obstruction try a nasopharyngeal airway. Key points:

- Ensure the patient will not hurt themselves while fitting.
- Give oxygen 100% by reservoir mask.
- Check blood sugar. If below 4 mmol/L, give 50 mL of 50% dextrose i.v. or 1 mg i.m. glucagon.

First line: benzodiazepines

If intravenous access is available, use the doses as listed under 'Second line' below, otherwise give:

- midazolam 10 mg buccal *or*
- diazepam 10 mg rectal.

Second line: benzodiazepines

If the first dose of benzodiazepine has not terminated the seizure after 10 minutes, give a further dose of benzodiazepine:

- lorazepam 4 mg i.v. *or*
- diazepam 10 mg i.v.

If the patient is an alcoholic, give high-dose intravenous thiamine to prevent long-term brain damage.

Third line: anticonvulsant

Phenytoin (or the pro-drug fosphenytoin) is given as a loading dose over 30 minutes and then (if necessary) as a continuous infusion. Patients already taking phenytoin do not need a loading dose. Phenytoin is a sodium channel blocker with cardiac effects, so ECG and blood pressure must be monitored during use, and contraindications include cardiac conduction problems or significant heart failure.

Fourth line: sedation and intubation

A generalised seizure lasting over 30 minutes, or recurrent seizures within 30 minutes without return of consciousness, is described as status epilepticus. If such convulsions continue for more than 60 minutes despite treatment this is 'refractory status epilepticus', and the patient should be sedated and intubated to control the seizure, and transferred to the ICU.

After the seizure: the post-ictal period

After a generalised seizure has finished, it is normal for the patient to be unconscious for a few minutes, longer with high doses of benzodiazepines. When consciousness returns, it is common for the patient to be transiently confused, agitated and sometimes aggressive. Partial seizures may have little or no post-ictal period.

Search for a cause
Was it a seizure?

As with syncope, a good witness history taken as soon as possible after the event provides the most valuable evidence. Other likely differential diagnoses are:

- Syncope/collapse (Chapter 30).
- Hypoxia, metabolic causes – hyponatraemia, hypocalcaemia.
- Toxic causes – see opposite (Chapter 25).

Seizure vs pseudo-seizure

Pseudo-seizures ('non-epileptic attacks') can be very difficult to differentiate from generalised seizures: about 25% of patients intubated for 'seizures' are having a pseudo-seizure. Pseudo-seizures are more likely if there are asymmetric movements, pelvic thrusting, head rolling, resistance to eye opening or no post-ictal period. In pseudo-seizures, incontinence is unusual and tongue biting, if it occurs, involves the tip rather than the sides of the tongue that one would expect in a generalised seizure. The reasons for pseudo-seizures are usually complex and the labelling has significant risks, so should only be confirmed by a senior doctor.

Causes, triggers and auras

In a person with known epilepsy, common causes are non-compliance, changed dose of anticonvulsant, or drug interactions. Alcohol or benzodiazepine withdrawal causes seizures. *Triggers* are factors that may cause fits in people who are not normally prone to fits, e.g. lack of sleep, infections. An *aura* is the feeling that a patient with epilepsy has that warns them that a seizure is imminent.

Examination

Look for head trauma, injuries occurring as a result of the seizure, signs of sepsis/systemic illness or toxidromes (Chapter 24). Any suspicion of a rash or neck stiffness should prompt immediate antibiotics for meningitis (Chapters 38 and 41).

Cardiovascular examination is particularly important because cardiac causes are common differential diagnoses in the young (tachyarrhythmias, hypertrophic obstructive cardiomyopathy: HOCM) and the elderly (bradyarrhythmias, postural hypotension, valvular disease). Collapse due to cardiac causes may be accompanied by a few seconds of jerking limbs due to transient inadequate brain perfusion –'anoxic jerks', which can result in mis-labelling as 'seizures'.

Neurological examination after the post-ictal period is often normal, but if there are focal neurological signs, this should prompt further investigation, e.g. CT. Immediately after a generalised seizure, the plantar reflexes may be upgoing, and there may be ankle clonus. Todd's palsy is a transient unilateral weakness following a seizure that resolves over a few hours, but can be difficult to differentiate from a TIA/stroke.

Investigations
Bedside investigations

- Blood glucose, ECG.

Laboratory investigations

- FBC, U + E, calcium.
- Anticonvulsant levels – not always helpful but should be performed if toxicity suspected (e.g. patient is ataxic).
- Prolactin rises after a seizure: the sample should be taken between 10 and 20 minutes after the seizure, but should only be ordered if the diagnosis is unclear.

Imaging

- CT indicated for first seizure or abnormal neurology.

Disposal: who can go home?
Known epilepsy

Often a person with known epilepsy is brought to the Emergency Department just because they have had a (normal for the patient) seizure in public. If the seizure is within their normal pattern, they have a full recovery, and will be with a responsible adult, discharge is likely to be safe.

'First fit'

Patients not previously known to be epileptic should be observed for at least 4 hours. If no serious underlying cause is found and there are no complications, they may be discharged. On discharge they must be advised, *and this must be recorded in the notes*, to avoid any activity in which a further fit would be dangerous e.g. *driving*, operating machinery, climbing ladders, unsupervised swimming, until they have been reviewed by a specialist. Outpatient clinic follow-up should be organised following EEG and CT.

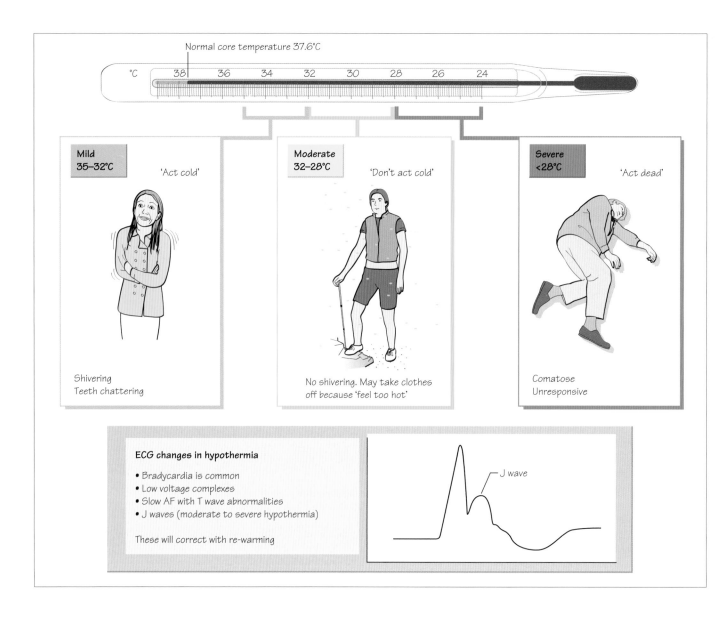

Normal core temperature 37.6°C

°C 38 36 34 32 30 28 26 24

Mild 35–32°C — 'Act cold'

Shivering
Teeth chattering

Moderate 32–28°C — 'Don't act cold'

No shivering. May take clothes off because 'feel too hot'

Severe <28°C — 'Act dead'

Comatose
Unresponsive

ECG changes in hypothermia

- Bradycardia is common
- Low voltage complexes
- Slow AF with T wave abnormalities
- J waves (moderate to severe hypothermia)

These will correct with re-warming

J wave

Hypothermia

Hypothermia is common in patients 'found on floor' in winter months. The elderly and alcoholics are at risk because of falls. Phenothiazines reduce hypothalamic sensitivity to temperature, and alcohol causes peripheral vasodilatation.

Conduction is the fastest way of losing heat, followed by convection and radiation. Under normal circumstances the hypothalamus responds to cold by directing the body to preserve core temperature by progressively shutting down blood supply to the outside shell – the skin, then the limbs. Muscle contractions are used to generate heat by shivering.

Diagnosing hypothermia

Core temperature is best measured with a nasopharyngeal or oesophageal temperature probe.

Primary assessment

- Remove wet clothing, nurse in a warm, well-monitored environment.
- Standard ABC assessment priorities apply.
- Avoid moving the patient in severe hypothermia, as this may precipitate ventricular fibrillation (VF).
- Consider rhabdomyolysis in patients 'found on floor' – measure creatine kinase (CK).

Rewarming

Deciding whether and how to rewarm is not always straightforward. Factors to consider are:

- Level of hypothermia.
- Rate of cooling.

- Age of the patient.
- Cardiac arrest.

Non-invasive rewarming

Patients with *mild hypothermia* need no special measures as they will generate their own heat – warm blankets are sufficient. Aluminium foil sheets are not effective.

Most patients with *moderate hypothermia*, and *stable* patients with *severe hypothermia*, can be effectively rewarmed at 1–2°C per hour using the combination of:
- Warmed humidified oxygen.
- Warm air blanket.

Warmed humidified oxygen uses the lungs as a heat exchanger and prevents the normal heat loss by evaporation from the lungs. The warm air blanket blows air at 43°C over the body.

Invasive rewarming

Patients with *severe hyperthermia* who are *unstable* may require invasive rewarming, either by filling a body cavity with warmed fluids, or directly heating the blood.

Infusing fluid warmed to 40°C into either the left hemithorax or peritoneum, draining and repeating can rewarm at up to 4°C per hour and is relatively simple to achieve using equipment available in any Emergency Department. The left hemithorax is preferred as it directly heats the heart and great vessels. Unfortunately the less invasive options, bladder or stomach washout, are not effective. The most rapid (1–2°C per 5 minutes) way of rewarming a patient is to use cardiac bypass, but this requires anticoagulation, and is not available in many centres.

Intravenous fluids Warmed fluids prevent further heat loss but are ineffective at rewarming. Practical experimentation with bathwater will demonstrate that adding 1 litre of water at 43°C does not significantly change the temperature of 70 litres of water at 28°C.

Shock may develop as rewarming occurs: intravenous fluids should be warmed to 43°C and given cautiously. In elderly patients, fluid overload may cause cardiac failure as the heart and kidneys may be unable to cope with the increased volume load.

Cardiac arrest

As the heart cools, charactistic 'J' waves are seen on ECG; atrial fibrillation, bradycardia and ventricular fibrillation may occur with progressive cooling, ending with asystole. Cardiac arrest is difficult to diagnose, as a very weak and slow pulse is difficult to detect: ECG and ultrasound are helpful to confirm.

The traditional maxim '*You're not dead until you're warm and dead*' holds true. Full normal recovery has been recorded in patients with prolonged periods of asystole. However, a common feature of patients who survive hypothermic cardiac arrest appears to be that they are not hypoxic while they are cooled.

Normal resuscitation protocols are followed, but defibrillation is often ineffective below 30°C, and is therefore not repeated until the temperature has been raised. Inability to provide invasive rewarming may make resuscitation futile. The decision to stop resuscitation is difficult, but some indicators are:
- A potassium level of more than 10 mmol/L.
- Patients with pre-existent organ failure that would preclude successful discharge from the ICU. Old age alone does not preclude survival.

Hyperthermia

Hyperthermia may be a result of environmental conditions, toxic effects of drugs or, very rarely, disease.

Heat stroke

This is when environmental conditions overwhelm the body's ability to lose heat, sometimes exacerbated by exercise in the heat. Heat exhaustion is a mild form of heat stroke.

The patient will have a temperature above 40°C, confusion/neurological abnormalities and (usually) absent sweating. Rhabdomyolysis and hepatic inflammation may be present, together with a raised white cell count (WCC).

Treatment is by cooling with cold intravenous fluids, tepid sponging and ice packs. Benzodiazepines and intubation may be necessary.

Drugs

Neuroleptic malignant syndrome is a rare side-effect of phenothiazine drugs (antipsychotics), which can present with rigidity, confusion and hyperthermia, usually soon after starting/increasing the drug.

Serotonin syndrome may present with a similar picture of rigidity, confusion and hyperthermia. This may occur in when a selective serotonin reuptake inhibitor (SSRI) drug interacts with another drug, often a monoamine oxidase inhibitor (MAOI). Users of amphetamines and related compounds such as MDMA ('ecstasy') also sometimes develop hyperthermia.

The treatment for all these conditions is benzodiazepines to reduce muscular rigidity, and cooling with cold fluids, tepid sponging and ice packs.

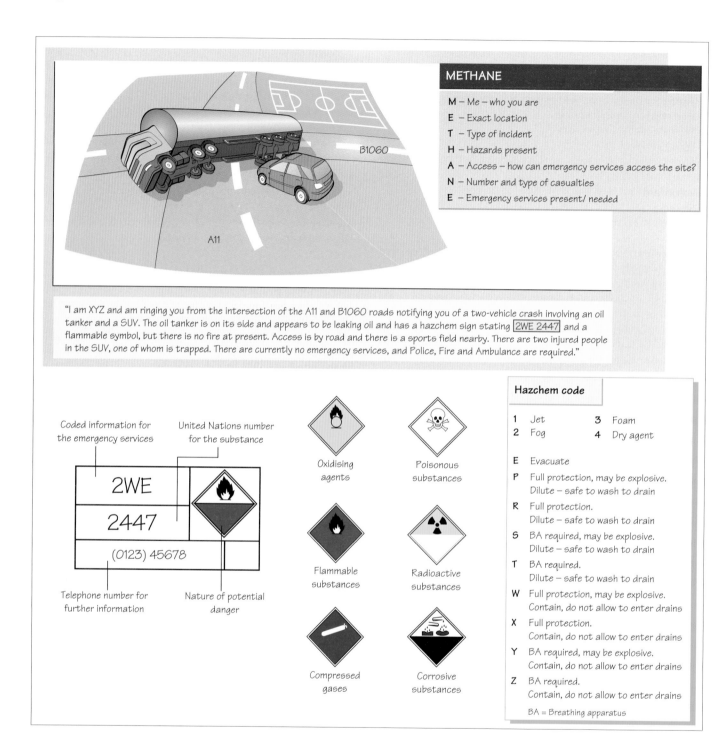

METHANE

M – Me – who you are
E – Exact location
T – Type of incident
H – Hazards present
A – Access – how can emergency services access the site?
N – Number and type of casualties
E – Emergency services present/ needed

"I am XYZ and am ringing you from the intersection of the A11 and B1060 roads notifying you of a two-vehicle crash involving an oil tanker and a SUV. The oil tanker is on its side and appears to be leaking oil and has a hazchem sign stating 2WE 2447 and a flammable symbol, but there is no fire at present. Access is by road and there is a sports field nearby. There are two injured people in the SUV, one of whom is trapped. There are currently no emergency services, and Police, Fire and Ambulance are required."

Coded information for the emergency services

United Nations number for the substance

2WE
2447
(0123) 45678

Telephone number for further information

Nature of potential danger

Oxidising agents

Poisonous substances

Flammable substances

Radioactive substances

Compressed gases

Corrosive substances

Hazchem code

1	Jet	3	Foam
2	Fog	4	Dry agent

E Evacuate
P Full protection, may be explosive.
   Dilute – safe to wash to drain
R Full protection.
   Dilute – safe to wash to drain
S BA required, may be explosive.
   Dilute – safe to wash to drain
T BA required.
   Dilute – safe to wash to drain
W Full protection, may be explosive.
   Contain, do not allow to enter drains
X Full protection.
   Contain, do not allow to enter drains
Y BA required, may be explosive.
   Contain, do not allow to enter drains
Z BA required.
   Contain, do not allow to enter drains

BA = Breathing apparatus

Pre-hospital and retrieval medicine are subspecialty areas within Emergency Medicine, and demand for these skills is increasing. Doctors with critical care skills in rapid-response vehicles or helicopters attend the scene of an incident or transfer patients from one healthcare facility to another that is better able to meet their needs.

Practising medicine out of a hospital environment is particularly challenging for a variety of reasons.

• Patients may be very distressed, which can make them more difficult to assess and treat.
• Technical reasons: monitoring equipment may be sensitive to vibration. Noise makes stethoscopes very difficult to use.
• Practical reasons: poor visibility, limited amount of equipment, cramped space or limited access.
• Personal reasons: out of 'comfort zone', motion sickness, extremes of heat and cold.

Despite this, doctors who do pre-hospital work tend to be particularly enthusiastic about it. When out of the normal hospital environment, it is particularly important to be appropriately dressed and equipped. Without a basic level of safety equipment, the Incident Officer will not allow you onto a potentially hazardous site.

Dress
- Strong footwear: boots with good soles and toecaps.
- High-visibility jacket/trousers with designation, e.g. 'doctor'.
- Safety helmet ± torch.
- Tabard/hat identifying role.
- Warm clothes.

Equipment
- Stethoscope.
- Trauma scissors.
- Pens and paper.
- Marker pen.
- Identity card.
- Mobile telephone.

If you are taking medical equipment, ensure you know what you have, and how it is packed. Ambulance staff keep a limited range of drugs.

At the scene
If possible, go past the crash and park on the same side. Leave plenty of space for emergency vehicles, leave hazard lights on and lock the car. Leave the keys with the police, if present.

Call the emergency services if this has not already been done. Put on any protective clothing you have.

Safety is the first priority – make sure all naked lights are extinguished and danger from other traffic is minimised. Do not put yourself in danger.

Who is in charge?
If Ambulance Service personnel are present at a incident, they will usually be responsible for medical resources, and you should report to the Ambulance Incident Officer. If it is a large incident there will be Police and Fire Services present, each of which will have their own Incident Officer and control structure. Fire Service takes control if hazardous substances are present; police if firearms may be involved.

The Incident Officer controls the scene by nominating people to perform tasks. Nothing should take place without their knowledge and, at the end of every task, staff should report back to the Incident Officer.

Aircraft
Helicopters are particularly useful in rural and remote areas with difficult vehicle access. In countries with well-developed trauma systems, helicopters allow rapid transfer of patients to major trauma centres, bypassing smaller centres that do not have the range of facilities to care for complex multi-trauma. The optimum range for helicopters is 50–200 kilometres (30–130 miles).

A helicopter weighing 3000 kg generates 3000 kg of downthrust: make sure there is no loose debris on the landing site, which should be 30×100 m. Keep well away from the landing site and wear eye protection. Do not shine lights on the landing surface or at the helicopter unless specifically requested to do so.

Do not approach a helicopter unless the rotors have stopped or you have been specifically bidden to approach by the pilot. The helicopter team will usually come to you. Only approach the helicopter from the front – the tail rotor spins at head height.

Fixed-wing aircraft are useful over longer distances, >200 km (120 miles), and have more space, but take longer to prepare.

Radio procedure
Radios are generally used to communicate at larger incidents. If you have to use one, you will be issued with a call sign. When you talk:
- remember to press the button;
- state who you are;
- end with 'over' to let the other party know you have finished speaking. ('Over and out' is only for movies!)

Phonetic alphabet

A	Alpha	M	Mike	Y	Yankee
B	Bravo	N	November	Z	Zulu
C	Charlie	O	Oscar	0	zero
D	Delta	P	Papa	1	wun
E	Echo	Q	Quebec	2	too
F	Foxtrot	R	Romeo	3	thu'ree
G	Golf	S	Sierra	4	fa'wer
H	Hotel	T	Tango	5	fy'vah
I	India	U	Uniform	6	six
J	Juliet	V	Victor	7	sev' en
K	Kilo	W	Whisky	8	ate
L	Lima	X	X-ray	9	niner

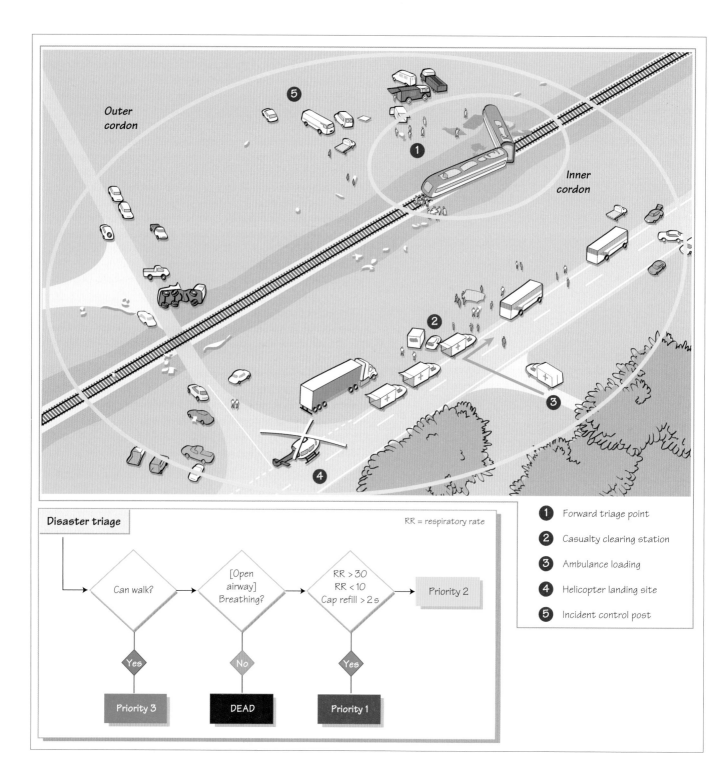

Outer cordon

Inner cordon

RR = respiratory rate

Disaster triage

Can walk? → [Open airway] Breathing? → RR > 30 RR < 10 Cap refill > 2 s → Priority 2

Yes → Priority 3

No → DEAD

Yes → Priority 1

1 Forward triage point
2 Casualty clearing station
3 Ambulance loading
4 Helicopter landing site
5 Incident control post

In medicine, it is normally assumed that there are sufficient resources and personnel to meet patients' needs. In a major incident this may not be the case, and there is a need for a system to ensure that limited resources are used in the most effective way.

Military-style command structures are used to ensure safety and clear lines of responsibility; orders from the scene controller must be obeyed by all on site.

Notification

METHANE is the mnemonic used for notifying a major incident. It is a standardised structure that tells the listener all the key information efficiently (Chapter 45).

Incident management

As the emergency services arrive, the police will take charge and cordon off the incident. The inner cordon contains the immediate area around the incident, and the outer cordon contains all the emergency services attending the incident. Each of the emergency services at an incident has their own separate control officer – a Bronze level controller. Only very large incidents would need high-level (Silver/Gold) controllers.

When the Fire Service has checked that the area is safe, healthcare personnel are allowed access to casualties in the inner cordon. There may be significant ongoing hazards, e.g. unsafe buildings, and in terrorist incidents secondary devices are commonly used to target rescuers.

The Ambulance Incident Officer (AIO) will request medical team(s) from hospitals if the incident is large or serious. Medical teams need to have safety clothing, identifying tabards, equipment and supplies relevant to the incident (Chapter 45). Several medical teams of one doctor and one nurse working together may be needed, together with a Medical Incident Officer to co-ordinate treatment and evacuation.

Incident management priorities

1 Command
2 Safety
3 Communication
4 Assessment
5 Triage
6 Treatment
7 Transport

Major incident triage

Triage is not about *treating* patients, but just *sorting* them so that subsequent medical care can be effectively targeted, and for this reason is best performed by nursing staff. Labels ensure that treatment teams can easily find the high-priority patients, and do not waste time reassessing dead patients. The categories of patient are P (= Priority) 1–3.

Triage in the context of a disaster is very different from normal hospital triage. It is sometimes described as reverse triage as the least ill patients, the walking wounded (P3), are separated first. These are patients who may have significant but not life-threatening injuries.

In a large incident, a forward triage point within the inner cordon allows stabilisation of patients before they are transported to the main casualty clearing station. Once patients arrive at the casualty clearing station, they are re-triaged and evacuated to hospitals according to their injuries and the specialised facilities that different hospitals can offer, e.g. trauma, burns, intensive care, neurosurgery.

The casualty clearing station is the nearest area to the inner cordon that has good transport access. Buildings offer shelter, power and light, which are useful if casualties will need to be held for any length of time.

At the hospital

Preparations start as soon as notification is received from the Ambulance Service of a major incident. Medical, nursing, support and administrative staff are notified by the hospital switchboard using a cascade system.

Security within the Emergency Department must be kept very tight ('lockdown') to ensure patient and staff safety, and a robust system of staff identification is essential. Preparations should be made to handle media and relatives away from the Emergency Department. The Emergency Department is cleared of all non-life-threatening emergencies. Inpatient teams conduct ward rounds to discharge all possible patients, and non-urgent operations are cancelled.

Patients are re-triaged on arrival at the Emergency Department and teams of doctors and nurses are allocated to deal with casualties (P1 and P2) in the Emergency Department. An area away from the main Emergency Department is used for 'walking wounded' (P3) patients. X-ray facilities and treatment rooms are necessary, so outpatient clinic areas are often used.

Emergency Department staff need physical and emotional support to cope with a disaster. Food, drink and rest are important for a sustained response, and measures should be taken to ensure that emotional support is available. A 'hot debrief' happens immediately after such an incident, followed up by a full debriefing meeting a few weeks later, so that all involved may discuss and learn from the experience, and the hospital's plans can be updated with this information.

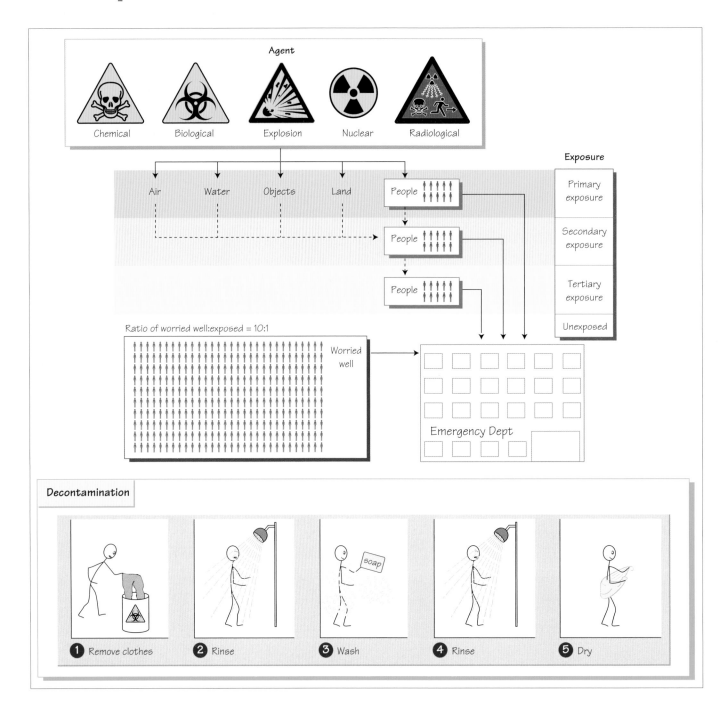

Hazardous materials are used in industrial and research facilities, and there is an ongoing risk of terrorist attacks in large urban areas. Health systems must be able to treat both the public and members of emergency services who may have been exposed to hazardous agents. This must be done without harming healthcare workers or other patients, as some agents have the potential for secondary harm. Rapid identification and treatment of these agents and use of standard life support protocols are effective.

Several factors determine the impact of hazards on health services.
- Toxicity: ability to kill or incapacitate.
- Latency of action: harmful effect may be delayed, e.g. phosgene gas which produces pulmonary oedema 24 hours after exposure.
- Persistence: resistance to degradation or decontamination (e.g. VX, a nerve agent, 'sticks' to people and objects).
- Transmissibility.

The major incident plan (Chapter 46) is a framework for dealing with a CBRNE incident, as even a small number of patients will impair an Emergency Department's ability to function normally. Toxicological advice is available from national centres listed in Chapter 24.

General approach
Security
Once a CBRNE incident is declared, all patients are considered 'dirty' (potentially contaminated); after screening ± decontamination, they become 'clean'. Clean and dirty areas must be clearly marked and physically separated. Hospital staff working in dirty areas must be protected with Personal Protective Equipment. This may range from gown, gloves, mask, glasses to full 'space suit' type of protection.

The hospital should have a 'lockdown' policy that can be rapidly implemented, limiting entrances – one for staff, the Emergency Department for patients. This minimises the risk of dirty patients putting other patients and staff at risk in clean areas.

Decontamination
Disaster planning often assumes a high degree of compliance – that all dirty patients are identified at the scene, obey officials, do not panic, wait patiently to be decontaminated at the scene and only then are transported to the hospital for medical care.

In reality, even assuming full co-operation by all casualties, there is a time lag between the incident and recognition that an incident may involve hazardous materials. In urban areas, patients may arrive at the Emergency Department before the hospital has been notified of the incident. Therefore all hospitals need facilities to decontaminate patients arriving at a hospital, and these should allow basic treatment of patients while being decontaminated.

Decontamination is managed by the Fire Service, with medical supervision being provided by hospital staff. Inflatable structures are used to provide shelter and a degree of privacy for those undergoing decontamination.

Decontamination involves patients:
1 Removing their clothes, which are bagged and treated as contaminated waste.
2 Rinsing to remove surface contamination.
3 Washing all over with soap and sponges.
4 Rinsing again.
5 Drying and putting on clean paper suit.

Failure to decontaminate patients before they enter the hospital results in contamination of other patients, staff and facilities. This is dangerous and necessitates shutting parts of the hospital for decontamination.

Chemical
Organophosphates
Organophosphates (OP) are used as pesticides and 'nerve agent' chemical weapons: exposure occurs due to ingestion or skin contact. OPs inhibit cholinesterase, resulting in rapid build-up of acetylcholine (ACh). The ubiquity of ACh as a neurotransmitter result in widespread nerve dysfunction.

- Muscarinic effects – DUMBELS (diarrhoea, urination, miosis – small pupil, bronchorrhoea and bronchospasm, emesis, lacrimation, salivation).
- Nicotinic effects – weakness, tremor, fasciculation and paralysis.
- CNS effects – agitation, seizures, coma.

Large doses of atropine are used to reverse the muscarinic effects, followed by pralidoxime to prevent cholinesterase irreversibly binding with the OP.

Cyanide
Cyanide binds to mitochondrial cytochromes to prevent aerobic respiration. Poisoning causes a profound lactic acidosis despite apparent good oxygenation. Without treatment there is rapidly progressive circulatory collapse and death.

Treatment depends on certainty of diagnosis and level of toxicity, but options are:
- chelation using cobalt EDTA;
- high-dose hydroxycobalamin to give cyanocobalamin (vitamin B_{12});
- sodium thiosulfate to produce thiocyanates.

Biological
Although bacterial contamination (e.g. anthrax) is always a possibility, the significant challenges in the immediate future are likely to be viral. The SARS (severe acute respiratory syndrome) infections in 2003 served as a warning about the rapid global spread of infectious disease in the modern age. The swine flu (H1N1) pandemic has proved very benign compared to predictions based on the avian flu (H5N1) influenza, but influenza viruses can combine and mutate.

Radiation
There are two groups of casualties to consider:
- Exposed to radiation;
- Contaminated with radioactive material.

The first group pose no risk to staff, whereas the latter needs careful decontamination, as outlined above. Decontamination should be monitored with a hand-held Geiger counter to ensure complete removal of all radioactive material, and staff should wear radiation dosimeters.

Radiation exposure can be fatal due to bone marrow toxicity and gastrointestinal failure. The time to develop vomiting is proportional to the patient's exposure, and therefore outcome – shorter times indicate higher exposure.

The 'worried well'
In real-life CBRNE incidents, large numbers of asymptomatic people present to Emergency Departments, concerned that they may have been exposed to a hazardous substance. The number of these people is usually much higher than those actually affected by the hazard. However, the former group may become inadvertently contaminated by those who have been exposed (secondary and tertiary exposure).

Depending on the material involved, the Emergency Department must rapidly develop and monitor a way of triaging the 'worried well' so that they can be reassured and swiftly discharged.

Case studies: questions

Case 1: Shortness of breath

A 40-year-old patient known to be asthmatic presents to the Emergency Department with increasing shortness of breath. For the last 2 days, this has been gradually increasing, and she is now using her salbutamol inhaler every 2 hours. She has a fever and productive cough with green sputum. Her chest hurts on the left when she coughs. On examination, she is alert, speaking a few words at a time. On listening to her chest, there is generalised wheeze, together with crackles heard over the left base. She has a peak expiratory flow rate (PEFR) of 190 mL/min, a respiratory rate of 40 breaths/minute, BP 130/80 mmHg, heart rate 110 bpm. A chest X-ray reveals left lower lobe pneumonia.

ABG on room air	Normal values
pH 7.30	pH = 7.35–7.45
PO_2 8.1 kPa (61 mmHg)	$PO_2 \approx 11.3$–13.3 kPa ($\approx$85–100 mmHg)
PCO_2 4.9 kPa (37 mmHg)	$PCO_2 \approx 4.8$–5.9 kPa ($\approx$36–44 mmHg)

1 *How severe is this patient's asthma?*
2 *How severe is this patient's pneumonia?*
3 *Comment on this patient's ABG result.*
4 *How should the asthma and pneumonia be treated?*
5 *What will you do for this patient when she is eventually discharged from hospital?*

Case 2: Acutely painful red eye

A 60-year-old female presents with a painful eye, blurred vision, headache and vomiting.

1 *Before you see the patient, list your differential diagnosis, with a brief comment to justify each diagnosis.*
2 *What other clinical findings would you expect if the diagnosis was glaucoma?*
3 *Describe the Emergency Department management of glaucoma.*
4 *If the patient had a painless loss of vision, what other conditions would be likely?*

Case 3: Arterial blood gas interpretation

An 18-year-old patient presents with vomiting due to 'possible gastroenteritis'. The presenting symptoms developed quickly, with fever and non-specific abdominal pain. On examination the patient appears unwell, slightly short of breath, heart rate 120 bpm, BP 90/60 mmHg, respiratory rate 32 breaths/minute, temperature 38.5°C, and no specific findings apart from diffusely tender abdomen.

1 *What does the blood gas on room air indicate?*

pH 7.17; PO_2 11.7 kPa (88 mmHg); PCO_2 2.7 kPa (20 mmHg).

Na^+ 135 mmol/L; K^+ 4.2 mmol/L;

Cl^- 105 mmol/L; HCO_3^- 6 mmol/L.

2 *What is the anion gap?*
3 *What are the differential diagnoses?*

The next patient is a 59-year-old smoker who has previously been treated for anxiety and depression, but has recently been bedbound following a knee operation. He presents to the Emergency Department feeling short of breath over the last day or so. On examination he has a respiratory rate of 32 breaths/minute, heart rate 100 bpm, BP 130/80 mmHg.

4 *(a) If this patient had the following ABG results, what acid–base disturbance would this be?*

pH 7.5; PO_2 10.6 kPa (79 mmHg); PCO_2 2.7 kPa (21 mmHg).

(b) If this patient has the following ABG results, what acid–base disturbance would this be?

pH 7.25; PO_2 7.2 kPa (54 mmHg); PCO_2 5.8 kPa (44 mmHg).

5 *Using the ABG results in 4(a), when this blood test was performed, the patient was breathing 35% oxygen by mask. What should the PO_2 be in a healthy patient with this inspired oxygen concentration, and what does the difference imply?*
6 *How should the patient with the ABG results in 4(b) above be managed?*

Case 4: Abdominal pain

A 57-year-old man presents to triage with abdominal pain. He is usually fairly well but overweight, and has high blood pressure. He had a sudden onset of right flank pain, which is constant, 9/10 severity. He is pacing around the room, and cannot sit still. He has a BP of 147/87 mmHg, heart rate 96 bpm.

1 *What are the differential diagnoses?*
2 *What bedside tests are helpful in differentiating between these diagnoses?*
3 *What imaging would you request?*
4 *Describe your treatment.*
5 *Your investigations show a 4 mm stone in the ureter. How will you decide if the patient is admitted or discharged?*

Case 5: Chest pain

A 40-year-old accountant presents to the Emergency Department with chest pain. He has known hypertension and has smoked 20 cigarettes per day for 20 years. He says the pain is tight across his chest, started three hours ago, and describes it as a 'pressure or tight feeling'. The pain radiates to his neck, and he feels nauseated and short of breath.

1 *List the differential diagnoses for this patient.*
2 *What initial investigations and treatment are appropriate?*
3 *What are the key treatments if the ECG confirms STEMI?*

A 24-year-old IT worker presents with left-sided chest pain, which came on suddenly earlier in the day. He is usually well, and is currently on an adventure holiday. His pain is worse on breathing and coughing. He is slightly short of breath, and has a recent cough and runny nose.

4 *What are the differential diagnoses for this patient?*
5 *A chest X-ray does not reveal a cause of his pain. What further test(s) is appropriate?*

Case 6: Bleed in early pregnancy

You have two patients in the Emergency Department with vaginal bleeding in early pregnancy. The first patient thinks she is having a miscarriage. Her period is 10 days late, and a urinary pregnancy test was positive a few days ago. However, today she started bleeding and she has lower abdominal pain, worse on the right.

She feels faint and her blood pressure is 80/50 mmHg.

1 *What are the differential diagnoses?*
2 *What immediate actions would you take?*
3 *What further management is needed?*

The second patient is 7 weeks pregnant. She has two children and has had a miscarriage in the past. She has had bleeding all day, with some dark discharge.

She has no abdominal pain. Her GP confirmed her pregnancy with a blood test and ultrasound 1 week previously, which showed an intrauterine gestational sac. An ultrasound is performed in the Emergency Department, demonstrating an empty uterus.

4 *How should this patient be managed?*

Case 7: Head injury

As a member of the trauma team you are helping looking after a patient with a head injury. Your patient is a 23-year-old man who intervened in an argument between an intoxicated man and his girlfriend. He was punched in the face and knocked to the ground, hitting his head on the ground. The man is brought to the Emergency Department semi-conscious, responding only to painful stimuli. Pupils are 4 mm wide, equal and reactive to light, and the patient smells of alcohol. Observations: BP 110/80 mmHg, heart rate 100 bpm, respiratory rate 24 breaths/minute and oxygen saturation 91%.

1 *Is the reduced consciousness state due to alcohol/drugs or head injury?*
2 *What other injuries should be considered?*
3 *What are the priorities in the first phase of stabilisation?*
4 *What features should be sought on further examination?*
5 *The patient has confused speech, opens eyes only to painful stimuli and when you press on the patient's left fingernail, the patient's right hand crosses the midline to try to remove the stimulus. What is the patient's score on Glasgow Coma Scale (GCS)?*

You review him 20 minutes later. He is now making incomprehensible sounds, eyes closed, withdraws from painful stimuli. He is snoring and his oxygen saturation is 94% on 15 L/minute by reservoir mask.

6 *What is the GCS now?*
7 *What should happen next?*

Case 8: Burns

A 33-year-old man is brought in by ambulance with burns. His neighbour heard a loud noise and found the patient unconscious at the bottom of the stairs. The patient has 20% partial thickness burns, including burns to the face. The neighbour is well despite dragging the patient out of the burning house and the thick smoke.

1 *What are the important things the ambulance crew may be able to tell you during handover of this patient?*
2 *Outline the initial assessment and resuscitation of this patient.*
3 *What things must not be overlooked in the resuscitation?*
4 *What analgesia will this patient require?*
5 *Describe the intravenous fluids that this patient is likely to require.*
6 *Should the patient be transferred to a burns centre?*

Case 9: Unconscious

An unconscious 19-year-old man is brought in by his university friends. They think that he has taken a lot of white tablets. One friend says he took an overdose because he had chronic pain and nothing was helping; another thought he was taking recreational pills. Another friend arrives saying he has just found five empty packets of paracetamol (acetaminophen) hidden under his bed, and one empty packet of antidepressants. On examination he has a patent airway, is breathing spontaneously, respiratory rate 12 breaths/minute, BP 90/50 mmHg and warm dry skin, heart rate 120 bpm. His GCS is 13, and he has large pupils, which are symmetrical and reactive to light. Respiratory examination is unremarkable. Abdominal examination reveals no bowel sounds, and a distended bladder.

1 *Describe the immediate management.*
2 *This patient's findings are consistent with which toxidrome pattern?*
3 *What drug is likely to have caused the toxidrome, and how should this be managed?*
4 *What other lethal overdose may be asymptomatic at this stage?*
5 *A colleague suggests giving this patient activated charcoal. Is this a good idea?*

Case 10: Vomiting

You are in the Emergency Department one afternoon when three patients present together with vomiting. The previous evening they all went out to a restaurant to celebrate their football team 'The Magpies' winning. The restaurant's popularity is based on cheap food and alcohol rather than scrupulous hygiene.

• Patient A is a 20-year-old male, who has diarrhoea, vomiting, a high fever, headache and muscle aches. Has vomited about ten times since 0400. He looks unwell and pale, with cool limbs and has mild non-localising abdominal pain: temp 38.5°C, BP 100/50 mmHg, heart rate 110 bpm.
• Patient B is a 23-year-old female. She has vomiting, high fever, and general aches and pains. She noticed a small amount of bright blood in the vomitus, after the third vomit, and it has continued as she has vomited often since 0400. She looks unwell and pale, with cool limbs: temp 38.7°C, BP 90/50 mmHg, heart rate 115 bpm.
• Patient C is a 22-year-old female. She has vomiting and no diarrhoea. The vomiting has been present for 5 days. She suggests that perhaps her housemates caught a bug from her, otherwise it must have been the food (or alcohol) from last night. Her vomiting is worse this morning. She looks well, and is apyrexial with BP 110/60 mmHg, heart rate 90 bpm.

1 *What possible diagnoses should be considered in these patients?*
2 *What tests are appropriate for patient A?*
3 *Outline your management of patient A.*
4 *What is the likely cause of the bleeding in patient B? What further information would you seek?*
5 *Patient C has had vomiting for longer than her housemates. What other diagnoses should be considered?*
6 *Patient A has been on oral prednisolone 50 mg for 2 weeks for asthma. How will this affect your management?*

Case 11: Weakness

A 57-year-old male patient presents to the Emergency Department after developing weakness of his right hand that lasted about 5 minutes. He now feels completely normal and thinks he is probably wasting your time coming in for a check-up. He has had no palpitations, chest pain or shortness of breath. He has a past history of high blood pressure and cholesterol, but says he is otherwise fit and well and has no previous medical history. He smokes 10 cigarettes per day and has a 40 pack-year history, takes no medication, and has no known allergies. On examination, BP is 150/95 mmHg, heart rate is 80 bpm and regular. There were no carotid bruits, murmurs or signs of cardiac failure. Neurological examination was unremarkable.

1 *What investigations will you perform?*
2 *Does this patient require admission to hospital?*
3 *What can be done to prevent stroke?*

The patient re-presents 3 days later with a recurrence of the same symptoms, but this time it lasts for 2 hours. You call the stroke team, arrange a CT head which is normal, and then the symptoms resolve, just as the stroke team arrive.

4 *What is your further management?*
5 *How might this be different if the symptoms are persistent?*
6 *What conditions can mimic ischaemic stroke, and what are the key clinical features of each? What investigations are useful in excluding stroke mimics?*

Case 12: Collapse

A 22-year-old man presents to the Emergency Department after an episode of collapse. The collapse did not happen during exercise and the patient does not remember collapsing. Similar episodes have happened before, and the patient now feels completely normal.

1 *What features are suggestive of seizures?*
2 *What features are suggestive of a cardiac cause?*

3 *Describe the patient's ECG (see below).*
4 *The patient is now asymptomatic. What further action would you take?*
5 *If this had been a 60-year-old man presenting with a collapse (with a normal ECG), what factors would influence you to admit the patient for observation and cardiac monitoring?*

Case 13: Headache

Two patients present to the Emergency Department with headache.

The first patient is a 27-year-old who was having sexual intercourse and had a sudden onset of severe occipital headache. It was the worst headache he has ever had. The headache has now gone and the man is reluctantly here with his girlfriend who wanted him 'checked up'.

1 *What is the most likely diagnosis?*
2 *What investigations will you perform?*

The second patient is a 51-year-old woman who has a long history of headaches. Today the headache is typical of her usual headache (unilateral, with visual symptoms, the light hurts her eyes), and she has nausea and vomiting. The left side of her face feels numb. Her GP is unavailable; he usually gives her an injection of pethidine (meperedine) and then she goes home to sleep it off.

3 *What is the most likely diagnosis?*
4 *What investigations will you perform?*
5 *What treatment is necessary?*

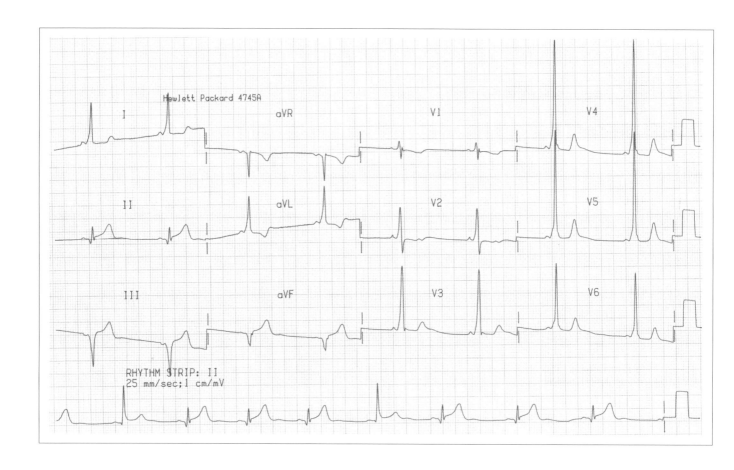

Case studies: answers

Case 1: Shortness of breath

1 The patient has severe asthma because they can only speak a few words at a time, and has increased heart and respiratory rates and hypoxia.

2 CURB-65 uses indicators of organ failure to predict mortality related to the pneumonia: one point each for:

- Confusion (neurological).
- Urea >7 mmol/L (renal).
- Respiratory rate >30 breaths/minute (lungs).
- Blood pressure <90 mmHg systolic or <60 mmHg diastolic (cardiovascular).
- Age 65 years or older.

While there are alternative, similar, predictive tools that could be used, as complexity increases, such tools become less reliable in 'real-life' practice. The CURB-65 has the advantage of being simple and memorable. The CURB score in this case is 1 (one point for respiratory rate), which puts her in the mild/low-risk group.

3 The patient has a mild acidosis: with hyperventilation one would expect the PCO_2 to be low, so the PCO_2 in the normal range is worrying. The symptoms have been present for 2 days, so the (relatively high) PCO_2 is likely to be a sign of relative hypoventilation due to tiredness.

4 A CURB-65 score of 1, on its own, suggests oral antibiotics without hospital admission; however, the severe asthma mandates admission. Therefore the treatment plan would be as follows:

(a) Asthma needs oxygen, continuous nebulisers of salbutamol (or in less severe cases, 12 puffs via spacer); intravenous corticosteroids (hydrocortisone 100 mg). Nebulised ipratropium bromide every 4 hours can be given, but the mainstays of treatment of asthma are β_2 agonists and steroids.

(b) Monitor with regular ABGs over the first few hours. If the patient deteriorates ($PO_2\downarrow$ and/or $PCO_2\uparrow$), magnesium, aminophylline and non-invasive ventilation may be used, depending on local protocols: early senior advice is necessary. Intubation is necessary for patients who present in extremis or who deteriorate despite other measures.

(c) Admission to hospital with appropriate monitoring, e.g. to high dependency unit (HDU).

(d) In view of the patient's level of illness, the first 24 hours of antibiotics should be intravenous.

5 When the patient is discharged, asthma education and an asthma plan are important, together with a letter to the GP, and a reducing course of steroids with enough medication to last until the next appointment. Inhaler technique should be checked, and the importance and benefit of use of spacers for aerosol puffers explained.

Learning points

- In a hyperventilating patient, expect a low PCO_2; if it is in the normal range (and is a true arterial rather than venous sample), this is a red flag warning of tiredness and impending deterioration.
- Scoring tools are helpful, but should not be used in isolation. It is important to consider the whole patient, together with their social circumstances before discharge is considered.

See Chapters 7 and 36.

Case 2: Acutely painful red eye

1 The important differential diagnoses are:

(a) Acute angle-closure glaucoma (correct age, eye symptoms and headache).

(b) Migraine headache (all common except the eye pain).

(c) Acute iritis/scleritis/episcleritis (unilateral red, painful eye, with loss of vision).

(d) Foreign body in eye (unilateral red eye with blurred vision, history, e.g. metal grinding without goggles).

(e) Retinal detachment (floaters and visual loss).

(f) Giant cell (temporal) arteritis in a patient over 50 years old.

2 The findings would include altered (reduced) visual acuity, a red eye, a cloudy cornea, dilated or mid-sized pupil that is unreactive or less reactive. Measurement of the intraocular pressure would reveal raised intraocular pressure.

3 Management of acute angle-closure glaucoma includes immediate ophthalmological referral and commencement of intravenous acetazolamide. Analgesia and antiemetics may also be necessary.

4 If the loss of vision is painless, central retinal artery occlusion or central retinal vein occlusion is likely.

Learning point

- Exclude the important threats to vision first: in this patient, glaucoma and giant cell arteritis.

See Chapter 22.

Case 3: Arterial blood gas interpretation

1 Metabolic acidosis. The pH is low, which means the patient is acidotic. The PCO_2 is low, because the patient is hyperventilating to try to compensate for the acidosis (excess H^+ ions) by moving the equilibrium of this equation to the left by expelling CO_2 from the body.

$$H_2O + CO_2 \Leftrightarrow H^+ + HCO_3^-$$

This patient has a metabolic acidosis with partial respiratory compensation: partial because the patient is still acidotic despite the low PCO_2. Patients with exhaustion, coma or respiratory problems may lose the ability to compensate in this way.

2 The anion gap measures the gap between positively and negatively charged ions in plasma.

$$\text{Anion gap} = (Na^+ + K^+) - (Cl^- + HCO_3^-)$$
$$(135 + 4) - (105 + 6) = 33 \text{ mmol/L}$$

The normal value is approximately 8 mmol/L.

3 Given that this is a raised anion gap metabolic acidosis, the main differential diagnoses are diabetic ketoacidosis, lactic acidosis, and renal failure. Given that the patient is febrile, lactic acidosis may be caused by dehydration/shock/sepsis. This clinical presentation is also consistent with diabetic ketoacidosis. An urgent bedside glucose test is essential. The level of acidosis here means the patient is significantly unwell and needs urgent senior review. In this case the diagnosis is not yet clear; the glucose and lactate should be available as soon as possible.

4 (a) Respiratory alkalosis. The pH is high, which means the patient has an alkalosis. The PCO_2 is low, which means the patient has a respiratory alkalosis. This is most likely due to hyperventilation due to anxiety. However, patients may hyperventilate to maintain oxygenation. The respiratory assessment should focus on excluding physical causes.

(b) Respiratory acidosis. The pH is low, which means the patient has an acidosis. The PCO_2 is high, which means the patient has a respiratory acidosis. It is likely the patient has respiratory failure.

5 The PO_2 is too low for someone on 35% oxygen (approximately double the normal concentration) unless there is some lung pathology that may be causing a ventilation/perfusion mismatch or poor gas diffusion in the alveoli.

The A-a gradient

In room air (21% oxygen) at sea level and with a PCO_2 of 40 mmHg (5.3 kPa),[1] the expected alveolar partial pressure of oxygen is:

$$P(\text{Alveolar } O_2) = P(\text{inspired oxygen}) - P(\text{Alveolar } H_2O)$$
$$- P(\text{Alveolar } CO_2)$$

$$PA_{O_2} = Pi_{O_2} - PH_2O - \frac{Pa_{CO_2}}{R} \, [R = \text{respiratory quotient} - \text{approx } 0.8]$$

$$PA_{O_2} = \frac{21}{100} \times (760 - 47) - \frac{40}{0.8}$$

$$PA_{O_2} \approx 100 \, mmHg \, (13.3 \, kPa)$$

The A-a gradient is the difference between this and the measured value.

The upper limit for the A-a gradient should be

$$= \frac{Age}{4} + 4 \text{ (in mmHg)}$$

---

[1] (1 kPa = 7.5 mmHg)

Predicted PA_{O_2} (alveolar oxygen) $= (35/100) \times (760 - 47) - (21/0.8)$
$$= 0.35 \times 713 - 26$$
$$= 250 - 26 = 224 \text{ mmHg}$$

This gives an A-a gradient of 224–79 = 145 mmHg.
Normal A-a gradient should be Age/4 + 4 = 56/4 + 4 = 19 + 4 = 23 mmHg (3.0 kPa)

This means that there is a significant ventilation/perfusion mismatch or oxygen diffusion problem in the lung. Bearing in mind his recent immobility, pulmonary embolus or pneumonia should be suspected.

6 Inspired oxygen concentration should be increased to a target oxygen saturation of 91% and a senior doctor should review the patient. Reversible causes of respiratory failure such as asthma or pneumonia should be treated; there should be close monitoring in a high dependency unit with repeat ABGs.
See Chapter 7.

Case 4: Abdominal pain

1 Renal colic vs leaking abdominal aortic aneurysm (AAA). 'Renal colic' type flank pain in a patient over the age of 50 is a leaking AAA until proven otherwise. Right upper quadrant (biliary) pain or pleuritic pain involving the right lower chest can also present as flank pain.

2 In this context, the critical intervention is to rule in or rule out AAA as:

AAA + pain = ruptured AAA.

- Hypotension or a pulsatile/expansile mass implies AAA.
- Blood in urine makes renal colic more likely but does not rule out AAA.
- Bedside ultrasound performed by a trained Emergency Department doctor gives an instant definitive diagnosis as to the presence or absence of an AAA, but cannot confirm or deny leakage.

3 Bedside ultrasound is quick, and does not interrupt resuscitation and is the 'gold standard' of care. In stable patients, CT with intravenous contrast provides greater anatomic detail and can demonstrate AAA location, leakage and potential complications, e.g. involvement of renal or spinal arteries. This is helpful in planning surgery/stent placement, and also demonstrates other abdominal pathology that may be present.

4 If leaking AAA, minimal fluid volume resuscitation should be used. Site 2 × large-bore (14 G or 16 G) cannulae, but do not give fluid if the patient is verbally responsive. Notify surgeon or radiologist (if stenting) and anaesthetist. Discuss with blood bank to arrange 6 units of cross-matched/type-specific blood, and give analgesia. Perform baseline blood tests: FBC, U+E, LFTs.

5 A 4 mm stone will most likely pass without intervention, provided:
- the pain has resolved;
- there are no complications such as obstruction, infection or renal failure;
- there are no social reasons requiring inpatient admission.

The patient should be appropriate for discharge if pain-free, or pain is easily managed with oral analgesics and outpatient urology review. Discharge with medication such as NSAIDs or alpha blockers (e.g. tamsulosin) to reduce the number of episodes of ureteric spasm and improve patient comfort.

Learning points
- 'Renal colic' in a patient over 50 is AAA until proven otherwise.
- CT is the diagnostic investigation of choice for 'renal colic'.
See Chapters 3, 19 and 20.

Case 5: Chest pain

1 Differential diagnoses include:
(a) Acute coronary syndrome
  (i) Myocardial infarction, STEMI vs non-STEMI
  (ii) Unstable angina.
(b) Aortic dissection.
(c) Pulmonary embolism.
(d) Upper gastrointestinal tract causes.
(e) Musculoskeletal pain.
2 Start with supportive treatment first:
(a) MONA: morphine, oxygen, nitrate (GTN), aspirin ± intravenous morphine.

(b) ECG within 5 minutes, to detect STEMI or other condition requiring immediate treatment.

(c) Work up to consider if reperfusion therapy is appropriate.

3 Mortality is reduced by:

(a) Antiplatelet therapy. Aspirin alone gives a similar benefit to thrombolysis with minimal risk; ensure aspirin has been given unless there is a real contraindication. Previous mild gastrointestinal upset is not a reason to withhold aspirin.

(b) Reperfusion options include primary percutaneous coronary angioplasty or thrombolysis. Primary angioplasty is the gold standard, but in situations where this is not possible for more than 90 minutes, thrombolysis with clot-dissolving drugs should be considered.

4 Differential diagnoses include:

(a) Pneumothorax.

(b) Pneumonia.

(c) Pulmonary embolism.

(d) Musculoskeletal.

5 A chest X-ray would show a pneumothorax or pneumonia, so a normal chest X-ray effectively excludes these conditions. As this person has a low pre-test probability of pulmonary embolism, a negative d-dimer test could rule out thromboembolism. However, this may not be necessary, and a senior medical review may confirm that this person is most likely to have musculoskeletal pain, probably a result of a cracked rib. X-ray examinations of the ribs are not necessary, as seeing a fracture will not change management.

Learning points

• ECG is the key diagnostic triage tool for patients with chest pain.

• A patient who has presented with chest pain should never be discharged without a senior review. These patients are a frequent cause of litigation.

See Chapters 34 and 35.

Case 6: Bleed in early pregnancy

1 Ruptured ectopic pregnancy or cervical shock. Ruptured ectopic pregnancy is rare, but can bleed faster than blood can be replaced. Simple miscarriage (inevitable abortion) does not cause hypotension, unless complicated by clot in the cervix, 'cervical shock', causing profound vagal drive resulting in bradycardia and hypotension.

2 Notify senior Emergency Department staff and the gynaecology service. Large-bore intravenous access should be obtained, e.g. 2 × 16G cannulae. Intravenous fluid administration should be guided by patient status, not blood pressure. Fluid should not be given while the patient is responsive (e.g. is talking), but if necessary small bolus of crystalloid (e.g. 500 mL) should be given up to a maximum of 2 litres when blood (cross-matched, type-matched or group O negative) should be used. An urgent speculum examination will determine whether the cervical os is open or not. Removal of any products of conception or clot from the cervical os using sponge forceps will resolve cervical shock.

3 Send bloods for FBC, clotting and cross-match at least two units of blood. Arrange immediate transfer to the operating theatre and notify anaesthetic staff. Arrange a urinary catheter. Check the patient's blood group: if rhesus-negative the patient will require anti-D immunoglobulin.

4 Given there was a previous normal ultrasound and the uterus is now empty, miscarriage (inevitable abortion) is likely. However, the Emergency Department ultrasound and the results reported by the patient must be verified. Perform a speculum examination to check the state of the cervical os. Verify the previous ultrasound and βhCG results, arrange a formal ultrasound and refer to the gynaecology team. If the results from these tests are equivocal, the gynaecology team may use serial quantitative βhCGs on an outpatient basis to clarify the situation. In a normal pregnancy, βhCG levels double every 48 hours: falling or stagnant results means failed pregnancy. The patient's blood group should be checked: if rhesus negative, anti-D is not always necessary in complete abortion before 12 weeks. Outpatient review and counselling should be offered.

Learning points

• Ruptured ectopic pregnancy is a life-threatening emergency.

• Do not forget to check for Rhesus status in obstetric or gynaecological emergencies.

See Chapter 23.

Case 7: Head injury

1 From the history, head injury is highly likely to be the cause of this clinical picture. To hit one's head on the ground implies loss of normal protective reflexes, i.e. unconscious while falling and/or a high degree of force. A history of alcohol or drug consumption should not change the management as it is dangerous to assume that the reduced consciousness state is due to alcohol. Therefore the patient must be assumed to have a significant head injury.

2 Cervical spine injury: any patient with a head injury should be assumed to have a cervical spine injury. Other traumatic injuries are also possible, e.g. fractured ribs, facial trauma, dental, nose, etc., but the cervical spine must be protected to prevent damage to the cord by movement of an unstable vertebral column.

3 Call the trauma team to ensure adequate numbers and skills of staff. The main treatment priorities are:

(a) Airway: ensure patent and protected.

(b) Cervical spine immobilisation: rigid cervical collar.

(c) Breathing: avoid hypoxia in head-injured patients.

(d) Circulation: avoid hypotension in head-injured patients.

(e) Check glucose.

(f) Imaging: chest X-ray, pelvis X-ray, ultrasound.

4 After the primary survey, continue to assess the patient:

(a) Disability: assess Glasgow Coma Scale (GCS) score and pupils, carry out neurological examination, looking for focal deficits.

(b) Exposure: remove clothing and log roll the patient.

(c) Full secondary survey.

(d) Document injuries.

5 The patient's score on the GCS is 11.

(a) Confused speech = 4

(b) Eyes open to pain = 2

(c) Localising pain = 5

6 The patient's score on the GCS is 7.

(a) Incomprehensible sounds = 2

(b) Eyes closed = 1

(c) Withdraws from pain = 4

7 A falling GCS >2 points or absolute value <9 is a neurosurgical emergency. This patient needs urgent intubation while cervical

spine protection is maintained, and urgent head CT to detect bleeding or raised intracranial pressure.

Learning points
• It is essential to avoid hypoxia or hypoventilation in head-injured patients.
• Make sure you can calculate the GCS quickly and correctly.
See Chapters 8–11.

Case 8: Burns
1 DeMIST:
   • Demographics: age, gender.
   • Mechanism of injury: fire, fall, smoke inhalation, possible blast injury.
   • Injuries sustained: from initial assessment.
   • Symptoms and signs, including vital signs.
   • Treatment given.

A structured handover is important to ensure transmission of all relevant information. Performing handover in a standardised way minimises communication errors, which are common in stressful situations. The team leader should repeat the key points of the handover back to the ambulance crew so that all present are aware of these, and to check understanding. In addition, details from the AMPLE history may also be available.
   • Allergies.
   • Medications.
   • Previous medical problems.
   • Last ate or drank.
   • Environment: any hazards, e.g. chemical/heat/cold.

2 Call the trauma team to ensure adequate numbers and skills of staff.

(a) Airway: look for evidence of inhalational burns, carbon/soot in nostrils, facial burns and singed eyebrows/eyelashes/nostril hairs, oropharyngeal redness, swelling, or stridor. Facial and airway burns swell massively in the hours following a burn, and risk occluding the airway. Expert assessment and early prophylactic intubation are necessary to avoid this. This patient is unconscious (i.e. GCS 3), therefore unable to protect his own airway from aspiration of vomit, therefore would need intubation anyway.

(b) Cervical spine protection: this patient has probably had a fall and is unconscious so cannot protect their cervical spine, so a collar is necessary.

(c) Breathing: give 100% oxygen, look for chest trauma.

(d) Circulation: look for shock. While burns alone may cause shock, this patient has other potential causes of shock due to the trauma, so other injuries must be sought.

(e) Disability: assess consciousness state and GCS.

(f) Exposure. initially, cool the burn, then warm the patient.

(g) Analgesia, usually morphine (see below), may require large doses.

(h) Secondary survey to follow, and an estimation of percentage of BSA of the burn, which is needed to calculate fluid resuscitation requirements.

3 Things that can easily be overlooked in a resuscitation situation are:
   (a) Airway burns.
   (b) Major trauma, electrical injury, inhalational exposure to CO or cyanide.

(c) Forensic issues: good documentation is important, as the police will often require a report.

(d) Deliberate self-harm: if possible, consider paracetamol levels/toxicological testing.

4 Early analgesia includes cooling the burn (but not the patient), dressings (e.g. cling film) and intravenous opiate analgesia.

5 Early intravenous fluids to treat shock:

(a) 20 mL/kg of crystalloid as a bolus if shocked. For an adult this will mean 1–2 litres immediately. Large-bore intravenous access is necessary, and blood/blood products often necessary.

(b) Using the Parkland Hospital formula: 2–4 mL/kg crystalloid × % burn × bodyweight in kg over 24 hours, half given in first 8 hours. This is *in addition* to normal maintenance fluids. Example: 3 mL × 70 kg × 20% burns = 4200 mL per 24 hours, which means 2100 mL over 8 hours then the rest over 16 hours. However, resuscitation should be titrated to adequate circulation/perfusion and urine output, and central venous monitoring may be necessary.

6 Yes. Factors for admission/transfer to a specialist burns centre will depend on local arrangements and policies, but usual reasons to transfer a patient include:
   • Full thickness burns.
   • Partial thickness burns >10% [burned area, not simple erythema]; or
   • Burns involving areas that are difficult to nurse: face/neck, hands, feet, perineum/genitalia/axilla; or
   • Circumferential burns: may require incision (escharotomy) to prevent limb ischaemia or allow respiratory movements if chest wall burns.
   • Inhalational burns (intubate before transport).
   • Electrical or chemical injury.

Learning point
• Severe burns are thankfully rare, but require meticulous assessment and treatment to avoid complications. Pay particular attention to those points that are 'easy to overlook' (question 3 above). *See Chapters 8, 9 and 13.*

Case 9: Unconscious
1 Resuscitation: the unconscious patient should be assessed and managed using the standard 'airway, breathing, circulation' protocol. Never forget glucose: hypoglycaemia is an easily treatable cause of unconsciousness that can cause great damage if untreated. Head injury or intracranial pathology should be considered.

2 Toxidromes are collections of symptoms or signs associated with certain toxic drugs/toxins. This patient has an *anticholinergic toxidrome*: tachycardia, altered state of consciousness, dry skin, dilated pupils, urinary retention and reduced bowel sounds are features of this syndrome.

3 A tricyclic antidepressant (TCA) overdose (e.g. amitryptiline), the second most common cause of death due to poisoning in the UK. It is important to recognise the toxidrome because these patients often deteriorate quickly. Recreational drugs such as amphetamines can cause some of these symptoms (wide pupil and tachycardia), but not usually the dry skin, dry mouth and urinary retention. TCA poisoning causes sodium channel blockade giving cardiac and neurological effects. The patient is at risk of ventricular arrhythmias, fitting and coma. If there are signs of serious

toxicity and acidosis, sodium bicarbonate should be given through a large peripheral or central vein.

4 Paracetamol (acetaminophen) is the commonest cause of death from poisoning, and is usually asymptomatic until the patient goes into liver failure 3–5 days after the overdose. *N*-acetylcysteine should be given now, as with five empty packets, it is likely the patient has taken a toxic dose (>150 mg/kg), and there is no clear time of ingestion from which to plot a paracetamol level on the graph.

5 Activated charcoal appears helpful if given soon after ingestion (within 1–2 hours). The patient needs a protected airway (i.e. is alert and drinks it voluntarily, or is intubated). This patient has a reduced GCS, increasing the risk of aspiration and therefore activated charcoal should not be given.

Learning points
• A clear understanding and chronology of events surrounding presentation are often not apparent when a patient first attends the Emergency Department. Assessment and treatment must 'cover all the bases', and so overdose must be considered in this situation.
• Always test for paracetamol, as by the time overdose is symptomatic, it is too late.
See Chapters 24 and 25.

Case 10: Vomiting
1 Differential diagnoses:
• Infectious gastroenteritis: *Salmonella, E. coli, Shigella, Campylobacter* (usually >48 hours).
• Toxin-mediated food poisoning: *Clostridium, Staphylococcus aureus, Bacillus cereus*
• Infectious gastroenteritis: viral.
• Alcoholic gastritis.
• Inflammatory bowel disease (unlikely in two patients at same time).

2 Bedside test: blood glucose.
Laboratory tests:
• FBC, U+E and amylase, to detect an elevated white cell count, assess dehydration and rule out acute pancreatitis.
• Blood cultures if clinically septic.
• Stool sample microbiology and culture if suspected food poisoning, as these are generally notifiable diseases due to public health and safety issues.

3 The patient appears to have toxin-mediated food poisoning. Management is supportive with antiemetics such as metoclopramide or prochlorperazine, and intravenous saline to treat dehydration. Patients can usually be discharged home safely when tolerating oral fluids and oral antiemetics.

4 Patient B probably has a Mallory-Weiss tear as there is a history of vomiting followed by subsequent blood-streaked vomits. Blood in the first vomit is much less likely to be Mallory-Weiss tear. Check for symptoms of peptic ulcer disease or reflux oesophagitis, such as indigestion or burning epigastric pain.
Use the Glasgow-Blatchford score to identify patients at low risk of further problems. A patient who fulfils the following criteria can be discharged safely, providing the patient has the resources to re-attend hospital if required.
• Haemoglobin level >12.9 g/dL (men) or >11.9 g/dL (women).
• Systolic blood pressure >109 mmHg.

• Pulse <100 bpm.
• Blood urea level <6.5 mmol/L (blood urea nitrogen level <18.2 mg/dL).
• No melaena or syncope.
• No past or present liver disease or heart failure.

5 Patient C has had symptoms for 5 days. This means that food poisoning from the previous night is unlikely to be the cause. The absence of diarrhoea despite this duration of illness means that other causes should be considered, including pregnancy (morning sickness), urinary tract infection, Addison's disease and medication side-effect.

6 Normal hypothalamic/adrenal function is suppressed by more than 5 days of exogenous steroids. Steroids provide immunosuppression that makes a patient more vulnerable to disease, and also suppress the body's normal inflammatory response to disease, potentially masking more serious presentations, e.g. sepsis. If steroids cannot be absorbed, e.g. due to vomiting, sudden withdrawal occurs, which may precipitate an Addisonian crisis. As this presentation may include a combination of dehydration, vomiting and low blood pressure, it can easily be missed. A short synacthen test is easy to perform in the Emergency Department, and then intravenous saline and steroids should be given.

Learning point
• Although it is tempting to reassure and discharge such patients, one must be alert to other, more serious, diseases that may also present with such common symptoms. That said, one must also avoid over-investigating patients with minor illnesses presenting to the Emergency Department.
See Chapters 38 and 40.

Case 11: Weakness
1 The following investigations should be performed:
• Bedside: ECG, looking specifically for atrial fibrillation or ischaemic heart disease; and a fingerprick blood glucose test to exclude hypoglycaemia.
• Blood tests include FBC, U+E and clotting.
• Chest X-ray to detect cardiac or respiratory disease.
• CT head, carotid Doppler and echocardiogram need to be performed within 1 week, based on the clinical information given. The use of early CT for transient ischaemic attack (TIA) is used mainly to detect stroke mimics, most of which do not have full resolution of symptoms.

2 The ABCD^2 score accurately predicts the risk of short-term stroke. Patients with ABCD^2 score >4 or crescendo (increasing) symptoms are at high risk (5%) of further ischaemic events within the next week. These patients need urgent investigation to identify and correct reversible factors. This patient has ABCD^2 score of 3:
• Age >60 years = 0 points
• BP >140/90 mmHg = 1 point
• Clinical features unilateral weakness = 2 points
• Duration of symptoms <10 minutes = 0 points
• No diabetes = 0 points
A patient with an ABCD^2 score of 3 should be reviewed by a specialist within 1 week.

3 Stroke can be prevented by:
(a) Aspirin or other antiplatelet agents (give to all patients unless contraindicated).
(b) Suppression of atrial fibrillation.

(c) Anticoagulation if there is persistent or paroxysmal atrial fibrillation or cardiac failure.

(d) Carotid enderarterctemy if carotid stenosis >70%.

4 The ABCD^2 score is now 5, by adding 2 points for duration of symptoms longer than 60 minutes. The recurrence of symptoms so soon after the initial episode suggests crescendo symptoms. Both of these mean that the patient should be admitted for treatment and urgent investigation including carotid Doppler and echocardiogram.

5 If the patient's symptoms persist, the likely diagnosis is ischaemic stroke. The patient is potentially eligible for thrombolytic therapy if stroke is confirmed by clinical symptoms and absence of bleeding on CT, and if less than 3 hours from symptom onset. After establishing absence of contraindications and obtaining informed consent, thrombolysis is performed with an infusion of tissue plasminogen activator (tPA).

6 A number of conditions can mimic stroke:

(a) *Hypoglycaemia*, which *must* be excluded in all patients on arrival.

(b) Space-occupying lesions or intracranial pathology:

  (i) Intracerebral abscess

  (ii) Brain tumours (primary or secondary)

  (iii) Intracerebral haemorrhage, especially if coagulopathy/anticoagulation medication

  (iv) Subdural haematoma (especially falls in elderly/alcoholic patients).

(c) Temporal arteritis: tender temporal artery with visual disturbance.

(d) Infective endocarditis and septic emboli: any patient with fever, murmur and TIA. Intravenous drug users at particularly high risk. Look for splinter haemorrhages.

(e) Post-ictal states: transient hemiplegia ('Todd's palsy') is reasonably common. Patients need a CT scan if they have a focal neurological deficit, new-onset seizures, or seizures that are not typical for them.

Learning point

• Stroke is a major cause of disability, and early aggressive investigation and treatment can effectively prevent strokes.
See Chapter 42.

Case 12: Collapse

1 A previous diagnosis of seizures makes seizure more likely, especially if there has been medication change, poor compliance or poor sleep, all of which may precipitate a seizure. A witness description of loss of consciousness, with a history describing the tonic and then clonic phase of a seizure, followed by altered state of consciousness, and gradual return to normal is classical for seizures. Biting of the tongue and incontinence are common.

2 A past history of cardiac disease or cardiac medication should be sought. A family history of cardiac problems or sudden death is important. A prodrome that is brief or absent suggests an arrhythmia. Collapse occurring on exertion can suggest a cardiac cause such as hypertrophic obstructive cardiomyopathy (HOCM) or arrhythmia.

3 There is a short PR interval (<120 ms), and slurred upstroke of the QRS delta (from the shape of the Greek letter Δ) wave. This ECG appearance is caused by an abnormal electrical connection between the atria and ventricles. Premature activation of the ven-

tricles (the delta wave) occurs because the conduction is not subject to the normal electrical delay that occurs in the atrioventricular (AV) node, hence the short P-R interval.

4 This is an important ECG to recognise: although the patient is now asymptomatic, it is likely that he is having episodic tachyarrhythmias. Treatment includes drug therapy and referral for ablation to a cardiologist specialising in electrophysiology.

5 High-risk features in patients presenting with collapse suggest need for admission for cardiac monitoring and further investigation. These include:

(a) History of heart failure (an important predictor) or ischaemic cardiac disease.

(b) Syncope on exertion, breathlessness.

(c) Abnormal ECG: long QT intervals, short QT interval.

(d) Hypotension.

(e) Age > 65 years, comorbidities, lack of social support.

(f) Family history of sudden death.

(g) Haematocrit <30%.

Learning points

• Collapse with loss of consciousness is always serious.
• Collapse occurring in patients with evidence of cardiac disease, especially heart failure, is associated with much higher mortality.
See Chapter 30.

Case 13: Headache

1 Subarachnoid haemorrhage (SAH): this presentation is consistent with a herald/sentinel/warning bleed. Although SAH is rare in young people, diagnosis at this stage, before a catastrophic rupture, can be life-saving.

2 If SAH is suspected, a CT brain is mandatory. High-resolution (64-slice) CT scanners are nearly 100% sensitive for SAH in the first 12 hours after onset of symptoms. If CT is normal, lumbar puncture should be performed at least 12 hours after onset of symptoms to detect xanthochromia. Xanthochromia is caused by bilirubin, a blood breakdown product, in the CSF. If these results are equivocal, MR scanning may be performed, which may pick up evidence of bleeding up to 2 weeks after symptoms.

3 Migraine headache. Other possibilities include tension headache, glaucoma or giant cell arteritis. Other serious illnesses such as meningitis and intracranial space-occupying lesions should be considered, but are unlikely if the headache is in the same pattern as previous migrainous headaches.

4 CT brain is not necessary if the pattern of symptoms is the same as has occurred previously in this patient.

5 Pethidine (meperidine) is a very poor choice of analgesic drug for this situation. It is a lipid-soluble opiate with a short duration of action and pethidine has a high risk of causing dependence/addiction. Better choices for treatment of severe acute migraine would be metoclopramide, prochlorperazine or chlorpromazine together with generous amounts (2 litres) of intravenous fluids. Triptans, e.g. sumatriptan, block 5HT 1B/1D receptors and can be helpful, but are expensive and have higher rates of rebound headache than the other treatments described. The doctor treating this patient should advise their senior doctor in the Emergency Department, who can contact the patient's GP to help ensure that the patient does not become habituated to opiates.
See Chapter 41.

Index

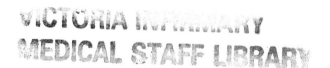

Keep up with critical fields

Would you like to receive up-to-date information on our books, journals and databases in the areas that interest you, direct to your mailbox?

Join the **Wiley e-mail service** - a convenient way to receive updates and exclusive discount offers on products from us.

Simply visit **www.wiley.com/email** and register online

We won't bombard you with emails and we'll only email you with information that's relevant to you. We will ALWAYS respect your e-mail privacy and NEVER sell, rent, or exchange your e-mail address to any outside company. Full details on our privacy policy can be found online.

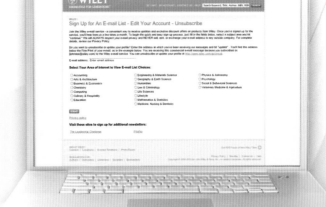

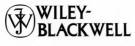
www.wiley.com/email

17841

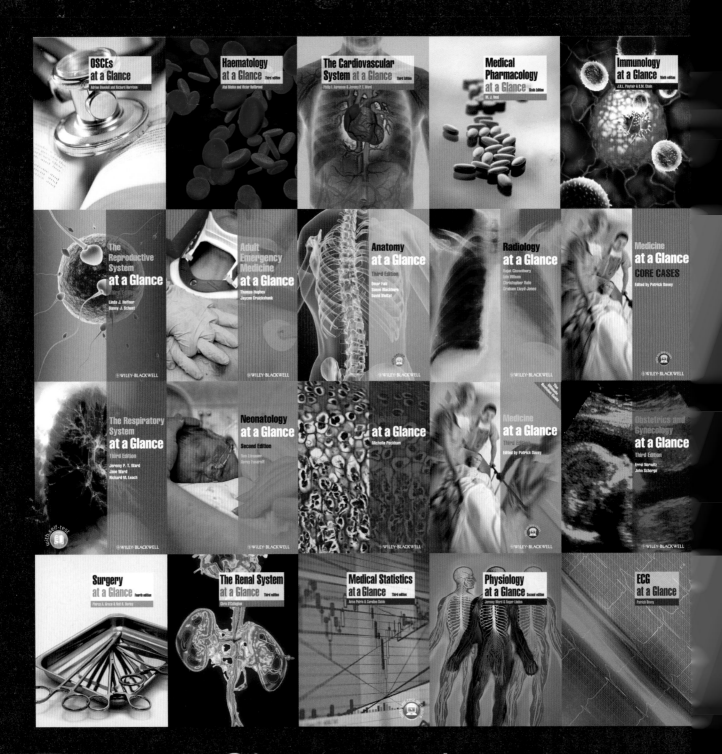
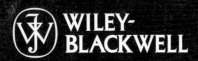

Cambridge IGCSE®

Modern World History

Option B: The 20th century

Cambridge IGCSE®

Modern World History

Option B: The 20th century

BEN WALSH

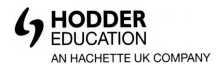

HODDER EDUCATION
AN HACHETTE UK COMPANY

® IGCSE is the registered trademark of Cambridge International Examinations.

The author and publisher would like to thank Mike Scott-Baumann and Terry Fiehn for their valuable contributions.

Every effort has been made to establish copyright and contact copyright holders prior to publication. If contacted, the publisher will be pleased to rectify any omissions or errors at the earliest opportunity.

Although every effort has been made to ensure that website addresses are correct at time of going to press, Hodder Education cannot be held responsible for the content of any website mentioned in this book. It is sometimes possible to find a relocated web page by typing in the address of the home page for a website in the URL window of your browser.

Hachette UK's policy is to use papers that are natural, renewable and recyclable products and made from wood grown in sustainable forests. The logging and manufacturing processes are expected to conform to the environmental regulations of the country of origin.

Orders: please contact Bookpoint Ltd, 130 Milton Park, Abingdon, Oxon OX14 4SB. Telephone: +44 (0)1235 827720. Fax: +44 (0)1235 400454. Lines are open 9.00–5.00, Monday to Saturday, with a 24-hour message answering service. Visit our website at www.hoddereducation.co.uk

©Ben Walsh 1996, 2001, 2009, 2013
This IGCSE edition first published in 2013 by
Hodder Education,
An Hachette UK Company
Carmelite House, 50 Victoria Embankment,
London EC4Y 0DZ

First edition published in 1996
Second edition published in 2001
Third edition published in 2009

Impression number   9
Year   2017

Cover photo © toa555–Fotolia
Illustrations by Oxford Designers & Illustrators and DC Graphic Design Ltd
Typeset in Garamond Light Condensed 10.5pt by DC Graphic Design Ltd
Printed in India

A catalogue record for this title is available from the British Library.

ISBN: 978 1 4441 6442 8

Also available:
- *GCSE Modern World History 1 International Relations Dynamic Learning* 978 1 4441 1760 8
- *GCSE Modern World History 2 Depth Studies Dynamic Learning* 978 1 4441 1777 6
- *GCSE Modern World History 3 Twentieth Century British History Dynamic Learning* 978 1 4441 1778 3

CONTENTS

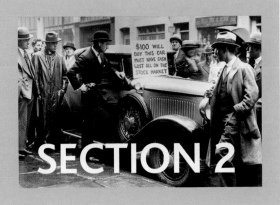

SOURCE 1

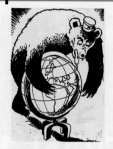

An American cartoon commenting on Stalin's take-over of eastern Europe. The bear represents the USSR.

Factfile

The League of Nations
➤ The League's home was in Geneva in Switzerland.
➤ Despite it being the brainchild of the US President, the USA was never a member of the League.

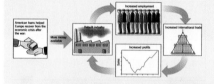

Think!

Revision Tip

Keywords

Chapter Summary

A) It will help you to learn the content

Is your main worry when you prepare for an exam that you won't know enough to answer the questions? Many people feel that way and it is true that there is a lot to learn in Cambridge IGCSE History. This book covers the Option B 20th century route for the Cambridge IGCSE syllabus. You will need good knowledge of the main events and the detail. This book will help you acquire both.

The **author text** explains all the key content clearly and comprehensively. But it does not just drone on about one thing after another. It helps you understand and investigate issues and establish links and relationships between topics.

It's full of brilliant **sources**. History is at its best when you can see what real people said, did, wrote, sang, watched on film, laughed about, cried over, and got upset about. Sources can really help you to understand the story better and remember it because they help you to see the big concepts and ideas in terms of what they meant to individuals at the time.

The **Factfiles** (key events) and **Profiles** (key people) are packed with hard facts and examples to use in your own work to support your arguments.

We use lots of **diagrams** and **timelines**. These help you to visualise, understand and remember topics. We also encourage you to draw your own diagrams – that is an even better way to learn.

For each topic there is a Focus Task (see opposite) that helps you organise the content. Many of the Focus Tasks deal with quite big issues that you will find easier if you have thought things through beforehand. So the **Think!** feature is designed to prepare you for the Focus Tasks. Sometimes they are literally steps en route to a Focus Task as in Chapter 4; at other times they simply ask you to think about an issue that is particularly important for understanding the period better.

There are **Revision Tips**. If the content seems overwhelming to you and you just don't know where to start this gives you an achievable target – just a couple of key points on each topic to identify and remember. Think of it as a 'First Aid' kit.

Keywords. Every subject and topic has its own vocabulary. If you don't know what these words mean you won't be able to write about the subject. So for each chapter we have provided a keyword list. These are the kind of words or terms that could be used in sources or an exam question without any explanation so you need to be able to understand them and use them confidently in your writing. They are all defined in the **glossary** on page 320. But we also want you to create your own keyword list – in a notebook or on your phone, write down each word with your own definitions.

Finally there is a content **Summary** at the end of every chapter or Key Question. This condenses all the content into a few points, which should help you to get your bearings in even the most complicated content.

B) It will help you to apply what you learn

The second big aim of this book is to help you to work with the content and think about it so that you are ready to apply what you learn. This is not an easy task. You will not suddenly develop this skill. You need to practise studying an issue, deciding what you think, and then selecting from all that you know the points that are really relevant to your argument.

The main way we help you with this is through the **Focus Tasks**

The title is a **Focus Point** or Key Question from the Cambridge IGCSE syllabus. Every Focus Point has its own Focus Task.

Often we ask you to create a comparative or a summary **chart or timeline** as in this example. The completed chart will also be perfect for revision purposes.

They help you to **apply your knowledge**. One of the most important skills in history is the ability to select, organise and deploy (use) knowledge to answer a particular question.

The structure of the task helps you to **focus on what is important** and ignore what is not. There are bullet points or charts to help you to **organise** your thinking.

Focus Task

How did the Bolsheviks consolidate their rule?

It is January 1924. Lenin is dead. Your task is to look back at the measures he used to consolidate Bolshevik rule.

1 Draw a timeline from 1917 to 1924, and mark on it the events of that period mentioned in the text.
2 Mark on the timeline:
   a) one moment at which you think Bolshevik rule was most threatened
   b) one moment at which you think it was most secure.
3 Write an explanation of how the Bolsheviks made their rule more secure. Mention the following:
   ♦ the power of the Red Army
   ♦ treatment of opposition
   ♦ War Communism
   ♦ the New Economic Policy
   ♦ the Treaty of Brest-Litovsk
   ♦ the victory in the Civil War
   ♦ the promise of a new society
   ♦ propaganda.

Revision Tip

And remember, to help you further, most Focus Tasks have a linked **Revision Tip** that gives you a more basic target – just a couple of key points that you will be able to apply in your answers.

C) It helps you prepare for your examination

If you read all the text and tackled all the Focus Tasks in this book we are sure you would also find you were well prepared for the challenges of the exam, but you will probably also want something more exam-focused – you will want to see the kind of questions you will face in an exam and how you might go about answering them. So:

Exam focus

Exam Focus appears on page 168 (for the core content) and page 316 (for the depth studies). These pages take you step by step through the exam requirements for Paper 1 and Paper 2, and show you the kinds of questions you might be asked. We also analyse and comment on some sample answers that help you to see what a good answer might look like. Components 3 and 4 are covered on page 319.

Exam Practice

Exam practice. At the end of every chapter there are some exam-style questions for you to practise. And in the Exam Focus sections there are plenty more examples of structured essays like in Paper 1 and questions on prescribed topics with sources and information like in Paper 2.

Source Analysis ▶

Source Analysis. Sources are an integral part of history. Historians use them to write history. We have used them to add colour and human detail to the stories of Modern World History. In Paper 2 of Cambridge IGCSE History you will also have to use sources to examine an issue when you will need to evaluate sources. So dotted throughout this book are Source Analysis questions that help you to evaluate sources – for example, thinking about their message, their purpose or their usefulness for a particular line of enquiry.

Text acknowledgements

Acknowledgements Laszlo Beke: extracts from *A Student's Diary: Budapest October 16 - November 1, 1956* (Hutchinson, 1957); Countee Cullen: 'For A Lady I Know' from *On These I Stand: An Anthology of the Best Poems of Countee Cullen* (Harper & Bros., 1947), copyrights held by Amistad Research Center, Tulane University, Administered by Thompson and Thompson; Adolf Hitler: extracts from *Mein Kampf*, translated by Ralph Manheim (Hutchinson, 1969), reproduced by permission of The Random House Group UK; Victor Klemperer: diary entries from *I Shall Bear Witness: The Diaries of Victor Klemperer, 1931-1941, Vol.1* (Phoenix, 1999), translation copyright © 1998 Martin Chalmers.

Every effort has been made to secure copyright permission prior to publication. If contacted, the publisher will be pleased to make any necessary revisions at the earliest opportunity.

Page 47, Source 12: the original caption was 'KEEPING HER GOING' *Doctors Eden and Delbos*. "I'm afraid her constitution isn't all it should be, but we mustn't give up hope yet."

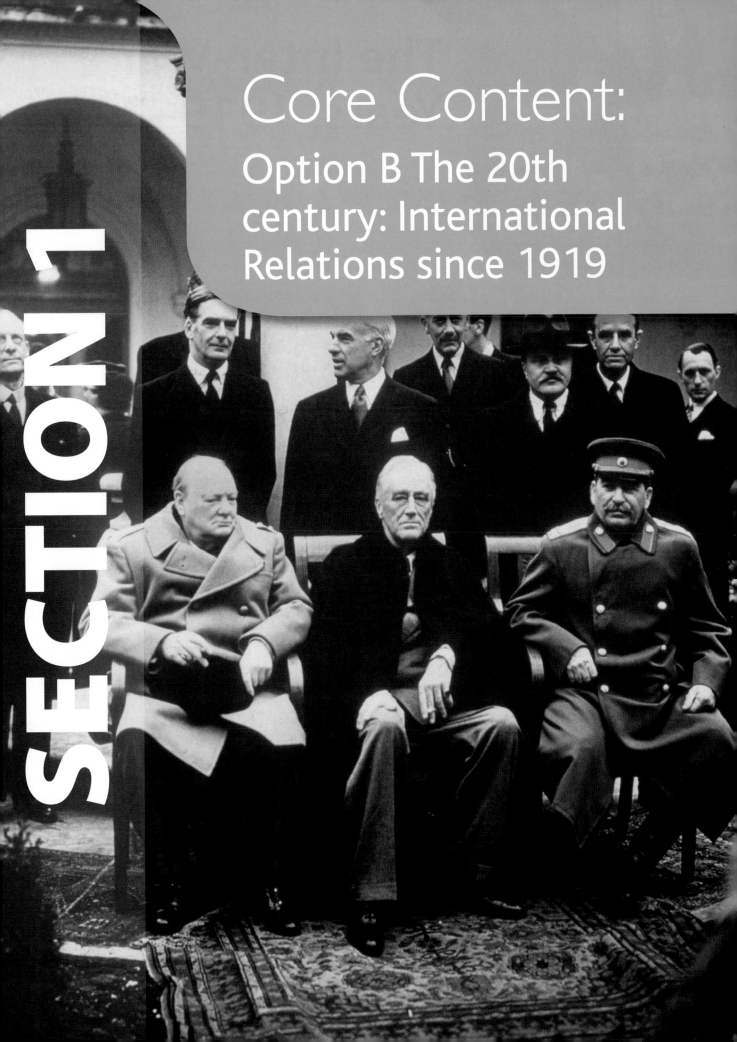

SECTION 1

Core Content:
Option B The 20th
century: International
Relations since 1919

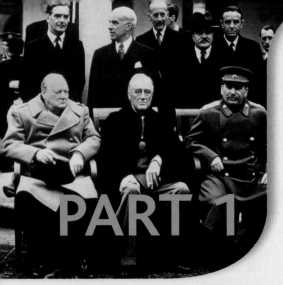

The Inter-War Years, 1919–39

PART 1

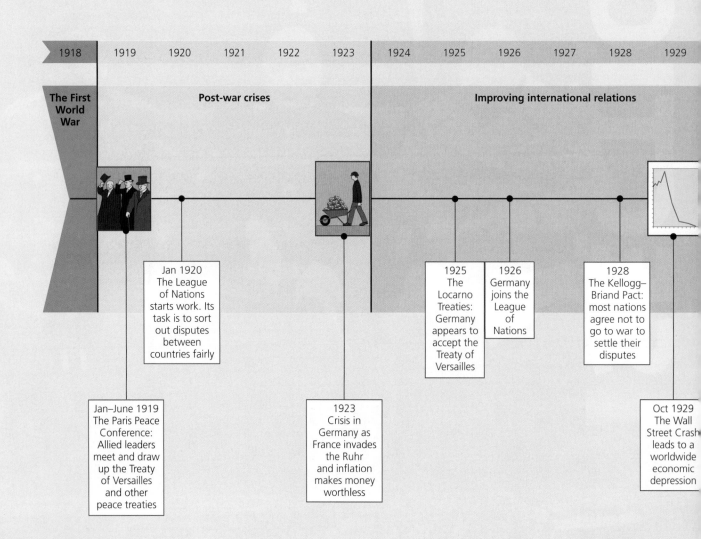

| 1918 | 1919 | 1920 | 1921 | 1922 | 1923 | 1924 | 1925 | 1926 | 1927 | 1928 | 1929 |

The First World War

Post-war crises

Improving international relations

Jan 1920
The League of Nations starts work. Its task is to sort out disputes between countries fairly

1925
The Locarno Treaties: Germany appears to accept the Treaty of Versailles

1926
Germany joins the League of Nations

1928
The Kellogg–Briand Pact: most nations agree not to go to war to settle their disputes

Jan–June 1919
The Paris Peace Conference: Allied leaders meet and draw up the Treaty of Versailles and other peace treaties

1923
Crisis in Germany as France invades the Ruhr and inflation makes money worthless

Oct 1929
The Wall Street Crash leads to a worldwide economic depression

Focus

Chapters 1–3 of this book cover a turbulent period of European history. After the trauma of the First World War, citizens of European countries were hoping for peace, prosperity and calm. Instead they got revolutions, economic depression, international disputes, dictatorships, and in the end a Second World War. How did this happen?

In Part 1:

♦ You will examine the peace treaties at the end of the First World War and consider whether they were fair (Chapter 1). Some would say that the peace treaties created problems for the future; others that they were the fairest they could have been given the very difficult situation after the First World War.

♦ The League of Nations was set up in 1920 to prevent war between countries. In Chapter 2 you will evaluate its successes (it did have many) and its failures (which tend to be remembered rather more than the successes) and reach your own view on how we should remember the League – as a success or a failure or something between.

♦ Finally in Chapter 3 you will examine the events of the 1930s which finally tipped Europe back into war. It is common to blame Hitler and his foreign policy for this slide to war but this chapter will help you to reach a balanced view that sees what other factors played a part.

The events in these chapters overlap in time. The timeline below gives you an overview of the main events you will be studying. It would be helpful if you made your own copy and added your own notes to it as you study.

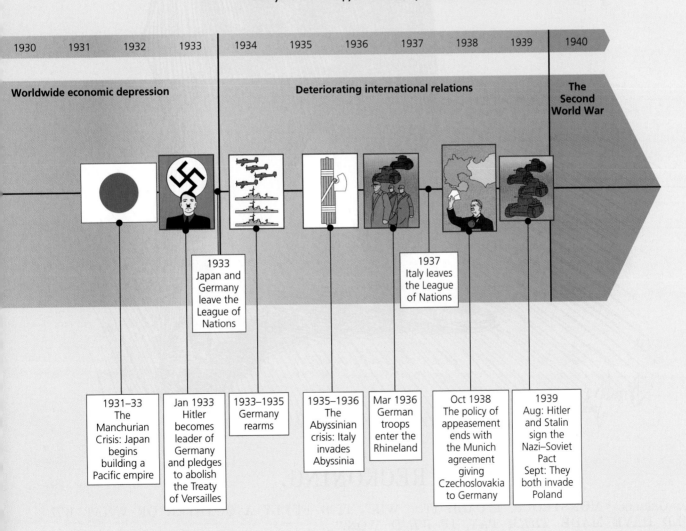

| 1930 | 1931 | 1932 | 1933 | 1934 | 1935 | 1936 | 1937 | 1938 | 1939 | 1940 |

Worldwide economic depression

Deteriorating international relations

The Second World War

1933 Japan and Germany leave the League of Nations

1937 Italy leaves the League of Nations

1931–33 The Manchurian Crisis: Japan begins building a Pacific empire

Jan 1933 Hitler becomes leader of Germany and pledges to abolish the Treaty of Versailles

1933–1935 Germany rearms

1935–1936 The Abyssinian crisis: Italy invades Abyssinia

Mar 1936 German troops enter the Rhineland

Oct 1938 The policy of appeasement ends with the Munich agreement giving Czechoslovakia to Germany

1939 Aug: Hitler and Stalin sign the Nazi–Soviet Pact Sept: They both invade Poland

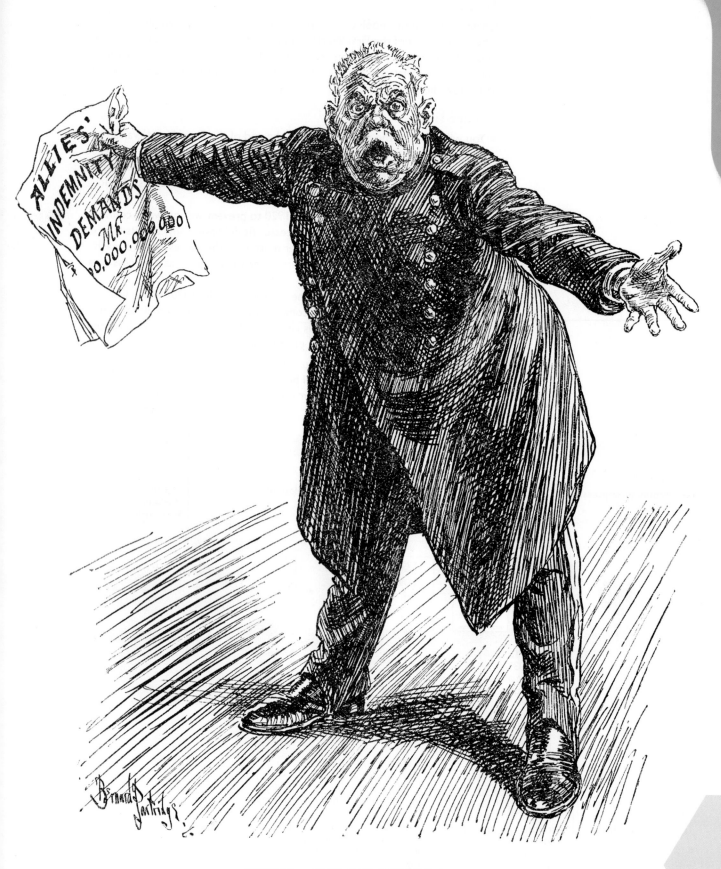

THE RECKONING.

PAN-GERMAN. "MONSTROUS, I CALL IT. WHY, IT'S FULLY A QUARTER OF WHAT *WE* SHOULD HAVE MADE *THEM* PAY, IF *WE'D* WON."

1 Were the peace treaties of 1919–23 fair?

FOCUS POINTS

- What were the motives and aims of the Big Three at Versailles?
- Why did all the victors not get everything they wanted?
- What was the impact of the peace treaty on Germany up to 1923?
- Could the treaties be justified at the time?

However long or violent a war is, eventually the opposing sides must make peace. But because war is destructive and leaves a bitter legacy, the peacemaking after a long conflict can be the hardest job of all.

The people who had that role in 1919 had a particularly hard task. The First World War involved more countries, using more powerful weapons, causing greater casualties and physical destruction, than any war before it. The war had bankrupted some countries. It led to revolutions in others. There was bitterness and resentment.

In this post-war atmosphere almost everyone agreed that part of the job of the peacemakers was to avoid another war like it – but no one agreed how to do that.

Any treaty is a balancing act. The peacemakers have to keep the victors happy but ensure that the defeated country accepts the terms of the peace. Was it really possible to produce a treaty which all sides would have seen as fair? That's the key question you will have to think about in this chapter.

You are going to investigate what happened when these peacemakers got together to draw up the peace treaties.

You will focus on

- what the peacemakers were hoping to achieve
- how they worked
- what they decided
- why they decided it.

Then you will reach conclusions about the key question – how 'fair' were the treaties they came up with, which means thinking about:

- whether people at the time thought the treaties were fair, and why or why not
- whether historians (with the benefit of hindsight) think they were fair.

And remember...

the peace process was not just about Germany. Between 1919 and 1923 the peacemakers drew up four treaties (one for each of the defeated powers) although in this chapter you are going to focus most on the Treaty which dealt with Germany: the Treaty of Versailles.

◄ This British cartoon was published in 1919 shortly after the terms of the Treaty of Versailles had been announced. A German man is holding the treaty terms saying that Germany has to pay for the damage caused by the war.

1 Does he think the Treaty is fair? Why or why not?
2 Does the cartoonist think the Treaty is fair? Why or why not?
3 What is the message of this cartoon?

**Woodrow Wilson
(President of the USA)**

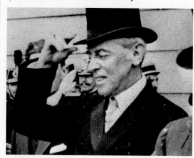

Background

♦ Born 1856.
♦ Became a university professor.
♦ First entered politics in 1910.
♦ Became President in 1912 and was re-elected in 1916.
♦ From 1914 to 1917 he concentrated on keeping the USA out of the war.
♦ Once the USA had joined the war in 1917, he drew up the **Fourteen Points** as the basis for ending the war fairly, so that future wars could be avoided.

Character

♦ An idealist and a reformer.
♦ As President, he had campaigned against corruption in politics and business. However, he had a poor record with regard to the rights of African Americans.
♦ He was obstinate. Once he made his mind up on an issue he was almost impossible to shift.

High hopes for peace

Looking back it may seem that the peacemakers in 1919 had an impossible job. But that is not how people saw it at the time. There was great optimism. One of the main reasons for these high hopes was the American President Woodrow Wilson.

In 1918 Wilson made a speech outlining **Fourteen Points** (see Factfile), which were to be the guidelines for a just and lasting peace treaty to end conflict.

When he arrived in Europe for the Paris Peace Conference, Wilson was seen almost as a saintly figure. Newspaper reports described wounded soldiers in Italy trying to kiss the hem of his cloak and in France peasant families kneeling to pray as his train passed by.

Wilson's ideas

How did Wilson think the peacemakers could build a better and more peaceful world?

● **Don't be too harsh on Germany.** Wilson did believe Germany should be punished. But he also believed that if Germany was treated harshly, some day it would recover and want revenge. He was also concerned that extremist groups, especially communists, might exploit Germans' resentment and communists might even seize power in Germany as they had in Russia in 1917.

● **Strengthen democracy in defeated countries.** For Wilson the key to peace in Europe was to strengthen democracy in the defeated nations so that their people would not let their leaders cause another war.

● **Give self-determination to small countries that had once been part of the European empires.** He wanted the different peoples of eastern Europe (for example, Poles, Czechs and Slovaks) to rule themselves rather than be part of Austria–Hungary's empire.

● **International co-operation.** Wilson also believed that nations should co-operate to achieve world peace. This would be achieved through a 'League of Nations'. Wilson believed this was the most important of his Fourteen Points.

You can see from these principles that Wilson was an idealist. However he was not a politician who could be pushed around. For example, he refused to cancel the debts owed to the USA by Britain and its Allies so that he could put pressure on them to accept his ideas.

Focus Task

What were the motives and aims of the Big Three at Versailles?

Using the information and sources on pages 6–9, fill out a chart like the one below summarising the aims of the three leaders at the Paris Peace Conference. Leave the fifth column blank. You will need it for a later task.

Leader	Country	Attitude towards Germany	Main aim(s)	
Wilson				
Lloyd George				
Clemenceau				

Revision Tip

Your completed chart should be perfect for revision on this topic. The basic requirement is to be sure you can name:

♦ each of the Big Three
♦ one priority for each of them at the peace talks
♦ two issues that they disagreed about.

SOURCE **1**

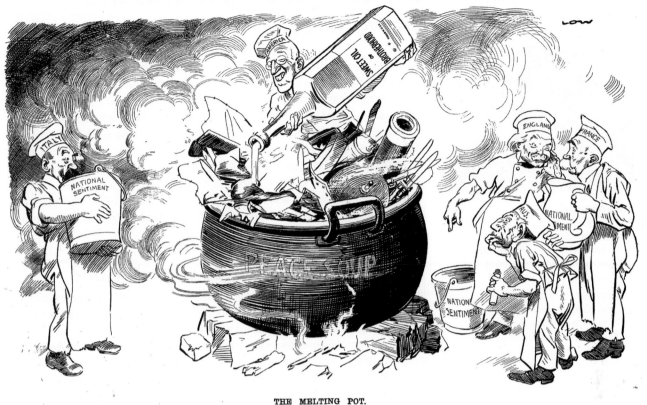

THE MELTING POT.

A cartoon published in 1919 in an Australian newspaper.

Source Analysis ▲

1 Study the main features of Source 1. Who is making the soup? Who is helping him? What are they adding to the mix? What is already in there?

2 Would you say Source 2 is optimistic about the prospects for peace? Make sure you can explain your answer by referring to specific features of the cartoon.

Factfile

THE FOURTEEN POINTS
(a summary)

1 No secret treaties.
2 Free access to the seas in peacetime or wartime.
3 Free trade between countries.
4 All countries to work towards disarmament.
5 Colonies to have a say in their own future.
6 German troops to leave Russia.
7 Independence for Belgium.
8 France to regain Alsace–Lorraine.
9 Frontier between Austria and Italy to be adjusted.
10 Self-determination for the peoples of eastern Europe (they should rule themselves and not be ruled by empires).
11 Serbia to have access to the sea.
12 Self-determination for the people in the Turkish empire.
13 Poland to become an independent state with access to the sea.
14 League of Nations to be set up.

Factfile

The Paris Peace Conference, 1919–20

➤ The Conference took place in the Palace of Versailles (a short distance from Paris).
➤ It lasted for twelve months.
➤ Thirty-two nations were supposed to be represented, but no one from the defeated countries was invited.
➤ Five treaties were drawn up at the Conference. The main one was the Treaty of Versailles, which dealt with Germany. The other treaties dealt with Germany's allies (see Factfile on page 19).
➤ All of the important decisions on the fate of Germany were taken by Clemenceau (Prime Minister of France), Lloyd George (Prime Minister of Britain) and Wilson (President of the USA) who together were known as 'The Big Three'.
➤ The Big Three were supported by a huge army of diplomats and expert advisers, but the Big Three often ignored their advice.

Profile

David Lloyd George
(Prime Minister of Britain)

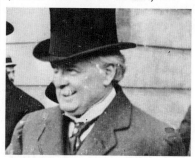

Background
➤ Born 1863.
➤ First entered politics in 1890.
➤ He was a very able politician who became Prime Minister in 1916 and remained in power until 1922.

Character
A realist. As an experienced politician, he knew there would have to be compromise. Thus he occupied the middle ground between the views of Wilson and Clemenceau.

Did everyone share Wilson's viewpoint?

Not surprisingly, when Wilson talked about lasting peace and justice other leaders agreed with him. After all, who would want to stand up in public and say they were *against* a just and lasting peace?!

However, many were doubtful about Wilson's ideas for achieving it. For example 'self-determination': it would be very difficult to give the peoples of eastern Europe the opportunity to rule themselves because they were scattered across many countries. Some people were bound to end up being ruled by people from another group with different customs and a different language. Some historians have pointed out that while Wilson talked a great deal about eastern and central Europe, he did not actually know very much about the area.

There were other concerns as well. So let's look at the aims and views of the other leaders at the Paris Peace Conference: David Lloyd George (from Britain) and Georges Clemenceau (from France).

Did Lloyd George agree with Wilson?

In public Lloyd George praised Wilson and his ideas. However, in private he was less positive. He complained to one of his officials that Wilson came to Paris like a missionary to rescue the European savages with his little sermons and lectures.

He agreed with Wilson on many issues, particularly that Germany should be punished but not too harshly. He did not want Germany to seek revenge in the future and possibly start another war.

Like Wilson he was deeply concerned that a harsh treaty might lead to a communist revolution like the one in Russia in 1917. He also wanted Britain and Germany to begin trading with each other again. Before the war, Germany had been Britain's second largest trading partner. British people might not like it, but the fact was that trade with Germany meant jobs in Britain.

However, unlike Wilson, Lloyd George had the needs of the British empire in mind. He wanted Germany to lose its navy and its colonies because they threatened the British empire.

SOURCE 2

We want a peace which will be just, but not vindictive. We want a stern peace because the occasion demands it, but the severity must be designed, not for vengeance, but for justice. Above all, we want to protect the future against a repetition of the horrors of this war.

Lloyd George speaking to the House of Commons before the Peace Conference.

SOURCE 3

If I am elected, Germany is going to pay . . . I have personally no doubt we will get everything that you can squeeze out of a lemon, and a bit more. I propose that every bit of [German-owned] property, movable and immovable, in Allied and neutral countries, whether State property or private property, should be surrendered by the Germans.

Sir Eric Geddes, a government minister, speaking to a rally in the general election campaign, December 1918.

Source Analysis ▲

1 In what ways are Sources 2 and 3 different?
2 Are there any ways in which they are similar?

Profile

Georges Clemenceau
(Prime Minister of France)

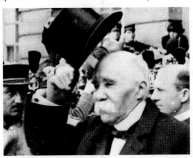

Background

➤ Born 1841 (he was aged 77 when the Paris Conference began).
➤ First entered French politics in 1871.
➤ Was Prime Minister of France from 1906 to 1909.
➤ From 1914 to 1917 he was very critical of the French war leaders. In November 1917 he was elected to lead France through the last year of the war.

Character

A hard, tough politician with a reputation for being uncompromising. He had seen his country invaded twice by the Germans, in 1870 and in 1914. He was determined not to allow such devastation ever again.

Pressures on Lloyd George

Lloyd George faced huge public pressures at home for a harsh treaty (see Source 2). People in Britain were not sympathetic to Germany in any way. They had suffered over 1 million casualties in the fighting as well as food shortages and other hardships at home. They had been fed anti-German propaganda for four years. They had also seen how Germany had treated Russia in 1918 when Russia surrendered. Under the Treaty of Brest-Litovsk Germany had stripped Russia of 25 per cent of its population and huge areas of Russia's best agricultural land.

Lloyd George had just won the 1918 election in Britain by promising to 'make Germany pay', even though he realised the dangers of this course of action. So Lloyd George had to balance these pressures at home with his desire not to leave Germany wanting revenge.

Think!

One of the ideas put forward at the Paris Conference was that Germany should lose some of its key industrial areas. How would you expect Lloyd George to react to a proposal like this? You could present your answer as a short speech by Lloyd George or in a paragraph of text.

Did Clemenceau agree with Wilson?

In public, Clemenceau of course agreed with Wilson's aim for a fair and lasting peace. However, he found Wilson very hard to work with. While he did not publicly criticise the Fourteen Points, Clemenceau once pointed out that even God had only needed Ten Commandments!

The major disagreement was over Germany. Clemenceau and other French leaders saw the Treaty as an opportunity to cripple Germany so that it could not attack France again.

Pressures on Clemenceau

France had suffered enormous damage to its land, industry, people – and self-confidence. Over two-thirds of the men who had served in the French army had been killed or injured. The war affected almost an entire generation.

By comparison, Germany seemed to many French people as powerful and threatening as ever. German land and industry had not been as badly damaged as France's. France's population (around 40 million) was in decline compared to Germany's (around 75 million).

The French people wanted a treaty that would punish Germany and weaken it as much as possible. The French President (Poincaré) even wanted Germany broken up into a collection of smaller states, but Clemenceau knew that the British and Americans would not agree to this.

Clemenceau was a realist and knew he would probably be forced to compromise on some issues. However, he had to show he was aware of public opinion in France.

Think!

Here are some extracts from the demands made by France before the Peace Conference started:
  a) German armed forces to be banned from the bank of the River Rhine (which bordered France).
  b) Germany to pay compensation for damage done by German forces in lands they occupied during the war.
  c) Germany's armed forces to be severely limited.
Which of these terms do you think made it into the final Treaty? Give each term a percentage chance and keep a note of your guesses. You will find out if you were right later in the chapter.

How did the peace-making process actually work?

In theory, the major issues like borders and reparations (compensation for war damage) were discussed in detail by all the delegates at the conference (see Source 4) – over 32 leaders with all their officials and advisers! As Source 5 shows, it quickly became impossible to consult everyone.

SOURCE 4

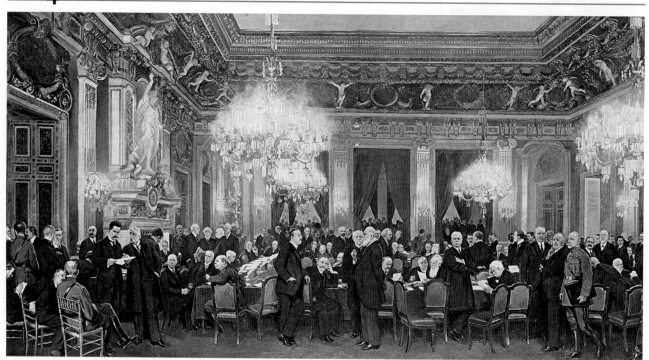

An official painting showing the delegates at the Paris Peace Conference at work.

SOURCE 5

'Wilson the Just' quickly disappointed expectations. Everything about him served to disillusion those he dealt with. All too soon the President was qualifying the Fourteen Points with 'Four Principles' and modifying them with 'Five Particulars'. Finding that one principle conflicted with another, he made compromising declarations about both. The Big Three abandoned Wilson's principle of open covenants openly arrived at, consulting others only when they needed expert advice. They were occasionally to be seen crawling round their maps on the hearth rug. Sometimes they agreed and, according to one British official 'were so pleased with themselves for doing so that they quite forgot to tell anyone what the agreement was'. Sometimes they almost came to blows. Lloyd George made rapid, quick fire points but they were ineffective against Clemenceau's granite obstinacy. Even Wilson's self-important confidence crashed against the rock of Clemenceau ... Clemenceau was delighted when the American President fell ill. He suggested that Lloyd George should bribe Wilson's doctor to make the illness last.

Historian Piers Brendon writing in 2006.

It soon became clear it would be impossible to agree terms that everyone would agree about.

- **Clemenceau clashed with Wilson over many issues**. The USA had not suffered nearly as badly as France in the war. Clemenceau resented Wilson's more generous attitude to Germany. They disagreed over what to do about Germany's Rhineland and coalfields in the Saar. In the end, Wilson had to give way on these issues. In return, Clemenceau and Lloyd George did give Wilson what he wanted in eastern Europe, despite their reservations about his idea of self-determination. However, this mainly affected the other four treaties, not the Treaty of Versailles.

- **Clemenceau also clashed with Lloyd George**, particularly over Lloyd George's desire not to treat Germany too harshly. For example, Clemenceau said that 'if the British are so anxious to appease Germany they should look overseas and make colonial, naval or commercial concessions'. Clemenceau felt that the British were quite happy to treat Germany fairly in Europe, where France rather than Britain was most under threat. However, they were less happy to allow Germany to keep its navy and colonies, which would be more of a threat to Britain.

- **Wilson and Lloyd George did not always agree either**. Lloyd George was particularly unhappy with point 2 of the Fourteen Points, allowing all nations access to the seas. Similarly, Wilson's views on people ruling themselves were somewhat threatening to the British government, for the British empire ruled millions of people all across the world from London.

Think!

Who said what about whom?

Here are some statements that were made by the Big Three at the Paris Peace Conference. Your task is to decide which leader made the statement and also who he was talking about. You will need to be able to explain your answer.

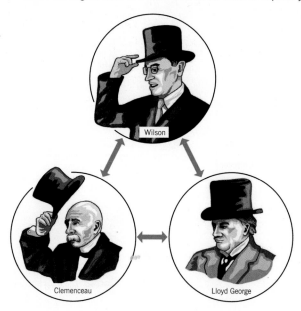

a) He is too anxious to preserve his empire to want self-determination for colonies.

b) His country has been ruling the waves for too long to accept the need for freedom of the seas.

c) He wants to wreck a country which in a few years could be a valuable trading partner and a source of vital jobs.

d) Freedom of the seas is all very well but who or what will protect my country's ships and trade?

e) What does he know about colonies and how they should be ruled? He probably doesn't know where most of them are!

f) How can I work with a man who thinks he is the first leader in 2000 years who knows anything about peace?

g) If he is so anxious to make concessions to the Germans then they should look overseas and make naval or colonial concessions.

h) He is stuck in the past. If he gets his way Germany will be left bitter and vengeful and there will be another war in a few years.

i) He is very happy to give concessions to Germany in areas which do not threaten his country.

j) If you carry on annoying me I am going to punch you!

k) There are new, better ways of making a peace agreement. He should accept that all states should disarm

l) He must make concessions to the Germans, perhaps over the Rhineland or Alsace–Lorraine.

The terms of the Treaty of Versailles

None of the Big Three was happy with the eventual terms of the Treaty. After months of negotiation, each of them had to compromise on some of their aims, otherwise there would never have been a treaty. The main terms can be divided into five areas.

1 War guilt
This clause was simple but was seen by the Germans as extremely harsh. Germany had to accept the blame for starting the war.

2 Reparations
The major powers agreed, without consulting Germany, that Germany had to pay reparations to the Allies for the damage caused by the war. The exact figure was not agreed until 1921 when it was set at £6,600 million – an enormous figure. If the terms of the payments had not later been changed under the Young Plan in 1929 (see page 236), Germany would not have finished paying this bill until 1984.

3 German territories and colonies
a) **Germany's European borders** were very extensive, and the section dealing with German territory in Europe was a complicated part of the Treaty. You can see the detail in Source 6.
In addition to these changes, the Treaty also forbade Germany to join together (Anschluss) with its former ally Austria.

SOURCE 6

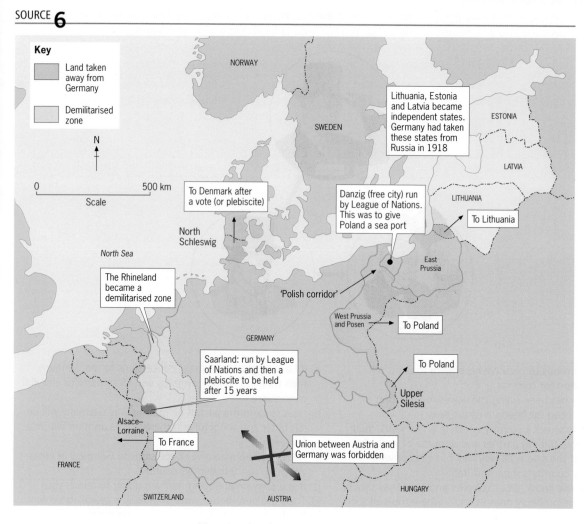

Key
- Land taken away from Germany
- Demilitarised zone

NORWAY

Lithuania, Estonia and Latvia became independent states. Germany had taken these states from Russia in 1918

ESTONIA

SWEDEN

LATVIA

To Denmark after a vote (or plebiscite)

Danzig (free city) run by League of Nations. This was to give Poland a sea port

LITHUANIA

To Lithuania

North Schleswig

North Sea

East Prussia

The Rhineland became a demilitarised zone

'Polish corridor'

West Prussia and Posen

To Poland

GERMANY

To Poland

Saarland: run by League of Nations and then a plebiscite to be held after 15 years

Upper Silesia

Alsace–Lorraine

To France

Union between Austria and Germany was forbidden

FRANCE

SWITZERLAND

AUSTRIA

HUNGARY

N

0   500 km
Scale

Map showing the impact of the Treaty of Versailles on the borders of Europe.

b) Germany's overseas empire was taken away. It had been one of the causes of bad relations between Britain and Germany before the war. Former German colonies such as Cameroon became mandates controlled by the League of Nations, which effectively meant that France and Britain controlled them.

4 Germany's armed forces

The size and power of the German army was a major concern, especially for France. The Treaty therefore restricted German armed forces to a level well below what they had been before the war.

- The army was limited to 100,000 men.
- Conscription was banned – soldiers had to be volunteers.
- Germany was not allowed armoured vehicles, submarines or aircraft.
- The navy could have only six battleships.
- The Rhineland became a demilitarised zone. This meant that no German troops were allowed into that area. The Rhineland was important because it was the border area between Germany and France (see Source 6).

5 League of Nations

- Previous methods of keeping peace had failed and so the League of Nations was set up as an international 'police force'. (You will study the League in detail in Chapter 2.)
- Germany was not invited to join the League until it had shown that it was a peace-loving country.

Focus Task A

Why did the victors not get everything they wanted?

1 Work in threes. Look back at the profiles of Clemenceau, Wilson and Lloyd George on pages 6, 8 and 9. Choose one each. Study the terms of the Treaty on these two pages. Think about:
- ♦ which terms of the Treaty would please your chosen leader and why
- ♦ which terms would displease him and why
- ♦ how far he seemed to have achieved his aims.

Report your findings to your partners.

2 Look back at the chart you compiled on page 6. There should be a blank fifth column. Put the heading 'How they felt about the Treaty' and fill it in for each leader with a one-sentence summary.

3 a) Choose one of the following phrases to finish off this sentence:
   The victors did not all get what they wanted because . . .
   - ♦ Clemenceau bullied Wilson and Lloyd George into agreeing to a harsh treaty.
   - ♦ the leaders' aims were too different – they could not all have got what they wanted and someone was bound to be disappointed.
   - ♦ public opinion in their home countries affected the leaders' decisions.
   b) Write a paragraph to explain why you chose that phrase.
   c) Write two more paragraphs to explain whether there is evidence to support the other two.

Revision Tip

The more you know about the Treaty of Versailles, the more it will help you. Make sure you can remember one or two key points under each of these headings: Blame, Reparations, Arms, Territory.

Focus Task B

Was the Treaty of Versailles fair?

It is important to make up your own mind about this key question and be able to back up your view with evidence and arguments. So place yourself on this scale and write some sentences to explain your position. This is provisional. You will return to it again.

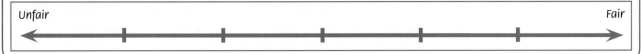

Unfair ←———|———|———|———|———|———→ *Fair*

How did Germans react to the Treaty?

The terms of the Treaty were announced on 7 May to a horrified German nation.

War guilt and reparations

Germany had to accept the blame for starting the war and therefore had to pay reparations.

- This 'war guilt' clause was particularly hated. Germans did not feel they had started the war. They felt at the very least that blame should be shared.
- They were bitter that Germany was expected to pay for all the damage caused by the war even though the German economy was severely weakened.

Disarmament

The German army was reduced to 100,000 men. It could have no air force, and only a tiny navy.

Germans felt these terms were very unfair. An army of 100,000 was very small for a country of Germany's size and the army was a symbol of German pride.

Also, despite Wilson's Fourteen Points calling for disarmament, none of the Allies were being asked or forced to disarm in the same way.

German territories

Germany certainly lost a lot of territory.
- 10 per cent of its land in Europe
- All of its overseas colonies
- 12.5 per cent of its population
- 16 per cent of its coalfields and almost half of its iron and steel industry.

This was a major blow to German pride, and to its economy. Both the Saar and Upper Silesia were important industrial areas.

Meanwhile, as Germany was losing colonies, the British and French were increasing their empires by taking control of German territories in Africa.

GERMAN REACTIONS

The Fourteen Points and the League of Nations

- To most Germans, the treatment of Germany was not in keeping with Wilson's Fourteen Points. For example, while self-determination was given to countries such as Estonia, Latvia and Lithuania, German-speaking peoples were being hived off into new countries such as Czechoslovakia to be ruled by non-Germans. *Anschluss* (union) with Austria was forbidden.
- Germany felt further insulted by not being invited to join the League of Nations.

Non-representation

Germans were angry that their government was not represented at the peace talks and that they were being forced to accept a harsh treaty without any choice or even comment. Germans did not feel they had lost the war so they should not have been treated as a defeated country.

The government that took Germany to war in 1914 was overthrown in a revolution and the new democratic government in Germany was hoping for fair and equal treatment from the Allies. When the terms were announced the new German government refused to sign the Treaty and the German navy sank its own ships in protest. At one point, it looked as though war might break out again. But what could the German leader Friedrich Ebert do? Germany would quickly be defeated if it tried to fight. Reluctantly, Ebert agreed to accept the terms of the Treaty and it was signed on 28 June 1919.

SOURCE 8

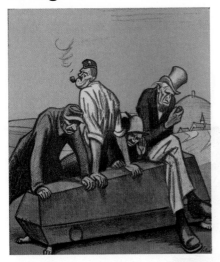

Cartoon from the German magazine *Simplicissimus*, June 1919. The caption in the magazine read: 'The Allies are burying Germany with the peace terms'.

Source Analysis ▲

Study Source 8. If you did not know this source was German would you be able to work this out? Explain how.

Focus Task

What was the impact of the peace treaty on Germany up to 1923?

Summarise the impact of the Treaty under each of these headings:
a) Political
b) Economic
c) Morale

Revision Tip

There are two problems Germany faced in the period 1919–23:
♦ political violence, and
♦ hyperinflation.
Make sure you can explain how each one was linked to the Treaty of Versailles.

The impact of the Treaty on Germany

The Treaty of Versailles had a profound effect on Germany for the next ten years and more. The Treaty was universally resented. The historian Zara Steiner contends that hatred of the Versailles Treaty was almost the only issue which all Germans in this period agreed on.

Political violence

Right-wing opponents of Ebert's government could not bear the Treaty. In 1920 they attempted a revolution. This rising, called the Kapp Putsch, was defeated by a general strike by Berlin workers which paralysed essential services such as power and transport. It saved Ebert's government but it added to the chaos in Germany – and the bitterness of Germans towards the Treaty.

Although Kapp was defeated, political violence remained a constant threat. There were numerous political assassinations or attempted assassinations. In the summer of 1922 Germany's foreign minister Walther Rathenau was murdered by extremists. Then in November 1923 Adolf Hitler led an attempted rebellion in Munich, known as the Munich Putsch (see page 239). Hitler's rebellion was defeated but he was got off lightly when he was put on trial and it was clear many Germans shared his hatred of Versailles. Over the next ten years he exploited German resentment of the Treaty of Versailles to gain support for himself and his Nazi party.

Conflict in the Ruhr

Under the Treaty Germany agreed to pay £6,600 million in reparations to the Allies. The first instalment of £50 million was paid in 1921, but in 1922 nothing was paid. Ebert tried to negotiate concessions from the Allies, but the French ran out of patience. In 1923 French and Belgian soldiers entered the Ruhr region and simply took what was owed to them in the form of raw materials and goods. This was quite legal under the Treaty of Versailles.

The results of the occupation of the Ruhr were disastrous for Germany. The German government ordered the workers to go on strike so that they were not producing anything for the French to take. The French reacted harshly, killing over 100 workers and expelling over 100,000 protesters from the region. More importantly, the strike meant that Germany had no goods to trade, and no money to buy things with. This in turn led to hyperinflation (see below).

There is much debate about the developments in the Ruhr. Most Germans believed that the crisis arose because the reparations were too high and Germany was virtually bankrupted. Many commentators at the time (including the British and French leaders) claimed that Germany was quite able to afford reparations, it just did not want to pay! Some historians argue that Germany stopped paying reparations in order to create a crisis and force the international community to revise the terms of the Treaty. The debate goes on, but there is no doubt that most Germans at the time believed the Treaty was responsible for the crisis and that the reparations were far too high.

Hyperinflation

The government solved the problem of not having enough money by simply printing extra money, but this caused a new problem – hyperinflation. The money was virtually worthless so prices shot up. The price of goods could rise between joining the back of a queue in a shop and reaching the front (see page 234)! Wages began to be paid daily instead of weekly.

Some Germans gained from this disaster. The government and big industrialists were able to pay off their huge debts in worthless marks. But others, especially pensioners, were practically wiped out. A prosperous middle-class family would find that their savings, which might have bought a house in 1921, by 1923 would not even buy a loaf of bread.

Germany eventually recovered from this disaster, but it left a bitter memory. The bitterness was directed towards the Treaty of Versailles. It is no coincidence that when Germany faced economic problems again in 1929 many Germans believed Hitler's claims that the Treaty was to blame and they should support his plans to overturn it.

Summary

While the treaty did cause some genuine problems for Germany the important thing to realise is that many Germans blamed it for other problems which had little to do with it. This resentment was then in turn exploited by extreme groups in Germany to gain power and influence for themselves.

How was the Treaty seen at the time?

> **It was unfair!**

None of the Big Three was happy with the Treaty (although for different reasons) and some of the diplomats who helped shape the Treaty were dissatisfied.

Some commentators at the time believed that the Treaty was unfair and unjust (see Source 9 for example).

SOURCE 9

Cannon fodder – a reference to the millions of men mown down by guns in the First World War.

Italy's leader Orlando (Italy).

The Big Three: Lloyd George (Britain); Clemenceau (France); Wilson (USA).

The child is the class of 1940 – children like him will be the ones who will fight in a future war because of the Treaty.

The Tiger is Clemenceau – he is so blinkered that he cannot see why the child is weeping.

PEACE AND FUTURE CANNON FODDER

The Tiger: "Curious! I seem to hear a child weeping!"

A cartoon published in the socialist newspaper *The Daily Herald* in 1919.

SOURCE 10

The historian, with every justification, will come to the conclusion that we were very stupid men . . . We arrived determined that a Peace of justice and wisdom should be negotiated; we left the conference conscious that the treaties imposed upon our enemies were neither just nor wise.

Harold Nicolson, a British official who attended the talks.

Source 9 is probably the most famous cartoon produced about the Treaty of Versailles. The artist, Will Dyson, thought that the peacemakers were blind and selfish and as a result they produced a disastrous treaty that would cause another terrible war. It is a powerful cartoon. Because history proved it right (the cartoonist even gets the date of the Second World War almost right) this cartoon has been reproduced many times ever since, including in millions of school textbooks.

Another powerful critic of the Treaty was a British economist, John Maynard Keynes. He wrote a very critical book called *The Economic Consequences of The Peace* published in 1919. This book was widely read and accepted and has influenced the way people have looked at the Treaty.

It is easy to think that everyone felt this way about the Treaty – but they did not!

It was fair!

SOURCE 11

The Germans have given in … They writhe at the obligation imposed on them to confess their guilt … Some of the conditions, they affirm, are designed to deprive the German people of its honour … They thought little of the honour of the nations whose territories they defiled with their barbarous and inhuman warfare for more than three awful years.

British newspaper *The Times*, 24 June 1919.

SOURCE 13

TERMS OF TREATY BETTER THAN GERMANY DESERVES
WAR MAKERS MUST BE MADE TO SUFFER

Germany's chickens are coming home to roost, and she is making no end of a song about it. That was expected, but it will not help her much … If Germany had her deserts, indeed, there would be no Germany left to bear any burden at all; she would be wiped off the map of Europe … Stern justice would demand for Germany a punishment 10 times harder than any she will have to bear …

The feeling in this country is not that Germany is being too hardly dealt by, but that she is being let off too lightly.

From the British newspaper *The People*, May 1919.

Source Analysis

1 Study Source 12. On your own copy, analyse Source 12 the way we have analysed Source 9 on page 16.
2 What does Source 13 reveal about British opinions on the Treaty?

At the time German complaints about the Treaty mostly fell on deaf ears. There were celebrations in Britain and France. If ordinary people in Britain had any reservations about the Treaty it was more likely to be that it was not harsh enough.

● Many people felt that the Germans were themselves operating a double standard. Their call for fairer treatment did not square with the harsh way they had treated Russia in the Treaty of Brest-Litovsk in 1918. Versailles was a much less harsh treaty than Brest-Litovsk.

● There was also the fact that Germany's economic problems, although real, were partly self-inflicted. Other states had raised taxes to pay for the war. The Kaiser's government had not done this. It had simply allowed debts to mount up because it had planned to pay Germany's war debts by extracting reparations from the defeated states.

SOURCE 12

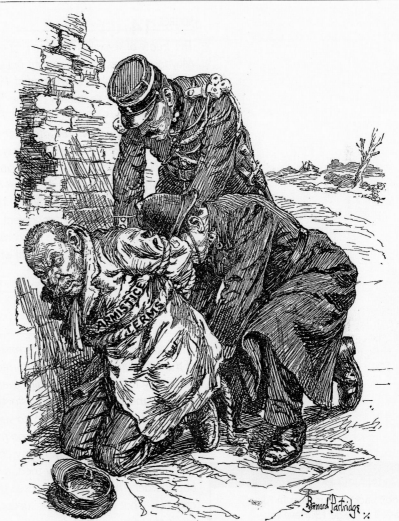

PUNCH, OR THE LONDON CHARIVARI.—February 19, 1919.

GIVING HIM ROPE?

German Criminal (*to Allied Police*). "HERE, I SAY, STOP! YOU'RE HURTING ME! [*Aside*] IF I ONLY WHINE ENOUGH I MAY BE ABLE TO WRIGGLE OUT OF THIS YET."

A British cartoon published in 1919.

How has the Treaty been seen with hindsight?

Looking back at the Treaty from the present day we know that it helped to create the cruel Nazi regime in Germany and helped cause the Second World War. We call this hindsight – when you look back at a historical event and judge it knowing its consequences. You would expect hindsight to affect historians' attitudes to the Treaty and it has – but maybe not exactly as you might expect.

Some historians side with critics of the Treaty and its makers. Others point out that the majority of people outside Germany thought that the Treaty was fair and that a more generous treaty would have been totally unacceptable to public opinion in Britain and France. They highlight that the peacemakers had a very difficult job balancing public opinion in their own countries with visions of a fairer future. Some say that the Treaty may have been the best that could be achieved in the circumstances.

SOURCE 14

The Treaty of Versailles has been repeatedly pilloried, most famously in John Maynard Keynes' pernicious but brilliant The Economic Consequences of the Peace, *published at the end of 1919 and still the argument underpinning too many current textbooks ... The Treaty of Versailles was not excessively harsh. Germany was not destroyed. Nor was it reduced to a second rank power or permanently prevented from returning to great power status ... With the disintegration of Austria-Hungary and the collapse of Tsarist Russia it left Germany in a stronger strategic position than before the war ... The Versailles Treaty was, nonetheless, a flawed treaty. It failed to solve the problem of both punishing and conciliating a country that remained a great power despite the four years of fighting and a military defeat. It could hardly have been otherwise, given the very different aims of the peacemakers, not to speak of the multiplicity of problems that they faced, many of which lay beyond their competence or control.*

Historian Zara Steiner writing in 2004.

SOURCE 15

The peacemakers of 1919 made mistakes, of course. By their offhand treatment of the non-European world they stirred up resentments for which the West is still paying today. They took pains over the borders in Europe, even if they did not draw them to everyone's satisfaction, but in Africa they carried on the old practice of handing out territory to suit the imperialist powers. In the Middle East they threw together peoples, in Iraq most notably, who still have not managed to cohere into a civil society. If they could have done better, they certainly could have done much worse. They tried, even cynical old Clemenceau, to build a better order. They could not foresee the future and they certainly could not control it. That was up to their successors. When war came in 1939, it was a result of twenty years of decisions taken or not taken, not of arrangements made in 1919.

Historian Margaret MacMillan writing in Peacemakers, 2001.

Focus Task

Look back at your work in Focus Task B on page 13. Have you changed your views after reading the information and sources on these three pages?

The other peace settlements

The Treaty of Versailles dealt with Germany, but Germany had allies in the First World War (Austria–Hungary, Bulgaria and Turkey) and there were four other treaties which dealt with them.

The Versailles Treaty usually gets the most attention but these other treaties were important, too. They set out what Europe and the Middle East would look like for the next few decades and in many ways these treaties still have a powerful impact on the world today. Looking at the other treaties may also help you to decide whether you think the Treaty of Versailles was fair. To help with this, we are going to look in more detail at just one other treaty, the Treaty of Sevres.

The Treaty of Sevres 1920

This Treaty was signed in August 1920. As you can see from Source 16, Turkey lost a substantial amount of territory and its original empire was broken up. Most historians agree it was a harsh treaty. As well as losing the territories shown in Source 16 parts of Turkey were defined as zones of influence controlled by the British, French or Italians. Armenia and Kurdistan became independent regions. Turkey's tax system, finances and budget were to be controlled by the Allies. Turkey had long been a great and proud empire and Turks were angered and humiliated by the terms.

What were the Allies trying to achieve?

SOURCE **16**

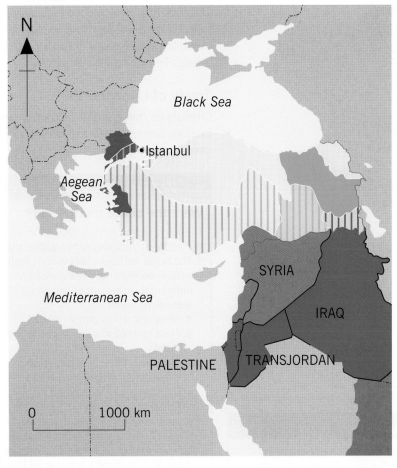

Treaty of Sevres (1920)
- Remaining Turkish territory
- Possible Kurdish territory

Territory ceded to:
- Armenia
- Greece
- France (France also took Tunisia and Morocco in Western North Africa)
- Britain

Zones of influence
- France
- Britain
- Italy
- International control, demilitarised

The impact of the Treaty of Sevres on Turkey.

19

What the Allies said **in public**:	What was going on **behind the scenes**:
<ul><li>All of the Big Three agreed that Turkey's time as a great power had to end.</li><li>Turkey had been unstable for some time. Many of its people (including Greeks, Armenians and Arab peoples) wanted independence so the Treaty should try to establish stable new states in Eastern Europe and the Middle East.</li><li>They agreed that Turkey would be punished for supporting Germany in the war.</li><li>President Wilson was keen for Armenia to become an independent state and that Armenians should rule themselves.</li></ul>	<ul><li>Italy essentially wanted Turkish territory as a reward for supporting the Allies in the First World War.</li><li>France and Britain wanted to strengthen or extend their empires and especially their commercial interests. France, Britain and Italy actually signed a secret Tripartite Agreement in August 1920 in which they effectively protected their commercial interests. Britain was particularly interested in the oilfields of Iraq and already had a large involvement in the oil industry of neighbouring Iran.</li><li>Britain had made promises to Arab peoples in return for their help in the war but was effectively unable or unwilling to honour these promises.</li></ul>

Did the Treaty bring peace and stability?

The simple answer is no!

Originally the Turkish government intended to accept the Treaty even though almost all Turks were outraged by its terms. However, Turkish nationalists under Mustafa Kemal Pasha set up a new Grand Assembly. They stopped the government signing the treaty and began to reverse the Treaty terms by force. The nationalists were unable to restore the Turkish empire's territories but they drove the Greeks out of Smyrna and forced the French to negotiate withdrawing from Turkish territory. They reached terms with the British over access to the Straits.

Wilson was unable to get support at home for his policies on Armenia. Armenia was forced to abandon its hope of becoming an independent state and opted to become part of the Soviet Union rather than be forced to become part of Turkey. There were many alleged atrocities in the fighting, such as the burning of Smyrna. However, the most controversial was the forced movement and mass killing of Armenians, which today is regarded as genocide by Armenians and most historians although Turkey rejects this claim bitterly.

Treaty of Lausanne 1923

Eventually the changes that the Turks had brought about were recognised in the Treaty of Lausanne. Smyrna, Anatolia and parts of Thrace became Turkish lands. Turkey's borders were fixed more or less as they are today.

Focus Task

Were the peace treaties fair?

The key question for this topic is 'Were the peace treaties fair?' If you compare the Treaty of Versailles with another treaty it should help you reach a judgement.

1 The bullet list below lists various features of the Treaty of Sevres. Make a table with three headings: 'Feature of Sevres'; 'Fair? (Give reasons)'; and 'Similar or different to treatment of Germany? (Give examples)'. Consider the following features of Sevres:

- Allies wanted to punish Turkey
- Allies wanted to achieve peace and stability
- Allies had differing aims and also looked after their own interests
- Treaty terms were imposed on Turkish government
- Strict controls on Turkish military
- Control of Turkey's finances
- Loss of territories
- Loss of empire
- Foreign forces controlling areas of Turkey
- Resentment of Turkish people
- Violent resistance against terms
- Renegotiated.

Work in pairs or small groups and discuss the features and fill out the centre column of your table to judge whether you think this feature was fair. Use a score of 1–5 where 1 is not at all fair; 5 is very fair.

2 Now think about the Treaty of Versailles. See if you can agree on whether Turkey was treated in a similar way to Germany.

3 Now reach your judgement: do you think that the Treaty of Sevres was more or less fair than the Treaty of Versailles? Make sure you can give reasons.

Revision Tip

It will help you answer questions about the period if you can name at least one of the treaties; who it affected; plus one way it was similar and one way it was different from the Treaty of Versailles.

Keywords

Make sure you know what these terms mean and be able to define them confidently.

Essential

- Anschluss
- Big Three
- demilitarised zone
- democracy
- disarmament
- Fourteen Points
- hyperinflation
- idealist/realist
- Kapp Putsch
- League of Nations
- mandates
- Paris Peace Conference
- reparations
- Rhineland
- Ruhr
- Saar
- self-determination
- Treaty of Brest-Litovsk
- Treaty of Versailles
- war guilt
- Young Plan

Useful

- co-operation
- conscription
- free trade
- general strike
- hindsight
- public opinion
- right-wing
- secret treaties
- territories

Chapter Summary

The peace treaties after the First World War

1. The Paris Peace Conference was set up to sort out what would happen to the defeated countries after the First World War.
2. The Conference was dominated by 'The Big Three': Wilson, Clemenceau and Lloyd George representing the USA, France and Britain (the countries that won the war).
3. The Big Three did not agree on many things. In particular they disagreed on how to treat Germany, the League of Nations and Wilson's Fourteen Points.
4. There were a number of Treaties – one for each of the defeated countries. The Treaty of Versailles was the treaty that dealt with Germany.
5. The main terms of the Treaty of Versailles were that Germany accepted blame for starting the war; had to pay reparations; lost land, industry, population and colonies; and was forced to disarm.
6. People in Germany were appalled by the Treaty but Germany had no choice but to sign it.
7. Germany had many post-war problems such as attempted revolutions and hyperinflation, which they blamed on the Treaty. But the Treaty was not the sole reason for these problems.
8. The Treaty also set up a League of Nations whose role was to enforce the Treaty of Versailles and to help prevent another war.
9. Opinion on the Treaty of Versailles varied at the time: some people thought it was too lenient on Germany, others that it was too harsh and would lead to Germany wanting revenge.
10. The other treaties dealt with Germany's allies and were built on similar principles to the Treaty of Versailles.

Exam Practice

See pages 168–175 and pages 316–319 for advice on the different types of questions you might face.

1. (a) What were the main terms of the Treaty of Versailles? **[4]**
   (b) What impact did the Treaty of Versailles have on Germany up to 1923? **[6]**
   (c) 'The Treaty of Versailles was fair on Germany.' How far do you agree with this statement? Explain your answer. **[10]**
2. Study Source 12 on page 17. What is the message of the cartoonist? Explain your answer by using details of the source and your own knowledge. **[7]**
3. Study Source 13 on page 17. Does this source prove that the Versailles settlement was fair to Germany? Explain your answer by using details of the source and your own knowledge. **[7]**

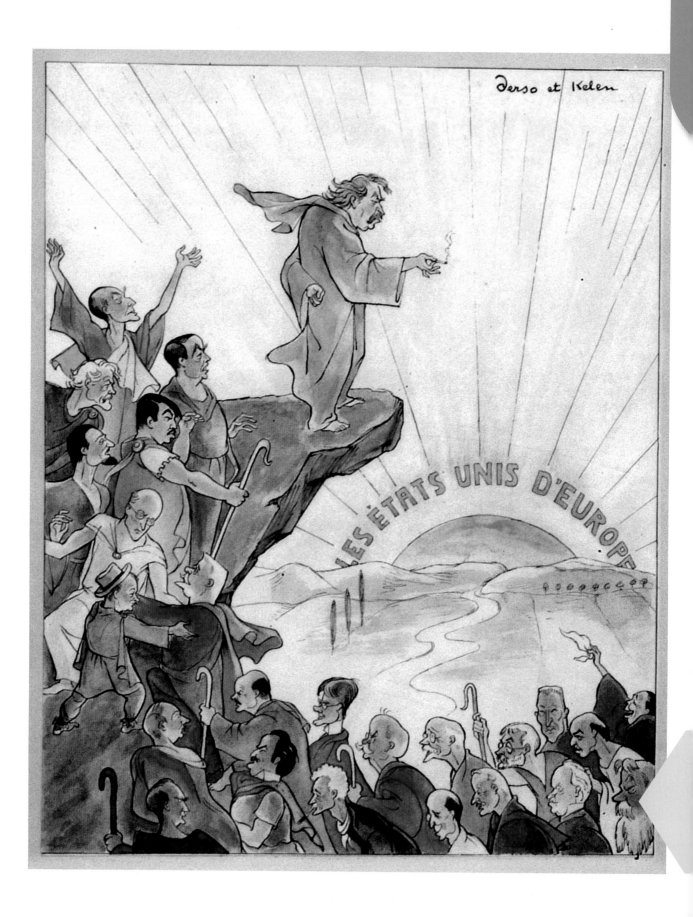

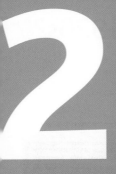

To what extent was the League of Nations a success?

FOCUS POINTS

- How successful was the League in the 1920s?
- How far did weaknesses in the League's organisation make failure inevitable?
- How far did the Depression make the work of the League more difficult?
- How successful was the League in the 1930s?

You saw in Chapter 1 that setting up a League Nations was one of Woodrow Wilson's key ideas for preventing another war. He saw the League as an organisation that would solve international disputes. He hoped that if the Great Powers had to talk to each other they would no longer need or even want to make secret alliances as they did before the First World War. He thought the League would protect smaller nations from aggression – if they had concerns then the League would be a place where their case would be heard by the world.

Without spoiling the story Wilson's original plan for the League never happened! This chapter will explain why. However, a scaled-down version of the League was created. How well did it do?

On the one hand people argue that the League achieved a lot.

- Its humanitarian agencies helped the sick, the poor and the homeless.
- Its financial agencies helped to stabilise several economies after the war.
- The League handled 66 major international disputes between the wars and was successful in half of them.

However, the League was unsuccessful in the larger international disputes involving the major powers. The League failed to stop the Japanese invasion of Manchuria in 1931 and Italy's invasion of Abyssinia in 1935, which had disastrous consequences for international relations in Europe.

So your key question in this chapter is to judge **to what extent** the League succeeded. This is not a question with a 'Yes' or 'No' answer. To tackle a 'to what extent' question you need to:

- weigh the League's successes against its failures
- compare the aims of the League with what it actually achieved
- assess whether the failures were the fault of the League or other factors and particularly:
  - how far the League's **organisation** weakened it
  - how far the League was let down by its own **members** and the other Great Powers
  - how far the League's work was hampered by the worldwide economic **Depression** that made the 1930s a dark and dangerous time.

This chapter takes you step by step through those questions so you can reach your own view on this key question: '**To what extent** was the League of Nations a success?'

◀ This picture was used as the menu card for a League of Nations banquet in the 1930s. It shows Briand (one of the most influential figures in the League) as Moses leading the statesmen of the world towards the 'Promised Land'. The sunrise is labelled 'The United States of Europe'. Discuss:

1 What impression does this picture give you of the League?
2 Does this picture surprise you? Why or why not?

2.1 How successful was the League in the 1920s?

The birth of the League

SOURCE 1

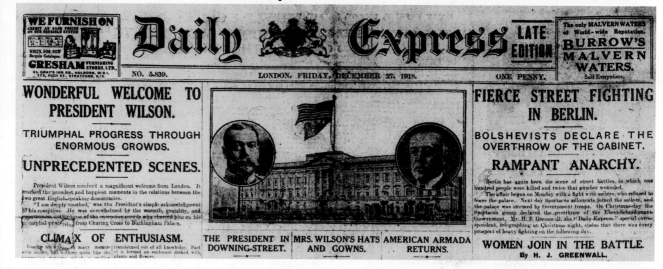

The front page of the *Daily Express*, 27 December 1918. Following the Allied victory in the First World War, President Woodrow Wilson was given a rapturous reception by ordinary people wherever he went in Europe.

SOURCE 2

Merely to win the war was not enough. It must be won in such a way as to ensure the future peace of the world.

President Woodrow Wilson, 1918.

Think!

Which of the three kinds of League proposed by the Allies do you think would be the best at keeping peace?
♦ a world parliament
♦ a simple organisation for emergencies only
♦ strong with its own army.

SOURCE 3

[If the European powers] had dared to discuss their problems for a single fortnight in 1914 the First World War would never have happened. If they had been forced to discuss them for a whole year, war would have been inconceivable.

President Wilson speaking in 1918.

After the First World War everyone wanted to avoid repeating the mass slaughter of the war that had just ended. They also agreed that a League of Nations – an organisation that could solve international problems without resorting to war – would help achieve this. However, there was disagreement about what kind of organisation it should be.

● President Wilson wanted the League of Nations to be like a **world parliament** where representatives of all nations could meet together regularly to decide on any matters that affected them all.

● Many British leaders thought the best League would be a **simple organisation** that would just get together in emergencies. An organisation like this already existed. It was called the Conference of Ambassadors.

● France proposed **a strong League with its own army**.

It was President Wilson who won. He insisted that discussions about a League should be a major part of the peace treaties and in 1919 he took personal charge of drawing up plans for the League. By February he had drafted a very ambitious plan.

All the major nations would join the League. They would disarm. If they had a dispute with another country, they would take it to the League. They promised to accept the decision made by the League. They also promised to protect one another if they were invaded. If any member did break the Covenant (see page 28) and go to war, other members promised to stop trading with it and to send troops if necessary to force it to stop fighting. Wilson's hope was that citizens of all countries would be so much against another conflict that this would prevent their leaders from going to war.

The plan was prepared in a great hurry and critics suggested there was some woolly thinking. Some people were angered by Wilson's arrogant style. He acted as if only he knew the solutions to Europe's problems. Others were worried by his idealism. Under threat of war, would the public really behave in the way he suggested? Would countries really do what the League said? Wilson glossed over what the League would do if they didn't.

Even so, most people in Europe were prepared to give Wilson's plans a try. They hoped that no country would dare invade another if they knew that the USA and other powerful nations of the world would stop trading with them or send their armies to stop them. In 1919 hopes were high that the League, with the United States in the driving seat, could be a powerful peacemaker.

SOURCE 4

For the first time in history the counsels of mankind are to be drawn together and concerted for the purpose of defending the rights and improving the conditions of working people – men, women, and children – all over the world. Such a thing as that was never dreamed of before, and what you are asked to discuss in discussing the League of Nations is the matter of seeing that this thing is not interfered with. There is no other way to do it than by a universal league of nations, and what is proposed is a universal league of nations.

Extract from a speech by President Woodrow Wilson to an American audience in 1919.

SOURCE 5A

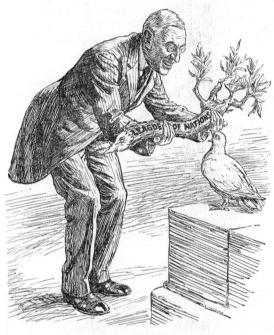

OVERWEIGHTED.

PRESIDENT WILSON. "HERE'S YOUR OLIVE BRANCH. NOW GET BUSY."
DOVE OF PEACE. "OF COURSE I WANT TO PLEASE EVERYBODY; BUT ISN'T THIS A BIT THICK?"

SOURCE 5B

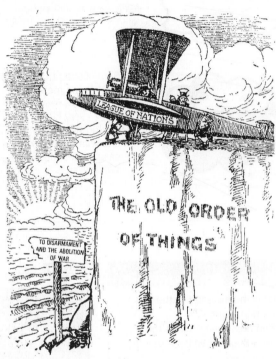

READY TO START.

Two British cartoons from 1919/1920.

Source Analysis ▲

Work in pairs. One of you work with Source 5A and the other work with Source 5B.

1 What is the message of your cartoon? Make sure that you explain what details in the cartoon help to get this message across.
2 Is your cartoon optimistic or pessimistic about the League of Nations? Give reasons.
3 Compare your ideas with your partner's, then write a paragraph comparing the two cartoons.

Focus Task

How successful was the League of Nations in the 1920s?

Your prediction

You may already have formed an opinion on the League of Nations – but if you haven't, even better! Make your prediction as to how successful you think the League will be *in the 1920s*. For example, how successful do you think it will be in settling the problems left over from the First World War?

50% Successes

50% Failures

To record your prediction, make your own copy of this diagram, but with one difference. Redraw the segments to show how successful *you* think it is going to be.
Draw your own diagram large and put it somewhere you can refer to it again as you will be asked to check back a number of times to reconsider your prediction.

A body blow to the League

Back in the USA, however, Woodrow Wilson had problems. Before the USA could even join the League, let alone take a leading role, he needed the approval of his Congress (the American 'Parliament'). And in the USA the idea of a League was not at all popular, as you can see from Source 6.

SOURCE 6

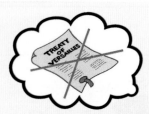

The league was supposed to enforce the Treaty of Versailles yet some Americans, particularly the millions who had German ancestors, hated the Treaty itself.

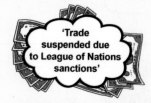

If the League imposed sanctions (e.g. stopping trade with a country that was behaving aggressively) it might be American trade and business that suffered most!

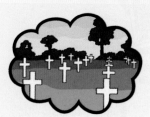

Some feared that joining the League meant sending US soldiers to settle every little conflict around the world. No one wanted that after casualties of the First World War.

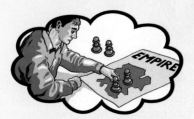

Some feared that the League would be dominated by Britain or France – and would be called to help defend their empires! Many in the US were anti-empires.

Reasons for opposition to the League in the USA.

SOURCE 7

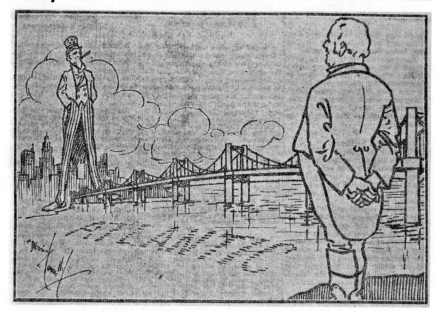

An American cartoon reprinted in the British newspaper the *Star*, June 1919.

Together, the critics of Wilson's plans (see Source 6) put up powerful opposition to the League. They were joined by Wilson's many other political opponents. Wilson's Democratic Party had run the USA for eight troubled years. Its opponents saw the League as an ideal opportunity to defeat him. Wilson toured the USA to put his arguments to the people, but when Congress voted in 1919 he was defeated.

In 1920 Wilson became seriously ill after a stroke. Despite that, he continued to press for the USA to join the League. He took the proposal back to Congress again in March 1920, but they defeated it by 49 votes to 35.

SOURCE **8**

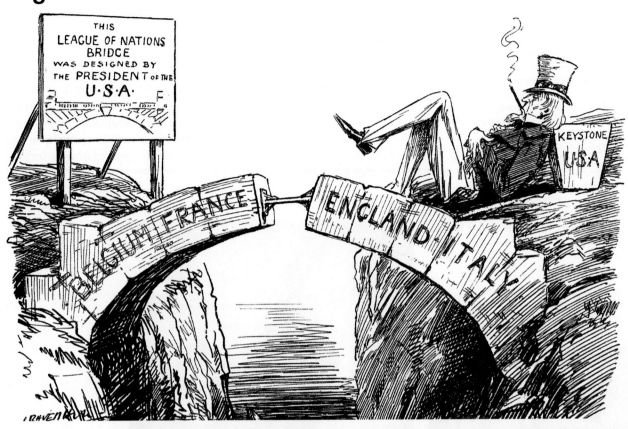

A British cartoon from 1920. The figure in the white top hat represents the USA.

Look back to your prediction from the Focus Task on page 25.

Source Analysis ▲

Source 8 is one of the most famous cartoons about the League of Nations. On your own copy of the cartoon add annotations to explain the key features. Then write your own summary of the message of the cartoonist.

Still the Democrats did not give up. They were convinced that if the USA did not get involved in international affairs, another world war might follow. In the 1920 election Wilson could not run for President – he was too ill – but his successor made membership of the League a major part of the Democrat campaign. The Republican candidate, Warren Harding, on the other hand, campaigned for America to be isolationist (i.e. not to get involved in international alliance but follow its own policies and self-interest). His slogan was to 'return to normalcy', by which he meant life as it was before the war, with the USA isolating itself from European affairs. The Republicans won a landslide victory.

So when the League opened for business in January 1920 the American chair was empty. The USA never joined. This was a personal rebuff for Wilson and the Democrats, but it was also a body blow to the League.

Think!

Look back to your prediction from the Focus Task on page 25. Do you want to change your prediction in light of the fact that the USA has not joined the league?

Revision Tip

Be sure you can remember:
♦ at least two reasons why some Americans were opposed to the USA joining the League (see Source 6)
♦ what isolationism means and how it affected the USA's decision.

The aims of the League

A Covenant set out the aims of the League of Nations. These were:

● to discourage aggression from any nation
● to encourage countries to co-operate, especially in business and trade
● to encourage nations to disarm
● to improve the living and working conditions of people in all parts of the world.

Article 10

The Covenant set out 26 Articles or rules, which all members of the League agreed to follow. Probably the most important Article was Article 10. 'The members of the League undertake to preserve against external aggression the territory and existing independence of all members of the League. In case of threat of danger the Council [of the League] shall advise upon the means by which this obligation shall be fulfilled.' Article 10 really meant **collective security**. By acting together (collectively), the members of the League could prevent war by defending the lands and interests of all nations, large or small.

SOURCE 9

The five giants represent the five continents of the Earth. The giants are standing firm together.

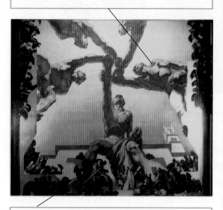

At the giants' feet, leaders of all the nations are working, reading and talking together. The League's members come from all five continents. The League believed that strength came from unity.

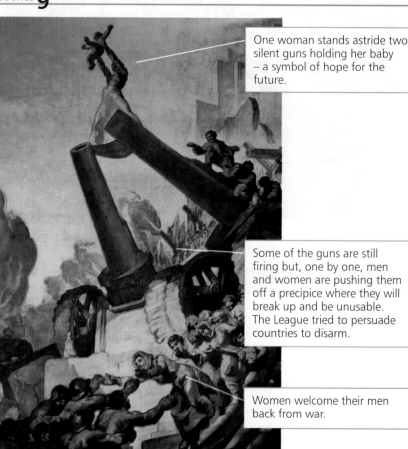

One woman stands astride two silent guns holding her baby – a symbol of hope for the future.

Some of the guns are still firing but, one by one, men and women are pushing them off a precipice where they will break up and be unusable. The League tried to persuade countries to disarm.

Women welcome their men back from war.

Wall paintings by the famous Spanish artist José Maria Sert that decorate the Assembly Chamber in the League's Headquarters in Geneva, Switzerland. They were designed to show the aims and values of the League.

Revision Tip

Make sure you can remember the four aims of the League. The initial letters may help you as they spell out AC/DC.

Think!

The League had four main aims:
◆ Discourage aggression
◆ Encourage co-operation
◆ Encourage disarmament
◆ Improve living conditions.

As you work through the chapter note down examples that you think could be used as
◆ Evidence of success
◆ Evidence of failure in each of the aims. You could record your evidence in a table.

Membership of the League

In the absence of the USA, Britain and France were the most powerful countries in the League. Italy and Japan were also permanent members of the Council, but throughout the 1920s and 1930s it was Britain and France who usually guided policy. Any action by the League needed their support.

However, both countries were poorly placed to take on this role. Both had been weakened by the First World War. Neither country was quite the major power it had once been. Neither of them had the resources to fill the gap left by the USA. Indeed, some British politicians said that if they had foreseen the American decision, they would not have voted to join the League either. They felt that the Americans were the only nation with the resources or influence to make the League work. In particular, they felt that trade sanctions would only work if the Americans applied them.

For the leaders of Britain and France the League posed a real problem. They were the ones who had to make it work, yet even at the start they doubted how effective it could be.

SOURCE 10

The League of Nations is not set up to deal with a world in chaos, or with any part of the world which is in chaos. The League of Nations may give assistance but it is not, and cannot be, a complete instrument for bringing order out of chaos.

Arthur Balfour, chief British representative at the League of Nations, speaking in 1920.

Both countries had other priorities.

- British politicians, for example, were more interested in rebuilding British trade and looking after the British empire than in being an international police force.
- France's main concern was still Germany. It was worried that without an army of its own the League was too weak to protect France from its powerful neighbour. It did not think Britain was likely to send an army to help it. This made France quite prepared to bypass the League if necessary in order to strengthen its position against Germany.

SOURCE 11

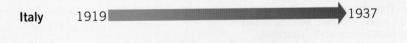
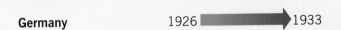
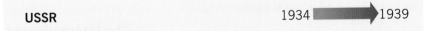

France	1919	1945
Britain	1919	1945
Italy	1919	1937
Japan	1919	1933
Germany	1926	1933
USSR	1934	1939
USA	never joined	

Membership of the League of Nations. This chart shows only the most powerful nations. More than 50 other countries were also members.

1 Study the diagram. Which part of the League would deal with the following problems:
   a) an outbreak of a new infectious disease
   b) a border dispute between two countries
   c) accidents caused by dangerous machinery in factories
   d) complaints from people in Palestine that the British were not running the mandated territory properly?

Organisation of the League

The Covenant laid out the League's structure and the rules for each of the bodies within it – see the diagram below.

The Council

- The Council was a smaller group than the Assembly, which met more often, usually about five times a year or more often in case of emergency. It included:
  - permanent members. In 1920 these were Britain, France, Italy and Japan.
  - temporary members. They were elected by the Assembly for three-year periods. The number of temporary members varied between four and nine at different times in the League's history.
- Each of the permanent members of the Council had a **veto**. This meant that one permanent member could stop the Council acting even if all other members agreed.
- The main idea behind the Council was that if any disputes arose between members, the members brought the problem to the Council and it was sorted out through discussion before matters got out of hand. However, if this did not work, the Council could use a range of powers:
  - **Moral condemnation**: they could decide which country was 'the aggressor', i.e. which country was to blame for the trouble. They could condemn the aggressor's action and tell it to stop what it was doing.
  - **Economic and financial sanctions**: members of the League could refuse to trade with the aggressor.
  - **Military force**: the armed forces of member countries could be used against an aggressor.

The Assembly

- The Assembly was the League's Parliament. Every country in the League sent a representative to the Assembly.
- The Assembly could recommend action to the Council and could vote on:
  - admitting new members to the League
  - appointing temporary members of the Council
  - the budget of the League
  - other ideas put forward by the Council.
- The Assembly only met **once a year**.
- Decisions made by the Assembly had to be **unanimous** – they had to be agreed by all members of the Assembly.

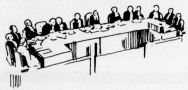

The Permanent Court of International Justice

- This was meant to play a key role in the League's work of settling disputes between countries peacefully.
- The Court was based at the Hague in the Netherlands and was made up of judges from the member countries.
- If it was asked, the Court would give a decision on a border dispute between two countries.
- It also gave legal advice to the Assembly or Council.
- However, the Court had no way of making sure that countries followed its rulings.

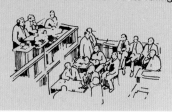

The Secretariat

- The Secretariat was a sort of civil service.
- It kept records of League meetings and prepared reports for the different agencies of the League.
- The Secretariat had specialist sections covering areas such as health, disarmament and economic matters.

The International Labour Organisation (ILO)

- The ILO brought together employers, governments and workers' representatives once a year.
- Its aim was to improve the conditions of working people throughout the world.
- It collected statistics and information about working conditions and it tried to persuade member countries to adopt its suggestions.

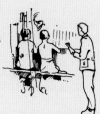

The League of Nations Commissions

As well as dealing with disputes between its members, the League also attempted to tackle other major problems. This was done through agencies, commissions or committees. The table below sets out the aims of some of these agencies and the scale of some of the problems facing them.

The Mandates Commissions

The First World War had led to many former colonies of Germany and her allies ending up as League of Nations mandates ruled by Britain and France on behalf of the League. The Mandates Commission was made up of teams of expert advisers whose job was to report to the League on how people in the mandates were being treated. The aim of the Commission was to make sure that Britain or France acted in the interests of the people of that territory, not its own interests. The Commission also took charge of the welfare of minority groups within other states, particularly the new territories created by the Peace Treaties of 1919–23.

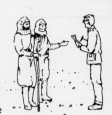

The Refugees Committee

At the end of the First World War there were hundreds of thousands of refugees who had fled from the areas of conflict. Some were trying to get back to their homes; others had no homes to go to. The most pressing problems were in former Russian territories: the Balkans, Greece, Armenia and Turkey. In 1927 the League reported that there were 750 000 refugees from former Russian territories and 168 000 Armenians. The League appointed the famous explorer Fridtjof Nansen to oversee the efforts to return refugees to their homes or help refugees to settle and find work in new countries. It was a mammoth task.

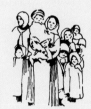

The Slavery Commission

This Commission worked to abolish slavery around the world. It was a particular issue in East Africa but slavery was also a major concern in many other parts of the world. And there were also many workers who were not technically slaves but were treated like slaves.

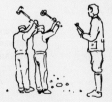

The Health Committee

The Health Committee attempted to deal with the problem of dangerous diseases and to educate people about health and sanitation. The First World War had brought about rapid developments in medicine and ideas about public health and disease prevention. The Health Committee worked with charities and many other independent agencies to collect statistics about health issues, to spread the new ideas and to develop programmes to fight disease.

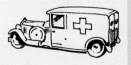

Were there weaknesses in the League's organisation?

Here is a conversation which might have taken place between two diplomats in 1920.

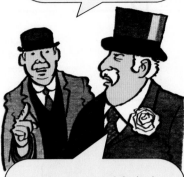

> Peace at last! The League of Nations will keep large and small nations secure.

> I'm not sure. It might look impressive but I think there are weaknesses in the League.

1 Work in pairs. Choose one statement each and write out the reasons each diplomat might give for his opinion. In your answer make sure you refer to:
   ♦ the membership of the League
   ♦ what the main bodies within the League can do
   ♦ how each body will make decisions
   ♦ how the League will enforce its decisions.
2 Go back to your diagram from page 25 and see if you want to change your predictions about how successful the League will be.

This is quite a complex chart. Your main aim is to be sure you know the difference between the League's Council and its Assembly.

Five of the problems shown in Source 12 are described on pages 33–4. They are highlighted in bold text on the map on this page. As you read about each one, score the League's success on a scale of −5 (a total failure) to +5 (a great success).

The League and border disputes in the 1920s

The treaties signed at the Paris Peace Conference had created new states and changed the borders of others. Inevitably this led to disputes and was the job of the League to sort out border disputes. From the start there was so much to do that some disputes were handled by the Conference of Ambassadors. Strictly this was not a body of the League of Nations. But it was made up of leading politicians from the main members of the League — Britain, France and Italy — so it was very closely linked to the League. As you can see from Source 12 the 1920s was a busy time.

SOURCE 12

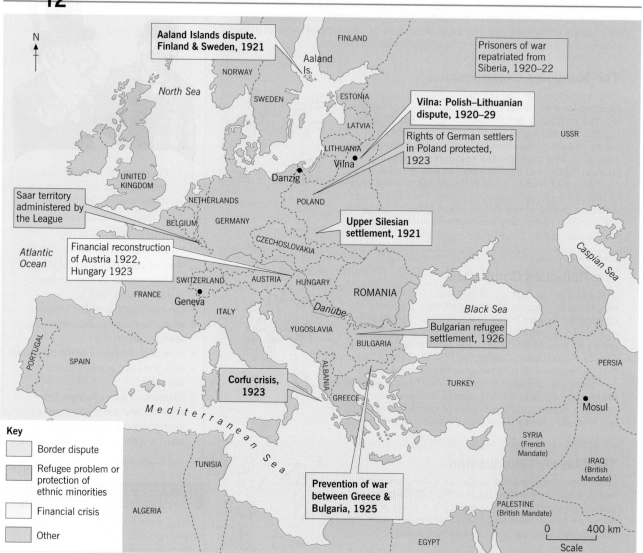

Problems dealt with by the League of Nations or the Conference of Ambassadors in the 1920s. The problems in bold text are described on pages 33–4.

This map actually shows only a few of the disputes which involved the League in this period. We have highlighted some of the more important ones. For example:

- In 1920 Poland effectively took control of the Lithuanian capital Vilna. Lithuania appealed to the League and the League protested to Poland but the Poles did not pull out. France and Britain were not prepared to act.
- In 1921 a dispute broke out between Germany and Poland over the Upper Silesia region. In the end, the League oversaw a peaceful plebiscite (vote) and divided the region between Germany and Poland. Both countries accepted the decision.
- Also in 1921, the League ruled on a dispute between Finland and Sweden over the Aaland Islands. Both sides were threatening to go to war but in the end Sweden accepted the League's ruling that the islands should belong to Finland.

We are now going to look at two other disputes in more detail.

SOURCE **13**

The League had been designed to deal with just such a dangerous problem as this. It had acted promptly and fairly and it had condemned the violence of the Italians. But it had lost the initiative. The result was that a great power had once again got away with using force against a small power.

Historians Gibbons and Morican referring to the Corfu crisis in *The League of Nations and the UNO*, 1970.

SOURCE **14**

The settlement of the dispute between Italy and Greece, though not strictly a League victory, upheld the principles on which it was based.

From J and G Stokes, *Europe and the Modern World*, 1973.

Source Analysis ▲

1 Sources 13 and 14 are referring to the same event. How do their interpretations differ?
2 Could they both be right? Explain your answer.
3 'The main problem in the Corfu crisis was not the League's organisation but the attitude of its own members.' Explain whether you agree.

Corfu, 1923

One of the boundaries that had to be sorted out after the war was the border between Greece and Albania. The Conference of Ambassadors was given this job and it appointed an Italian general called Tellini to supervise it. On 27 August, while they were surveying the Greek side of the frontier area, Tellini and his team were ambushed and killed. The Italian leader Mussolini was furious and blamed the Greek government for the murder. On 29 August he demanded that it pay compensation to Italy and execute the murderers. The Greeks, however, had no idea who the murderers were. On 31 August Mussolini bombarded and then occupied the Greek island of Corfu. Fifteen people were killed. Greece appealed to the League for help. The situation was serious. It seemed very like the events of 1914 that had triggered the First World War. Fortunately, the Council was already in session, so the League acted swiftly. Articles 12 and 15 of the League of Nations were designed for exactly this situation. Under these articles, when League members were in dispute and there was a danger of war, members could take their dispute to the Council and get a judgement. By 7 September it had prepared its judgement. It condemned Mussolini's actions. It also suggested that Greece pay compensation but that the money be held by the League. This money would then be paid to Italy if, and when, Tellini's killers were found.

However, Mussolini refused to let the matter rest. He insisted that this dispute had to be settled by the Council of Ambassadors because the Council of the League was not competent to deal with the issue. Mussolini would probably have failed if the British and French had stood together. Records from the meetings of the British government show that the British did not accept the Italian case and that the British were prepared to intervene to force Mussolini out of Corfu. However, the French completely disagreed and backed the Italians, probably because their forces were tied up in the Ruhr at this time (see pages 00–00) and could not tackle a dispute with Italy as well. The British could have acted alone, possibly by imposing sanctions or sending naval forces to Corfu. Article 16 of the League Covenant said that actions could be taken if one side committed an act of war. But the British were not prepared to act without the French and argued that Mussolini's actions did not constitute an act of war.

In the end Mussolini got his way and the Council of ambassadors made the final ruling on the dispute. A Commission was set up consisting of British, French, Italian and Japanese representatives. The Italian Commissioner was the only one to blame the Greeks in the dispute. Despite this the Council's ruling was changed and the Greeks had to apologise and pay compensation directly to Italy. On 27 September, Mussolini withdrew from Corfu boasting of his triumph.

There was much anger in the League over the Council's actions and League lawyers challenged the legality of the decision. However, the ruling was never changed. As historian Zara Steiner says: 'the dispute showed that the weakest of the great powers could get its way when Britain and France agreed to sacrifice justice for co-operation'.

The Geneva Protocol

The Corfu incident demonstrated how the League of Nations could be undermined by its own members. Britain and France drew up the Geneva Protocol in 1924, which said that if two members were in dispute they would have to ask the League to sort out the disagreement and they would have to accept the Council's decision. They hoped this would strengthen the League. But before the plan could be put into effect there was a general election in Britain. The new Conservative government refused to sign the Protocol, worried that Britain would be forced to agree to something that was not in its own interests. So the Protocol, which had been meant to strengthen the League, in fact weakened it.

SOURCE **15**

Make only slight resistance. Protect the refugees. Prevent the spread of panic. Do not expose the troops to unnecessary losses in view of the fact that the incident has been laid before the Council of the League of Nations, which is expected to stop the invasion.

A telegram from the Bulgarian Ministry of War in Sofia to its army commanders, 22 October 1925.

Source Analysis

1 Read Source 15. Why do you think Bulgaria was so optimistic about the League?
2 Look at Source 16. What impression of the League does this cartoon give you?

Focus Task

Did the weaknesses in the League's organisation make failure inevitable?

Can you find evidence to support or challenge each of the following criticisms of the League's organisation:

♦ that it would be slow to act
♦ that members would act in their own interests, not the League's
♦ that without the USA it would be powerless?

Use a table like this to record your answers:

Criticism	Evidence for	Evidence against

Focus first on the Bulgarian and Corfu crises. These will be most useful for your exam. Then look for evidence from the other crises.

Keep your table safe. You will add to it in a later task on page 37.

Once you have completed your table look at the balance of evidence. Does this suggest to you that the League could have succeeded, or not?

Bulgaria, 1925

Two years after Corfu, the League was tested yet again. In October 1925, Greek troops invaded Bulgaria after an incident on the border in which some Greek soldiers were killed. Bulgaria appealed for help. It also sent instructions to its army (see Source 15).

The secretary-general of the League acted quickly and decisively, calling a meeting of the League Council in Paris. The League demanded both sides stand their forces down and Greek forces withdraw from Bulgaria. Britain and France solidly backed the League's judgement (and it is worth remembering they were negotiating the Locarno Treaties at the same time – see the Factfile on page 36). The League sent observers to assess the situation and judged in favour of the Bulgarians. Greece had to pay £45,000 in compensation and was threatened with sanctions if it did not follow the ruling.

The Greeks obeyed, although they did complain that there seemed to be one rule for the large states (such as Italy) and another for the smaller ones (such as themselves). Nevertheless the incident was seen as a major success for the League and many observers seemed to forget the shame of the Corfu incident as optimism about the effectiveness of the League soared. Few pointed out that it was not so much the effectiveness of the machinery of League in this dispute but the fact that the great powers were united on their decision.

SOURCE **16**

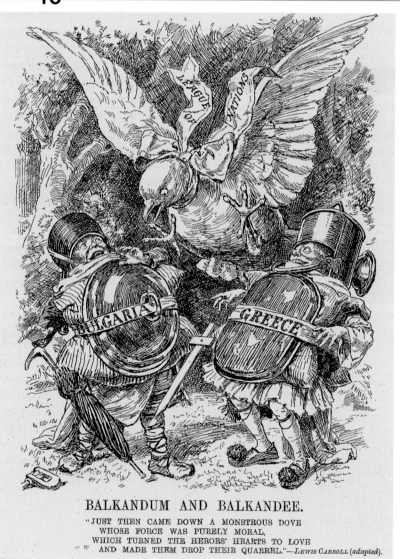

BALKANDUM AND BALKANDEE.

"JUST THEN CAME DOWN A MONSTROUS DOVE
WHOSE FORCE WAS PURELY MORAL,
WHICH TURNED THE HEROES' HEARTS TO LOVE
AND MADE THEM DROP THEIR QUARREL."—LEWIS CARROLL (*adapted*).

A cartoon about the Bulgarian crisis in *Punch*, 11 November 1925. The characters are based on Tweedledee and Tweedledum, from the children's book *Alice's Adventures in Wonderland*, who were always squabbling.

SOURCE **17**

A

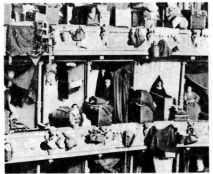

B

Two League of Nations' projects.

1 Study Sources 17A and 17B. What aspects of the League's work do you think they show?
2 Why do you think the founders of the League wanted it to tackle social problems?
3 The work of the League's commissions affected hundreds of millions of people, yet historians write very little about this side of its work. Why do you think this is?

Revision Tip

Border disputes

Make sure you can:
♦ describe one success in the 1920s and explain why it was a success
♦ describe one failure in the 1920s and explain why it was a failure
and as a bonus:
♦ describe and explain one **partial** success or failure.

The commissions

Make sure you can remember two specific examples of work done by the League's commissions or committees. Choose the ones that you think affected the most people.

How did the League of Nations work for a better world?

The League of Nations had set itself a wider task than simply waiting for disputes to arise and hoping to solve them. Through its commissions or committees (see page 31), the League aimed to fight poverty, disease and injustice all over the world.

● **Refugees**   The League did tremendous work in getting refugees and former prisoners of war back to their homelands. Head of the Refugees Committee Fridtjof Nansen introduced a document which became known as the 'Nansen Passport'. This made it much easier for genuine refugees to travel across borders to return home or resettle in new lands. It is estimated that in the first few years after the war, about 400,000 prisoners were returned to their homes by the League's agencies. When war led to a refugee crisis hit Turkey in 1922, hundreds of thousands of people had to be housed in refugee camps. The League acted quickly to stamp out cholera, smallpox and dysentery in the camps. However, the Refugee Committee was constantly short of funds and Nansen spent much of his time trying to raise donations. Its work became more difficult in the 1930s as the international situation became more tense and the authority of the League declined.

● **Working conditions**   The International Labour Organisation was successful in banning poisonous white lead from paint and in limiting the hours that small children were allowed to work. It also campaigned strongly for employers to improve working conditions generally. It introduced a resolution for a maximum 48-hour week, and an eight-hour day, but only a minority of members adopted it because they thought it would raise industrial costs. Like the Refugees Commission, the ILO was also hampered by lack of funds and also because it could not do much more than 'name and shame' countries or organisations that broke its regulations or generally mistreated workers. Nevertheless it was influential and it was a step forward in the sense that many abuses were not even known about before the ILO exposed them.

● **Health**   The Health Committee produced some important achievements. As well as collecting statistical information and spreading good practice it sponsored research into infectious diseases with institutes in Singapore, London and Denmark. These institutes were important in helping to develop vaccines and other medicines to fight deadly diseases such as leprosy and malaria. It started the global campaign to exterminate mosquitoes, which greatly reduced cases of malaria and yellow fever in later decades. Even the USSR, which was otherwise opposed to the League, took Health Committee advice on preventing plague in Siberia. The Health Committee is generally regarded as one of the most successful of the League's organisations and its work was continued by the United Nations Organisation after 1945 in the form of the World Health Organisation.

● **Transport**   The League made recommendations on marking shipping lanes and produced an international highway code for road users.

● **Social problems**   The League blacklisted four large German, Dutch, French and Swiss companies which were involved in the illegal drug trade. It brought about the freeing of 200,000 slaves in British-owned Sierra Leone. It organised raids against slave owners and traders in Burma. It challenged the use of forced labour to build the Tanganyika railway in Africa, where the death rate among the African workers was a staggering 50 per cent. League pressure brought this down to four per cent, which it said was 'a much more acceptable figure'.

Even in the areas where it could not remove social injustice the League kept careful records of what was going on and provided information on problems such as drug trafficking, prostitution and slavery.

Factfile

International agreements of the 1920s

➤ **1921 Washington Conference:** USA, Britain, France and Japan agreed to limit the size of their navies.

➤ **1922 Rapallo Treaty:** The USSR and Germany re-established diplomatic relations.

➤ **1924 The Dawes Plan:** to avert a terrible economic crisis in Germany, the USA lent money to Germany to help it to pay its reparations bill (see this page).

➤ **1925 Locarno treaties:** Germany accepted its western borders as set out in the Treaty of Versailles. This was greeted with great enthusiasm, especially in France. It paved the way for Germany to join the League of Nations.

➤ **1928 Kellogg–Briand Pact:** 65 nations agreed not to use force to settle disputes. This is also known as the Pact of Paris.

➤ **1929 Young Plan:** reduced Germany's reparations payments.

Source Analysis ▶

1 What is Source 18 commenting on?
2 Is the cartoonist praising or criticising someone or something in Source 18? Explain your answer.

Disarmament

In the 1920s, the League largely failed in bringing about disarmament. At the Washington Conference in 1921 the USA, Japan, Britain and France agreed to limit the size of their navies, but that was as far as disarmament ever got.

The failure of disarmament was particularly damaging to the League's reputation in Germany. Germany had disarmed. It had been forced to. But no other countries had disarmed to the same extent. They were not prepared to give up their own armies and they were certainly not prepared to be the first to disarm.

Even so, in the late 1920s, the League's failure over disarmament did not seem too serious because of a series of international agreements that seemed to promise a more peaceful world (see Factfile).

SOURCE 18

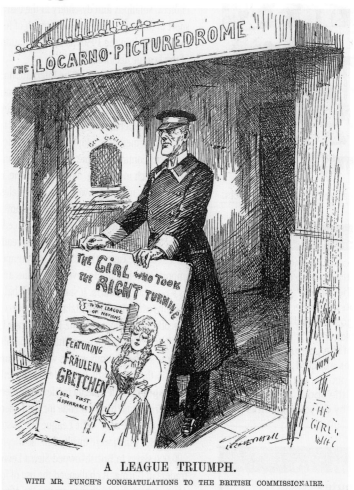

A LEAGUE TRIUMPH.
WITH MR. PUNCH'S CONGRATULATIONS TO THE BRITISH COMMISSIONAIRE.

A *Punch* cartoon from 1925. The woman on the billboard represents Germany.

SOURCE 19

There was a tendency for nations to conduct much of their diplomacy outside the League of Nations and to put their trust in paper treaties. After the USA assisted Europe financially there seemed to be more goodwill which statesmen tried to capture in pacts and treaties. Many of them, however, were of little value. They represented no more than the hopes of decent men.

Written by historian Jack Watson in 1984.

Economic recovery

Another reason for optimism in 1928 was that, after the difficult days of the early 1920s, the economies of the European countries were once again recovering. The Dawes Plan of 1924 had helped to sort out Germany's economic chaos and had also helped to get the economies of Britain and France moving again (see Source 20). The recovery of trading relationships between these countries helped to reduce tension. That is why one of the aims of the League had been to encourage trading links between the countries. When countries were trading with one another, they were much less likely to go to war with each other.

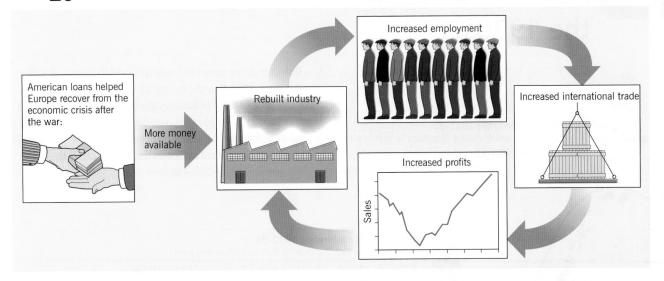

How the Dawes Plan helped economic recovery in Europe.

How far did the League succeed in the 1920s?

Although Wilson's version of the League never happened, the League still achieved a lot in the 1920s. It helped many sick, poor and homeless people. It stabilised several economies after the war. Perhaps most important of all, the League became one of the ways in which the world sorted out international disputes (even if it was not the only way). Historian Zara Steiner has said that 'the League was very effective in handling the "small change" of international diplomacy'. The implication, of course, is that the League could not deal with 'big' issues but it was not tested in this way in the 1920s.

Some historians believe that the biggest achievement of the League was the way it helped develop an 'internationalist mindset' among leaders – in other words it encouraged them to think in terms of collaborating rather than competing. One way in which the League did this was simply by existing! Great and small powers felt that it was worth sending their ministers to League meetings throughout the 1920s and 1930s, so they would often talk when they might not have done so otherwise. Even when the Great Powers acted on their own (for example, over Corfu) it was often after their ministers had discussed their plans at League meetings!

Focus task

How successful was the League in the 1920s?

It is now time to draw some conclusions to this key question.

Stage 1: Recap your work so far

1 Look back at your table from page 34. What evidence have you found of success or failure in each objective?
2 Look back to your predictions for the League for the 1920s (page 25). Has the League performed better or worse than you predicted? Redraw your prediction to show the balance of success and failure in the 1920s.

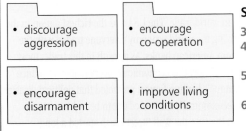

Stage 2: Evaluate the successes and failures

3 Create four file cards like this – one for each of the League's objectives.
4 Put the objective you think was achieved to the greatest extent at the top, and that which was achieved to the least extent at the bottom.
5 Write a paragraph to explain your order and support it with evidence from this chapter.
6 Suggest one change the League could make to be more effective in each of its objectives. Explain how the change would help.

Stage 3: Reach a judgement

7 Which of the following statements do you most agree with?
 ♦ 'The League of Nations was a great force for peace in the 1920s.'
 ♦ 'Events of the 1920s showed just how weak the League really was.'
 ♦ 'The League's successes in the 1920s were small-scale, its failures had a higher profile.'
Explain why you have chose your statement, and why you rejected the others.

2.2 How successful was the League of Nations in the 1930s?

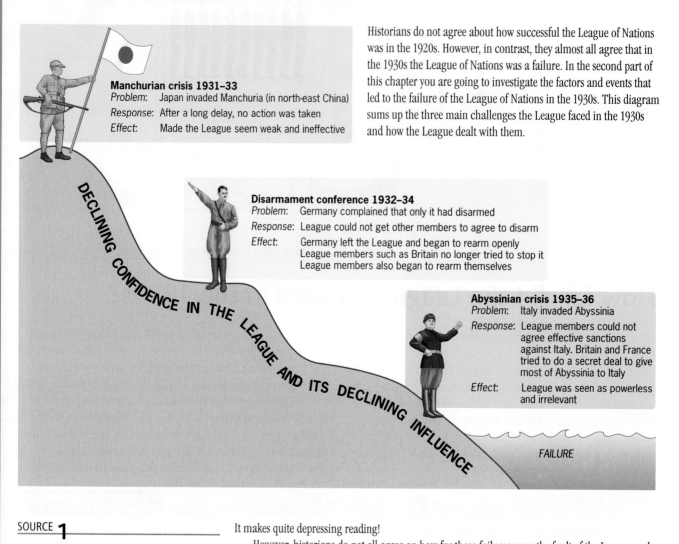

Manchurian crisis 1931–33
Problem: Japan invaded Manchuria (in north-east China)
Response: After a long delay, no action was taken
Effect: Made the League seem weak and ineffective

Disarmament conference 1932–34
Problem: Germany complained that only it had disarmed
Response: League could not get other members to agree to disarm
Effect: Germany left the League and began to rearm openly
League members such as Britain no longer tried to stop it
League members also began to rearm themselves

Abyssinian crisis 1935–36
Problem: Italy invaded Abyssinia
Response: League members could not agree effective sanctions against Italy. Britain and France tried to do a secret deal to give most of Abyssinia to Italy
Effect: League was seen as powerless and irrelevant

DECLINING CONFIDENCE IN THE LEAGUE AND ITS DECLINING INFLUENCE

FAILURE

Historians do not agree about how successful the League of Nations was in the 1920s. However, in contrast, they almost all agree that in the 1930s the League of Nations was a failure. In the second part of this chapter you are going to investigate the factors and events that led to the failure of the League of Nations in the 1930s. This diagram sums up the three main challenges the League faced in the 1930s and how the League dealt with them.

SOURCE 1

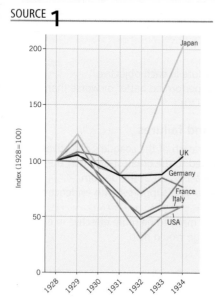

The rise and fall in industrial production in selected countries, 1928–34.

It makes quite depressing reading!

However, historians do not all agree on how far these failures were the fault of the League and how far other factors that the League could not control were more important. The biggest of these was the economic depression so let's start with that.

The economic depression

In the late 1920s there had been a boom in world trade. The USA was the richest nation in the world. American business was the engine driving the world economy. Everyone traded with the USA. Most countries also borrowed money from American banks. As a result of this trade, most countries were getting richer. You saw on page 37 how this economic recovery helped to reduce international tension. However, one of the League's leading figures predicted that political disaster might follow if countries did not co-operate economically. He turned out to be right.

In 1929 economic disaster did strike. In the USA the Wall Street Crash started a long depression that quickly caused economic problems throughout the world (see page 41). It damaged the trade and industry of all countries (see Source 1). It affected relations between countries and it also led to important political changes within countries (see diagram on page 39).

In the 1930s, as a result of the Depression much of the goodwill and the optimism of the late 1920s evaporated.

● As US loans dried up, businesses in many countries went bust, leading to unemployment.
● Some countries tried to protect their own industries by bringing in tariffs to stop imports. But this just meant their trading partners did the same thing and trade got even worse, leading to more businesses going bust and more unemployment.
● Many countries (including Germany, Japan, Italy and Britain) started to rearm (build up their armed forces) as a way of trying to get industries working and giving jobs to the unemployed.
● As their neighbours rearmed, many states began to fear that their neighbours might have other plans for their new armies so they built up their own forces.

The internationalist spirit of the 1920s was replaced by a more nationalist 'beggar my neighbour' approach in the 1930s.

The USA
One way that the League of Nations could stop one country invading another was to use economic sanctions. But the Depression made the USA unwilling to help in this because economic sanctions would make its own economy even worse.

Top priority – sort out US economy. Low priority – help sort out international disputes.

Britain
Britain was one of the leaders of the League of Nations. But, like the USA, it was unwilling to help sort out international disputes while its economy was bad. For example, when Japan invaded Machuria it did nothing – it did not support economic sanctions against Japan and did not send troops to protect Machuria.

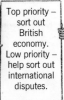

Top priority – sort out British economy. Low priority – help sort out international disputes.

Japan
The Depression threatened to bankrupt Japan. Its main export was silk to the USA, gut the USA was buying less silk. So Japan had less money to buy food and raw materials. Its leaders were all army general. They decided to build an empire by taking over weaker countries that had the raw materials Japan needed. They started by invading Machuria (part of China) in 1931.

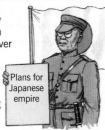

Plans for Japanese empire

Germany
The Depression hit Germany badly. There was unemployment, poverty and chaos. Germany's weak leaders seemed unable to do anything. As a result, Germans elected Adolf Hitler to lead them. He was not good news for international peace. He openly planned to invade Germany's neighbours and to win back land that Germany had lost in the Great War.

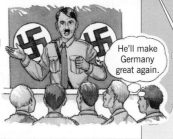

He'll make Germany great again.

Italy
In Italy economic problems encouraged Mussolini to try and build an overseas empire to distract people's attention from the difficulties the government faced.

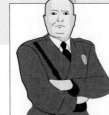

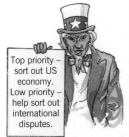

Focus task

How did the Depression make the work of the League harder?

Study these statements:
a) 'I have not worked since last year.'
b) 'I will support anyone who can get the country back to work.'
c) 'If we had our own empire we would have the resources we need. Economic depressions would not damage us so much.'
d) 'Reparations have caused this mess.'
e) 'The bank has closed. We've lost everything!'
f) 'We need tough leaders who will not be pushed around by the League of Nations or the USA.'
g) 'We should ban all foreign goods. That will protect the jobs of our workers.'

1 Suggest which country (or countries) they could have been made in during the Depression – USA, Britain, France, Germany, Japan or Italy
2 Suggest why these views would worry the League of Nations.

How did the Manchurian crisis weaken the League?

The first major test for the League came when the Japanese invaded Manchuria in 1931.

SOURCE 2

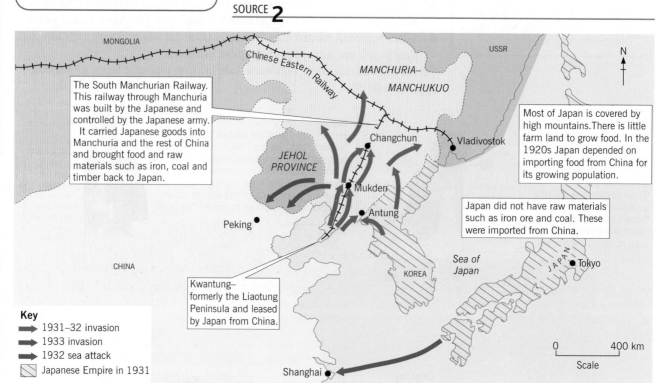

The railways and natural resources of Manchuria.

Map labels and annotations:

The South Manchurian Railway. This railway through Manchuria was built by the Japanese and controlled by the Japanese army. It carried Japanese goods into Manchuria and the rest of China and brought food and raw materials such as iron, coal and timber back to Japan.

Most of Japan is covered by high mountains. There is little farm land to grow food. In the 1920s Japan depended on importing food from China for its growing population.

Japan did not have raw materials such as iron ore and coal. These were imported from China.

Kwantung— formerly the Liaotung Peninsula and leased by Japan from China.

Key
➡ 1931–32 invasion
➡ 1933 invasion
➡ 1932 sea attack
▨ Japanese Empire in 1931

Place names: MONGOLIA, USSR, Chinese Eastern Railway, MANCHURIA–MANCHUKUO, Changchun, Vladivostok, JEHOL PROVINCE, Mukden, Antung, Peking, CHINA, KOREA, Sea of Japan, JAPAN, Tokyo, Shanghai

0 — 400 km Scale

Background

Since 1900 Japan's economy and population had been growing rapidly. By the 1920s Japan was a major power with a powerful military, strong industries and a growing empire (see Source 2). But the Depression hit Japan badly as China and the USA put up tariffs (trade barriers) against Japanese goods. Army leaders in Japan were in no doubt about the solution to Japan's problems – Japan would not face these problems if it had an empire to provide resources and markets for Japanese goods.

Invasion 1, 1931

In 1931 an incident in Manchuria gave them an ideal opportunity. The Japanese army controlled the South Manchurian Railway (see Source 2). When Chinese troops allegedly attacked the railway the Japanese armed forces used this as an excuse to invade and set up a government in Manchuoko (Manchuria), which they controlled. Japan's civilian government protested but the military were now in charge.

China appeals

China appealed to the League. The Japanese argued that China was in such a state of anarchy that they had to invade in self-defence to keep peace in the area. For the League of Nations this was a serious test. Japan was a leading member of the League. It needed careful handling. What should the League do?

SOURCE 3

I was sad to find everyone [at the League] so dejected. The Assembly was a dead thing. The Council was without confidence in itself. Beneš [the Czechoslovak leader], who is not given to hysterics, said [about the people at the League] 'They are too frightened. I tell them we are not going to have war now; we have five years before us, perhaps six. We must make the most of them.'

The British elder statesman Sir Austen Chamberlain visited the League of Nations late in 1932 in the middle of the Manchurian crisis. This is an adapted extract from his letters.

The League investigates

There was now a long and frustrating delay. The League's officials sailed round the world to assess the situation in Manchuria for themselves. This was well before the days of instant communication by satellite. There was not even reliable air travel. It was September 1932 – a full year after the invasion – before they presented their report. It was detailed and balanced, but the judgement was very clear. Japan had acted unlawfully. Manchuria should be returned to the Chinese.

Invasion 2, 1933

However, in February 1933, instead of withdrawing from Manchuria the Japanese announced that they intended to invade more of China. They still argued that this was necessary in self-defence. On 24 February 1933 the report from the League's officials was approved by 42 votes to 1 in the Assembly. Only Japan voted against. Smarting at the insult, Japan resigned from the League on 27 March 1933. The next week it invaded Jehol (see Source 2).

The League responds

The League was powerless. It discussed economic sanctions, but without the USA, Japan's main trading partner, they would be meaningless. Besides, Britain seemed more interested in keeping up a good relationship with Japan than in agreeing to sanctions. The League also discussed banning arms sales to Japan, but the member countries could not even agree about that. They were worried that Japan would retaliate and the war would escalate.

There was no prospect at all of Britain and France risking their navies or armies in a war with Japan. Only the USA and the USSR would have had the resources to remove the Japanese from Manchuria by force and they were not even members of the League.

Consequences

All sorts of excuses were offered for the failure of the League. Japan was so far away. Japan was a special case. Japan did have a point when it said that China was itself in the grip of anarchy. However, the significance of the Manchurian crisis was obvious. As many of its critics had predicted, the League was powerless if a strong nation decided to pursue an aggressive policy and invade its neighbours. Japan had committed blatant aggression and got away with it. Back in Europe, both Hitler and Mussolini looked on with interest. Within three years they would both follow Japan's example.

Source Analysis

1 Source 4 is a comment on this Manchurian crisis. On your own copy of this cartoon add annotations to explain:
   a) the key features
   b) the message
   c) what the cartoonist thinks of the League.
2 Read Source 3. Does Beneš share the same view of the League as the cartoonist in Source 4?

Think!

1 Why did it take so long for the League to make a decision over Manchuria?
2 Did the League fail in this incident because of the way it worked or because of the attitude of its members?

SOURCE 4

A cartoon by David Low, 1933. Low was one of the most famous cartoonists of the 1930s. He regularly criticised both the actions of dictators around the world and the ineffectiveness of the League of Nations.

To make myself perfectly clear, I would ask: is there anyone within or without Germany who honestly considers the present German regime to be peaceful in its instincts . . . Germany is inhibited from disturbing the peace of Europe solely by its consciousness of its present military inferiority.

Professor William Rappard speaking to the League in 1932.

Why did disarmament fail in the 1930s?

The next big failure of the League of Nations was over disarmament. As you saw on page 00, the League had not had any success in this area in the 1920s either, but at that stage, when the international climate was better, it had not seemed to matter as much. In the 1930s, however, there was increased pressure for the League to do something about disarmament. The Germans had long been angry about the fact that they had been forced to disarm after the First World War while other nations had not done the same. Many countries were actually spending more on their armaments than they had been before the First World War.

Disarmament Conference

In the wake of the Manchurian crisis, the members of the League realised the urgency of the problem. In February 1932 the long-promised Disarmament Conference finally got under way. By July 1932 it had produced resolutions to prohibit bombing of civilian populations, limit the size of artillery, limit the tonnage of tanks, and prohibit chemical warfare. But there was very little in the resolutions to show how these limits would be achieved. For example, the bombing of civilians was to be prohibited, but all attempts to agree to abolish planes capable of bombing were defeated. Even the proposal to ban the manufacture of chemical weapons was defeated.

German disarmament

It was not a promising start. However, there was a bigger problem facing the Conference – what to do about Germany. The Germans had been in the League for six years. Most people now accepted that they should be treated more equally than under the Treaty of Versailles. The big question was whether everyone else should disarm to the level that Germany had been forced to, or whether the Germans should be allowed to rearm to a level closer to that of the other powers. The experience of the 1920s showed that the first option was a non-starter. But there was great reluctance in the League to allow the second option.

This is how events relating to Germany moved over the next 18 months.

July 1932: Germany tabled proposals for all countries to disarm down to its level. When the Conference failed to agree the principle of 'equality', the Germans walked out.

September 1932: The British sent the Germans a note that went some way to agreeing equality, but the superior tone of the note angered the Germans still further.

December 1932: An agreement was finally reached to treat Germany equally.

January 1933: Germany announced it was coming back to the Conference.

February 1933: Hitler became Chancellor of Germany at the end of January. He immediately started to rearm Germany, although secretly.

May 1933: Hitler promised not to rearm Germany if 'in five years all other nations destroyed their arms'.

June 1933: Britain produced an ambitious disarmament plan, but it failed to achieve support at the Conference.

October 1933: Hitler withdrew from the Disarmament Conference, and soon after took Germany out of the League altogether.

> ## Source Analysis ▼
>
> 1 What is the message of Source 6?
> 2 Why might this cartoon have been published in Germany in July 1933?

Mariannes Papagei
Le perroquet de Marianne | Madame La France's Parrot | Il pappagallo di Marianna

A German cartoon from July 1933. The parrot represents France. It is calling for more security.

By this stage, all the powers knew that Hitler was secretly rearming Germany already. They also began to rebuild their own armaments. Against that background the Disarmament Conference struggled on for another year but in an atmosphere of increasing futility. It finally ended in 1934.

SOURCE 7

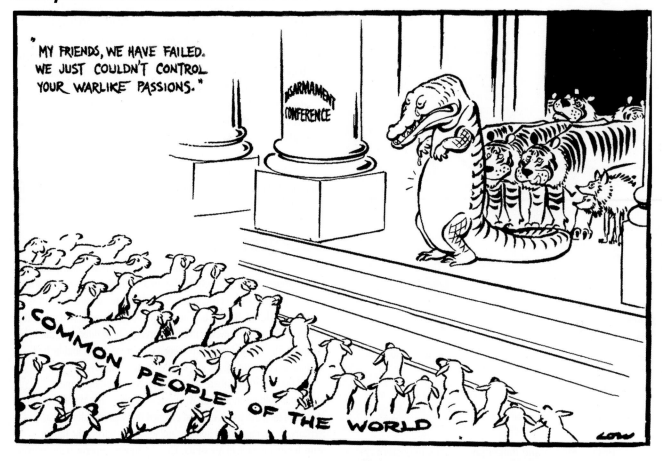

"MY FRIENDS, WE HAVE FAILED. WE JUST COULDN'T CONTROL YOUR WARLIKE PASSIONS."

DISARMAMENT CONFERENCE

COMMON PEOPLE OF THE WORLD

LOW

David Low's cartoon commenting on the failure of the Disarmament Conference in 1934.

Reasons for failure

The Conference failed for a number of reasons. Some say it was all doomed from the start. No one was very serious about disarmament anyway. But there were other factors at work.

It did not help that Britain and France were divided on this issue. By 1933 many British people felt that the Treaty of Versailles was unfair. In fact, to the dismay of the French, the British signed an agreement with Germany in 1935 that allowed Germany to build up its navy as long as it stayed under 35 per cent of the size of the British navy. Britain did not consult either its allies or the League about this, although it was in violation of the Treaty of Versailles.

It seemed that each country was looking after itself and ignoring the League.

How did Mussolini's invasion of Abyssinia damage the League?

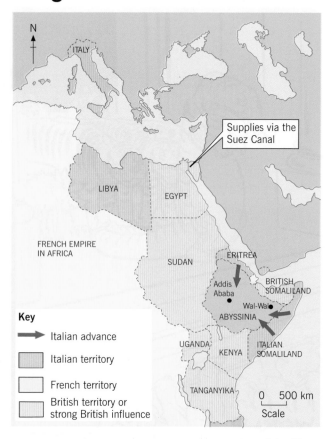

Key

→ Italian advance

▨ Italian territory

▢ French territory

▨ British territory or strong British influence

British, French and Italian possessions in eastern Africa.

The fatal blow to the League came when the Italian dictator Mussolini invaded Abyssinia in 1935. There were both similarities with and differences from the Japanese invasion of Manchuria.

● **Like Japan**, Italy was a leading member of the League. Like Japan, Italy wanted to expand its empire by invading another country.
● However, **unlike Manchuria**, this dispute was on the League's doorstep. Italy was a European power. It even had a border with France. Abyssinia bordered on the Anglo-Egyptian territory of Sudan and the British colonies of Uganda, Kenya and British Somaliland. Unlike events in Manchuria, the League could not claim that this problem was in an inaccessible part of the world.

Some argued that Manchuria had been a special case. Would the League do any better in this Abyssinian crisis?

Background

The origins of this crisis lay back in the previous century. In 1896 Italian troops had tried to invade Abyssinia but had been defeated by a poorly equipped army of tribesmen. Mussolini wanted revenge for this humiliating defeat. He also had his eye on the fertile lands and mineral wealth of Abyssinia. However, most importantly, he wanted glory and conquest. His style of leadership needed military victories and he had often talked of restoring the glory of the Roman Empire.

In December 1934 there was a dispute between Italian and Abyssinian soldiers at the Wal-Wal oasis – 80 km inside Abyssinia. Mussolini took this as his cue and claimed this was actually Italian territory. He demanded an apology and began preparing the Italian army for an invasion of Abyssinia. The Abyssinian emperor Haile Selassie appealed to the League for help.

Think!

To help you analyse these events draw a timeline, from December 1934 to May 1936, down the middle of a piece of paper and use the text to mark the key events on it. On one side put the actions of Mussolini or Hitler, on the other the actions of Britain, France and the League.

Phase 1: the League plays for time

From January 1935 to October 1935, Mussolini was supposedly negotiating with the League to settle the dispute. However, at the same time he was shipping his vast army to Africa and whipping up war fever among the Italian people.

To start with, the British and the French failed to take the situation seriously. They played for time. They were desperate to keep good relations with Mussolini, who seemed to be their strongest ally against Hitler. They signed an agreement with him early in 1935 known as the Stresa Pact which was a formal statement against German rearmament and a commitment to stand united against Germany. At the meeting to discuss this, they did not even raise the question of Abyssinia. Some historians suggest that Mussolini believed that Britain and France had promised to turn a blind eye to his exploits in Abyssinia in return for his joining them in the Stresa Pact.

However, as the year wore on, there was a public outcry against Italy's behaviour. A ballot was taken by the League of Nations Union in Britain in 1934–35. It showed that a majority of British people supported the use of military force to defend Abyssinia if necessary. Facing an autumn election at home, British politicians now began to 'get tough'. At an assembly of the League, the British Foreign Minister, Hoare, made a grand speech about the value of collective security, to the delight of the League's members and all the smaller nations. There was much talking and negotiating. However, the League never actually did anything to discourage Mussolini.

On 4 September, after eight months' deliberation, a committee reported to the League that neither side could be held responsible for the Wal-Wal incident. The League put forward a plan that would give Mussolini some of Abyssinia. Mussolini rejected it.

Phase 2: sanctions or not?

In October 1935 Mussolini's army was ready. He launched a full-scale invasion of Abyssinia. Despite brave resistance, the Abyssinians were no match for the modern Italian army equipped with tanks, aeroplanes and poison gas.

This was a clear-cut case of a large, powerful state attacking a smaller one. The League was designed for just such disputes and, unlike in the Manchurian crisis, it was ideally placed to act.

There was no doubting the seriousness of the issue either. The Covenant (see Factfile, page 28) made it clear that sanctions must be introduced against the aggressor. A committee was immediately set up to agree what sanctions to impose.

Sanctions would only work if they were imposed quickly and decisively. Each week a decision was delayed would allow Mussolini to build up his stockpile of raw materials. The League banned arms sales to Italy; banned loans to Italy; banned imports from Italy. It also banned the export to Italy of rubber, tin and metals. However, the League delayed a decision for two months over whether to ban oil exports to Italy. It feared the Americans would not support the sanctions. It also feared that its members' economic interests would be further damaged. In Britain, the Cabinet was informed that 30,000 British coal miners were about to lose their jobs because of the ban on coal exports to Italy.

More important still, the Suez Canal, which was owned by Britain and France, was not closed to Mussolini's supply ships. The canal was the Italians' main supply route to Abyssinia and closing it could have ended the Abyssinian campaign very quickly. Both Britain and France were afraid that closing the canal could have resulted in war with Italy. This failure was fatal for Abyssinia.

SOURCE 9

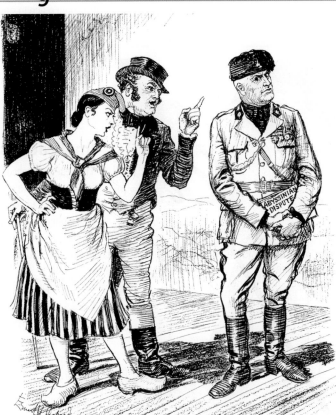

THE AWFUL WARNING.

FRANCE AND ENGLAND
(together ?).

"WE DON'T WANT YOU TO FIGHT,
BUT, BY JINGO, IF YOU DO,
WE SHALL PROBABLY ISSUE A JOINT MEMORANDUM
SUGGESTING A MILD DISAPPROVAL OF YOU."

A cartoon from *Punch*, 1935, commenting on the Abyssinian crisis. *Punch* was usually very patriotic towards Britain. It seldom criticised British politicians over foreign policy.

Source Analysis ▶

1 Study Source 9. At what point in the crisis do you think this might have been published? Use the details in the source and the text to help you decide.
2 Here are three possible reasons why this cartoon was drawn:
   ♦ To tell people in Britain what British and French policy was
   ♦ To criticise British and French policy
   ♦ To change British and French policy.
Which do you think is the best explanation?

45

The Hoare–Laval Pact

Equally damaging to the League was the secret dealing between the British and the French that was going on behind the scenes. In December 1935, while sanctions discussions were still taking place, the British and French Foreign Ministers, Hoare and Laval, were hatching a plan. This aimed to give Mussolini two-thirds of Abyssinia in return for his calling off his invasion! Laval even proposed to put the plan to Mussolini before they showed it to either the League of Nations or Haile Selassie. Laval told the British that if they did not agree to the plan, then the French would no longer support sanctions against Italy.

However, details of the plan were leaked to the French press. It proved quite disastrous for the League. Haile Selassie demanded an immediate League debate about it. In both Britain and France it was seen as a blatant act of treachery against the League. Hoare and Laval were both sacked. But the real damage was to the sanctions discussions. They lost all momentum. The question about whether to ban oil sales was further delayed. In February 1936 the committee concluded that if they did stop oil sales to Italy, the Italians' supplies would be exhausted in two months, even if the Americans kept on selling oil to them. But by then it was all too late. Mussolini had already taken over large parts of Abyssinia. And the Americans were even more disgusted with the ditherings of the French and the British than they had been before and so blocked a move to support the League's sanctions. American oil producers actually stepped up their exports to Italy.

The outcomes

On 7 March 1936 the fatal blow was delivered. Hitler, timing his move to perfection, marched his troops into the Rhineland, an act prohibited by the Treaty of Versailles (see page 12). If there had been any hope of getting the French to support sanctions against Italy, it was now dead.

The French were desperate to gain the support of Italy and were now prepared to pay the price of giving Abyssinia to Mussolini.

Italy continued to defy the League's orders and by May 1936 had taken the capital of Abyssinia, Addis Ababa. On 2 May, Haile Selassie was forced into exile. On 9 May, Mussolini formally annexed the entire country.

Implications for the League

The League watched helplessly. Collective security had been shown up as an empty promise. The League of Nations had failed. If the British and French had hoped that their handling of the Abyssinian crisis would help strengthen their position against Hitler, they were soon proved very wrong. In November 1936 Mussolini and Hitler signed an agreement of their own called the Rome–Berlin Axis.

SOURCE **10**

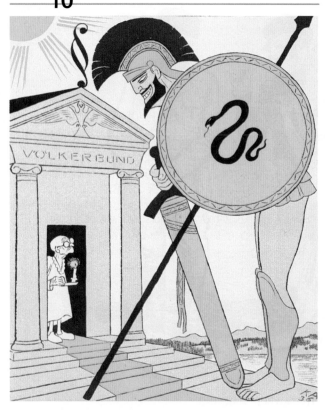

A German cartoon from the front cover of the pro-Nazi magazine Simplicissimus, 1936. The warrior is delivering a message to the League of Nations (the 'Völkerbund'): 'I am sorry to disturb your sleep but I just wanted to tell you that you should no longer bother yourselves about this Abyssinian business. The matter has been settled elsewhere.'

SOURCE **11**

Could the League survive the failure of sanctions to rescue Abyssinia? Could it ever impose sanctions again? Probably there had never been such a clear-cut case for sanctions. If the League had failed in this case there could probably be no confidence that it could succeed again in the future.

Anthony Eden, British Foreign Minister, expressing his feelings about the crisis to the British Cabinet in May 1936.

SOURCE **12**

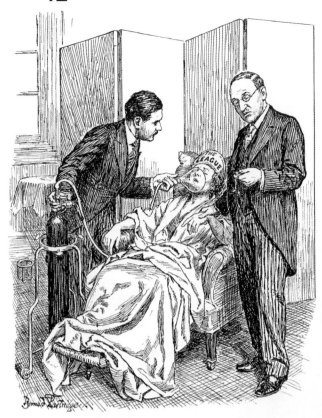

A cartoon from *Punch*, 1938. The doctors represent Britain and France.

Think!

Write a caption for the cartoon in Source 12, showing people's feelings about the League after the Abyssinian crisis. The real caption is on page viii.

Focus Task

How far did weaknesses in the League's organisation make failure inevitable?

1 When the League was set up its critics said there were weaknesses in its organisation that would make it ineffective. On page 34 you drew up a table to analyse the effect of these weaknesses in the 1920s. Now do a similar analysis for the 1930s.
What evidence is there in the Manchurian crisis, the disarmament talks and the Abyssinian crisis of the following criticisms of the League:
♦ that it would be slow to act
♦ that members would act in their own interests
♦ that without the USA it would be powerless?
2 'The way the League was set up meant it was bound to fail.' Explain how far you agree with this statement. Support your answer with evidence from the tables you have compiled for this Focus Task and the one on page 34.

A disaster for the League and for the world

Historians often disagree about how to interpret important events. However, one of the most striking things about the events of 1935 and 1936 is that most historians seem to agree about the Abyssinian crisis: it was a disaster for the League of Nations and had serious consequences for world peace.

SOURCE **13**

The implications of the conquest of Abyssinia were not confined to East Africa. Although victory cemented Mussolini's personal prestige at home, Italy gained little or nothing from it in material terms. The damage done, meanwhile, to the prestige of Britain, France and the League of Nations was irreversible. The only winner in the whole sorry episode was Adolf Hitler.

Written by historian TA Morris in 1995.

SOURCE **14**

After seeing what happened first in Manchuria and then in Abyssinia, most people drew the conclusion that it was no longer much use placing their hopes in the League . . .

Written by historian James Joll in 1976.

SOURCE **15**

The real death of the League was in 1935. One day it was a powerful body imposing sanctions, the next day it was an empty sham, everyone scuttling from it as quickly as possible. Hitler watched.

Written by historian AJP Taylor in 1966.

SOURCE **16**

Yes, we know that World War began in Manchuria fifteen years ago. We know that four years later we could easily have stopped Mussolini if we had taken the sanctions against Mussolini that were obviously required, if we had closed the Suez Canal to the aggressor and stopped his oil.

British statesman Philip Noel Baker speaking at the very last session of the League in April 1946.

Focus task A

Why did the League of Nations fail in the 1930s?

Here is a diagram summarising reasons for the failure of the League of Nations in the 1930s. Complete your own copy of the diagram to explain how each weakness affected the League's actions in Manchuria and Abyssinia. We have filled in some points for you. There is one weakness that you will not be able to write about – you will find out about it in Chapter 3.

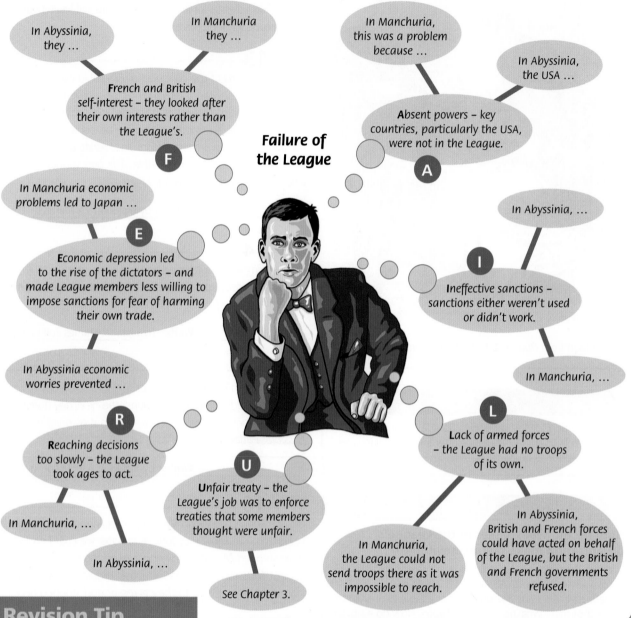

In Abyssinia, they …

In Manchuria they …

In Manchuria, this was a problem because …

In Abyssinia, the USA …

French and British self-interest – they looked after their own interests rather than the League's.
F

Absent powers – key countries, particularly the USA, were not in the League.
A

Failure of the League

In Manchuria economic problems led to Japan …

Economic depression led to the rise of the dictators – and made League members less willing to impose sanctions for fear of harming their own trade.
E

In Abyssinia, …

Ineffective sanctions – sanctions either weren't used or didn't work.
I

In Manchuria, …

In Abyssinia economic worries prevented …

Reaching decisions too slowly – the League took ages to act.
R

Lack of armed forces – the League had no troops of its own.
L

In Manchuria, …

Unfair treaty – the League's job was to enforce treaties that some members thought were unfair.
U

In Abyssinia, …

See Chapter 3.

In Manchuria, the League could not send troops there as it was impossible to reach.

In Abyssinia, British and French forces could have acted on behalf of the League, but the British and French governments refused.

Revision Tip

The memory aid FAILURE should help you remember these key points for an exam.

Focus Task B

To what extent was the League of Nations a success?

The last few pages have been all about failure. But remember there were successes too. Look back over the whole chapter.
1 The League and its aims: give the League a score out of 5 on how far it achieved its aims. Make sure you can support your score with examples.
2 Other factors which led to success: give these a score out of 5 to show their importance – remember the examples.
3 Other factors which led to failure: Repeat step 2.
4 Weigh successes against failures: how does the League score out of 100?
5 Write a short paragraph explaining your mark out of 100.

Keywords

Make sure you know what these terms mean and are able to define them confidently.

Essential

- Abyssinian crisis
- Disarmament
- Economic depression
- Isolationism
- Manchurian crisis
- Trade sanctions
- Wall Street Crash
- Article 10
- Assembly
- Collective security
- Commissions
- Conference of Ambassadors
- Council
- Covenant
- Military force
- Moral condemnation
- Secretariat
- Unanimous

Useful

- Normalcy
- Tariffs

Chapter Summary

The League of Nations

1 The League of Nations was set up to solve problems between countries before they led to war.

2 Its methods were mainly diplomacy (talking), trade sanctions, or if necessary using the armies of their members.

3 It was the big idea of President Wilson but his own country the USA never joined but returned to its isolationist policy.

4 The leading members were Britain and France but they had their own interests and bypassed the League when it suited them.

5 The League's structure made it slow to take decisions, which made it less effective in settling international disputes, but it did have some successes in the 1920s.

6 The League's agencies (committees and commissions) were set up to solve social problems such as post-war refugee crises, health problems and slavery/forced labour. It had many successes throughout the 1920s and 1930s.

7 The League was supposed to encourage disarmament but failed to get any countries to disarm.

8 In the 1930s the League's work was made much harder by the economic depression, which made countries less willing to co-operate and helped turn previously democratic countries such as Germany into dictatorships.

9 In 1931–32 the League condemned the Japanese invasion of Manchuria and China but was helpless to do anything to stop it.

10 In 1936–37 the League tried to prevent Italy invading Abyssinia but it could not agree what to do and never even enforced trade sanctions.

11 From 1936 the League was seen as irrelevant to international affairs although its agencies continued its humanitarian work.

Exam Practice

See pages 168–175 and pages 316–319 for advice on the different types of questions you might face.

1 (a) Describe the main powers available to the League to sort out international disputes. **[4]**

(b) Explain why the League of Nations did not impose sanctions against Italy during the Abyssinian crisis. **[6]**

(c) 'The League of Nations had failed before the Abyssinian crisis even started.' How far do you agree with this statement? Explain your answer. **[10]**

2 Study Source 17 on page 35. How useful are these two photographs for finding out about the League of Nations? Explain your answer by using details of the source and your own knowledge. **[7]**

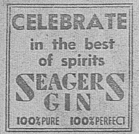

DAILY SKETCH

No. 9,177   SATURDAY, OCTOBER 1, 1938   ONE PENNY

PREMIER SAYS 'PEACE FOR OUR TIME'—P. 3

Give Thanks In Church To-morrow

TO-MORROW is Peace Sunday.

Hardly more than a few hours ago it seemed as if it would have been the first Sunday of the most senseless and savage war in history.

The "Daily Sketch" suggests that the Nation should attend church to-morrow and give thanks.

THE fathers and mothers who might have lost their sons, the young people who would have paid the cost of war with their lives, the children who have been spared the horror of modern warfare—let them all attend Divine Service and kneel in humility and thankfulness.

To-morrow should not be allowed to pass without a sincere and reverent recognition of its significance.

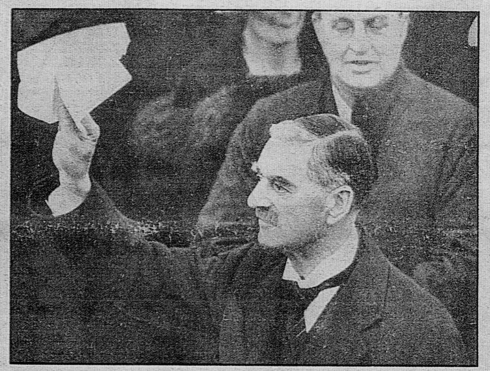

MR. CHAMBERLAIN shows the paper that represents his great triumph for European peace to the thousands who gave him such a thunderous welcome at Heston yesterday. It is the historic Anglo-German Pact signed by himself and the Fuehrer, Herr Hitler.

'Determined To Ensure Peace'

WHEN Mr. Chamberlain arrived at Heston last night he said:

"This morning I had another talk with the German Chancellor, Herr Hitler. Here is a paper which bears his name as well as mine. I would like to read it to you:

"'We, the German Fuehrer and Chancellor and the British Prime Minister, have had a further meeting to-day and are agreed in recognising that the question of Anglo-German relations is of the first importance for the two countries and for Europe.

"'We regard the agreement signed last night and the Anglo-German Naval Agreement as symbolic of the desire of our two peoples never to war with one another again.

"'We are resolved that the method of consultation shall be the method adopted to deal with any other questions that may concern our two countries and we are determined to continue our efforts to remove possible sources of difference and thus to contribute to the assurance of peace in Europe.'"

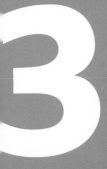

Why had international peace collapsed by 1939?

FOCUS POINTS

- What were the long-term consequences of the peace treaties of 1919–23?
- What were the consequences of the failures of the League in the 1930s?
- How far was Hitler's foreign policy to blame for the outbreak of war in 1939?
- Was the policy of appeasement justified?
- How important was the Nazi–Soviet Pact?
- Why did Britain and France declare war on Germany in September 1939?

The image on the opposite page represents the most famous moment of Appeasement – the policy followed by Britain and France towards Hitler through the 1930s. The British Prime Minister has returned from a meeting with Hitler having agreed to give him parts of Czechoslovakia, in return for which Hitler promised peace.

If you know the story already then you will know that this agreement proved totally empty – 'not worth the paper it was written on' as they say! Hitler did not keep his word, and probably never meant to.

But just forget hindsight for a moment and try to join with the people of Britain welcoming back a leader who seemed to be doing his best to preserve a crumbling peace.

You can see from the newspaper there is a genuine desire to believe in the possibility of peace. Chamberlain had not given up on the possibility of peace; nor had the British people. They did not think that war was inevitable – even in 1938. They did all they could to avoid it.

In this chapter your task is to work out why, despite all the efforts of international leaders, and all the horrors of war, international peace finally collapsed in 1939.

Here are some of the factors you will consider. They are all relevant and they are all connected. Your task will be to examine each one, then see the connections and weigh the importance of these different factors.

1. Treaties after the First World War particularly the Treaty of Versailles	2. The failures of the League of Nations	3. The worldwide economic depression
4. The policy of Appeasement	5. The Nazi-Soviet pact	6. Hitler's actions and particularly his foreign policy

◀ Opposite is the front page of the *Daily Sketch*, 1 October 1938. Read it carefully and select one or two phrases which suggest or prove that:

- the British people thought Chamberlain was a hero
- the newspaper approves of Chamberlain
- people in Britain genuinely feared a war was imminent in 1938
- Hitler was respected
- Hitler could be trusted
- this agreement would bring lasting peace.

Hitler's war

Between 1918 and 1933 Adolf Hitler rose from being an obscure and demoralised member of the defeated German army to become the all-powerful Führer, dictator of Germany, with almost unlimited power and an overwhelming ambition to make Germany great once again. His is an astonishing story which you can read about in detail in Chapter 9. Here you will be concentrating on just one intriguing and controversial question: how far was Hitler responsible for the outbreak of the Second World War.

Hitler's plans

Hitler was never secretive about his plans for Germany. As early as 1924 he had laid out in his book *Mein Kampf* what he would do if the Nazis ever achieved power in Germany.

Abolish the Treaty of Versailles!

Like many Germans, Hitler believed that the Treaty of Versailles was unjust.

He hated the Treaty and called the German leaders who had signed it 'The November Criminals'. The Treaty was a constant reminder to Germans of their defeat in the First World War and their humiliation by the Allies. Hitler promised that if he became leader of Germany he would reverse it (see Source 1).

By the time he came to power in Germany, some of the terms had already been changed. For example, Germany had stopped making reparations payments altogether. However, most points were still in place. The table on page 53 shows the terms of the Treaty that most angered Hitler.

Expand German territory!

The Treaty of Versailles had taken away territory from Germany. Hitler wanted to get that territory back. He wanted Germany to unite with Austria. He wanted German minorities in other countries such as Czechoslovakia to rejoin Germany. But he also wanted to carve out an empire in eastern Europe to give extra *Lebensraum* or 'living space' for Germans (see Source 2).

Defeat Communism!

A German empire carved out of the Soviet Union would also help Hitler in one of his other objectives – the defeat of Communism or Bolshevism. Hitler was anti-Communist. He believed that Bolsheviks had helped to bring about the defeat of Germany in the First World War. He also believed that the Bolsheviks wanted to take over Germany (see Source 3).

SOURCE 1

We demand equality of rights for the German people in its dealings with other nations, and abolition of the Peace Treaties of Versailles and St Germain.

From Hitler's *Mein Kampf*, 1923–24.

SOURCE 2

We turn our eyes towards the lands of the east . . . When we speak of new territory in Europe today, we must principally think of Russia and the border states subject to her. Destiny itself seems to wish to point out the way for us here.

Colonisation of the eastern frontiers is of extreme importance. It will be the duty of Germany's foreign policy to provide large spaces for the nourishment and settlement of the growing population of Germany.

From Hitler's *Mein Kampf*.

SOURCE 3

We must not forget that the Bolsheviks are blood-stained. That they overran a great state [Russia], and in a fury of massacre wiped out millions of their most intelligent fellow-countrymen and now for ten years have been conducting the most tyrannous regime of all time. We must not forget that many of them belong to a race which combines a rare mixture of bestial cruelty and vast skill in lies, and considers itself specially called now to gather the whole world under its bloody oppression.

The menace which Russia suffered under is one which perpetually hangs over Germany. Germany is the next great objective of Bolshevism. All our strength is needed to raise up our nation once more and rescue it from the embrace of the international python . . . The first essential is the expulsion of the Marxist poison from the body of our nation.

From Hitler's *Mein Kampf*.

Think!

It is 1933. Write a briefing paper for the British government on Hitler's plans for Germany. Use Sources 1–3 to help you.

Conclude with your own assessment on whether the government should be worried about Hitler and his plans.

In your conclusion, remember these facts about the British government:

♦ Britain is a leading member of the League of Nations and is supposed to uphold the Treaty of Versailles, by force if necessary.
♦ The British government does not trust the Communists and thinks that a strong Germany could help to stop the Communist threat.

Hitler's actions

This timeline shows how, between 1933 and 1939, Hitler turned his plans into actions.

DATE	ACTION
1933	Took Germany out of the League of Nations; began rearming Germany
1934	Tried to take over Austria but was prevented by Mussolini
1935	Held massive rearmament rally in Germany
1936	Reintroduced conscription in Germany; sent German troops into the Rhineland; made an anti-Communist alliance with Japan
1937	Tried out Germany's new weapons in the Spanish Civil War; made an anti-Communist alliance with Italy
1938	Took over Austria; took over the Sudetenland area of Czechoslovakia
1939	Invaded the rest of Czechoslovakia; invaded Poland; war

War

SOURCE 4

Any account of the origins and course of the Second World War must give Hitler the leading part. Without him a major war in the early 1940s between all the world's great powers was unthinkable.

British historian Professor Richard Overy, writing in 1996.

Other factors

When you see events leading up to the war laid out this way, it makes it seem as if Hitler planned it all step by step. In fact, this view of events was widely accepted by historians until the 1960s. In the 1960s, however, the British historian AJP Taylor came up with a new interpretation. His view was that Hitler was a gambler rather than a planner. Hitler simply took the logical next step to see what he could get away with. He was bold. He kept his nerve. As other countries gave in to him and allowed him to get away with each gamble, so he became bolder and risked more. In Taylor's interpretation it is Britain, the Allies and the League of Nations who are to blame for letting Hitler get away with it — by not standing up to him. In this interpretation it is other factors that are as much to blame as Hitler himself:

- the wordwide economic depression
- the weaknesses of the post-war treaties
- the actions of the leading powers — Britain, France, the USA and the USSR.

As you examine Hitler's actions in more detail, you will see that both interpretations are possible. You can make up your own mind which you agree with.

Revision Tip

The details in this chart will be a very useful revision aid. So add pictures and highlights to help you learn the information.

Think!

Hitler and the Treaty of Versailles

1. Draw up a table like this one to show some of the terms of the Treaty of Versailles that affected Germany.
2. As you work through this chapter, fill out the other columns of this 'Versailles chart'.

Terms of the Treaty of Versailles	What Hitler did and when	The reasons he gave for his action	The response from Britain and France
Germany's armed forces to be severely limited			
The Rhineland to be a demilitarised zone			
Germany forbidden to unite with Austria			
The Sudetenland taken into the new state of Czechoslovakia			
The Polish Corridor given to Poland			

SOURCE **6**

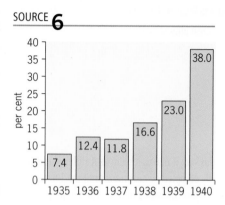

The proportion of German spending that went into armaments, 1935–40.

Source Analysis

How far do Sources 6 and 7 prove Source 5 to be wrong?

Think!

1 Fill out the first row of your 'Versailles chart' on page 53 to summarise what Hitler did about rearmament.
2 What factors allowed Hitler to get away with rearming Germany? Look for:
   a) the impact of the Despression
   b) the Treaty of Versailles
   c) the League of Nations
   d) the actions of Britain and France.

Rearmament

Hitler came to power in Germany in 1933. One of his first steps was to increase Germany's armed forces. Thousands of unemployed workers were drafted into the army. This helped him to reduce unemployment, which was one of the biggest problems he faced in Germany. But it also helped him to deliver on his promise to make Germany strong again and to challenge the terms of the Treaty of Versailles.

Hitler knew that German people supported rearmament. But he also knew it would cause alarm in other countries. He handled it cleverly. Rearmament began in secret at first. He made a great public display of his desire not to rearm Germany – that he was only doing it because other countries refused to disarm (see page 42). He then followed Japan's example and withdrew from the League of Nations.

In 1935 Hitler openly staged a massive military rally celebrating the German armed forces. In 1936 he even reintroduced conscription to the army. He was breaking the terms of the Treaty of Versailles, but he guessed correctly that he would get away with rearmament. Many other countries were using rearmament as a way to fight unemployment. The collapse of the League of Nations Disarmament Conference in 1934 (see pages 42–43) had shown that other nations were not prepared to disarm.

Rearmament was a very popular move in Germany. It boosted Nazi support. Hitler also knew that Britain had some sympathy with Germany on this issue. Britain believed that the limits put on Germany's armed forces by the Treaty of Versailles were too tight. The permitted forces were not enough to defend Germany from attack. Britain also thought that a strong Germany would be a good buffer against Communism.

Britain had already helped to dismantle the Treaty by signing a naval agreement with Hitler in 1935, allowing Germany to increase its navy to up to 35 per cent of the size of the British navy. The French were angry with Britain about this, but there was little they could do. Through the rest of the 1930s Hitler ploughed more and more spending into armaments (see Sources 6 and 7).

SOURCE **7**

	Warships	Aircraft	Soldiers
1932	(30)	(36)	(100,000)
1939	(95)	(8,250)	(950,000)

German armed forces in 1932 and 1939.

The Saar plebiscite

The Saar region of Germany had been run by the League of Nations since 1919 (see page 32).

In 1935 the League of Nations held the promised plebiscite for people to vote on whether their region should return to German rule. Hitler was initially wary as many of his opponents had fled to the Saar. The League, however, was determined that the vote should take place and Hitler bowed to this pressure. So it seemed that the League was being firm and decisive with Hitler. The vote was an overwhelming success for Hitler. His propaganda minister Joseph Goebbels mounted a massive campaign to persuade the people of the Saar to vote for the Riech. Around 90 per cent of the population voted to return to German rule. This was entirely legal and within the terms of the Treaty. It was also a real morale booster for Hitler. After the vote Hitler declared that he had 'no further territorial demands to make of France'.

SOURCE **8**

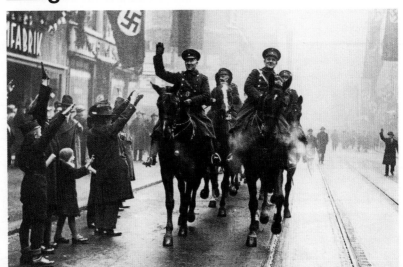

Following the plebiscite in 1935, people and police express their joy at returning to the German Reich by giving the Nazi salute.

Source Analysis

1 Explain in your own words what is happening in Source 8. For example, who are the people on horseback? Why are people saluting?
2 Do you trust Source 8 to be an accurate portrayal of the feelings of the people of the Saar in January 1935?
3 What is the message of the cartoon in Source 9? Explain your answer using details of the source and your knowledge.

SOURCE **9**

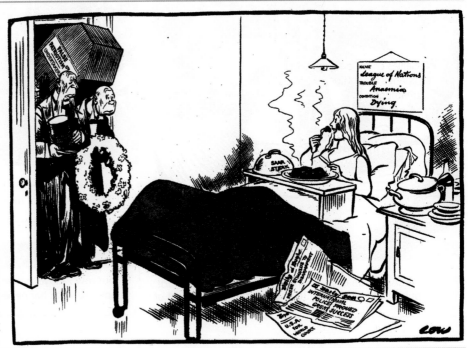

A British cartoon published in January 1935, soon after the Saar plebiscite. The figure in bed is the League of Nations. The caption was 'Sitting up and taking nourishment'.

Remilitarisation of the Rhineland

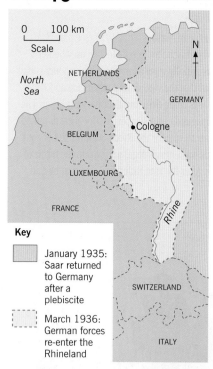

The Rhineland.

Key

- January 1935: Saar returned to Germany after a plebiscite

- March 1936: German forces re-enter the Rhineland

In March 1936, Hitler took his first really big risk by moving troops into the Rhineland area of Germany. The Rhineland was the large area either side of the River Rhine that formed Germany's western border with France and Belgium.

The demilitarisation of the Rhineland was one of the terms of the Treaty of Versailles. It was designed to protect France from invasion from Germany. It had also been accepted by Germany in the Locarno Treaties of 1925. Hitler was taking a huge gamble. If he had been forced to withdraw, he would have faced humiliation and would have lost the support of the German army (many of the generals were unsure about him, anyway). Hitler knew the risks, but he had chosen the time and place well.

- **France** had just signed a treaty with the USSR to protect each other against attack from Germany (see Source 11). Hitler used the agreement to claim that Germany was under threat. He argued that in the face of such a threat he should be allowed to place troops on his own frontier.

- Hitler knew that many people in **Britain** felt that he had a right to station his troops in the Rhineland and he was fairly confident that Britain would not intervene. His gamble was over France. Would France let him get away with it?

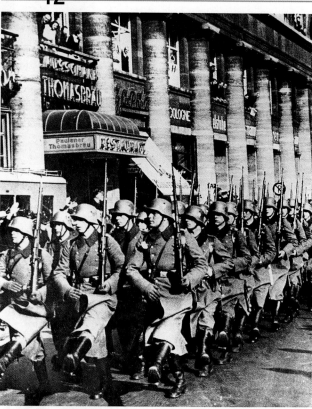

German troops marching through the city of Cologne in March 1936. This style of marching with high steps was known as goose-stepping.

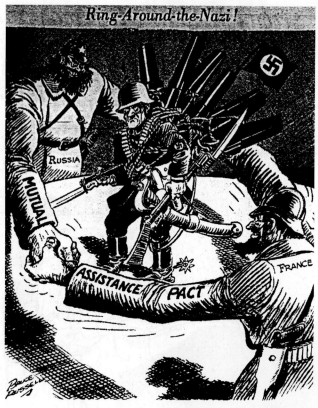

An American cartoon entitled 'Ring-Around-the-Nazi!' published in March 1936 showing the encirclement of Germany by France and the USSR.

Think!

Fill out row 2 of your 'Versailles chart' on page 53 to summarise what happened in the Rhineland.

SOURCE 13

At that time we had no army worth mentioning . . . If the French had taken any action we would have been easily defeated; our resistance would have been over in a few days. And the Air Force we had then was ridiculous – a few Junkers 52s from Lufthansa and not even enough bombs for them . . .

Hitler looks back on his gamble over the Rhineland some years after the event.

SOURCE 14

Hitler has got away with it. France is not marching. No wonder the faces of Göring and Blomberg [Nazi leaders] were all smiles.

Oh, the stupidity (or is it the paralysis?) of the French. I learnt today that the German troops had orders to beat a hasty retreat if the French army opposed them in any way.

Written by William Shirer in 1936. He was an American journalist in Germany during the 1930s. He was a critic of the Nazi regime and had to flee from Germany in 1940.

As the troops moved into the Rhineland, Hitler and his generals sweated nervously. They had orders to pull out if the French acted against them. Despite the rearmament programme, Germany's army was no match for the French army. It lacked essential equipment and air support. In the end, however, Hitler's luck held.

The attention of the League of Nations was on the Abyssinian crisis which was happening at exactly the same time (see pages 44–47). The League condemned Hitler's action but had no power to do anything else. Even the French, who were most directly threatened by the move, were divided over what to do. They were about to hold an election and none of the French leaders was prepared to take responsibility for plunging France into a war. Of course, they did not know how weak the German army was. In the end, France refused to act without British support and so Hitler's big gamble paid off. Maybe next time he would risk more!

SOURCE 15

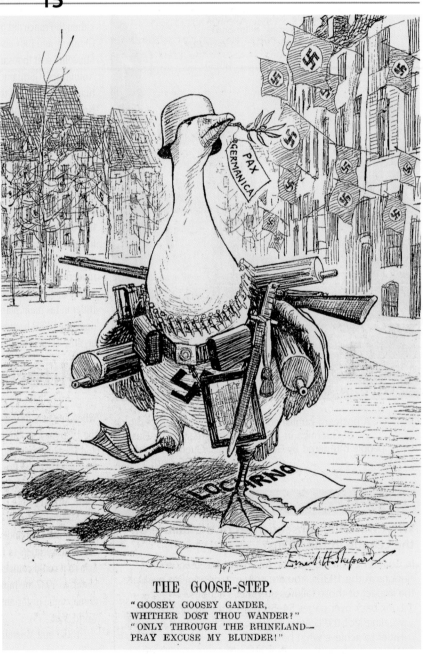

THE GOOSE-STEP.

"GOOSEY GOOSEY GANDER,
WHITHER DOST THOU WANDER?"
"ONLY THROUGH THE RHINELAND—
PRAY EXCUSE MY BLUNDER!"

A British cartoon about the reoccupation of the Rhineland, 1936. *Pax Germanica* is Latin and means 'Peace, German style'.

Source Analysis

1 Does Source 11 prove that Hitler was correct when he argued that Germany was under threat? Explain your answer.
2 What do Sources 13 and 14 disagree about? Why might they disagree about it?
3 Why has the cartoonist in Source 15 shown Germany as a goose?
4 Look at the equipment being carried by the goose. What does this tell you about how the cartoonist saw the new Germany?
5 Would you regard reoccupation of the Rhineland as a success for Hitler or as a failure for the French and the British? Explain your answer by referring to the sources.

SOURCE 16

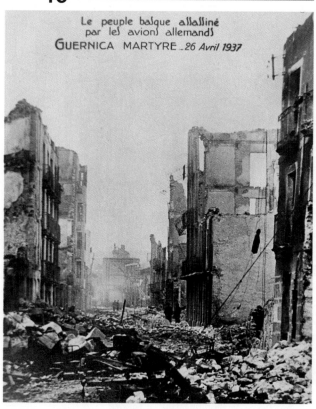

Le peuple basque assassiné par les avions allemands
GUERNICA MARTYRE _ 26 Avril 1937

A postcard published in France to mark the bombing of Guernica in 1937. The text reads 'The Basque people murdered by German planes. Guernica martyred 26 April 1937'.

The Spanish Civil War

In 1936 a civil war broke out in Spain between supporters of the Republican government and right-wing rebels under General Franco. A civil war in a European state would have been an important event anyway, but this one became extremely significant because it gained an international dimension.

Stalin's USSR's supported the Republican government (in the form of weapons, aircraft and pilots). Thousands of volunteers from around 50 countries joined International Brigades to support the Republicans. At the same time, Hitler and Mussolini declared their support for General Franco. He seemed to be a man who shared their world view.

The governments of Britain and France refused to intervene directly although France did provide some weapons for the Republicans. Germany and Italy also agreed not to intervene but then blatantly did so. Mussolini sent thousands of Italian troops, although officially they were 'volunteers'. Germany sent aircraft and pilots who took part in most of the major campaigns of the war. They helped transport Franco's forces from North Africa to Spain. Later they took part in bombing raids on civilian populations in Spanish cities (see Source 16 for example). Thanks partly to Hitler's help the Nationalists won the war and a right-wing dictatorship ruled Spain for the next 36 years.

The conflict had important consequences for peace in Europe. It gave combat experience to German and Italian forces. It strengthened the bonds between Mussolini and Hitler. Historian Zara Steiner argues that Britain's non-intervention in Spain convinced Hitler that he could form an alliance with Britain or persuade them (and France) to remain neutral in a future war. At the same time the devastating impact of modern weapons convinced Chamberlain and many others that war had to be avoided at all costs. Thus, the Spanish Civil War further encouraged Hitler in his main plan to reverse the Treaty of Versailles. At the same time, the USSR became increasingly suspicious of Britain and France because of their reluctance to get involved in opposing fascism.

Militarism and the Axis

When he wrote his memoirs in later years Winston Churchill described the 1930s as a 'Gathering Storm'. Many shared his gloomy view. Hitler and Mussolini had shown that their armed forces were effective and that they were ready to use them. Mussolini had triumphed in Abyssinia and was aggressively trying to assert his authority in the Mediterranean and North Africa.

Meanwhile in the east Japan was under the control of hardline nationalist commanders such as General Tojo. They also had the support of business leaders in Japan. They wanted to extend Japan's empire across Asia so it could compete with other world powers, particularly the United States. In 1937 the Japanese took their next big step with the invasion of China. Some historians regard this as the first campaign of the Second World War.

Hitler and Mussolini saw that they had much in common with the military dictatorship in Japan. In 1936, Germany and Japan signed an Anti-Comintern Pact, to oppose Communism. Comintern was the USSR's organisation for spreading Communism to other countries. In 1937, Italy also signed it. The new alliance was called the Axis alliance.

Anschluss with Austria, 1938

Think!

Complete row 3 of your 'Versailles chart' on page 53, summarising what Hitler did about Austria.

Source Analysis ▼

Work in pairs. Take either Source 17 or Source 18.

1 For your source work out:
   a) which character in the cartoon represents Mussolini and which Hitler
   b) what your cartoon suggests about the relationship between Hitler and Mussolini
   c) what is the cartoonist's opinion of the *Anschluss*. Find details in the source to support your view.

2 Compare your answers with your partner's and discuss any points of agreement or disagreement.

3 Write your own paragraph in answer to this question: How far do Sources 17 and 18 agree about the *Anschluss*?

With the successes of 1936 and 1937 to boost him, Hitler turned his attention to his homeland of Austria. The Austrian people were mainly German, and in *Mein Kampf* Hitler had made it clear that he felt that the two states belonged together as one German nation. Many in Austria supported the idea of union with Germany, since their country was so economically weak. Hitler was confident that he could bring them together into a 'greater Germany'. In fact, he had tried to take over Austria in 1934, but on that occasion Mussolini had stopped him. Four years later, in 1938, the situation was different. Hitler and Mussolini were now allies.

There was a strong Nazi Party in Austria. Hitler encouraged the Nazis to stir up trouble for the government. They staged demonstrations calling for union with Germany. They caused riots. Hitler then told the Austrian Chancellor Schuschnigg that only *Anschluss* (political union) could sort out these problems. He pressurised Schuschnigg to agree to *Anschluss*. Schuschnigg appealed for some kind of gesture of support such as threatening sanctions against Hitler or issuing a strong statement. France and Britain failed to provide this support so Schuschnigg felt he had no option but to call a plebiscite (a referendum), to see what the Austrian people wanted. Hitler was not prepared to risk this – he might lose! He simply sent his troops into Austria in March 1938, supposedly to guarantee a trouble-free plebiscite. Under the watchful eye of the Nazi troops, 99.75 per cent voted for *Anschluss*.

Anschluss was completed without any military confrontation with France and Britain. Chamberlain, the British Prime Minister, felt that Austrians and Germans had a right to be united and that the Treaty of Versailles was wrong to separate them. Britain's Lord Halifax had even suggested to Hitler before the *Anschluss* that Britain would not resist Germany uniting with Austria.

Once again, Hitler's risky but decisive action had reaped a rich reward – Austria's soldiers, weapons and its rich deposits of gold and iron ore were added to Germany's increasingly strong army and industry. Hitler was breaking yet another condition of the Treaty of Versailles, but the pattern was becoming clear. The Treaty itself was seen as suspect. Britain and France were not prepared to go to war to defend a flawed treaty.

SOURCE **17**

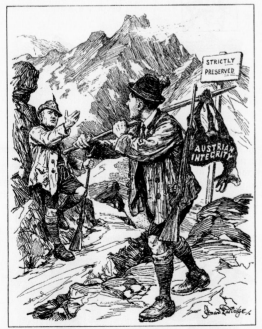

GOOD HUNTING

Mussolini. "All right, Adolf—I never heard a shot."

A British cartoon commenting on the *Anschluss*.

SOURCE **18**

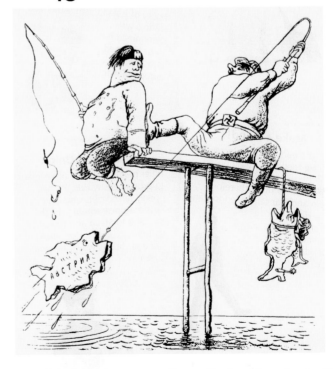

A Soviet cartoon commenting on the *Anschluss* showing Hitler catching Austria.

Appeasement: for and against!

If Britain and France were not prepared to defend the Treaty of Versailles, would they let Hitler have more of his demands? The short answer is yes, and Britain's policy at this time is known as Appeasement. Neville Chamberlain is the man most associated with this policy (see Profile page 63) although he did not become Prime Minister until 1937. Many other British people (probably the majority), including many politicians, were also in favour of this policy. However, there were some at the time who were very critical. Here are the main arguments for and against.

Trusting Hitler

After each new move he made Hitler said this was all he wanted. Yet he often went back on those promises. Appeasement was based on the mistaken idea that Hitler was trustworthy.

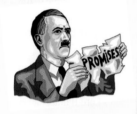

Fear of Communism

Hitler was not the only concern of Britain and its allies. He was not even their main worry. They were more concerned about the spread of Communism and particularly the dangers to world peace posed by Stalin, the new leader in the USSR. Many saw Hitler as the buffer to the threat of spreading Communism.

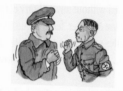

Memories of the Great War

Both British and French leaders, and much of their population, vividly remembered the horrific experiences of the First World War. They wished to avoid another war at almost any cost.

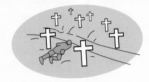

German arms

Germany was rearming publicly and quickly year by year. Hitler claimed he was trying to catch up with other countries, but others could see that Germany was better armed than Britain or France.

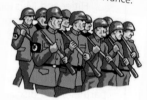

British arms

The British government believed that the armed forces were not ready for war against Hitler. Britain only began rearming in 1935 and intelligence suggested the British were some way behind the Germans.

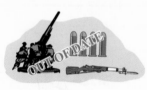

The USA

American support had been vital to Britain's success in the First World War. Britain could not be sure it could face up to Germany without the guarantee of American help. But since 1919 the USA had followed a policy of isolationism. American leaders were determined not to be dragged into another European war.

The British empire

For Britain to fight a war against Germany it needed to be sure it had the support of the countries in its empire or Commonwealth. It was not a guaranteed certainty that they would all support a war.

The Treaty of Versailles

Many felt that the Treaty of Versailles was unfair to Germany. Some of Hitler's demands were not unreasonable. They assumed that once these wrongs were put right then Germany would become a peaceful nation again.

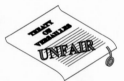

Make a stand!

Hitler the gambler took increasing risks. He tried something out to see if there would be any comeback. At some point therefore Britain and France needed to stand up to Hitler to prevent a later bigger and more dangerous move.

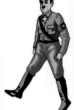

The Soviet Union

Hitler made no secret of his plans to expand eastwards. He had openly talked of taking land in Russia. Appeasement sent the message to Stalin and the USSR that Britain and France would not stand in Hitler's way if he invaded Russia.

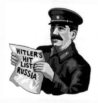

Hitler's allies

Hitler had already observed how his allies, particularly the right-wing dictatorships in Japan and Italy, had got away with acts of aggression.

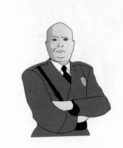

Economic problems

Britain and France had large debts (many still left over from fighting the First World War) and huge unemployment as a result of the Depression. They could not afford a war.

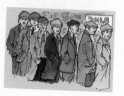

Focus Task

Why did Britain and France follow a policy of Appeasement?

The cards on page 60 show various arguments that were advanced for or against Appeasement. Study the cards, then:

1 Sort them into arguments for and arguments against Appeasement. If there are any you are not sure about leave them aside as you can come back to them.
2 On each card write a 'for' or 'against'.
3 Sort the cards into those that:
   a) would have been obvious to British and French leaders at the time
   b) would only be clear with hindsight.

4 Make notes under the following headings to summarise why Britain followed a policy of appeasement:
   a) military reasons
   b) economic reasons
   c) fear
   d) public opinion
5 Use your notes to write a short paragraph to explain in your own words why the British government followed a policy of Appeasement.

Think!

Most people in Britain supported the policy of Appeasement. Write a letter to the London *Evening Standard* justifying Appeasement and pointing out why the cartoonist is wrong. Your letter should be written in either 1936 or 1938 and it will need to be different according to which source you pick. You can use some of the arguments from the Focus Task on page 53 in your letter.

Revision Tip

Make sure you can explain:
◆ what Appeasement was
◆ two examples of Appeasement in action.
Be sure you can describe:
◆ one reason why Chamberlain followed the policy of Appeasement
◆ one reason why people criticised the policy.

One of the most famous critics was David Low, cartoonist with the popular newspaper the London *Evening Standard*. You have seen many of Low's cartoons in this book already. Low was a fierce critic of Hitler, but also criticised the policy of Appeasement. Source 19 shows one of his cartoons on the issue, but if you visit the British Cartoon Archive web site you can see all of Low's cartoons.

SOURCE 19

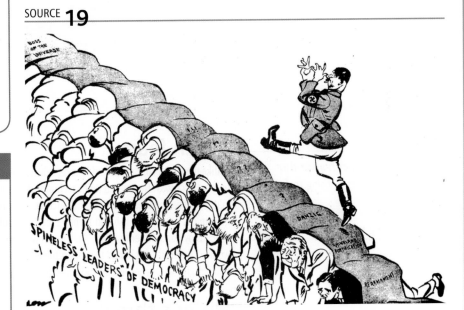

A cartoon by David Low from the London *Evening Standard*, 1936. This was a popular newspaper with a large readership in Britain.

Source Analysis ▲

Fill out a table like this to analyse Source 19. On page 64, fill out a second column to analyse Source 27 in the same way.

	Source 19	Source 27
Date published		
Critical or supportive?		
Of what/whom?		
How can we tell?		
Why was the cartoon published at this time?		

The Sudetenland, 1938

After the Austrian *Anschluss*, Hitler was beginning to feel that he could not put a foot wrong. But his growing confidence was putting the peace of Europe in increasing danger.

SOURCE **20**

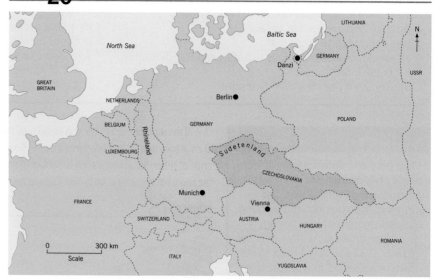

Central Europe after the *Anschluss*.

SOURCE **21**

I give you my word of honour that Czechoslovakia has nothing to fear from the Reich.

Hitler speaking to Chamberlain in 1938.

Czech fears

Unlike the leaders of Britain and France, Edvard Beneš, the leader of Czechoslovakia, was horrified by the *Anschluss*. He realised that Czechoslovakia would be the next country on Hitler's list for takeover. It seemed that Britain and France were not prepared to stand up to Hitler. Beneš sought guarantees from the British and French that they would honour their commitment to defend Czechoslovakia if Hitler invaded. The French were bound by a treaty and reluctantly said they would. The British felt bound to support the French. However, Chamberlain asked Hitler whether he had designs on Czechoslovakia and was reassured by Hitler's promise (Source 21).

Hitler's threats

Despite what he said to Chamberlain, Hitler did have designs on Czechoslovakia. This new state, created by the Treaty of Versailles, included a large number of Germans — former subjects of Austria–Hungary's empire — in the Sudetenland area. Henlein, who was the leader of the Nazis in the Sudetenland, stirred up trouble among the Sudetenland Germans and they demanded to be part of Germany. In May 1938, Hitler made it clear that he intended to fight Czechoslovakia if necessary. Historians disagree as to whether Hitler really meant what he said. There is considerable evidence that the German army was not at all ready for war. Even so the news put Europe on full war alert.

Preparations for war

Unlike Austria, Czechoslovakia would be no walk-over for Hitler. Britain, France and the USSR had all promised to support Czechoslovakia if it came to war. The Czechs themselves had a modern army. The Czechoslovak leader, Beneš, was prepared to fight. He knew that without the Sudetenland and its forts, railways and industries, Czechoslovakia would be defenceless.

All through the summer the tension rose in Europe. If there was a war, people expected that it would bring heavy bombing of civilians as had happened in the Spanish Civil War, and in cities around Britain councils began digging air-raid shelters. Magazines carried advertisements for air-raid protection and gas masks.

Think!

Write a series of newspaper headlines for different stages of the Sudetenland crisis, for example:
◆ March 1938
◆ May 1938
◆ early September 1938
◆ 30 September 1938.
Include headlines for:
◆ a Czech newspaper
◆ a British newspaper
◆ a German newspaper.

SOURCE 22

How horrible, fantastic, incredible it is that we should be digging trenches and trying on gas masks here because of a quarrel in a far away country between people of whom we know nothing. I am myself a man of peace to the depths of my soul.

From a radio broadcast by Neville Chamberlain, September 1938.

Profile
Neville Chamberlain

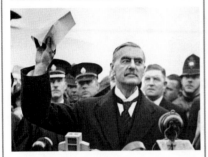

- Born 1869.
- He was the son of the famous radical politician Joseph Chamberlain.
- He was a successful businessman in the Midlands before entering politics.
- During the First World War he served in the Cabinet as Director General of National Service. During this time he saw the full horrors of war.
- After the war he was Health Minister and then Chancellor. He was noted for his careful work and his attention to detail. However, he was not good at listening to advice.
- He was part of the government throughout the 1920s and supported the policy of Appeasement towards Hitler. He became Prime Minister in 1937, although he had little experience of foreign affairs.
- He believed that Germany had real grievances – this was the basis for his policy of Appeasement.
- He became a national hero after the Munich Conference of 1938 averted war.
- In 1940 Chamberlain resigned as Prime Minister and Winston Churchill took over.

SOURCE 23

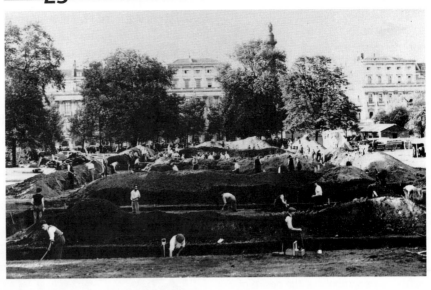

Digging air raid defences in London, September 1938.

Crisis talks

In September the problem reached crisis point. In a last-ditch effort to avert war, Chamberlain flew to meet Hitler on 15 September. The meeting appeared to go well. Hitler moderated his demands, saying he was only interested in parts of the Sudetenland – and then only if a plebiscite showed that the Sudeten Germans wanted to join Germany. Chamberlain thought this was reasonable. He felt it was yet another of the terms of the Treaty of Versailles that needed to be addressed. Chamberlain seemed convinced that, if Hitler got what he wanted, he would at last be satisfied.

On 19 September the French and the British put to the Czechs their plans to give Hitler the parts of the Sudetenland that he wanted. However, three days later at a second meeting, Hitler increased his demands. He said he 'regretted' that the previously arranged terms were not enough. He wanted all the Sudetenland.

SOURCE 24

The Sudetenland is the last problem that must be solved and it will be solved. It is the last territorial claim which I have to make in Europe.

The aims of our foreign policy are not unlimited . . . They are grounded on the determination to save the German people alone . . . Ten million Germans found themselves beyond the frontiers of the Reich . . . Germans who wished to return to the Reich as their homeland.

Hitler speaking in Berlin, September 1938.

To justify his demands, he claimed that the Czech government was mistreating the Germans in the Sudetenland and that he intended to 'rescue' them by 1 October. Chamberlain told Hitler that his demands were unreasonable. The British navy was mobilised. War seemed imminent.

The Munich Agreement

With Mussolini's help, a final meeting was held in Munich on 29 September. While Europe held its breath, the leaders of Britain, Germany, France and Italy decided on the fate of Czechoslovakia.

On 29 September they decided to give Hitler what he wanted. They announced that Czechoslovakia was to lose the Sudetenland. They did not consult the Czechs, nor did they consult the USSR. This is known as the Munich Agreement. The following morning Chamberlain and Hitler published a joint declaration (Source 26) which Chamberlain said would bring 'peace for our time'.

SOURCE 25

People of Britain, your children are safe. Your husbands and your sons will not march to war. Peace is a victory for all mankind. If we must have a victor, let us choose Chamberlain, for the Prime Minister's conquests are mighty and enduring – millions of happy homes and hearts relieved of their burden.

The *Daily Express* comments on the Munich Agreement, 30 September 1938.

SOURCE 26

We regard the Agreement signed last night . . . as symbolic of the desire of our two peoples never to go to war with one another again. We are resolved that we shall use consultation to deal with any other questions that may concern our two countries, and we are determined to continue our efforts to assure the peace of Europe.

The joint declaration of Chamberlain and Hitler, 30 September 1938.

SOURCE 28

By repeatedly surrendering to force, Chamberlain has encouraged aggression . . . our central contention, therefore, is that Mr Chamberlain's policy has throughout been based on a fatal misunderstanding of the psychology of dictatorship.

The *Yorkshire Post*, December 1938.

Source Analysis

1 Study Sources 25–29. Sort them into the categories:
   a) those that support the Munich Agreement
   b) those that criticise the Munich Agreement.
2 List the reasons why each source supports or criticises the agreement.
3 Imagine you are a teacher setting a test.
   ◆ Which of Sources 25–29 would work well for an 'Are you surprised?' question?
   ◆ Which of Sources 25–29 would work well for a 'How useful is this source?' question? Explain your answers.

Consequences

Hitler had gambled that the British would not risk war. He spoke of the Munich Agreement as 'an undreamt-of triumph, so great that you can scarcely imagine it'. The prize of the Sudetenland had been given to him without a shot being fired. On 1 October German troops marched into the Sudetenland. At the same time, Hungary and Poland helped themselves to Czech territory where Hungarians and Poles were living.

The Czechs had been betrayed. Beneš resigned. But the rest of Europe breathed a sigh of relief. Chamberlain received a hero's welcome back in Britain, when he returned with the 'piece of paper' – the Agreement – signed by Hitler (see Profile, page 63).

SOURCE 27

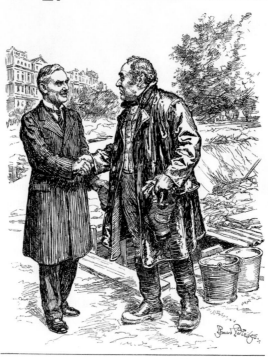

A GREAT MEDIATOR

John Bull. "I've known many Prime Ministers in my time, Sir, but never one who worked so hard for security in the face of such terrible odds."

A British cartoon published in 1938 at the time of the Munich Agreement. John Bull represents Britain. You can find many more cartoons about the Agreement at the British Cartoon Archive website.

SOURCE 29

We have suffered a total defeat … I think you will find that in a period of time Czechoslovakia will be engulfed in the Nazi regime. We have passed an awful milestone in our history. This is only the beginning of the reckoning.

Winston Churchill speaking in October 1938. He felt that Britain should resist the demands of Hitler. However, he was an isolated figure in the 1930s.

Triumph or sell-out?

What do you think of the Munich Agreement? Was it a good move or a poor one? Most people in Britain were relieved that it had averted war, but many were now openly questioning the whole policy of Appeasement. Even the public relief may have been overstated. Opinion polls in September 1938 show that the British people did not think Appeasement would stop Hitler. It simply delayed a war, rather than preventing it. Even while Chamberlain was signing the Munich Agreement, he was approving a massive increase in arms spending in preparation for war.

Think!

Complete row 4 of your 'Versailles chart' on page 53.

The end of Appeasement

Czechoslovakia, 1939

Although the British people welcomed the Munich Agreement, they did not trust Hitler. In an opinion poll in October 1938, 93 per cent said they did not believe him when he said he had no more territorial ambitions in Europe. In March 1939 they were proved right. On 15 March, with Czechoslovakia in chaos, German troops took over the rest of the country.

SOURCE **30**

Key

- October 1938 Teschen taken by Poland
- November 1938 to March 1939 Slovak border areas and Ruthenia taken by Hungary
- October 1938 Sudetenland region given to Germany in the Munich Agreement
- March 1939 Remainder of Czechoslovakia taken under German control
- German border in 1939

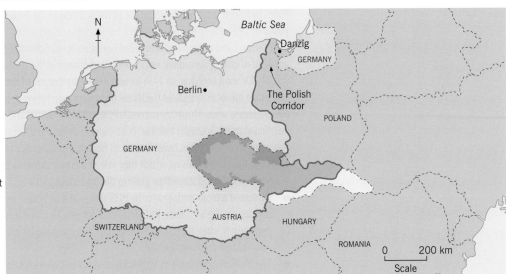

The take-over of Czechoslovakia by 1939.

SOURCE **31**

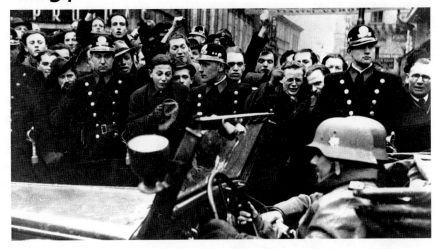

German troops entering Prague, the capital of Czechoslovakia, in March 1939.

There was no resistance from the Czechs. Nor did Britain and France do anything about the situation. However, it was now clear that Hitler could not be trusted. For Chamberlain it was a step too far. Unlike the Sudeten Germans, the Czechs were not separated from their homeland by the Treaty of Versailles. This was an invasion. If Hitler continued unchecked, his next target was likely to be Poland. Britain and France told Hitler that if he invaded Poland they would declare war on Germany. The policy of Appeasement was ended. However, after years of Appeasement, Hitler did not actually believe that Britain and France would risk war by resisting him.

Think!

1 Choose five words to describe the attitude of the crowd in Source 31.
2 Why do you think that there was no resistance from the Czechs?
3 Why do you think Britain and France did nothing in response to the invasion?

The Nazi–Soviet Pact, 1939

Look at your 'Versailles chart' from page 53. You should have only one item left. As Hitler was gradually retaking land lost at Versailles, you can see from Source 31 that logically his next target was the strip of former German land in Poland known as the Polish Corridor. He had convinced himself that Britain and France would not risk war over this, but he was less sure about Stalin and the USSR. Let's see why.

Stalin's fears

Stalin had been very worried about the German threat to the Soviet Union ever since Hitler came to power in 1933. Hitler had openly stated his interest in conquering Russian land. He had denounced Communism and imprisoned and killed Communists in Germany. Even so, Stalin could not reach any kind of lasting agreement with Britain and France in the 1930s. From Stalin's point of view, it was not for want of trying. In 1934 he had joined the League of Nations, hoping the League would guarantee his security against the threat from Germany. However, all he saw at the League was its powerlessness when Mussolini successfully invaded Abyssinia, and when both Mussolini and Hitler intervened in the Spanish Civil War. Politicians in Britain and France had not resisted German rearmament in the 1930s. Indeed, some in Britain seemed even to welcome a stronger Germany as a force to fight Communism, which they saw as a bigger threat to British interests than Hitler.

Stalin's fears and suspicions grew in the mid 1930s.

- He signed a treaty with France in 1935 that said that France would help the USSR if Germany invaded the Soviet Union. But Stalin was not sure he could trust the French to stick to it, particularly when they failed even to stop Hitler moving his troops into the Rhineland, which was right on their own border.

- The Munich Agreement in 1938 increased Stalin's concerns. He was not consulted about it. Stalin concluded from the agreement that France and Britain were powerless to stop Hitler or, even worse, that they were happy for Hitler to take over eastern Europe and then the USSR.

SOURCE 32

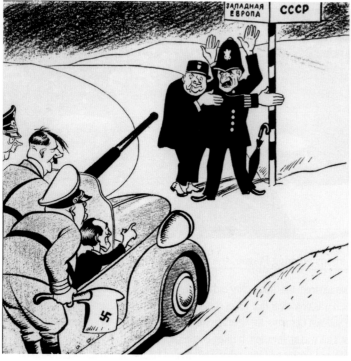

A Soviet cartoon from 1939. CCCP is Russian for USSR. The French and the British are directing Hitler away from western Europe and towards the USSR.

Stalin's negotiations

Despite his misgivings, Stalin was still prepared to talk with Britain and France about an alliance against Hitler. The three countries met in March 1939, but Chamberlain was reluctant to commit Britain. From Stalin's point of view, France and Britain then made things worse by giving Poland a guarantee that they would defend it if it was invaded. Chamberlain meant the guarantee as a warning to Hitler. Stalin saw it as support for one of the USSR's potential enemies.

Negotiations between Britain, France and the USSR continued through the spring and summer of 1939. However, Stalin also received visits from the Nazi foreign minister Ribbentrop. They discussed a rather different deal, a Nazi–Soviet Pact.

Stalin's decision

In August, Stalin made his decision. On 23 August 1939, Hitler and Stalin, the two arch enemies, signed the Nazi–Soviet Pact and announced the terms to the world. They agreed not to attack one another. Privately, they also agreed to divide Poland between them.

SOURCE **33**

It will be asked how it was possible that the Soviet government signed a non-aggression pact with so deceitful a nation, with such criminals as Hitler and Ribbentrop . . . We secured peace for our country for eighteen months, which enabled us to make military preparations.

Stalin, in a speech in 1941.

Why did Stalin sign the Pact?

It was clear what Hitler gained from the Pact. He regarded it as his greatest achievement. It gave him half of Poland and ensured he would not face a war on two fronts if he invaded Poland. He had promised the Russians they could have the rest of Poland as well as the Baltic states but he never intended to allow Stalin to keep these territories.

It is also clear what Stalin gained from it. It gave him some territory that had once been part of Russia, but that was not the main point. The real benefit was time! Stalin did not expect Hitler to keep his word. He knew he was Hitler's number one target. But he did not trust Britain and France either. He did not think they were strong enough or reliable enough as allies against Hitler. He expected to have to fight Hitler alone at some point. So it was important to get his forces ready. So what he most needed was time to build up his forces to protect the USSR from the attack he knew would come.

Consequences

The Pact cleared the way for Hitler to invade Poland. On 1 September 1939 the Germany army invaded Poland from the west, where they met little resistance. Britain and France demanded he withdraw from Poland or they would declare war. After the experience of the past three years Hitler was certain Britain and France would not actually do anything about this. If he was planning ahead at all, then in his mind the next move would surely be an attack against his temporary ally, the USSR. However Hitler was in for a surprise. Britain and France kept their pledge. On 3 September they declared war on Germany.

SOURCE 35

The Gathering Storm has been one of the most influential books of our time. It is no exaggeration to claim that it has strongly influenced the behaviour of Western politicians from Harry S. Truman to George W. Bush.

… It is a good tale, told by a master story-teller, who did, after all, win the Nobel prize for literature; but would a prize for fiction have been more appropriate?

Professor John Charmley of the University of East Anglia writing about Churchill's account of the 1930s called *The Gathering Storm*.

Was Appeasement justified?

Chamberlain certainly believed in Appeasement. In June 1938 he wrote in a letter to his sister: 'I am completely convinced that the course I am taking is right and therefore cannot be influenced by the attacks of my critics.' He was not a coward or a weakling. When it became obvious that he had no choice but to declare war in 1939 he did.

On page 60 you studied the main reasons Chamberlain followed this policy and the reasons why people opposed him. However, remember that Chamberlain was not alone. There were many more politicians who supported him in 1938 than opposed him. It looked pretty clear to them in 1938 that the balance fell in favour of Appeasement.

Yet when Hitler broke his promises and the policy did not stop war, the supporters of Appeasement quickly turned against the policy, some claiming that they had been opposed all along. Appeasers were portrayed as naïve, foolish or weak – Source 34 is one of hundreds of examples which parody the policy and the people who pursued it. Historians since then and popular opinion too have judged Chamberlain very harshly. Chamberlain's 'Peace for our time' speech is presented as self-deception and a betrayal. Chamberlain and his cabinet are seen as 'second-rate politicians' who were out of their depth as events unfolded before them. On the other hand the opponents of Appeasement such as Winston Churchill are portrayed as realists who were far-sighted and brave.

SOURCE 34

'*Remember . . . One More Lollypop, and Then You All Go Home!*'

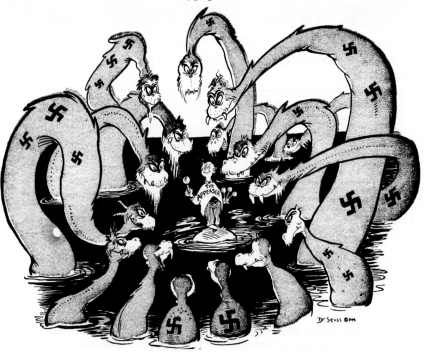

A cartoon by the American artist Dr Seuss published on 13 August 1941 (before the USA entered the Second World War).

It really has been a very one-sided debate. Yet this debate matters because the failure of Appeasement to stop Hitler has had a profound influence on British and American foreign policy ever since. It is now seen as the 'right thing' to stand up to dictators. You will find an example of this in Chapter 7 when you study the Gulf War. This is a lesson that people have learned from history. One of the reasons why people study history is to avoid making the same mistakes from the past but before we leap so quickly to judgement on this issue, let's run this argument through two different checks.

SOURCE 36

So how did my pre-emptive strategy stand up to a computer stress test? Not as well as I had hoped, I have to confess. The Calm & the Storm made it clear that lining up an anti-German coalition in 1938 might have been harder than I'd assumed. To my horror, the French turned down the alliance I proposed to them. It also turned out that, when I did go to war with Germany, my own position was pretty weak. The nadir [low point] was a successful German invasion of England, a scenario my book rules out as militarily too risky.

Professor Niall Ferguson in an article for the *New York Magazine*, 16 October 2006.

Think!

Study graphs A–C in Source 37.
1 What evidence do they provide to support the view that Britain's armed forces caught up with Germany's between 1938 and 1939?
2 What evidence do they provide to oppose this view?

Check 1: If Chamberlain had stood up to Hitler in 1938 what would have happened?

The historian Professor Niall Ferguson of Harvard University has set out some 'counter-factual' scenarios – suggesting what might have happened if particular policies were followed. In particular, he has argued that confronting Hitler in 1938 instead of appeasing him 'would have paid handsome dividends. Even if it had come to war over Czechoslovakia, Germany would not have won. Germany's defences were not yet ready for a two-front war.'

Professor Ferguson then had the chance to test his scenario by playing a computer game! *The Calm & the Storm* is a powerful simulation which allows users to make decisions and then computes the possible impact of those decisions. You can read his conclusions in Source 36.

Professor Ferguson believes that using computer simulations could help leaders of the future make key decisions in times of crisis. Maybe you don't trust a computer game to teach you anything about history! But you might trust some hard statistics. So try check 2.

Check 2: Did Appeasement buy time for Chamberlain to rearm Britain?

One of the strongest arguments for Appeasement was that in 1938 Britain simply was not equipped to fight a war with Germany. So did Appeasement allow Britain to catch up?

In the 1960s British historian AJP Taylor argued that Chamberlain had an exaggerated view of Germany's strength. Taylor believed that German forces were only 45 per cent of what British intelligence reports said they were.

But Taylor was writing in 1965 – not much help to Chamberlain in the 1930s. Britain had run down its forces in the peaceful years of the 1920s. The government had talked about rearmament since 1935 but Britain only really started rearming when Chamberlain became Prime Minister in 1937. Chamberlain certainly thought that Britain's armed forces were not ready for war in 1938. His own military advisers and his intelligence services told him this.

So did Appeasement allow Britain the time it needed to rearm? Source 37 will help you to decide.

SOURCE 37

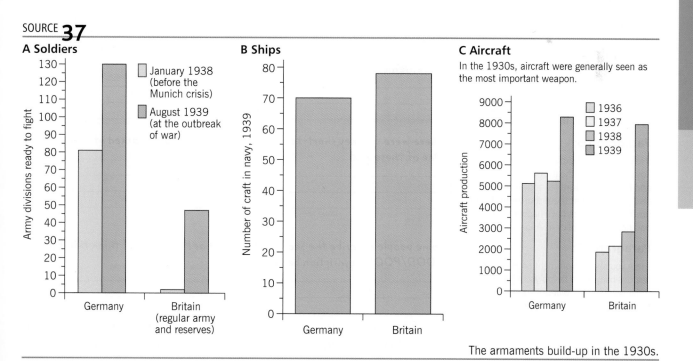

A Soldiers

January 1938 (before the Munich crisis)

August 1939 (at the outbreak of war)

Army divisions ready to fight — Germany, Britain (regular army and reserves)

B Ships

Number of craft in navy, 1939 — Germany, Britain

C Aircraft

In the 1930s, aircraft were generally seen as the most important weapon.

1936, 1937, 1938, 1939

Aircraft production — Germany, Britain

The armaments build-up in the 1930s.

Focus Task

Why had international peace collapsed by 1939?

You have covered a lot of material in the last two chapters. In this task you are going to make sure that you have the important events and developments clear in your mind.

1 Work in groups of six. Each take a blank sheet of paper and write a heading like the ones on the right. On your sheet summarise the ways in which this factor helped to bring about the war.

2 Now come back together as a group and write your own summary of how the war broke out. You can use this structure, but set yourself a word limit of 75 words per paragraph, less if you can.

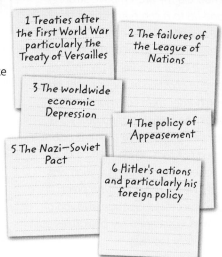

1 Treaties after the First World War particularly the Treaty of Versailles

2 The failures of the League of Nations

3 The worldwide economic Depression

4 The policy of Appeasement

5 The Nazi–Soviet Pact

6 Hitler's actions and particularly his foreign policy

Paragraph 1:

(This is the place to explain how resentment against the Versailles Treaty brought Hitler to power in the first place and guided his actions in the 1930s.)

Paragraph 2:

(Here you should explain how the failure of the League encouraged Hitler and made him think he could achieve his aims.)

Paragraph 3:

(Here you should explain how the Depression was an underlying cause of the failure of the League, Japan's aggression and Hitler's rise to power.)

Paragraph 4:

(Here you should briefly describe what Appeasement was, and how instead of stopping Hitler it encouraged him. You could also point out the links between Appeasement and the Depression.)

Paragraph 5:

(Here you should explain how the Nazi–Soviet Pact led to the invasion of Poland and how that in turn led to war. You could also point out that these short-term factors probably could not have happened if there had not been a policy of Appeasement.)

Paragraph 6:

(Here you should comment on Hitler's overall responsibility. How far do you agree that Hitler wanted war, planned for it, and if so does that mean he caused the war?)

Paragraph 7:

(Here you should indicate which factor(s) you think were most important. This is where you should bring in any of the factors you discussed in stage 5 of the Focus Task.)

There were important long-term factors which help to explain why war broke out in 1939. One factor was the Versailles Treaty. It was important because . . .

_____

_____

_____

The failure of the League of Nations in the 1930s also contributed towards the outbreak of war. This was because . . .

_____

_____

_____

Economic factors also played an important role. The worldwide economic Depression . . .

_____

_____

_____

Another factor which helps to explain the outbreak of war was the policy of Appeasement. Appeasement . . .

_____

_____

_____

There were also key short-term factors which actually sparked off the war. One of these was . . .

_____

_____

_____

Some people describe the Second World War as Hitler's war. I think this is a GOOD/POOR description because . . .

_____

_____

_____

All of these factors played important roles. However, [INSERT YOUR CHOICE OF FACTOR(S)] was / were particularly important because . . .

_____

_____

_____

Chapter Review Focus Task

Reaching a judgement

Almost there! In the last task you wrote a clear explanation of the various reasons why peace collapsed by 1939. However, you need to go further. You also need to be able to compare the importance of these reasons (or factors) and see the links between them. For example, if you were asked this question:

*'The Nazi Soviet Pact of 1939 was more important than the policy of Appeasement in causing the Second World War.'
How far do you agree with this statement?*

what would you say? Most students find it hard to explain what they think and end up **giving information about each factor** (describing events) rather than **making a judgement and supporting it**. This review task helps you to overcome this problem.

Stage 1: Understand and evaluate each factor

There are six major factors. The cards analyse why each one might be seen as:

♦ a **critical** factor (i.e. the war probably would not have happened without it) or just

♦ one of several **important** factors (i.e. the war could still possibly have happened without it).

a) Read the cards carefully to make sure you understand the arguments.

b) For each of the 'killer sources' 1-6 (on page 72) decide whether this supports the argument that this factor was critical or just one of several important factors.

Factor 1: The Treaty of Versailles

♦ **Critical?** Versailles and the other Treaties created a situation in Europe which made war inevitable. It was only a matter of time before Germany tried to seek revenge, overturn the Treaty and start another war. Many commentators felt at the time that it was only a question of when war might come not **whether** it would.

♦ **Important?** The Treaties contributed to the tensions of the time but they did not create them. Politicians in the 1930s could have defended the treaties or changed them. It was political choices in the 1930s which caused war not the treaties.

Factor 2: The failure of the League of Nations

♦ **Critical?** The League of Nations' job was to make sure that disputes were sorted out legally. In the 1920s it created a spirit of cooperation. But, in Manchuria 1931 and Abyssinia 1935–36 the League completely failed to stand up to aggression by Japan and Italy. This encouraged Hitler's aggression from 1936 onwards since he believed no one would try to stop him.

♦ **Important?** The League never really fulfilled the role of peacekeeper – even in the 1920s it gave in to Italy over Corfu. The failure of the League in the 1930s was important because it encouraged Hitler but even if the League had been stronger Hitler would still have tried to overturn the Treaty of Versailles and to destroy Communism.

Factor 3: The worldwide economic Depression

♦ **Critical?** The Depression critically weakened the League of Nations. It destroyed the spirit of international cooperation which had built up in the 1920s and set countries against each other. Without the Depression leading to these problems there could not have been a war.

♦ **Important?** The Depression was certainly important – it made Japan and Italy invade Manchuria and Abyssinia. It brought Hitler to power in Germany and started German rearmament. However it is linked to all the other factors – it did not cause the war in itself. Even with the Depression Hitler could have been stopped if Britain and France had had the will to resist him. The Depression did not make war inevitable.

Factor 4: The policy of Appeasement

♦ **Critical?** Appeasement was critical because it made Hitler think he could get away with anything. Britain and France could have stopped Hitler in 1936 when he marched troops into the Rhineland but their nerve failed. From this point on Hitler felt he could not lose and took gamble after gamble. As a result of appeasement he did not even believe Britain would fight him when he invaded Poland in 1939.

♦ **Important?** The policy of Appeasement only came about because, without the USA, the League of Nations, and its leading members, Britain and France, were not strong enough to keep peace. The Depression so weakened Britain and France that they did not have the money to oppose Hitler. The policy of appeasement would not have been followed without these other factors.

Factor 5: The Nazi–Soviet Pact

♦ **Critical?** Although Hitler thought that Britain and France would not fight him he was not sure about the Soviet Union. So the Soviet Union was the only country that stood in the way of his plans. Without the Nazi–Soviet Pact Hitler would not have taken the gamble to invade Poland and war would never have begun.

♦ **Important?** The Pact allowed Hitler to invade Poland, but war was already inevitable before that – due to Hitler's actions and his hatred of Communism. Hitler had made clear his plans to take land from the USSR. Plus which it was the policy of Appeasement that drove Stalin to sign the Pact because he thought he could not rely on the support of Britain or France to oppose Hitler.

Factor 6: Hitler's actions

♦ **Critical?** There could have been no war without Hitler. It was Hitler's vision of Lebensraum, his hatred of Communism and his determination to reverse the Versailles settlement which led to war. He consciously built up Germany's army and weapons with the intention of taking it to war. At each stage of the road to war from 1936 to 1939 it was Hitler's beliefs or actions or decisions that caused the problem.

♦ **Important?** Hitler was the gambler. He only did what he could get away with. So without the weakness of the League of Nations, or the reluctance of Britain, France, or the Soviet Union to stand up to him; without the flawed Treaties; without the economic problems of the 1930s Hitler would not have got anywhere. He would have been forced to follow a more peaceful foreign policy and there would have been no war.

Stage 2: Investigate connections between factors

From Stage 1 it should be clear to you that these factors are connected to each other. Let's investigate these connections.

a) Make six simple cards with just the factor heading.

b) Display your cards on a large sheet of paper and draw lines connecting them together. Some links are already mentioned on the cards on page 71 but you may be able to think of many more.

c) Write an explanation along each link. For example between 'the policy of Appeasement' and 'The Nazi-Soviet Pact' you might write:

'The policy of Appeasement helped cause the Nazi-Soviet Pact. It alarmed Stalin so that he felt he had to make his own deal with Hitler thinking that France and Britain would just give him whatever he wanted.'

d) Take a photo of your finished chart.

Stage 3: Rank the factors

Which of these factors is most important? In Stage 2 you will already have started to draw your own conclusions about this. It will be really helpful when you come to answering questions about relative importance if you have already decided what you think! Remember there is no right answer to which is most important but whatever your view you must be able to support it with key points and with evidence. So:

a) Take your cards and put them in a rank order of importance.

b) To justify your order, in the space between each card you need to be able to complete this sentence:

'X was more important than Y because…'

Stage 4: Compare two factors

Back to the question we started with:

'The Nazi Soviet Pact of 1939 was more important than the policy of Appeasement in causing the Second World War.' How far do you agree with this statement?

With all the thinking that you have done you should have already made up your mind on what you think, but to help you structure and support your argument you could complete a chart like this. NB if you can include the killer source in your written answer all the better.

	Reasons more important	**Reasons less important**
Policy of Appeasement		
Nazi-Soviet Pact		

Killer sources and quotations

SOURCE 1

When war came in 1939, it was a result of twenty years of decisions taken or not taken, not of arrangements made in 1919.

Historian Margaret Macmillan writing in 2001

SOURCE 2

The failure of the World Disarmament Conference not only crushed the hopes of many supporters of the League of Nations and the disarmament movements but also strengthened the ranks of those who opted for appeasement or some form of pacifism. Pressures for collective action gave way to policies of self-defence, neutrality and isolation. Against such a background, the balance of power shifted steadily away from the status quo nations in the direction of those who favoured its destruction. The reconstruction of the 1920s was not inevitably doomed to collapse by the start of the 1930s. Rather, the demise of the Weimar Republic and the triumph of Hitler proved the motor force of destructive systemic change.

Historian Zara Steiner writing in 2011

SOURCE 3

If new accounts by historians show that statesmen were able to use the League to ease tensions and win time in the 1920s, no such case appears possible for the 1930s. Indeed, the League's processes may have played a role in that deterioration. Diplomacy requires leaders who can speak for their states; it requires secrecy; and it requires the ability to make credible threats. The Covenant's security arrangements met none of those criteria.

Historian Susan Pedersen writing in 2007

SOURCE 4

We turn our eyes towards the lands of the east . . . When we speak of new territory in Europe today, we must principally think of Russia and the border states subject to her. Destiny itself seems to wish to point out the way for us here. Colonisation of the eastern frontiers is of extreme importance. It will be the duty of Germany's foreign policy to provide large spaces for the nourishment and settlement of the growing population of Germany.

Adolf Hitler, *Mein Kampf*, 1923

SOURCE 5

The vindictiveness of British and French peace terms helped to pave the way for Nazism in Germany and a renewal of hostilities. World War 2 resulted from the very silly and humiliating punitive peace imposed on Germany after World War 1.

Historian George Kennan writing in 1984

SOURCE 6

By repeatedly surrendering to force, Chamberlain has encouraged aggression… our central contention, therefore, is that Mr Chamberlain's policy has throughout been based on a fatal misunderstanding of the psychology of dictatorship.

The Yorkshire Post, December 1938.

SOURCE 7

The effects of the depression encouraged not only the emergence of authoritarian and interventionist governments but led to the shattering of the global financial system. Most European states followed 'beggar-thy-neighbour' tactics. Germany, Hungary, and most of the East European states embarked on defensive economic policies – often at cost to their neighbours.

Historian Zara Steiner writing in 2011

Exam Practice

See pages 168–175 and pages 316–319 for advice on the different types of questions you might face.

1 (a) What was the policy of Appeasement? **[4]**
  (b) What was the significance of the Munich Agreement of 1938? **[6]**
  (c) 'Appeasement was a wise policy that delayed war until Britain was ready.' How far do you agree with this statement? Explain your answer. **[10]**
2 Study Source 27 on page 64. What is the message of the cartoonist? Use details of the source and your own knowledge to explain your answer.

Keywords

Make sure you know what these terms mean and are able to define them confidently.

Essential

♦ *Anschluss*
♦ Anti-Comintern Pact
♦ Appeasement
♦ Bolshevism
♦ Communism
♦ *Lebensraum*
♦ *Mein Kampf*
♦ Rearmament
♦ Remilitarisation
♦ Spanish Civil War
♦ Sudetenland
♦ The Munich Agreement
♦ The Nazi–Soviet Pact
♦ The Polish Corridor

Useful

♦ Conscription
♦ Mobilised
♦ Radical
♦ 'The November Criminals'

Chapter Summary

The collapse of international peace

1 The late 1920s had been a time of hope for international relations with a series of agreements that seemed to make the world a more peaceful place with countries co-operating and trading with each other.
2 The Great Depression of the 1930s led to political turmoil in many countries and the rise of the dictators such as Hitler in Germany. Hitler formed alliances with other right-wing regimes in Italy and Japan.
3 Germany was still unhappy about its treatment under the Treaty of Versailles and Hitler set out to challenge the terms of the Treaty of Versailles, first of all by rearming Germany (secretly from 1933, then publicly from 1935).
4 He also challenged the Treaty, for example by sending troops into the demilitarised zone of the Rhineland in 1936.
5 The League of Nations and Britain and France did not try to stop Hitler doing these things. This policy was called Appeasement – giving Hitler what he wanted in the hope he would not ask for more.
6 The most famous act of Appeasement was over the Sudetenland – an area of Czechoslovakia that Hitler wanted to take over.
7 In the Munich Agreement (October 1938) Britain and France let Hitler have the Sudetenland as long as he did not try to take over the rest of Czechoslovakia. When Hitler invaded the rest of Czechoslovakia in early 1939 it marked the end of the policy of Appeasement and they told Hitler that any further expansion would lead to war.
8 Although Hitler was very anti-Communist and saw Stalin and the USSR as his enemy he signed a Pact with Stalin in 1939 to not attack each other but to divide Poland between them.
9 When Hitler invaded Poland in September 1939 Britain declared war on Germany.
10 Hitler's foreign policy played a major role in causing the Second World War but historians argue that there were other very important factors that contributed as well, particularly the economic Depression, the failures of the League of Nations and the unfairness of the post-First World War peace treaties.

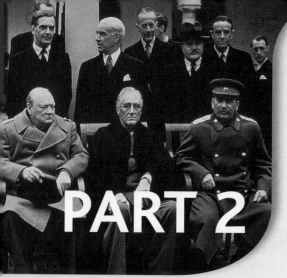

The Cold War and the Gulf, 1945–2000

PART 2

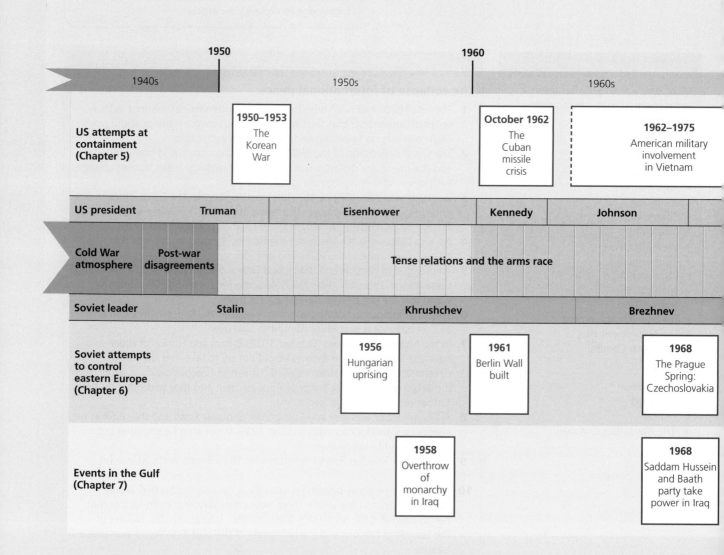

	1950		**1960**	
1940s		1950s		1960s

US attempts at containment (Chapter 5)	**1950–1953** The Korean War		**October 1962** The Cuban missile crisis	**1962–1975** American military involvement in Vietnam
US president	Truman	Eisenhower	Kennedy	Johnson
Cold War atmosphere	Post-war disagreements	Tense relations and the arms race		
Soviet leader	Stalin	Khrushchev		Brezhnev
Soviet attempts to control eastern Europe (Chapter 6)		**1956** Hungarian uprising	**1961** Berlin Wall built	**1968** The Prague Spring: Czechoslovakia
Events in the Gulf (Chapter 7)		**1958** Overthrow of monarchy in Iraq		**1968** Saddam Hussein and Baath party take power in Iraq

Focus

The Second World War led to a decisive change in the balance of power around the world. The countries that had dominated European affairs from 1919 to 1939 such as France, Britain or Germany were now much poorer or less powerful. World history was much more affected by what the leaders of the new 'superpowers' (the USA and the USSR) believed and did. So the big story of Part 2 is how the superpowers became enemies, how they clashed (directly or indirectly) during the Cold War and how they tried to influence the affairs of other countries.

♦ In Chapter 4 you will examine the short-term causes of the Cold War. Why did the USA and the USSR, who had fought together as allies against Hitler, fall out and enter a 40-year period of tension and distrust?

♦ One of the USA's obsessions in this Cold War period was to hold back the spread of Communism. Chapter 5 examines why they so feared the spread of Communism, how they tried to contain it and helps you to judge how successful they were.

♦ While the USA was trying to contain Communism, the Soviet Union was trying to shore it up in its east European neighbours. This was no easy task. They faced frequent protests and problems. In Chapter 6 you will consider how they did this, how far they succeeded and why in the end it all came crashing down with the demolition of the Berlin Wall and the collapse of the Soviet Union itself.

♦ Finally, in Chapter 7 you will shift your focus to the Persian Gulf and the intertwined fates of two countries Iraq and Iran. You will examine how they developed in the period 1970–2000 and why they came into conflict with each other and with the western powers.

The events in these chapters overlap. The timeline below gives you an overview of the main events you will be studying. It would be helpful if you made your own copy and added your own notes to it as you study.

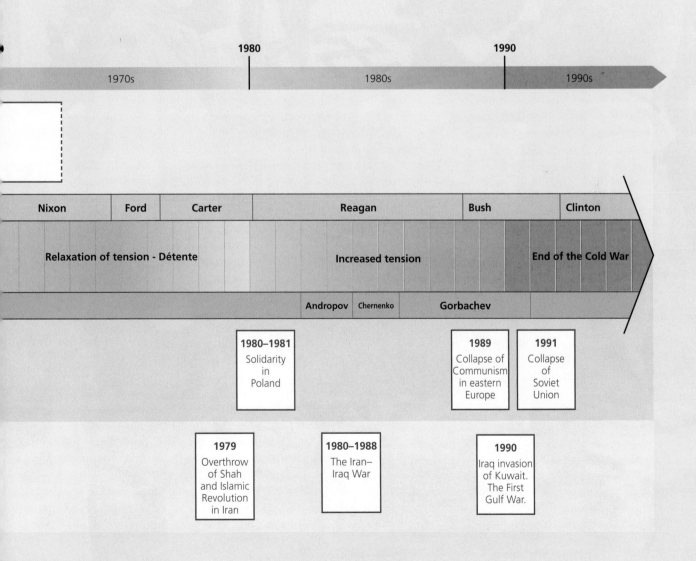

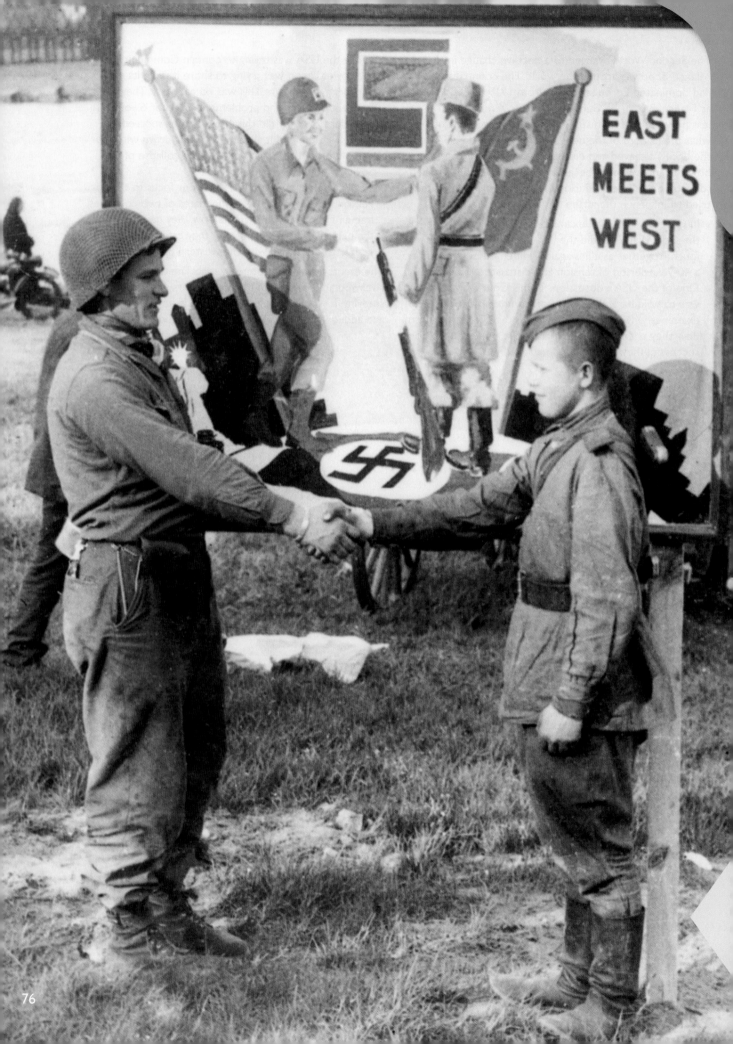

Who was to blame for the Cold War?

FOCUS POINTS

- Why did the USA–USSR alliance begin to break down in 1945?
- How had the USSR gained control of eastern Europe by 1948?
- How did the USA react to Soviet expansionism?
- What were the consequences of the Berlin Blockade?
- Who was the more to blame for starting the Cold War: the USA or the USSR?

In May 1945 American troops entered Berlin from the west, as Russian troops moved in from the east. They met and celebrated victory together. Yet three years later these former allies were arguing over Berlin and war between them seemed a real possibility.

What had gone wrong?

In this chapter you will consider:

- how the wartime alliance between the USA and the USSR broke down
- how the Soviet Union gained control over eastern Europe and how the USA responded
- the consequences of the Berlin Blockade in 1948.

The key question you will be returning to at the end is who is most to blame for this increasing tension (which became known as 'The Cold War').

- Was it the USSR and Stalin with his insistence on taking over and controlling eastern Europe?
- Or was it the USA and President Truman with the Truman Doctrine and Marshall Aid?
- Or should they share the blame? In the post-war chaos in Europe they both saw it as their role to extend their influence, to proclaim the benefits of their own political system and denounce the other side. So maybe they should share the blame.
- Or was the Cold War inevitable – beyond the control of either country?

Here are some of the factors that you will study in this chapter. At the end you will be asked to become an expert in one of them so you could help yourself by making notes about each one as you read the chapter.

The situation before the Second World War	The personal relationships between various leaders	The conflicting beliefs of the superpowers
The war damage suffered by the USSR	Stalin's take-over of eastern Europe	Marshall Aid for Europe
The Berlin Blockade		

◀ It is not just cartoons that can have messages. Photos can too. This photo shows American and Soviet soldiers shaking hands in April 1945.

1 What is the message of the photo?
2 How far do you trust it to show relations between the USA and the USSR in 1945?

Think!

Create your own version of the timeline on pages 74–75. You will be adding events and comments to it throughout the chapter to help you in your final Focus Task.

To start, extend the timeline back to 1917 and use the information on these two pages to mark any events or developments that might affect relationships between the USA and the Soviet Union.

Source Analysis

1 Cartoons often criticise particular people or their actions. Sometimes they praise. Sometimes they simply comment on a situation. Would you say Source 1 is criticising, praising or commenting? Explain how the points in the cartoon helped you to decide.
2 Spot the loaded language! What words and phrases in Source 2 tell us that this source is hostile to Communism and the USSR?

Allies against Hitler

During the Second World War the Allies produced many images showing friendly co-operation between American, British and Soviet forces and peoples. In fact the real story is rather different. Hitler was the common danger which united President Roosevelt (USA), Winston Churchill (Britain) and Communist leader Josef Stalin of the Soviet Union (the USSR). This is shown in Source 1. It was a strategic wartime alliance not a bond of brotherhood. This becomes clear when we look back further into history.

SOURCE **1**

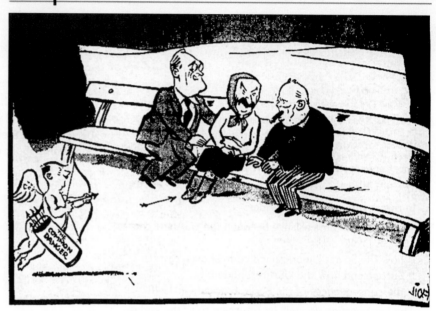

A British cartoon from 1941, with the caption 'Love conquers all'.

The two sides were enemies long before they were allies. The USSR had been a Communist country for more than 30 years. The majority of politicians and business leaders in Britain and the USA hated and feared Communist ideas (see the Factfiles on page 79). In the past they had helped the enemies of the Communists. This made the USSR wary of Britain and the USA. And Britain and the USA were just as wary of the USSR. In the **1920s** suspected Communists had been persecuted in a 'Red Scare'. In **1926** the British government reacted harshly to a General Strike partly because it was convinced that the Strike was the work of agents of the USSR.

- Relations between Britain and the USSR were harmed in the **1930s** by the policy of Appeasement (see page 60). It seemed to Stalin that Britain was happy to see Germany grow in power so that Hitler could attack him.
- Stalin responded by signing a pact with Hitler (see page 66) – they promised not to attack each other, and divided Poland between them! To the western nations this seemed like a cynical act on Stalin's part.

So in many ways the surprising thing is that the old enemies managed a war-time alliance at all. But they did and the course of the war in Europe was decisively altered when Germany invaded the USSR in 1941. The Soviets mounted a fierce defence of their country against the power of the German forces from 1941 to 1945. It was Soviet determination and Soviet soldiers that turned the tide of the European war against Germany. Churchill and Roosevelt admired the Soviets and sent vital supplies but tension remained. Stalin wanted his allies to launch a second military front against Germany and was bitter that this did not happen until June 1944.

SOURCE **2**

Like a prairie-fire, the blaze of revolution was sweeping over every American institution of law and order a year ago. It was eating its way into the homes of the American workmen . . . crawling into the sacred corners of American homes . . .

Robbery, not war, is the ideal of Communism . . . Obviously it is the creed of any criminal mind, which acts always from motives impossible to understand for those with clean thoughts.

Extract from a statement by Mitchell Palmer, Attorney General of the USA, April 1920.

Factfile

A clash of ideologies

The USA	The USSR
The USA was capitalist. Business and property were privately owned.	The USSR was Communist. All industry was owned and run by the state.
It was a democracy. Its government was chosen in free democratic elections.	It was a one-party dictatorship. Elections were held, but all candidates belonged to the Communist Party.
It was the world's wealthiest country. But as in most capitalist countries, there were extremes – some great wealth and great poverty as well.	It was an economic superpower because its industry had grown rapidly in the 1920s and 1930s, but the general standard of living in the USSR was much lower than in the USA. Even so, unemployment was rare and extreme poverty was rarer than in the USA.
For Americans, being free of control by the government was more important than everyone being equal.	For Communists, the rights of individuals were seen as less important than the good of society as a whole. So individuals' lives were tightly controlled.
Americans firmly believed that other countries should be run in the American way.	Soviet leaders believed that other countries should be run in the Communist way.
People in the USA were alarmed by Communist theory, which talked of spreading revolution.	Communism taught that the role of a Communist state was to encourage Communist revolutions worldwide. In practice, the USSR's leaders tended to take practical decisions rather than be led by this ideology.
Americans generally saw their policies as 'doing the right thing' rather than serving the interests of the USA.	Many in the USSR saw the USA's actions as selfishly building its economic empire and political influence.

Revision Tip

You need to know these things so make your own copies of the diagrams on the right and then use the Factfile to make notes around them summarising the two systems.

USSR

 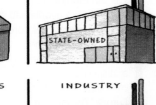 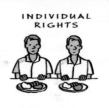

USA

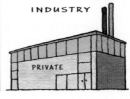 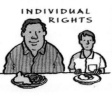

Superpowers

The USA and the USSR had emerged from the war as the two 'superpowers'. After the Second World War powers like Britain and France were effectively relegated to a second division. US leaders felt there was a responsibility was attached to being a superpower. In the 1930s, the USA had followed a policy of isolation – keeping out of European and world affairs. The Americans might have disapproved of Soviet Communism, but they tried not to get involved. However, by the 1940s the US attitude had changed. Roosevelt had set the Americans firmly against a policy of isolation and this effectively meant opposing Communism. In March 1945 he said to the American Congress that America 'will have to take the responsibility for world collaboration or we shall have to bear the responsibilities for another world conflict'. There would be no more appeasement of dictators. From now on, every Communist action would meet an American reaction.

Revision Tip

Make sure you can remember at least two examples of agreement at Yalta and one (the main!) disagreement.

The Yalta Conference, February 1945

In February 1945 it was clear that Germany was losing the European war, so the Allied leaders met at Yalta in the Ukraine to plan what would happen to Europe after Germany's defeat. The Yalta Conference went well. Despite their differences, the Big Three – Stalin, Roosevelt and Churchill – agreed on some important matters.

It seemed that, although they could not all agree, they were still able to negotiate and do business with one another.

Agreements

✔ Japan
Stalin agreed to enter the war against Japan once Germany had surrendered.

✔ Germany
They agreed that Germany would be divided into four zones: American, French, British and Soviet.

✔ Elections
They agreed that as countries were liberated from occupation by the German army, they would be allowed to hold free elections to choose the government they wanted.

✔ United Nations
The Big Three all agreed to join the new United Nations Organisation, which would aim to keep peace after the war.

✔ War criminals
As Allied soldiers advanced through Germany, they were revealing the horrors of the Nazi concentration camps. The Big Three agreed to hunt down and punish war criminals who were responsible for genocide.

✔ Eastern Europe
The Soviet Union had suffered terribly in the war. An estimated 20 million Soviet people had died. Stalin was therefore concerned about the future security of the USSR and specifically the risk of another invasion from Europe. The Big Three agreed that eastern Europe should be seen as a 'Soviet sphere of influence'.

Disagreements

✘ Poland
The only real disagreement was about Poland.
- Stalin wanted the border of the USSR to move westwards into Poland. Stalin argued that Poland, in turn, could move its border westwards into German territory.
- Churchill did not approve of Stalin's plans for Poland, but he also knew that there was not very much he could do about it because Stalin's Red Army was in total control of both Poland and eastern Germany.
- Roosevelt was also unhappy about Stalin's plan, but Churchill persuaded Roosevelt to accept it, as long as the USSR agreed not to interfere in Greece where the British were attempting to prevent the Communists taking over. Stalin accepted this.

SOURCE 3

We argued freely and frankly across the table. But at the end on every point unanimous agreement was reached … We know, of course, that it was Hitler's hope and the German war lords' hope that we would not agree – that some slight crack might appear in the solid wall of allied unity … But Hitler has failed. Never before have the major allies been more closely united – not only in their war aims but also in their peace aims.

Extract from President Roosevelt's report to the US Congress on the Yalta Conference.

SOURCE 4

I want to drink to our alliance, that it should not lose its . . . intimacy, its free expression of views . . . I know of no such close alliance of three Great Powers as this . . . May it be strong and stable, may we be as frank as possible.

Stalin, proposing a toast at a dinner at the Yalta Conference, 1945.

Think!

1 The photo on page 1 of this book shows the Big Three at the Yalta Conference. Imagine you were describing the scene in this photo for a radio audience in 1945. Describe for the listeners:
◆ the obvious points (such as people you can see)
◆ the less obvious points (such as the mood of the scene)
◆ the agreements and disagreements the Big Three had come to.

Source Analysis

Behind the scenes at Yalta

The war against Hitler had united Roosevelt, Stalin and Churchill and at the Yalta Conference they appeared to get on well. But what was going on behind the scenes? Sources 5–10 will help you decide.

SOURCE 5

In the hallway [at Yalta] we stopped before a map of the world on which the Soviet Union was coloured in red. Stalin waved his hand over the Soviet Union and exclaimed, 'They [Roosevelt and Churchill] will never accept the idea that so great a space should be red, never, never!'

Milovan Djilas writing about Yalta in 1948.

SOURCE 6

I have always worked for friendship with Russia but, like you, I feel deep anxiety because of their misinterpretation of the Yalta decisions, their attitude towards Poland, their overwhelming influence in the Balkans excepting Greece, the difficulties they make about Vienna, the combination of Russian power and the territories under their control or occupied, coupled with the Communist technique in so many other countries, and above all their power to maintain very large Armies in the field for a long time. What will be the position in a year or two?

Extract from a telegram sent by Prime Minister Churchill to President Truman in May 1945.

SOURCE 7

Perhaps you think that just because we are the allies of the English we have forgotten who they are and who Churchill is. There's nothing they like better than to trick their allies. During the First World War they constantly tricked the Russians and the French. And Churchill? Churchill is the kind of man who will pick your pocket of a kopeck! [A kopeck is a low value Soviet coin.] And Roosevelt? Roosevelt is not like that. He dips in his hand only for bigger coins. But Churchill? He will do it for a kopeck.

Stalin speaking to a fellow Communist, Milovan Djilas, in 1945. Djilas was a supporter of Stalin.

SOURCE 8

The Soviet Union has become a danger to the free world. A new front must be created against her onward sweep. This front should be as far east as possible. A settlement must be reached on all major issues between West and East in Europe before the armies of democracy melt.

Churchill writing to Roosevelt shortly after the Yalta Conference. Churchill ordered his army leader Montgomery to keep German arms intact in case they had to be used against the Russians.

SOURCE 9

Once, Churchill asked Stalin to send him the music of the new Soviet Russian anthem so that it could be broadcast before the summary of the news from the Soviet German front. Stalin sent the words [as well] and expressed the hope that Churchill would set about learning the new tune and whistling it to members of the Conservative Party. While Stalin behaved with relative discretion with Roosevelt, he continually teased Churchill throughout the war.

Written by Soviet historian Sergei Kudryashov after the war.

SOURCE 10

[At Yalta] Churchill feared that Roosevelt was too pro-Russian. He pressed for a French zone to be added to the other three to add another anti-Russian voice to the armies of occupation.

Written by Christopher Culpin in a school textbook, *The Modern World*, 1984.

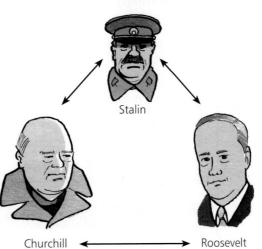

1 Draw a simple diagram like this and use Sources 5–10 to summarise what each of the leaders thought of the other.
2 How do Sources 5–10 affect your impression of the Yalta Conference?
3 How far do you trust these sources to tell you what the leaders actually thought of each other?

SOURCE 11

SOURCE 11

This war is not as in the past; whoever occupies a territory also imposes on it his own social system. Everyone imposes his own system as far as his army has power to do so. It cannot be otherwise.

Stalin speaking, soon after the end of the Second World War, about the take-over of eastern Europe.

SOURCE 12

Unless Russia is faced with an iron fist and strong language another war is in the making. Only one language do they understand – 'how many [army] divisions have you got?' ... I'm tired of babying the Soviets.

President Truman, writing to his Secretary of State in January 1946.

Think!

1 Read Source 11. At Yalta, Churchill and Roosevelt had agreed with Stalin that eastern Europe would be a Soviet 'sphere of influence'. Do you think Source 11 is what they had in mind?

2 Explain how each of the three developments described in the text might affect relationships at Potsdam.

3 What is your overall impression of Source 12:
♦ a reasonable assessment of Stalin based on the facts
♦ an overreaction to Stalin based on fear and prejudice against the USSR?
Use extracts from the source to support your view.

Focus Task

Why did the USA–USSR alliance begin to break down in 1945?

Under the following headings, make notes to summarise why the Allies began to fall out in 1945:
♦ Personalities
♦ Actions by the USA
♦ Actions by the USSR
♦ Misunderstandings

The Potsdam Conference, July–August 1945

In May 1945, three months after the Yalta Conference, Allied troops reached Berlin. Hitler committed suicide. Germany surrendered. The war in Europe was won.

A second conference of the Allied leaders was arranged for July 1945 in the Berlin suburb of Potsdam. However, in the five months since Yalta a number of changes had taken place which would greatly affect relationships between the leaders.

1 Stalin's armies were occupying most of eastern Europe

Soviet troops had liberated country after country in eastern Europe, but instead of withdrawing his troops Stalin had left them there. Refugees were fleeing out of these countries fearing a Communist take-over. Stalin had set up a Communist government in Poland, ignoring the wishes of the majority of Poles. He insisted that his control of eastern Europe was a defensive measure against possible future attacks.

2 America had a new president

On 12 April 1945, President Roosevelt died. He was replaced by his Vice-President, Harry Truman. Truman was a very different man from Roosevelt. He was much more anti-Communist than Roosevelt and was very suspicious of Stalin. Truman and his advisers saw Soviet actions in eastern Europe as preparations for a Soviet take-over of the rest of Europe.

3 The Allies had tested an atomic bomb

On 16 July 1945 the Americans successfully tested an atomic bomb at a desert site in the USA. At the start of the Potsdam Conference, Truman informed Stalin about it.

The Potsdam Conference finally got under way on 17 July 1945. Not surprisingly, it did not go as smoothly as Yalta.

To change the situation further still, in July there was an election in Britain. Churchill was defeated, so half way through the conference he was replaced by a new Prime Minister, Clement Attlee. In the absence of Churchill, the conference was dominated by rivalry and suspicion between Stalin and Truman. A number of issues arose on which neither side seemed able to appreciate the other's point of view.

Disagreements at Potsdam

✗ Germany	✗ Reparations	✗ Eastern Europe
Stalin wanted to cripple Germany completely to protect the USSR against future threats. Truman did not want to repeat the mistake of the Treaty of Versailles.	Twenty million Russians had died in the war and the Soviet Union had been devastated. Stalin wanted compensation from Germany. Truman, however, was once again determined not to repeat the mistakes at the end of the First World War and resisted this demand.	At Yalta, Stalin had won agreement from the Allies that he could set up pro-Soviet governments in eastern Europe. He said, 'If the Slav [the majority of east European] people are united, no one will dare move a finger against them'. Truman became very unhappy about Russian intentions and soon adopted a 'get tough' attitude towards Stalin.

Revision Tip

Your notes from the Focus Task will be useful for revision. Make sure you can remember one example of each.

Source Analysis ▼

1 How do Sources 13 and 14 differ in their interpretation of Stalin's actions?
2 Explain why they see things so differently.
3 How do Sources 15 and 16 differ in their interpretation of Churchill?
4 Explain why there are differences.

The 'iron curtain'

The Potsdam Conference ended without complete agreement on these issues. Over the next nine months, Stalin achieved the domination of eastern Europe that he was seeking. By 1946 Poland, Hungary, Romania, Bulgaria and Albania all had Communist governments which owed their loyalty to Stalin. Churchill described the border between Soviet-controlled countries and the West as an iron curtain (see Source 13). The name stuck.

SOURCE 13

A shadow has fallen upon the scenes so lately lighted by the Allied victory. From Stettin on the Baltic to Trieste on the Adriatic, an iron curtain has descended. Behind that line lie all the states of central and eastern Europe. The Communist parties have been raised to power far beyond their numbers and are seeking everywhere to obtain totalitarian control. This is certainly not the liberated Europe we fought to build. Nor is it one which allows permanent peace.

Winston Churchill speaking in the USA, in the presence of President Truman, March 1946.

SOURCE 14

The following circumstances should not be forgotten. The Germans made their invasion of the USSR through Finland, Poland and Romania. The Germans were able to make their invasion through these countries because, at the time, governments hostile to the Soviet Union existed in these countries. What can there be surprising about the fact that the Soviet Union, anxious for its future safety, is trying to see to it that governments loyal in their attitude to the Soviet Union should exist in these countries?

Stalin, replying to Churchill's speech (Source 13).

SOURCE 15

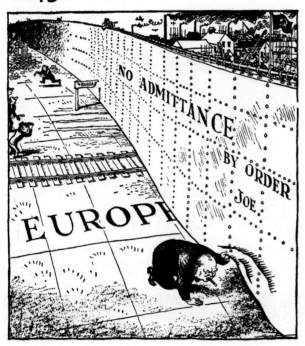

A British cartoon commenting on Churchill's 'iron curtain' speech, in the *Daily Mail*, 6 March 1946.

SOURCE 16

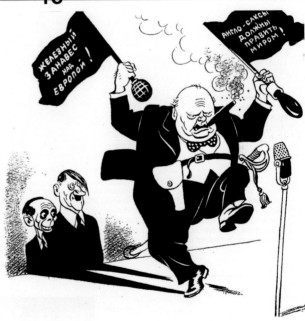

A Soviet cartoon. Churchill is shown with two flags, the first proclaiming that 'Anglo-Saxons must rule the world' and the other threatening an 'iron curtain'. Notice who is formed by his shadow!

Think!

Some historians say that Churchill is as much to blame for the post-war distrust between the Soviet Union and the West as Roosevelt, Truman or Stalin. What evidence is there on pages 80–83 to support or challenge this view?

Stalin strengthens his grip

Source 17 shows how Stalin extended Soviet power across eastern Europe. With Communist governments established throughout eastern Europe, Stalin gradually tightened his control in each country. The secret police imprisoned anyone who opposed Communist rule.

SOURCE **17**

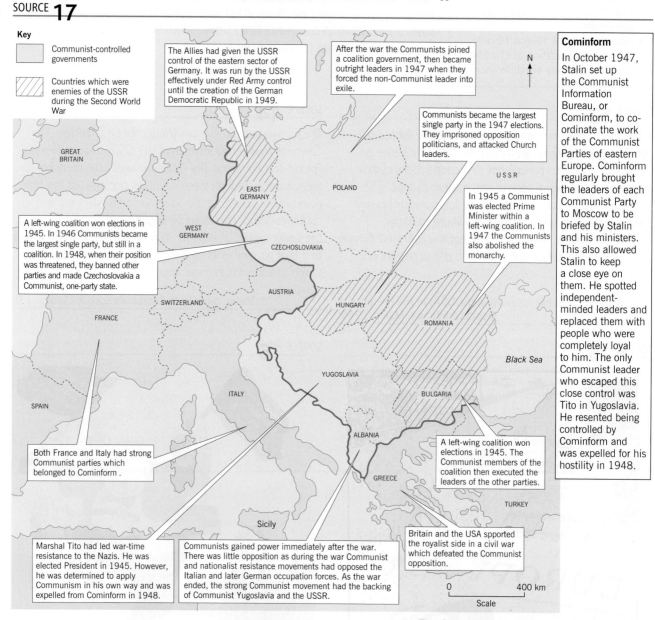

Key

Communist-controlled governments

Countries which were enemies of the USSR during the Second World War

The Allies had given the USSR control of the eastern sector of Germany. It was run by the USSR effectively under Red Army control until the creation of the German Democratic Republic in 1949.

After the war the Communists joined a coalition government, then became outright leaders in 1947 when they forced the non-Communist leader into exile.

Communists became the largest single party in the 1947 elections. They imprisoned opposition politicians, and attacked Church leaders.

In 1945 a Communist was elected Prime Minister within a left-wing coalition. In 1947 the Communists also abolished the monarchy.

A left-wing coalition won elections in 1945. In 1946 Communists became the largest single party, but still in a coalition. In 1948, when their position was threatened, they banned other parties and made Czechoslovakia a Communist, one-party state.

Both France and Italy had strong Communist parties which belonged to Cominform .

A left-wing coalition won elections in 1945. The Communist members of the coalition then executed the leaders of the other parties.

Marshal Tito had led war-time resistance to the Nazis. He was elected President in 1945. However, he was determined to apply Communism in his own way and was expelled from Cominform in 1948.

Communists gained power immediately after the war. There was little opposition as during the war Communist and nationalist resistance movements had opposed the Italian and later German occupation forces. As the war ended, the strong Communist movement had the backing of Communist Yugoslavia and the USSR.

Britain and the USA spported the royalist side in a civil war which defeated the Communist opposition.

0 — 400 km
Scale

The Communists in eastern Europe, 1945–48.

Cominform

In October 1947, Stalin set up the Communist Information Bureau, or Cominform, to co-ordinate the work of the Communist Parties of eastern Europe. Cominform regularly brought the leaders of each Communist Party to Moscow to be briefed by Stalin and his ministers. This also allowed Stalin to keep a close eye on them. He spotted independent-minded leaders and replaced them with people who were completely loyal to him. The only Communist leader who escaped this close control was Tito in Yugoslavia. He resented being controlled by Cominform and was expelled for his hostility in 1948.

Focus Task

How did the USSR gain control of eastern Europe?

1 Study Source 17. Find examples of the Communists:
  a) banning other parties
  b) killing or imprisonng opponents
  c) winning democratic elections
2 Find examples of how these factors helped the USSR take control
  a) the Red Army
  b) Communist involvement in resistance movements
  c) agreements at Yalta
3 'The only important factor in the Communist take-over of eastern Europe was armed force.' How far do you agree with this statement? Explain your answer carefully.

The reaction of the USA

The Western powers were alarmed by Stalin's take-over of eastern Europe. Roosevelt, Churchill and their successors had accepted that Soviet security needed friendly governments in eastern Europe. They had agreed that eastern Europe would be a Soviet 'sphere of influence' and that Stalin would heavily influence this region. However, they had not expected such complete Communist domination. They felt it should have been possible to have governments in eastern Europe that were both democratic and friendly to the USSR. Stalin saw his policy in eastern Europe as making himself secure, but Truman could only see the spread of Communism.

SOURCE 18

After all the efforts that have been made and the appeasement that we followed to try and get a real friendly settlement, not only is the Soviet government not prepared to co-operate with any non-Communist government in eastern Europe, but it is actively preparing to extend its hold over the remaining part of continental Europe and, subsequently, over the Middle East and no doubt the Far East as well. In other words, physical control of Europe and Asia and eventual control of the whole world is what Stalin is aiming at – no less a thing than that. The immensity of the aim should not betray us into thinking that it cannot be achieved.

Extract from a report by the British Foreign Secretary to the British Cabinet in March 1948. The title of the report was 'The Threat to Civilisation'.

SOURCE 19

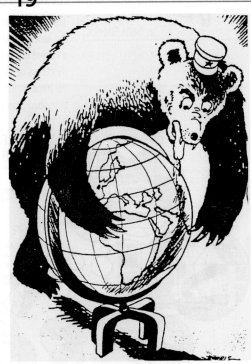

An American cartoon commenting on Stalin's take-over of eastern Europe. The bear represents the USSR.

By 1948, Greece and Czechoslovakia were the only eastern European countries not controlled by Communist governments. It seemed to the Americans that not only Greece and Czechoslovakia but even Italy and France were vulnerable to Communist take-over. Events in two of these countries were to have a decisive effect on America's policy towards Europe.

Greece, 1947

When the Germans retreated from Greece in 1944, there were two rival groups – the monarchists and the Communists – who wanted to rule the country. Both had been involved in resistance against the Nazis. The Communists wanted Greece to be a Soviet republic. The monarchists wanted the return of the king of Greece. Churchill sent British troops to Greece in 1945 supposedly to help restore order and supervise free elections. In fact, the British supported the monarchists and the king was returned to power.

In 1946, the USSR protested to the United Nations that British troops were a threat to peace in Greece. The United Nations took no action and so the Communists tried to take control of Greece by force. A civil war quickly developed. The British could not afford the cost of such a war and announced on 24 February 1947 that they were withdrawing their troops. Truman stepped in. Paid for by the Americans, some British troops stayed in Greece. They tried to prop up the king's government. By 1950 the royalists were in control of Greece, although they were a very weak government, always in crisis.

SOURCE 20

I believe that it must be the policy of the United States to support free peoples who are resisting attempted subjugation by armed minorities or by outside pressures . . . The free peoples of the world look to us for support in maintaining those freedoms.
If we falter in our leadership, we may endanger the peace of the world.

President Truman speaking on 12 March 1947, explaining his decision to help Greece.

The Truman Doctrine

American intervention in Greece marked a new era in the USA's attitude to world politics, which became known as 'the Truman Doctrine' (see Source 20).

Under the Truman Doctrine, the USA was prepared to send money, equipment and advice to any country which was, in the American view, threatened by a Communist take-over. Truman accepted that eastern Europe was now Communist. His aim was to stop Communism from spreading any further. This policy became known as containment.

Others thought containment should mean something firmer. They said that it must be made clear to the Soviet Union that expansion beyond a given limit would be met with military force.

The Marshall Plan

Truman believed that Communism succeeded when people faced poverty and hardship. He sent the American General George Marshall to assess the economic state of Europe. What he found was a ruined economy. The countries of Europe owed $11.5 billion to the USA. There were extreme shortages of all goods. Most countries were still rationing bread. There was such a coal shortage in the hard winter of 1947 that in Britain all electricity was turned off for a period each day. Churchill described Europe as 'a rubble heap, a breeding ground of hate'.

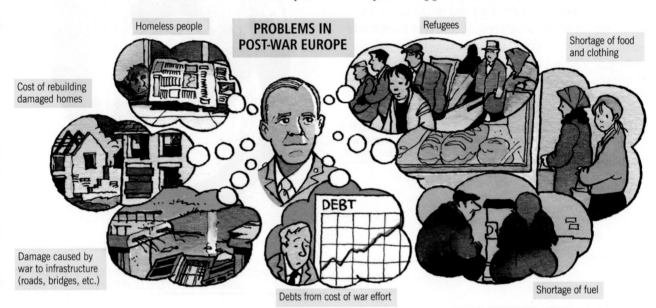

Marshall suggested that about $17 billion would be needed to rebuild Europe's prosperity. 'Our policy', he said, 'is directed against hunger, poverty, desperation and chaos.'

In December 1947, Truman put his plan to Congress. For a short time, the American Congress refused to grant this money. Many Americans were becoming concerned by Truman's involvement in foreign affairs. Besides, $17 billion was a lot of money!

Czechoslovakia, 1948

Americans' attitude changed when the Communists took over the government of Czechoslovakia. Czechoslovakia had been ruled by a coalition government which, although it included Communists, had been trying to pursue policies independent of Moscow. The Communists came down hard in March 1948. Anti-Soviet leaders were purged. One pro-American Minister, Jan Masaryk, was found dead below his open window. The Communists said he had jumped. The Americans suspected he'd been pushed. Immediately, Congress accepted the Marshall Plan and made $17 billion available over a period of four years.

Think!

Explain how events in
a) Greece
b) Czechoslovakia
affected American policy in Europe.

Think!

1 Draw a diagram to summarise the aims of Marshall Aid. Put political aims on one side and economic aims on the other. Draw arrows and labels to show how the two are connected.

2 Which of the problems in post-war Europe do you think would be the most urgent for Marshall Aid to tackle. Explain your choice.

Marshall Aid

On the one hand, Marshall Aid was an extremely generous act by the American people. On the other hand, it was also motivated by American self-interest. They wanted to create new markets for American goods. The Americans remembered the disastrous effects of the Depression of the 1930s and Truman wanted to do all he could to prevent another worldwide slump.

Stalin viewed Marshall Aid with suspicion. After expressing some initial interest, he refused to have anything more to do with it. He also forbade any of the eastern European states to apply for Marshall Aid. Stalin's view was that the anti-Communist aims behind Marshall Aid would weaken his hold on eastern Europe. He also felt that the USA was trying to dominate as many states as possible by making them dependent on dollars.

SOURCE 21

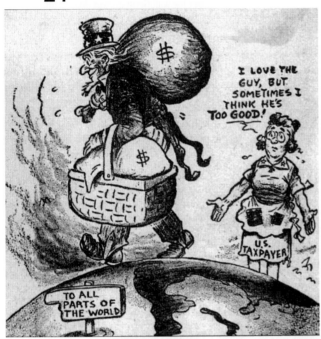

An American cartoon, 1949.

SOURCE 22

A Soviet cartoon commenting on Marshall Aid. The rope spells out the words 'Marshall Plan' and the lifebelt magnet is labelled 'Aid to Europe'.

Source Analysis ▲

1 Do Sources 21 and 22 support or criticise Marshall Aid?

2 Do you think the sources give a fair impression of Marshall Aid? Explain your answer.

Revision Tip

Stalin and Truman saw Marshall Aid differently. Try to sum up each view in a sentence.

Focus Task

How did the USA react to Soviet expansion?

1 Work in pairs and write two accounts of US policy in Europe. One of you should write from the point of view of the Americans; the other should write from the point of view of the Soviets. The sources and text on these two pages will help you.
You should include reference to:
a) US actions in the Greek Civil War in 1947
b) the Truman Doctrine
c) Soviet action in Czechoslovakia in 1948
d) the Marshall Plan and Marshall Aid.
As you consider each event, try to use it to make one side look reasonable or the other side unreasonable – or both!

2 Was the distrust between the USA and the USSR a problem of action (what each side is actually doing) or interpretation (how things are seen)?

The Berlin Blockade

By 1948 the distrust between the USA and the USSR was so great that leaders were talking in public about the threat of war between the two countries. Instead of running down arms expenditure, as you would expect them to after a war, the two sides actually increased their stock of weapons.

Each side took every opportunity to denounce the policies or the plans of the other. A propaganda war developed. Despite all the threatening talk, the two sides had never actually fired on one another. But in 1948 they came dangerously close to war.

SOURCE 23

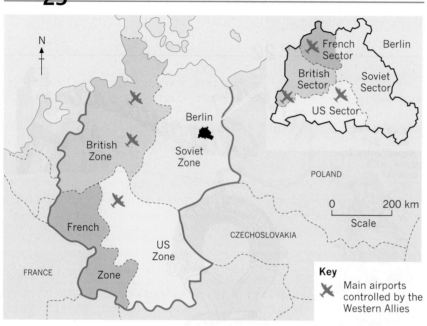

Germany in 1948.

The Western zones recover

After the war, Germany was divided into four zones (see Source 23). Germany had become a real headache for the Western Allies. After the destruction of war, their zones were in economic chaos. Stalin feared a recovering Germany and wanted to keep it crippled. But it was clear to the Allies that Germany could not feed its people if it was not allowed to rebuild its industries. Although they themselves were wary of rebuilding Germany too quickly, Britain, France and the USA combined their zones in 1946 to form one zone which was called Trizonia to start with but became known in 1949 as West Germany. In 1948 they reformed the currency and within months there were signs that Germany was recovering.

SOURCE 24

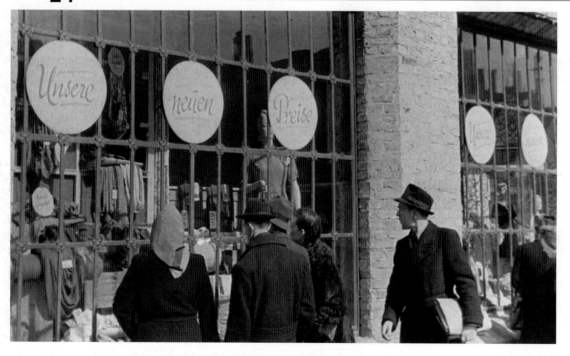

Berlin shoppers look at goods in shop windows a few days after the new currency was brought in. The notices say 'Our new prices'. Before the new currency, shops had few goods on display and there had been a thriving black market.

SOURCE **25**

On 23 June the Soviet authorities suspended all traffic into Berlin because of alleged technical difficulties . . . They also stopped barge traffic on similar grounds. Shortly before midnight, the Soviet authorities issued orders to . . . disrupt electric power from Soviet power plants to the Western sectors. Shortage of coal was given as a reason for this measure.

US Government report, June 1948.

SOURCE **26**

The crisis was planned in Washington, behind a smokescreen of anti-Soviet propaganda. In 1948 there was danger of war. The conduct of the Western powers risked bloody incidents. The self-blockade of the Western powers hit the West Berlin population with harshness. The people were freezing and starving. In the Spring of 1949 the USA was forced to yield . . . their war plans had come to nothing, because of the conduct of the USSR.

A Soviet commentary on the crisis.

Source Analysis

1 Read Source 25. What reasons did the Soviet Union give for cutting off West Berlin?
2 Why do you think the USA did not believe these were genuine reasons?
3 How do Sources 26 and 27 differ in their interpretation of the blockade?
4 What is the message of the cartoon in Source 28?
5 Which source do you think gives the most reliable view of the blockade?

The blockade

Stalin felt that the USA's handling of western Germany was provocative. He could do nothing about the reorganisation of the western zones, or the new currency, but he felt that he could stamp his authority on Berlin. It was deep in the Soviet zone and was linked to the western zones of Germany by vital roads, railways and canals. In June 1948, Stalin blocked all these supply lines, cutting off the two-million strong population of West Berlin from western help. Stalin believed that this would force the Allies out of Berlin and make Berlin entirely dependent on the USSR.

It was a clever plan. If US tanks did try to ram the road-blocks or railway blocks, Stalin would see it as an act of war. However, the Americans were not prepared to give up. They saw West Berlin as a test case. If they gave in to Stalin on this issue, the western zones of Germany might be next. Truman wanted to show that he was serious about his policy of containment. He wanted Berlin to be a symbol of freedom behind the Iron Curtain.

The Berlin airlift

The only way into Berlin was by air. So in June 1948 the Allies decided to air-lift supplies. As the first planes took off from their bases in West Germany, everyone feared that the Soviets would shoot them down, which would have been an act of war. People waited anxiously as the planes flew over Soviet territory, but no shots were fired. The planes got through and for the next ten months West Berlin was supplied by a constant stream of aeroplanes (three per minute) bringing in everything from food and clothing to oil and building materials. It made life possible in the western sectors, although there were enormous shortages and many Berliners decided to leave the city altogether. By May 1949, however, it was clear that the blockade of Berlin would not make the Western Allies give up Berlin, so Stalin reopened communications.

SOURCE **27**

We refused to be forced out of the city of Berlin. We demonstrated to the people of Europe that we would act and act resolutely, when their freedom was threatened. Politically it brought the people of Western Europe closer to us. The Berlin blockade was a move to test our ability and our will to resist.

President Truman, speaking in 1949.

SOURCE **28**

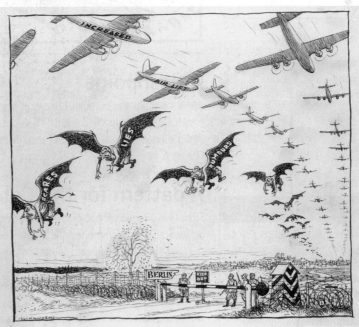

A cartoon by Leslie Illingworth from the *Daily Mail*, 20 April 1949.

SOURCE **29**

The Berlin air-lift was a considerable achievement but neither side gained anything from the confrontation. The USSR had not gained control of Berlin. The West had no guarantees that land communications would not be cut again. Above all confrontation made both sides even more stubborn.

Historian Jack Watson writing in 1984.

The consequences of the Berlin Blockade

A divided Germany

As a result of the Berlin Blockade, Germany was firmly divided into two nations. In May 1949, the British, French and American zones became the Federal Republic of Germany (known as West Germany). The Communist eastern zone was formed into the German Democratic Republic (or East Germany) in October 1949.

A powerful symbol

Germany would stay a divided country for 41 years. Throughout that time Berlin would remain a powerful symbol of Cold War tensions – from the American point of view, an oasis of democratic freedom in the middle of Communist repression; from the Soviet point of view, an invasive cancer growing in the workers' paradise of East Germany.

SOURCE **30**

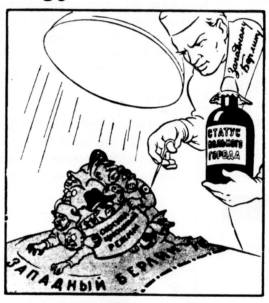

A 1958 Soviet cartoon. A Soviet doctor is injecting the cancer (the 'Occupation regime' of the Western Allies) with a medicine called 'Free City Status for West Berlin'.

Think!

It is difficult to give an exact date for when the Cold War actually started.
♦ Some might say that it was at Yalta, as Stalin, Churchill and Roosevelt argued over Poland.
♦ Others might say that it started in 1948 with the Berlin Blockade.
♦ There are other possible starting dates as well between 1945 and 1948.

What do you think? As a class, list all the possible starting dates you can think of. Then choose three to compare. Whatever your choice, support it with evidence from this chapter.

A flashpoint

Berlin was more than a symbol, however. It was also a potential flashpoint. As you study the story of the Cold War, you will find that the USA's and the USSR's worries about what might happen in Berlin affected their policies in other areas of the world. You will pick up the story of Berlin again in Chapter 6, page 133.

A pattern for the Cold War

Since 1946 some people had been using the term 'Cold War' to describe the tense relationships between the Western powers and the Soviet Union. The Berlin Blockade helped demonstrate what this Cold War actually consisted of. It set out a pattern for Cold War confrontations.

● On the one hand, the two superpowers and their allies had shown how suspicious they were of each other; how they would obstruct each other in almost any way they could; how they would bombard each other with propaganda.
● On the other hand, each had shown that it was not willing to go to war with the other.

The Berlin Blockade established a sort of tense balance between the superpowers that was to characterise much of the Cold War period.

Revision Tip

For the topic of the Berlin Blockade, aim to be able to explain (with examples):
♦ how the Allies started to rebuild Germany
♦ one reason this alarmed Stalin
♦ two important consequences of the blockade.

SOURCE **31**

Article 3: To achieve the aims of this Treaty, the Parties will keep up their individual and collective capacity to resist armed attack.

Article 5: The Parties agree that an armed attack against one or more of them in Europe or North America shall be considered an attack against them all.

Extracts from the NATO Charter.

NATO and the Warsaw Pact

During the Berlin Blockade, war between the USSR and the USA seemed a real possibility. At the height of the crisis, the Western powers met in Washington and signed an agreement to work together. The new organisation they formed in April 1949 was known as NATO (North Atlantic Treaty Organisation). Source 33 shows the main terms of the NATO alliance, and Source 34 shows Stalin's reaction to it.

Although the USSR was critical of NATO it took no further action until 1955 when the NATO powers allowed West Germany to join NATO. This brought back terrible reminders of the Second World War. In response the USSR and the main Communist states in Eastern Europe (including Poland, East Germany, Czechoslovakia, Romania and Hungary) formed the Warsaw Pact alliance. The members of the alliance promised to defend each other if any one member was attacked. They also promised not to interfere in the internal affairs of each member state and asserted the independence of each member of the alliance. In reality of course the USSR had huge influence over the independence and internal affairs of each of the member states.

SOURCE **32**

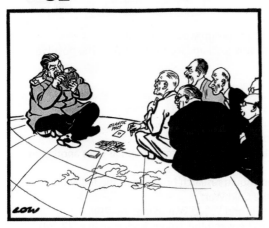

A cartoon by David Low, 1949, entitled 'Your play, Joe'. Western leaders wait to see how Stalin will react to the formation of NATO.

SOURCE **33**

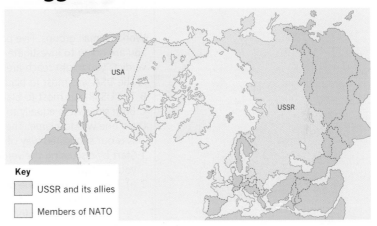

Key

USSR and its allies

Members of NATO

NATO and the Soviet satellites of eastern Europe. With the establishment of NATO, Europe was once again home to two hostile armed camps, just as it had been in 1914.

SOURCE **34**

The Soviet government did everything it could to prevent the world from being split into two military blocks. The Soviet Union issued a special statement analysing the grave consequences affecting the entire international situation that would follow from the establishment of a military alliance of the Western powers. All these warnings failed, however, and the North Atlantic Alliance came into being.

Stalin commenting on the formation of NATO, 1949.

Source Analysis

1 What evidence is there in Sources 31–34 to indicate that NATO was a purely defensive alliance?

2 Read Source 34. What 'grave consequences' do you think Stalin had in mind?

Focus Task

What were the consequences of the Berlin Blockade?

Here are some consequences of the Berlin Blockade.

◆ The Soviet Union and the West both claimed a victory.
◆ The Western Allies set up a military alliance called NATO.
◆ Many westerners left Berlin for good.
◆ The airlift showed the West's commitment to Berlin.
◆ The airlift kept Berlin working.
◆ Berlin became a symbol of Cold War tension.
◆ It ended the four-power administration of Germany and Berlin and split Germany into two blocs. Germany remained a divided country for 40 years.
◆ There was no fighting – the dispute ended peacefully.
◆ It heightened fear of the Soviet Union in the west.
◆ The airlift improved relations between Germans and the Allies (who had so recently been at war).

Write each consequence on a card then:

    a) divide the cards into short-term and long-term consequences

    b) choose two which you think are the most significant consequences and explain your choice.

Focus Task

Who was more to blame for the Cold War?

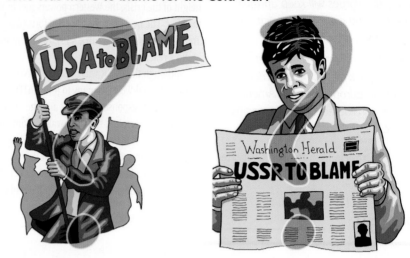

Work in small groups. Five people per group would be ideal.

You are going to investigate who was to blame for the Cold War. The possible verdicts you might reach are:

A The USA was most to blame.

B The USSR was most to blame.

C Both sides were equally to blame.

D No one was to blame. The Cold War was inevitable.

This is our suggested way of working.

1 Start by discussing the verdicts together. Is one more popular than another in your group?

2 a) Each member of the group should research how one of the following factors helped to lead to the Cold War:

♦ the situation before the Second World War (pages 78–79).

♦ the personal relationships between the various leaders (pages 77–84).

♦ the conflicting beliefs of the superpowers (pages 83–84).

♦ the war damage suffered by the USSR (pages 80 and 83).

♦ Stalin's take-over of eastern Europe (pages 82–83).

♦ Marshall Aid for Europe (pages 86–87).

♦ the Berlin Blockade (pages 88–90)

You can start with the page numbers given. You can introduce your own research from other books or the internet if you wish.

b) Present your evidence to your group and explain which, if any, of the verdicts

A–D your evidence most supports.

3 As a group, discuss which of the verdicts now seems most sensible.

4 Write a balanced essay on who was to blame, explaining why each verdict is a possibility but reaching your own conclusion about which is best. The verdicts A–D give you a possible structure for your essay. Write a paragraph on each verdict, selecting relevant evidence for your group discussion. A final paragraph can explain your overall conclusion.

Revision Tip

It is useful to think about big questions like 'who was most to blame…' but it is also useful to think about the role of specific factors so turn your research for question 2 into revision cards and share them with your fellow students.

Make sure you know what these terms mean and are able to define them confidently.

- Atomic bomb
- Alliance
- Appeasement
- Berlin airlift
- Berlin Blockade
- Capitalism
- Cominform
- Communism
- Democracy
- Dictatorship
- Iron curtain
- Isolationism
- Marshall Aid
- Marshall Plan
- NATO
- Potsdam Conference
- Russia
- Soviet sphere of influence
- Superpower
- The Soviet Union
- The West/The Western Powers
- Truman Doctrine
- Yalta Conference

Chapter Summary

The beginnings of the Cold War

1 The USSR was a Communist country with a one-party state; the USA was a capitalist democracy. They had very different ideas about how a country should be run and had been enemies throughout the 1930s. However, because they had a shared enemy (Hitler) they were allies during the Second World War.

2 When it was clear that Germany was going to be defeated their leaders met together at Yalta (in the USSR) to plan what would happen after the war. The US and Soviet leaders, Roosevelt and Stalin, appeared to get on well, although behind the scenes there were tensions and disagreements.

3 They agreed that after the war Germany (and its capital Berlin) would be divided into four sectors run by Britain, the USA, France and the USSR, and that eastern Europe would be a Soviet 'sphere of influence'.

4 After the war ended the countries met again at Potsdam in Germany but by this time much had changed: Roosevelt had been replaced as President by Truman; Stalin's troops were occupying most of eastern Europe and the Americans had dropped an atomic bomb.

5 Relations between the USA and USSR quickly deteriorated and a Cold War started (a Cold War is the threat of war and deep mistrust but no outright fighting).

6 All the countries of eastern Europe elected or had forced on them a Communist government that was allied to the USSR. The division between Communist east and capitalist west became known as the iron curtain.

7 The USA wanted to stop Communism spreading – the Truman Doctrine said that America would help any country that was resisting outside pressure (by which Truman meant Communism). This marked a decisive end to US isolationism.

8 The USA offered financial help (Marshall Aid) to countries in western Europe to rebuild.

9 The USSR saw Marshall Aid and the Truman Doctrine as a threat to the USSR, which might lead to an attack on the USSR itself.

10 Berlin became the first focus of Cold War tension when it was blockaded by Stalin to prevent supplies getting into the US/British/French sectors. The western allies responded with the Berlin airlift.

Exam Practice

See pages 168–175 and pages 316–319 for advice on the different types of questions you might face.

1 (a) What was agreed by the Allied leaders at the Yalta Conference? **[4]**

(b) Why had relationships between the USA and the USSR changed by the time of the Potsdam Conference? **[6]**

(c) 'The Cold War was caused by the Soviet take-over of eastern Europe.' How far do you agree with this statement? Explain your answer. **[10]**

2 Study Source 3 on page 80 and Source 7 on page 81. Why are these sources so different? Explain your answer using the sources and your knowledge. **[7]**

3 Study Source 15 on page 83. What is the message of the cartoonist? Explain your answer. **[7]**

4 Study Sources 26, 27 and 28 on page 89. Which of Sources 26 or 27 would the cartoonist in Source 28 agree with? Explain your answer using the sources and your own knowledge. **[8]**

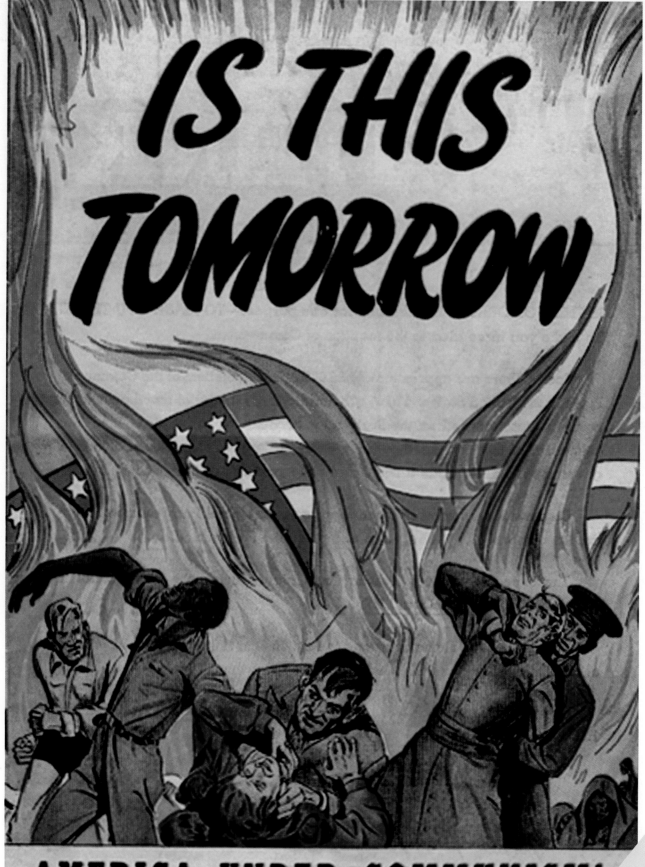

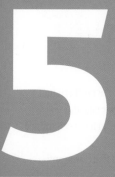

5 How effectively did the USA contain the spread of Communism?

FOCUS POINTS

This key question will be explored through case studies of the following:

- the Korean War, 1950–53
- the Cuban Missile Crisis of 1962
- US involvement in the Vietnam War

Although the USA was the world's most powerful nation, in 1950 it seemed to President Truman that events were not going America's way, particularly with regard to Communism.

- ◆ As you have seen in Chapter 4 most of eastern Europe had fallen under the influence of the Communist USSR 1945–48.
- ◆ China became Communist in 1949. The Americans had always regarded China as their strongest ally in the Far East. Between 1946 and 1949 they gave billions of dollars of aid to the Nationalist government in China, largely to prevent a Communist takeover. That had failed. Suddenly a massive new Communist state had appeared on the map.
- ◆ Also in 1949 the Soviet leader Stalin announced that the USSR had developed its own atomic bomb. The USA was no longer the world's only nuclear power.
- ◆ Furthermore American spies reported to President Truman that Stalin was using his network (Cominform) to help Communists win power in Malaya, Indonesia, Burma, the Philippines and Korea. The USA had visions of the Communists overrunning all of Asia, with country after country being toppled like a row of dominoes.

There was already a strong anti-Communist feeling in the USA. These developments made it stronger. There was no doubt in the minds of American leaders (indeed most American people) that this spread should be resisted. If they could have done, they would have liked to turn back the Communist advances but that was unrealistic. So from 1947 onwards the USA followed the policy of Containment – holding back Communism so it did not spread any further. But as the 1950s dawned this looked like a serious challenge.

In this chapter you will investigate:

- ◆ the different methods the USA used to try to contain the spread of Communism
- ◆ how successful these methods were during the Korean War, the Cuban Missile Crisis and the Vietnam War – using these case studies you will make up your own mind
- ◆ how successful the policy was in the years 1950–75: how effectively did the USA contain the spread of Communism?

◀ This is a cover of a comic book published in the United States in 1947.

1 What impression does this comic cover give you of:
   a) the USA?
   b) Communism?
2 What is the message of this picture?

Case study 1: The Korean War

Background

Korea had been ruled by Japan until 1945. At the end of the Second World War the northern half was liberated by Soviet troops and the southern half by Americans. When the war ended:

- **The North** remained Communist-controlled, with a Communist leader who had been trained in the USSR, and with a Soviet-style one-party system.
- **The South** was anti-Communist. It was not very democratic, but the fact that it was anti-Communist was enough to win it the support of the USA.

There was bitter hostility between the North's Communist leader, Kim Il Sung, and Syngman Rhee, President of South Korea. Reunification did not seem likely. In 1950 this hostility spilled over into open warfare. North Korean troops overwhelmed the South's forces. By September 1950 all except a small corner of south-east Korea was under Communist control (see Source 5, map 1).

As you have already seen in Chapter 4, US President Truman was determined to contain Communism – to stop it spreading further. In his view, Korea was a glaring example of how Communism would spread if the USA did nothing (see Source 2). Remember that for Truman and for many Americans, containment was not so much a policy they wanted as a policy they had to make do with. If they could have done they would have liked to turn back the spread of Communism but that would have risked an all-out war with the USSR. So from the US point of view, it was not so much that they believed in containment, it was that they believed that they could not accept anything less.

USA or United Nations?

President Truman immediately sent advisers, supplies and warships to the waters around Korea. But he was aware that if he was going to take action it would look better to the rest of the world if he had the support of other countries, especially if he had the support of the United Nations. In fact the ideal situation would be a UN intervention in Korea rather than an American one.

Truman put enormous pressure on the UN Security Council to condemn the actions of the North Koreans and to call on them to withdraw their troops. The USA was the single biggest contributor to the UN budget and was therefore in a powerful position to influence its decisions. However, this did not mean the USA always got its own way and it would probably have failed this time except for some unusual circumstances. In the Cold War atmosphere of 1950, each superpower always denounced and opposed the other. Normally, in a dispute such as this, the Soviet Union would have used its right of veto to block the call for action by the UN. However, the USSR was boycotting the UN at this time over another issue (whether Communist China should be allowed to join the UN). So when the resolution was passed the USSR was not even at the meeting to use its veto. So Truman was able to claim that this was a UN-sponsored operation, even if Soviet newspapers and other media claimed that the decision was not valid.

Under the resolution (see Source 1) the UN committed itself to using its members' armies to drive North Korean troops out of South Korea. Eighteen states (including Britain) provided troops or support of some kind, mostly allies of the USA. However, the overwhelming part of the UN force that was sent to Korea was American. The commander, General MacArthur, was also an American.

September 1950 – the UN force advances

United Nations forces stormed ashore at Inchon in September 1950 (see Source 5, map 1). At the same time, other UN forces and South Korean troops advanced from Pusan. The North Koreans were driven back beyond their original border (the 38th parallel) within weeks.

SOURCE **1**

The UN will render such assistance to the republic of Korea as may be necessary to restore international peace and security to the area.

Resolution 84 passed by the United Nations in 1950.

SOURCE **2**

Korea is a symbol to the watching world. If we allow Korea to fall within the Soviet orbit, the world will feel we have lost another round in our match with the Soviet Union, and our prestige and the hopes of those who place their faith in us will suffer accordingly.

The US State Department, 1950.

SOURCE **3**

If the UN is ever going to do anything, this is the time, and if the UN cannot bring the crisis in Korea to an end then we might as well just wash up the United Nations and forget it.

American Senator Tom Connally speaking in 1950. He was a Republican and strongly anti-Communist.

SOURCE 4

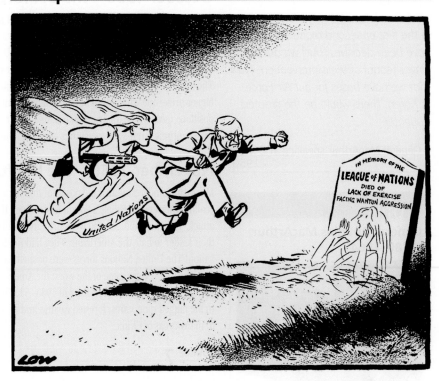

A cartoon by David Low, 1950.

SOURCE 5

Map 1: September 1950	Map 2: October 1950	Map 3: January 1951	Map 4: July 1953

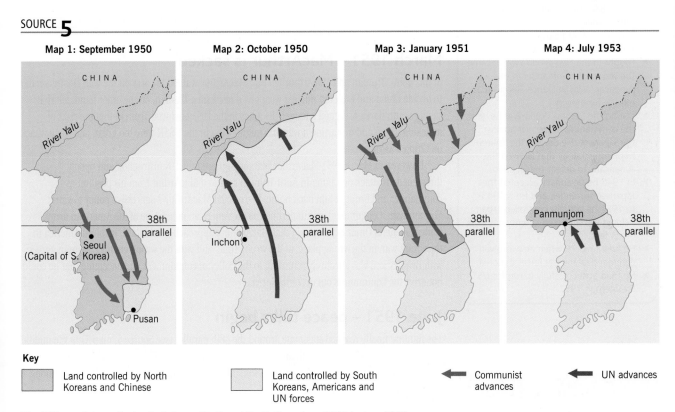

Key

☐ Land controlled by North Koreans and Chinese

☐ Land controlled by South Koreans, Americans and UN forces

← Communist advances

← UN advances

The 38th parallel was the border between North and South Korea from 1945 to June 1950.

The Korean War, 1950–53

Had they [the Chinese] intervened in the first or second months it would have been decisive, [but] we are no longer fearful of their intervention. Now that we have bases for our Air Force in Korea, there would be the greatest slaughter.

General MacArthur speaking in October 1950.

Profile

General Douglas MacArthur (1880–1964)

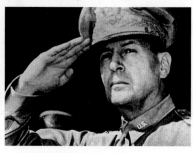

➤ Born 1880. His father was a successful army leader.

➤ Trained at West Point, the top American military academy.

➤ Fought in the First World War. Became the youngest commander in the American army in France. Received 13 medals for bravery.

➤ During the Second World War he was the commander of the war against the Japanese. He devised the 'island-hopping' strategy that allowed the Americans to defeat the Japanese.

➤ In 1945 he personally accepted the Japanese surrender, and from 1945 to 1951 he virtually controlled Japan, helping the shattered country get back on its feet.

➤ He was aged 70 when he was given command of the UN forces in Korea.

➤ He tried unsuccessfully to run for US President in 1952.

Think!

Use the text to write some extra bullet points for the Profile describing:

a) MacArthur's personality and beliefs

b) his actions in Korea.

October 1950 – the UN force presses on

MacArthur had quickly achieved the original UN aim of removing North Korean troops from South Korea. But the Americans did not stop. Despite warnings from China's leader, Mao Tse-tung, that if they pressed on China would join the war, the UN approved a plan to advance into North Korea. By October, US forces had reached the Yalu River and the border with China (see Source 5, map 2). The nature of the war had now changed. It was clear that MacArthur and Truman were after a bigger prize, one which went beyond containment. As the UN forces advanced and secured their positions (see Source 6), Truman and MacArthur saw an opportunity to remove Communism from Korea entirely. Even Mao's warnings were not going to put them off.

November 1950 – the UN force retreats

MacArthur underestimated the power of the Chinese. Late in October 1950, 200,000 Chinese troops (calling themselves 'People's Volunteers') joined the North Koreans. They launched a blistering attack. They had soldiers who were strongly committed to Communism and had been taught by their leader to hate the Americans. They had modern tanks and planes supplied by the Soviet Union. The United Nations forces were pushed back into South Korea.

Conditions were some of the worst the American forces had known, with treacherous cold and blinding snowstorms in the winter of 1950–51. The Chinese forces were more familiar with fighting in the jagged mountains, forested ravines and treacherous swamps – as the landscape was similar to many areas of China.

Even the reports to the UN were censored by [American] state and defence departments. I had no connection with the United Nations whatsoever.

From General MacArthur's memoirs.

March 1951 – MacArthur is sacked

At this point, Truman and MacArthur fell out. MacArthur wanted to carry on the war. He was ready to invade China and even use nuclear weapons if necessary. Truman, on the other hand, felt that saving South Korea was good enough. His allies in the UN convinced Truman that the risks of attacking China and of starting a war that might bring in the USSR were too great, and so an attack on China was ruled out.

However, in March 1951 MacArthur blatantly ignored the UN instruction and openly threatened an attack on China. In April Truman removed MacArthur from his position as commander and brought him back home. He rejected MacArthur's aggressive policy towards Communism. Containment was underlined as the American policy. One of the American army leaders, General Omar Bradley, said that MacArthur's approach would have 'involved America in the wrong war, in the wrong place, at the wrong time, and with the wrong enemy'. Truman agreed with Bradley and was effectively returning to the policy of containment and accepting that he could not drive the Communists out of North Korea.

June 1951 – peace talks begin

The fighting finally reached stalemate around the 38th parallel (see Source 5, map 3) in the middle of 1951. Peace talks between North and South Korea began in June 1951, although bitter fighting continued for two more years. The casualties on all sides were immense – but particularly among civilians (see Sources 8 and 9).

July 1953 – armistice

In 1952 Truman was replaced by President Eisenhower, who wanted to end the war. Stalin's death in March 1953 made the Chinese and North Koreans less confident. An armistice was finally signed in July 1953. The border between North and South Korea was much the same as it had been before war started in 1950.

SOURCE **8**

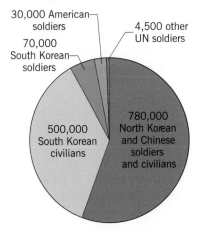

30,000 American soldiers
4,500 other UN soldiers
70,000 South Korean soldiers
500,000 South Korean civilians
780,000 North Korean and Chinese soldiers and civilians

Total killed: 1.4 million

Civilian and military deaths in the Korean War. American military fatalities per year of conflict were actually higher than the Vietnam War.

SOURCE **9**

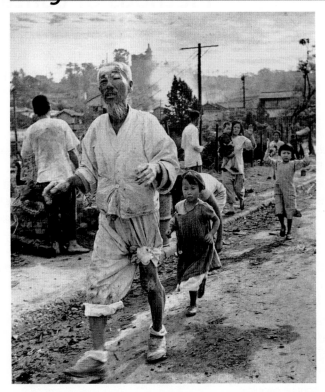

Civilian casualty in the early stages of the Korean War as South Koreans fled from the advancing North Koreans.

A success for containment?

In one sense the Korean War was a success for the USA. The cost and the casualties were high but it showed that the USA had the will and the means to contain Communism. South Korea remained out of Communist hands.

On the other hand it showed the limits of the policy. The USA had to accept that North Korea remained Communist. It also highlighted tensions among American leaders. Hardline anti-Communist politicians and military leaders wanted to go beyond containment – to push back Communism. They thought that Truman had shown weakness in not going for outright victory. More moderate politicians and commanders argued that this would not be worth the risk.

These tensions would affect US policy over the coming decades.

Focus Task

Was the Korean War a success for containment?

Draw up your own copy of this table. You will use it to compare the three case studies. At this stage, just focus on the Korean War. You are going to revisit this task at the end of the Cuban Missile Crisis and the Vietnam War as well. We have started it off for you. Your completed chart will be a useful revision tool.

Case study	Why were the Americans worried?	What methods did the Americans use to contain Communism?	What problems did they face?	What was the outcome?	Success or failure (out of 10) with reasons supported by evidence
Korea	Communist North Korea invaded capitalist South Korea				

Methods of containment

There was no doubt at all in the minds of American leaders that Communism had to be resisted. The question was how to do it. The Korean War showed the Americans that they could not just send their soldiers to fight a war whenever they saw a problem. It was too expensive and it did not really work very well. Containment needed other methods.

Alliances

The USA created a network of anti-Communist alliances around the world: SEATO in South East Asia and CENTO in central Asia and the Middle East. The USA gave money, advice and arms to these allies. In return, the leaders of these countries suppressed Communist influence in their own countries.

The USSR saw these alliances as aggressive. They accused the USA of trying to encircle the Communist world. In 1955 the Soviet Union set up the Warsaw Treaty Organisation, better known as the Warsaw Pact. This included the USSR and all the Communist east European countries except Yugoslavia.

SOURCE 10

We shall never have a secure peace and a happy world so long as Soviet Communism dominates one-third of all the world's people and is in the process of trying to extend its rule to many others. Therefore we must have in mind the liberation of these captive peoples. Now liberation does not mean war. Liberation can be achieved by processes short of war. A policy which only aims at containing Russia is an unsound policy … If our only policy is to stay where we are, we will be driven back.

JF Dulles, US Secretary of State, speaking on his appointment in 1952.

Think!

Read Source 10. What methods do you think Dulles had in mind to 'liberate captive peoples' without a war?

SOURCE 11

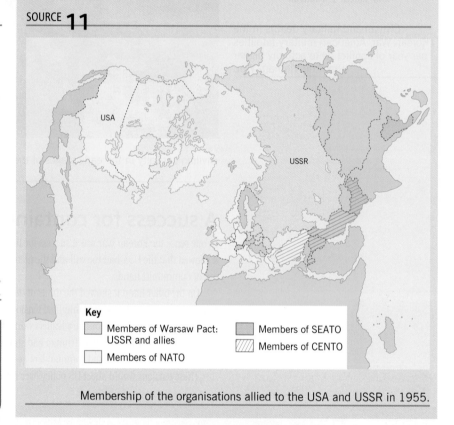

Key
- Members of Warsaw Pact: USSR and allies
- Members of NATO
- Members of SEATO
- Members of CENTO

Membership of the organisations allied to the USA and USSR in 1955.

Arms race

At the same time both the USSR and the USA were engaged in an 'arms race'.

The Americans had developed their first atomic bomb in 1945. They did not share the secret of their bomb with the USSR, even while they were still allies. When the USA dropped the first bombs on Hiroshima and Nagasaki in August 1945, 70,000 people were killed instantly. The awesome power of the explosions and the incredible destruction caused by the bombs made Japan surrender within a week. It was clear to both the USA and the USSR that atomic bombs were the weapons of the future.

Over the next decade the USA and USSR developed ever bigger, more deadly and more flexible weapons. They spent vast amounts of money on new weapons. They spied on one another to steal technological secrets. The USSR tended to use spies such as Rudolf Abel. He worked in New York until he was arrested in 1957. The USA favoured hi-tech spying such as the U2 plane – a spy plane which flew so high it could not be shot down but took incredibly detailed photos of the ground. It could read a newspaper from 14 miles up in the sky!

Each side perfected nuclear bombs that could be launched from submarines or planes. The USA placed short-range nuclear weapons in Turkey (one of their CENTO allies). Both sides developed ICBMs, which could travel from continent to continent in half an hour.

The impact of the arms race

The arms race was partly about **quality** – who had the most sophisticated weapons. The Soviets took the lead in technology in the 1950s, building on the achievements of their successful space programme. These technological advances by the USSR rocked public opinion in the USA. The Cold War was a propaganda war much more than a military war. You had to show that your system was superior; that your scientists were cleverer. To lose advantage to the Soviet Union was a blow to the USA.

However the arms race was also about **quantity**. The US public was alarmed to be told that the USSR had many more nuclear missiles than the USA. This so-called 'missile gap' was widely reported in the American media during the 1950s. We now know that the missile gap was a myth. The USA always had more missiles than the USSR. However:

● Khrushchev was not going to admit this because he would look foolish and it would aid his critics inside the USSR.

● At the same time, the American military commanders were happy to go along with the claims that there was a missile gap because it helped them to get funding from the government to pay for the development of new weapons systems.

● By the early 1960s Eisenhower also knew the missile gap was a myth because he had an important source in the Soviet military who had defected to the CIA. However, because this contact was still in the USSR, Eisenhower could not admit he knew how many missiles the Soviets actually had without revealing his source.

So, myth or not, the USA forged ahead with its own missile production programme to 'narrow the missile gap'.

Deterrence and MAD

The result was that by 1961, both of the superpowers had hundreds of missiles pointed at each other. The USA had more than the USSR, but the advantage did not really matter because both sides had enough to destroy each other many times over. On each side the theory was that such weapons made them more secure. The 'nuclear deterrent' meant the enemy would not dare attack first, because it knew that, if it did, the other would strike back before its bombs had even landed and it too would be destroyed. It would be suicidal. So having nuclear weapons deterred the other side from attacking first. This policy also became known as MAD (Mutually Assured Destruction). Surely no side would dare strike first when it knew the attack would destroy itself too.

Fear

Leaders might see their nuclear weapons as a deterrent, but others worried that the world was moving into a very dangerous time. For example, an American B-47 bomber crashed in Norfolk, England in 1957. The resulting fire came within minutes of setting off two nuclear bombs that would have devastated all of East Anglia. In 1962, a US radar station mistook one of its own satellites for an incoming Soviet missile and was minutes away from triggering a full nuclear 'response' attack on the USSR. Of course, governments did not tell their people about these incidents – both Soviet and US leaders were very secretive. But they could not hide the big issue – that the nuclear arms race seemed to have raised the stakes so high that one suicidal leader, one poor decision or (most worryingly of all) one small and innocent mistake could trigger a catastrophe that could destroy Europe, the USA and the Soviet Union within minutes.

Fear of 'the bomb' was a common feature of life in 1950s' and 1960s' America. The arms race was a topic of everyday conversation. Children were taught at school what do if there was a nuclear attack. Some people protested against the arms race. Robert Oppenheimer, the man who led the team that developed the atom bomb, opposed the H-bomb. He felt it was wrong to develop a more powerful bomb in peacetime. Others protested at the vast amounts being spent on weapons. But the most common feelings were of helplessness and fear. People wondered whether this was the end. Were they the last generation to walk this planet? Would nuclear warfare signal the end of the world?

It was against the background of the nuclear arms race that Cuba became the next major flashpoint of the Cold War.

Think!

Create a diagram that shows how the following facors were connected:
♦ alliances
♦ nuclear arms race
♦ propaganda
♦ spying.
The author recommends a Venn diagram but you might prefer a spider diagram or some other format. Or try different formats and see which works well for you.

Revision Tip

Make sure you can remember:
♦ one example of the USA creating an alliance to contain Communism
♦ one example of it using arms technology to contain Communism.

Case study 2: The Cuban Missile Crisis

SOURCE **12**

We considered it part of the United States practically, just a wonderful little country over there that was of no danger to anybody, as a matter of fact it was a rather important economic asset to the United States.

American TV reporter Walter Cronkite

SOURCE **13**

I believe there is no country in the world . . . whose economic colonisation, humiliation and exploitation were worse than in Cuba, partly as a consequence of US policy during the Batista regime. I believe that, without being aware of it, we conceived and created the Castro movement, starting from scratch.

President Kennedy speaking in 1963.

Source Analysis

1 How far do Sources 12 and 13 agree about Cuba's relationship with the USA before the revolution?
2 Apart from the caption in Russian, how else can you tell that the cartoon in Source 14 is a Soviet cartoon?
3 'The aim of the cartoonist in Source 14 was simply to tell people that the USA was forbidding Cuba to make friends with the USSR, nothing more.' Do you agree with this statement?

Revision Tip

From these two pages you should make sure you remember:
♦ one reason why the USA disliked Castro's government
♦ how the USA initially tried to contain Communism on Cuba.

The Cuban Revolution?

Cuba is a large island just 160 km from Florida in the southern USA. It had long been an American ally. Americans owned most of the businesses on the island and they had a huge naval base there (see Source 18 on page 104). The Americans also provided the Cuban ruler, General Batista, with economic and military support. Batista was a dictator. His rule was corrupt and unpopular. The Americans supported Batista primarily because he was just as opposed to Communism as they were.

Enter Fidel Castro

There was plenty of opposition to Batista in Cuba itself. In 1959, after a three-year campaign, Fidel Castro overthrew Batista. Castro was charming, clever and also ruthless. He quickly killed, arrested or exiled many political opponents. Castro was also a clever propagandist. He was very charismatic, and he had a vision for a better Cuba which won over the majority of Cubans.

The USA responds

The USA was taken by surprise at first and decided to recognise Castro as the new leader of Cuba. However, within a short period of time relations between the two countries grew worse. There were two important reasons:

● There were thousands of Cuban exiles in the USA who had fled from Castro's rule. They formed powerful pressure groups demanding action against Castro.
● Castro took over some American-owned businesses in Cuba, particularly the agricultural businesses. He took their land and distributed it to his supporters among Cuba's peasant farmer population.

SOURCE **14**

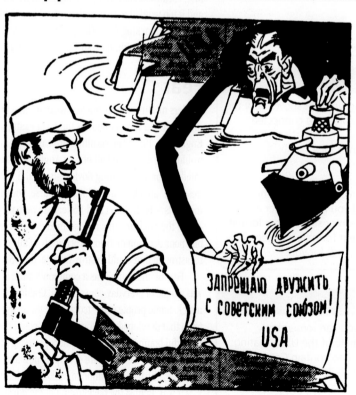

A 1960 Soviet cartoon. The notice held by the US Secretary of State says to Castro in Cuba: 'I forbid you to make friends with the Soviet Union.'

By October 1962 the historic friendship between Cuba and the USA was gone. Behind this change was the story of the betrayal of the Cuban people. It began with Fidel Castro triumphantly entering Havana in 1959. Castro promised democracy and freedom and for a time it appeared to most Cubans that they were liberated. But it soon became apparent that Castro had sold out to Premier Khrushchev of the Communists.

Commentary from an American TV programme made in 1962.

I think he [Khrushchev] did it [was so aggressive in the meeting] because of the Bay of Pigs. He thought that anyone who was so young and inexperienced as to get into that mess could be beaten; and anyone who got into it and didn't see it through had no guts. So he just beat the hell out of me.

If he thinks I'm inexperienced and have no guts, until we remove those ideas we won't get anywhere with him.

Kennedy speaking after a meeting with Khrushchev in 1961

Factfile

Bay of Pigs invasion

➤ Cuban exiles were funded and trained by CIA and supported by US air power.
➤ Plan originally devised by President Eisenhower's government but Kennedy approved it when he became President. Training began in April 1960.
➤ Cuban security services knew that the invasion was coming.
➤ Invasion took place on 17 April 1961. It was a complete failure. US intelligence which stated that Cuban people would rebel against Castro proved to be wrong.

Kennedy ordered extensive investigations into the disaster. Key failings included:

➤ lack of secrecy so that USA could not deny its involvement;
➤ poor links between various US departments;
➤ failure to organise resistance inside Cuba;
➤ insufficient Spanish-speaking staff.

As early as June 1960, US President Eisenhower authorised the US Central Intelligence Agency **(CIA)** to investigate ways of overthrowing Castro. The CIA provided support and funds to Cuban exiles. They also investigated ways to disrupt the Cuban economy, such as damaging sugar plantations. American companies working in Cuba refused to co-operate with any Cuban businesses which used oil or other materials which had been imported from the USSR. The American media also broadcast a relentless stream of criticism of Castro and his regime (see Source 15 for example).

Castro responded to US hostility with a mixed approach. He assured Americans living in Cuba that they were safe and he allowed the USA to keep its naval base. He said he simply wanted to run Cuba without interference. However, by the summer of 1960 he had allied Cuba with the Soviet Union. Soviet leader Khrushchev signed a trade agreement giving Cuba $100 million in economic aid. Castro also began receiving arms from the Soviet Union and American spies knew this.

To invade or not to invade, that is the question!

In January 1961 the USA's new President, John F Kennedy, broke off diplomatic relations with Cuba. Castro thought that the USA was preparing to invade his country. The Americans did not invade directly, but Kennedy was no longer prepared to tolerate a Soviet satellite in the USA's 'sphere of influence'. The plans to overthrow Castro which were begun under Eisenhower began to take shape.

The Bay of Pigs

Rather than a direct invasion, President Kennedy supplied arms, equipment and transport for 1,400 anti-Castro exiles to invade Cuba and overthrow him. In April 1961 the exiles landed at the Bay of Pigs. They were met by 20,000 Cuban troops, armed with tanks and modern weapons. The invasion failed disastrously. Castro captured or killed them all within days.

The impact of the invasion

The half-hearted invasion suggested to Cuba and the Soviet Union that, despite its opposition to Communism in Cuba, the USA was unwilling to get directly involved in Cuba. The Soviet leader Khrushchev was scornful of Kennedy's pathetic attempt to oust Communism from Cuba.

Historians too argue that the Bay of Pigs fiasco further strengthened Castro's position in Cuba. It suggested to the USSR that Kennedy was weak. It also made Castro and Khrushchev very suspicious of US policy.

Focus Task

How did the USA respond to the Cuban revolution?

1 The President has asked his advisers how he should deal with Cuba. Here are some suggestions they might have made:

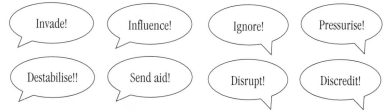

Record examples you can find of the USA doing any of these things. If you find examples of American actions that are not covered by these words record them too.

2 Place these actions on a 'containment continuum' like this:

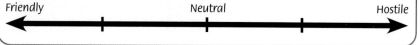

[Estimates were that the] missiles had an atomic warhead [power] of about half the current missile capacity of the entire Soviet Union. The photographs indicated that missiles were directed at certain American cities. The estimate was that within a few minutes of their being fired 80 million Americans would be dead.

President Kennedy's brother, Robert Kennedy, describing events on Thursday 18 October in the book he wrote about the crisis, *13 Days*.

Khrushchev arms Castro

After the Bay of Pigs fiasco, Soviet arms flooded into Cuba. In May 1962 the Soviet Union announced publicly for the first time that it was supplying Cuba with arms. By July 1962 Cuba had the best-equipped army in Latin America. By September it had thousands of Soviet missiles, plus patrol boats, tanks, radar vans, missile erectors, jet bombers, jet fighters and 5,000 Soviet technicians to help to maintain the weapons.

The Americans watched all this with great alarm. They seemed ready to tolerate conventional arms being supplied to Cuba, but the big question was whether the Soviet Union would dare to put **nuclear** missiles on Cuba. In September Kennedy's own Intelligence Department said that it did not believe the USSR would send nuclear weapons to Cuba. The USSR had not taken this step with any of its satellite states before and the US Intelligence Department believed that the USSR would consider it too risky to do it in Cuba. On 11 September, Kennedy warned the USSR that he would prevent 'by whatever means might be necessary' Cuba's becoming an offensive military base — by which, everyone knew, he meant a base for nuclear missiles. The same day the USSR assured the USA that it had no need to put nuclear missiles on Cuba and no intention of doing so.

The October crisis

On Sunday, 14 October 1962, an American spy plane flew over Cuba. It took amazingly detailed photographs of missile sites in Cuba. To the military experts two things were obvious — that these were nuclear missile sites, and that they were being built by the USSR.

More photo reconnaissance followed over the next two days. This confirmed that some sites were nearly finished but others were still being built. Some already supplied with missiles, others were awaiting them. The experts said that the most developed of the sites could be ready to launch missiles in just seven days. American spy planes also reported that twenty Soviet ships were currently on the way to Cuba carrying missiles.

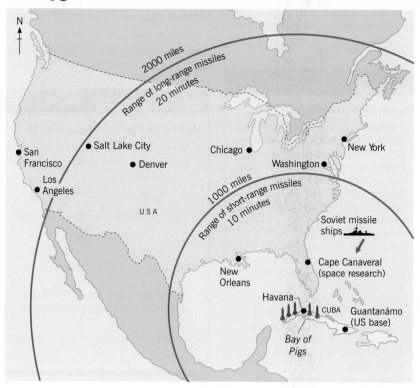

Map showing the location of Cuba and the range of the Cuban missiles.

Think!

How should President Kennedy deal with the Cuban crisis?

On Tuesday 16 October, President Kennedy was informed of the discovery. He formed a special team of advisers called Ex Comm.

They came up with several choices.

Work in groups. You are advisers to the President. You have to reduce Ex Comm's five options to just two for the President to choose between.

When you have made your decision explain why you have rejected the three you have.

Option 1 Do nothing?

For: The Americans still had a vastly greater nuclear power than the Soviet Union. The USA could still destroy the Soviet Union, so – the argument went – the USSR would never use these missiles. The biggest danger to world peace would be to overreact to this discovery.

Against: The USSR had lied about Cuban missiles. Kennedy had already issued his solemn warning to the USSR. To do nothing would be another sign of weakness.

Option 2 Surgical air attack?

An immediate selected air attack to destroy the nuclear bases themselves.

For: It would destroy the missiles before they were ready to use.

Against: 1 Destruction of all sites could not be guaranteed. Even one left undamaged could launch a counter-attack against the USA.
2 The attack would inevitably kill Soviet soldiers. The Soviet Union might retaliate at once.
3 To attack without advance warning was seen as immoral.

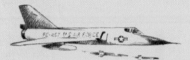

Option 3 Invasion?

All-out invasion of Cuba by air and sea.

For: An invasion would not only get rid of the missiles but Castro as well. The American forces were already trained and available to do it.

Against: It would almost certainly guarantee an equivalent Soviet response, either to protect Cuba, or within the Soviet sphere of influence – for example, a take-over of Berlin.

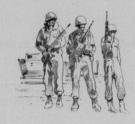

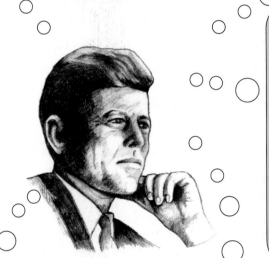

Option 4 Diplomatic pressures?

To get the United Nations or other body to intervene and negotiate.

For: It would avoid conflict.

Against: If the USA was forced to back down, it would be a sign of weakness.

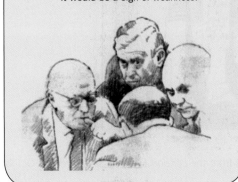

Option 5 Blockade?

A ban on the Soviet Union bringing in any further military supplies to Cuba, enforced by the US navy who would stop and search Soviet ships. And a call for the Soviet Union to withdraw what was already there.

For: It would show that the USA was serious, but it would not be a direct act of war. It would put the burden on Khrushchev to decide what to do next. The USA had a strong navy and could still take the other options if this one did not work.

Against: It would not solve the main problem – the missiles were already on Cuba. They could be used within one week. The Soviet Union might retaliate by blockading Berlin as it had done in 1948.

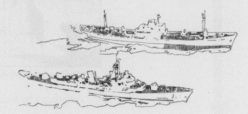

Tue 16 October ....

Sat 20 October ....

Mon 22 October ....

Source Analysis ▶

1 What words and phrases in Source 19 reveal how serious Kennedy believed the situation was in October 1962?
2 Kennedy was renowned as a skilled communicator. How did he convince his audience that he was in the right?

What happened next?

President Kennedy was informed of the missile build-up. Ex Comm formed.

Kennedy decided on a blockade of Cuba.

Kennedy announced the blockade and called on the Soviet Union to withdraw its missiles. He addressed the American people:

SOURCE 19

Good Evening, My Fellow Citizens:

This government, as promised, has maintained the closest surveillance of the Soviet military build-up on the island of Cuba. Within the past week, unmistakable evidence has established the fact that a series of offensive missile sites is now in preparation on that imprisoned island. The purpose of these bases can be none other than to provide a nuclear strike capability against the Western Hemisphere...

Acting, therefore, in the defence of our own security and of the entire Western Hemisphere, and under the authority entrusted to me by the Constitution as endorsed by the resolution of the Congress, I have directed that the following initial steps be taken immediately:

First: To halt this offensive build-up, a strict quarantine on all offensive military equipment under shipment to Cuba ... Second: I have directed the continued and increased close surveillance of Cuba and its military build-up. . . . I have directed the Armed Forces to prepare for any eventualities ... Third: It shall be the policy of this nation to regard any nuclear missile launched from Cuba against any nation in the Western Hemisphere as an attack on the United States, requiring a full retaliatory response upon the Soviet Union.

Extract from President Kennedy's TV broadcast to the American people on 22 October 1962.

Tue 23 October ....

Kennedy received a letter from Khrushchev saying that Soviet ships would not observe the blockade. Khrushchev did not admit the presence of nuclear missiles on Cuba.

Wed 24 October ....

The blockade began. The first missile-carrying ships, accompanied by a Soviet submarine, approached the 500-mile (800-km) blockade zone. Then suddenly, at 10.32 a.m., the twenty Soviet ships which were closest to the zone stopped or turned around.

Source Analysis ▶

1 Source 20 is a British cartoon. Pretend you did not know this. Explain why it is unlikely to be an American or Soviet cartoon.
2 What is its attitude to the two sides in the crisis?

SOURCE 20

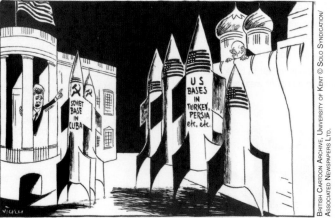

"INTOLERABLE HAVING YOUR ROCKETS ON MY DOORSTEP!"

BRITISH CARTOON ARCHIVE, UNIVERSITY OF KENT © SOLO SYNDICATION/ ASSOCIATED NEWSPAPERS LTD.

A cartoon by Vicky (Victor Weisz) from the *London Evening Standard*, 24 October 1962.

Thu 25 October .... **Despite the Soviet ships turning around,** intensive aerial photography revealed that work on the missile bases in Cuba was proceeding rapidly.

Fri 26 October .... **Kennedy received a long personal letter from Khrushchev.** The letter claimed that the missiles on Cuba were purely defensive, but went on: 'If assurances were given that the USA would not participate in an attack on Cuba and the blockade was lifted, then the question of the removal or the destruction of the missile sites would be an entirely different question.' This was the first time Khrushchev had admitted the presence of the missiles.

Sat 27 October a.m. .... **Khrushchev sent a second letter** – revising his proposals – saying that the condition for removing the missiles from Cuba was that the USA withdraw its missiles from Turkey.

An American U-2 plane was shot down over Cuba. The pilot was killed. The President was advised to launch an immediate reprisal attack on Cuba.

Sat 27 October p.m. .... **Kennedy decided to delay** an attack. He also decided to ignore the second Khrushchev letter, but accepted the terms suggested by Khrushchev on 26 October. He said that if the Soviet Union did not withdraw, an attack would follow.

SOURCE 21

It was a beautiful autumn evening, the height of the crisis, and I went up to the open air to smell it, because I thought it was the last Saturday I would ever see.

Robert McNamara talking about the evening of 27 October 1962. McNamara was one of Kennedy's closest advisers during the Cuban Crisis.

Sun 28 October .... **Khrushchev replied to Kennedy:** 'In order to eliminate as rapidly as possible the conflict which endangers the cause of peace . . . the Soviet Government has given a new order to dismantle the arms which you described as offensive and to crate and return them to the Soviet Union.'

SOURCE 22

Source Analysis ▶

Does Source 22 give the impression that either Khrushchev or Kennedy has the upper hand? Explain whether you think the events of the Crisis on these pages support that view.

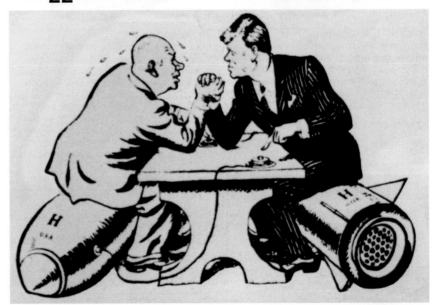

A cartoon from the British newspaper, the *Daily Mail*.

Think!

Kennedy described Wednesday 24 October and Saturday 27 October as the darkest days of the crisis. Use the information on this page to explain why.

Why did the Soviet Union place nuclear missiles on Cuba?

It was an incredibly risky strategy. The USSR had supplied many of its allies with conventional weapons but this was the first time that any Soviet leader had placed nuclear weapons outside Soviet territory. Why did Khrushchev take such an unusual step? The USSR must have known that it would cause a crisis. What's more, the USSR made no attempt at all to camouflage the sites, and even allowed the missiles to travel on open deck. This has caused much debate as to what Khrushchev was really doing. Historians have suggested various possible explanations.

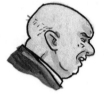

To bargain with the USA
If Khrushchev had missiles on Cuba, he could agree to remove them in return for some American concessions.

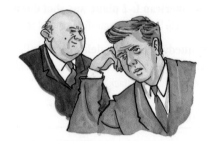

To test the USA
In the strained atmosphere of Cold War politics the missiles were designed to see how strong the Americans really were – whether they would back off or face up.

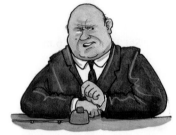

To trap the USA
Khrushchev wanted the Americans to find them and be drawn into a nuclear war. He did not even try to hide them.

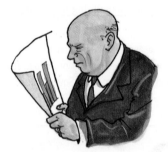

To close the missile gap
Khrushchev was so concerned about **the missile gap** between the USSR and the USA that he would seize any opportunity he could to close it. With missiles on Cuba it was less likely that the USA would ever launch a 'first strike' against the USSR.

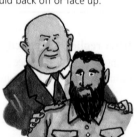

To defend Cuba
Cuba was the only Communist state in the Western hemisphere, and it had willingly become Communist rather than having become Communist as a result of invasion by the USSR. In addition, Cuba was in 'Uncle Sam's backyard'. As Castro himself put it: 'The imperialist cannot forgive that we have made a socialist revolution under the nose of the United States.' Just by existing, Castro's Cuba was excellent propaganda for the USSR.

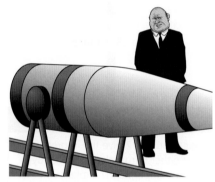

To strengthen his own position in the USSR
The superiority of the USA in nuclear missiles undermined Khrushchev's credibility inside the USSR. His critics pointed out that he was the one who had urged the USSR to rely on nuclear missiles. Now, could he show that the USSR really was a nuclear power?

Think!

1. Which of the explanations above do Sources 23 and 24 support?
2. Talking in private Khrushchev called the missiles 'a hedgehog in Uncle Sam's pants'. Which of the explanations does this statement support?
3. Which explanation do you think Khrushchev's actions on 26 and 27 October support (see page 107)?
4. Choose the explanation(s) that you think best fit what you have found out about the crisis. Explain your choice.

SOURCE 23

From the territory of the Soviet Union, the medium-range missiles couldn't possibly reach the territory of the USA, but deployed on Cuba they would become strategic nuclear weapons. That meant in practical terms we had a chance to narrow the differences between our forces.

General Anatoly Gribkov, commander, Soviet forces, Cuba.

SOURCE 24

In addition to protecting Cuba, our missiles would have equalized what the West likes to call the 'balance of power'. The Americans had surrounded our country with military bases and threatened us with nuclear weapons, and now they would learn just what it feels like to have enemy missiles pointing at you …

Khrushchev writing in his memoirs in 1971.

The outcomes ...

For Kennedy and the USA

- Kennedy came out of the crisis with a greatly improved reputation in his own country and throughout the West. He had stood up to Khrushchev and had made him back down.
- Kennedy had also successfully stood up to the hardliners in his own government. Critics of containment had wanted the USA to invade Cuba – to turn back Communism. However, the Cuban Missile Crisis highlighted the weakness of their case. Such intervention was not worth the high risk.
- On the other hand, he did secretly agree to remove the missiles from Turkey. This was slightly awkward for him as technically the decision to remove them was a decision for NATO. His NATO allies were unhappy that Kennedy had traded them during the Cuban Missile Crisis but clearly this was much better than a nuclear war.
- Kennedy also had to accept that Castro's Cuba would remain a Communist state in America's backyard. The USA still has trade and other economic restrictions in place against Cuba today.

For Khrushchev and the USSR

- In public Khrushchev was able to highlight his role as a responsible peacemaker, willing to make the first move towards compromise.
- There was no question that keeping Cuba safe from American action was a major achievement for the Soviets. Cuba was a valuable ally and proved a useful base to support Communists in South America.
- Khrushchev did also get the USA to withdraw its nuclear missiles from Turkey. However, Khrushchev had to agree that this withdrawal was to be kept secret so he was unable to use it for propaganda purposes.
- The crisis also exposed the USA to criticism amongst some of its allies. Newspaper articles in Britain, for example, felt that the USA was unreasonable to have missiles in Turkey and then object to Soviet missiles in Cuba.
- On the other hand, there was no denying the fact that Khrushchev had been forced to back down and remove the missiles. The Soviet military was particularly upset at the terms of the withdrawal. They were forced to put the missiles on the decks of their ships so the Americans could count them. They felt this was a humiliation.
- Khrushchev's actions in Cuba made no impact on the underlying problem of the Missile Gap. The USSR went on to develop its stockpile of ICBMs at a huge financial cost, but it never caught up with the USA.
- In 1964 Khrushchev himself was forced from power by his enemies inside the USSR. Many commentators believe that the Cuban Missile Crisis contributed to this.

For the Cold War

- Historians agree that the Cuban Missile Crisis helped to thaw Cold War relations between the USA and the USSR.
- Both leaders had seen how their game of brinkmanship had nearly ended in nuclear war. Now they were more prepared to take steps to reduce the risk of nuclear war.
- A permanent 'hot line' phone link direct from the White House to the Kremlin was set up.
- The following year, in 1963, they signed a Nuclear Test Ban Treaty. It did not stop the development of weapons, but it limited tests and was an important step forward.
- Although it was clear the USSR could not match US nuclear technology or numbers of weapons, it was also clear that this was not necessary. The Soviet nuclear arsenal was enough of a threat to make the USA respect the USSR. It is noticeable that for the rest of the Cold War the Superpowers avoided direct confrontation and fought through their allies where possible.

For Castro's Cuba

- Castro was very upset by the deal which Khrushchev made with America but he had little choice. He needed the support of the USSR.
- Cuba stayed Communist and highly armed. The nuclear missiles were removed but Cuba remained an important base for Communist supporters in South America. Cuban forces also intervened to help the Communist side in a civil war in Angola (in South-West Africa) in the 1970s.
- Castro also kept control of the American companies and other economic resources he nationalised during his revolution. This remains a source of dispute between Cuba and the USA today but Castro has never backed down.

Think!

1. Use the information on this page to fill out a table of positive and negative outcomes for the USA and the USSR.
2. Who do you think gained the most from the Cuban Missile Crisis?

Focus Task

Was the Cuban Missile Crisis a success for containment?

Look back at your table from page 99. Complete a second row for the Cuban Missile Crisis.

Revision Tip

Make sure you can remember from this case study:
- one reason that this might be seen as a success for containment
- one reason it might be seen as a failure.

Case study 3: The Vietnam War

Although Americans were relieved at the outcome of the Cuban Crisis it did not reduce their fear of Communism. Very soon they found themselves locked in a costly war in Vietnam, which put a massive question mark over the very policy of containment.

Origins of the Vietnam War

Vietnam had a long history of fighting outsiders.

Fighting the Japanese

Before the Second World War, Vietnam (or Indochina as it was called then) had been ruled by France. During the war the region was conquered by the Japanese. They treated the Vietnamese people savagely. As a result, a strong anti-Japanese resistance movement (the Viet Minh) emerged under the leadership of Communist Ho Chi Minh.

Ho was a remarkable individual. He had lived in the USA, Britain and France. In the 1920s he had studied Communism in the USSR. In 1930 he had founded the Indochinese Communist Party. He inspired the Vietnamese people to fight the Japanese.

When the Second World War ended, the Viet Minh entered the northern city of Hanoi in 1945 and declared Vietnam independent.

Fighting the French

The French had other ideas. In 1945 they came back wanting to rule Vietnam again, but Ho was not prepared to let this happen. Another nine years of war followed between the Viet Minh who controlled the north of the country and the French who controlled much of the south.

From 1949 Ho was supported by China, which had became a Communist state in 1949. You have already studied how the USA dealt with a similar situation in Korea (pages 96–99) so how would you expect the USA to react to this development? In this case rather than sending troops or getting a UN resolution the USA poured $500 million a year into the French war effort. Despite this the French were unable to hold on to the country and pulled out of Vietnam in 1954.

A peace conference was held in Geneva and the country was divided into North and South Vietnam until elections could be held to decide its future (see Source 25).

Why did US involvement escalate?

Under the terms of the ceasefire, elections were to be held within two years to reunite the country. You will remember how the USA criticised Stalin for not holding free elections in Soviet-controlled eastern Europe after the war (see pages 82–85). In Vietnam in 1954 the USA applied a different rule. It prevented the elections from taking place because it feared that the Communists would win (see Source 26).

Why did the Americans do this? Their policy was a strange combination of determination and ignorance. President Eisenhower and his Secretary of State JF Dulles were convinced that China and the USSR were planning to spread Communism throughout Asia. The idea was often referred to as the domino theory. If Vietnam fell to Communism, then Laos, Cambodia, Thailand, Burma and possibly even India might also fall – just like a row of dominoes. The Americans were determined to resist the spread of Communism in Vietnam, which they saw as the first domino in the row. However, their methods and policies showed their ignorance of the Vietnamese people and the region.

SOURCE 25

A poor feudal nation had beaten a great colonial power ... It meant a lot; not just to us but to people all over the world.

Viet Minh commander Vo Nguyen Giap commenting on the victory over France in 1954.

SOURCE 26

It was generally agreed that had an election been held, Ho Chi Minh would have been elected Premier ... at the time of the fighting, possibly 80 per cent of the population would have voted for the communist Ho Chi Minh as their leader.

President Eisenhower writing after the Vietnam War.

SOURCE 27

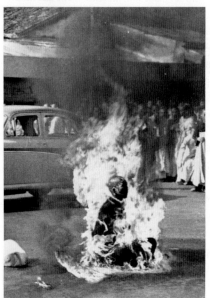

Quang Duc, a 73-year-old Buddhist priest, burns himself to death in protest against the attacks on Buddhist shrines by the government of South Vietnam in 1963

Think!

1 Many neutral observers in Vietnam were critical of US policy towards Diem's regime. Explain why.

2 Explain how US politicians would have defended their policies.

Financial support for Diem's regime

In 1955 the Americans helped Ngo Dinh Diem to set up the Republic of South Vietnam. They supported him because he was bitterly anti-Communist and was prepared to imprison or exile Communists. However, Diem's regime was very unpopular with the Vietnamese people.

- He belonged to the landlord class, which treated the Vietnamese peasants with contempt.
- He was a Christian and showed little respect for the Buddhist religion of most Vietnamese peasants (see Source 27).
- Diem's regime was also extremely corrupt. He appointed members of his family or other supporters to positions of power and refused to hold elections, even for local councils.

The Americans were concerned and frustrated by his actions, but as Dulles said, 'We knew of no one better.' The USA supported Diem's regime with around $1.6 billion in the 1950s. Diem was overthrown by his own army leaders in November 1963, but the governments that followed were equally corrupt. Even so, they also received massive US support.

The emergence of the Viet Cong

The actions of these anti-Communist governments increased support among the ordinary peasants for the Communist-led National Front for the Liberation of South Vietnam, which was set up in December 1960. This movement was usually called the Viet Cong. It included South Vietnamese opponents of the government, but also large numbers of Communist North Vietnamese taking their orders from Ho Chi Minh. Peasants who did not support the Viet Cong faced intimidation and violence from them.

The Viet Cong also started a guerrilla war against the South Vietnamese government. Using the Ho Chi Minh trail (see Source 28), the Viet Cong sent reinforcements and ferried supplies to guerrilla fighters. These fighters attacked South Vietnamese government forces, officials and buildings. They gradually made the countryside unsafe for government forces. They also attacked American air force and supply bases.

In response the South Vietnamese government launched their 'strategic hamlet' programme, which involved moving peasant villages from Viet Cong-controlled areas to areas controlled by the South Vietnamese government. The Americans helped by supplying building materials, money, food and equipment for the villagers to build improved farms and houses. In practice this policy backfired as the peasants resented it – and corrupt officials pocketed money meant to buy supplies for the villagers.

From 'advisers' to combat troops

By 1962 President Kennedy was sending military personnel (he always called them 'advisers') to help the South Vietnamese army fight the Viet Cong (see Source 29). However, Kennedy said he was determined that the USA would not 'blunder into war, unclear about aims or how to get out again'. He was a keen historian himself and had studied the USA's past successes and failures. He was well aware from the Korean war ten years earlier what could and could not be achieved by military intervention.

However President Kennedy was assassinated in 1963. His successor, Lyndon Johnson, was more prepared than Kennedy to commit the USA to a full-scale conflict in Vietnam to prevent the spread of Communism.

In August 1964, North Vietnamese patrol boats opened fire on US ships in the Gulf of Tonkin. In a furious reaction, the US Congress passed the Tonkin Gulf Resolution, which gave the President power to 'take all necessary measures to prevent further aggression and achieve peace and security'. It effectively meant that Johnson could take the USA into a full-scale war if he felt it was necessary, and very soon he did.

- **In February 1965 the US started** Operation Rolling Thunder – a gigantic bombing campaign against North Vietnamese cities, factories, army bases and the Ho Chi Minh Trail, which continued for three years.
- **On 8 March 1965**, 3,500 US marines, combat troops rather than advisers, came ashore at Da Nang.

The USA was now officially at war in Vietnam.

SOURCE **28**

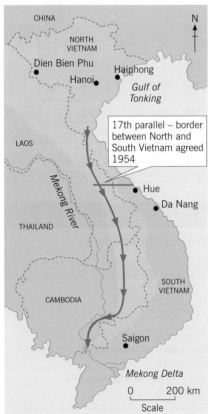

Key

Communist-controlled areas in the mid 1960s

→ Ho Chi Minh trail

Vietnam in the mid 1960s

First is the simple fact that South Vietnam, a member of the free world family, is striving to preserve its independence from Communist attack. Second, South East Asia has great significance in the forward defence of the USA. For Hanoi, the immediate object is limited: conquest of the south and national unification. For Peking, however, Hanoi's victory would only be a first step towards eventual Chinese dominance of the two Vietnams and South East Asia and towards exploitation of the new strategy in other parts of the world.

Robert McNamara, US Defence Secretary, explaining in 1964 why he supported the policy of sending US troops to Vietnam.

Source Analysis ▲

Compare Source 29 with Source 2 on page 96. How similar are the arguments used in 1964 about Vietnam to those used in 1950 about Korea?

Why did the US send troops to Vietnam?

The answer to this question may seem obvious! It was because of the policy of containment and the 'domino theory'. That is certainly how the President and his advisers explained it (see Source 29 for example). However there is a more controversial view held by some historians that powerful groups within the USA wanted a war.

In 1961 President Eisenhower himself warned that America had developed a powerful 'military–industrial complex'. The government gave huge budgets to the military commanders. These budgets were spent on weapons made by some of America's biggest companies. Thus, both the armed forces and business actually gained from conflict. Eisenhower did not accuse business and military leaders of anything, but in his last speech as President he warned the American people not to let these groups become too influential. Some historians believe that this was a factor in American involvement in Vietnam, but it is hotly disputed by others.

SOURCE **30**

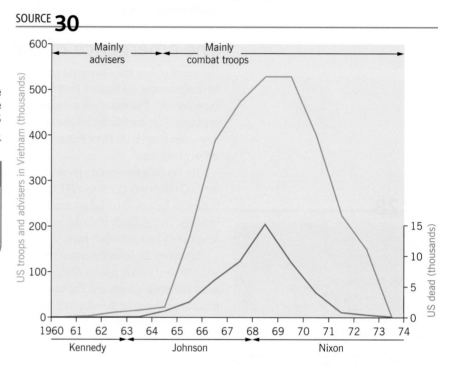

US troops and deaths in Vietnam, 1960–74. US troops were not the only foreign soldiers in the war. About 46,000 Australian and New Zealand troops fought too.

Revision Tip

Make sure you can recall:
♦ two reasons why Communism was becoming stronger in Vietnam
♦ two measures taken by the USA to resist the spread of Communism.

Focus Task A

Why did the USA get increasingly involved in Vietnam?

1 Draw a timeline of the period 1945–65.
2 Mark on it increasing American involvement using the following headings:
   ♦ No direct American involvement
   ♦ Financial support
   ♦ Political involvement
   ♦ Military involvement
3 Write annotations to show the date on which each of these phases started and what events triggered the increasing involvement.
4 Choose two events that you think were critical in increasing the USA's involvement in the war in Vietnam. Explain your choice.

Tactics and technology in the Vietnam War

With hindsight it is easy to see that the American decision to get fully involved in the war was a huge gamble. But political leaders did not have the benefit of hindsight. They made their decision on the basis of what they knew and believed at the time. They knew their technology and firepower was superior to the Viet Cong and they believed that would allow them to win the war.

However they were soon proved wrong. As time wore on it became clear that the USA needed more than money and technology to win this kind of war. On the next two pages you will find out why by comparing Viet Cong and US tactics. Focus Task B will direct your reading.

Focus Task B

Why couldn't the Americans win?

Stage 1 – Understand the tactics

1 Work in pairs. Take either the Viet Cong or the Americans. Use page 114 or 115 to find out about the your side's tactics. Create a diagram by following these steps:
   ♦ In the inner circle record the tactics.
   ♦ In the outer circle the reason for using those tactics.
   ♦ Draw lines to show how the tactics and reasons are connected.
   Compare your diagram with your partner's.

Stage 2 – Thinking it through

2 Make your own table like this, then using your research from stage 1 record in columns 2 and 4 how far each side had these qualities. You can add further rows if you think of other important qualities.

Qualities	The US army	⚖ or ⚖	Viet Cong
Well-trained soldiers			
The right technology			
Reliable supplies and equipment			
Effective tactics			
Support from the Vietnamese population			
Motivated and committed soldiers			
Other			

3 Next, in each row of column 3, draw some scales to show which way the balance falls for this quality. Did the USA or the Viet Cong have the advantage?
4 Now think about the overall picture – how the strengths and weaknesses work together.
   a) Were the armies finely balanced? Or was the balance strongly weighted to one side or the other?
   b) Which quality was most important in determining who won the war? Was one so important that being ahead in that area meant that other advantages or disadvantages did not matter?

Stage 3 – Explaining your conclusions

5 Now write up your answer. You could use this structure:
   a) Describe how the failure of the US army was a combination of its own weaknesses and Viet Cong strengths.
   b) Give balanced examples of US successes and failures.
   c) Give balanced examples of Viet Cong successes and failures.
   d) Choose one American weakness and one Viet Cong strength that you think were absolutely vital in preventing the USA from beating the Viet Cong and explain the significance of the points you have chosen.

Revision Tip

Find five reasons why the USA could not defeat the Viet Cong. Make sure you can recall:
♦ two or three strengths of the Viet Cong (with examples)
♦ two or three weaknesses of the USA (with examples).

Viet Cong tactics

In early 1965 the Viet Cong had about 170,000 soldiers. They were heavily outnumbered and outgunned. They were no match for the US and South Vietnamese forces in open warfare. In November 1965 in the Ia Dreng Valley, US forces killed 2,000 Viet Cong for the loss of 300 troops. However, this did not daunt Ho Chi Minh.

Guerilla warfare

Ho had been in China and seen Mao Tse-tung use guerrilla warfare to achieve a Communist victory. The principles of guerrilla warfare were simple: retreat when the enemy attacks; raid when the enemy camps; attack when the enemy tires; pursue when the enemy retreats. Ho had successfully used these guerrilla tactics himself to drive out the French.

Guerrilla warfare was a nightmare for the US army. Guerrillas did not wear uniform. They were hard to tell apart from the peasants in the villages. They had no known base camp or headquarters. They worked in small groups with limited weapons. They attacked then disappeared into the jungle, into the villages or into tunnels (see Source 32).

Guerrilla attacks aimed to wear down enemy soldiers and wreck their morale. US soldiers lived in constant fear of ambushes or booby traps such as pits filled with sharpened bamboo stakes. One of the least popular duties for US soldiers was going 'on point', which meant leading the patrol checking for booby traps – 11 per cent of US casualties were caused by booby traps. Another 51 per cent were from ambushes or hand-to-hand combat. The Viet Cong favoured close-quarter fighting because it knew that the Americans would not use their superior guns for fear of hitting their own troops. This was known as 'hanging on to the American belts'.

Civilians

Ho knew how important it was to keep the population on his side. The Viet Cong fighters were expected to be courteous and respectful to the Vietnamese peasants. They helped the peasants in the fields during busy periods. However, the Viet Cong could be ruthless – they were quite prepared to kill peasants who opposed them or who co-operated with their enemies. They also conducted a campaign of terror against the police, tax collectors, teachers and any other employees of the South Vietnamese government. Between 1966 and 1971 the Viet Cong killed an estimated 27,000 civilians.

Supplies

The Viet Cong depended on supplies from North Vietnam that came along the Ho Chi Minh trail. US and South Vietnamese planes bombed this constantly, but 40,000 Vietnamese worked to keep it open whatever the cost.

Commitment

The total of Viet Cong and North Vietnamese dead in the war has been estimated at 1 million – far higher than US losses. However, this was a price that Ho Chi Minh was prepared to pay. Whatever the casualties, there were replacement troops available. The greatest strength of the Viet Cong fighters was that they simply refused to give in.

Think!

1 One Viet Cong leader said: 'The people are the water. Our armies are the fish.' What do you think he meant?
2 Find evidence on pages 114–115 to support the view that:
   ◆ the VietCong had the support of the people
   ◆ they did not.

SOURCE 31

I remember sitting at this wretched little outpost one day with a couple of my sergeants. We'd been manning this thing for three weeks and running patrols off it. We were grungy and sore with jungle rot and we'd suffered about nine or ten casualties on a recent patrol. This one sergeant of mine said, 'You know, Lieutenant, I don't see how we're ever going to win this.' And I said, 'Well, Sarge, I'm not supposed to say this to you as your officer – but I don't either.' So there was this sense that we just couldn't see what could be done to defeat these people.

Philip Caputo, a lieutenant in the Marine Corps in Vietnam in 1965–66, speaking in 1997.

SOURCE 32

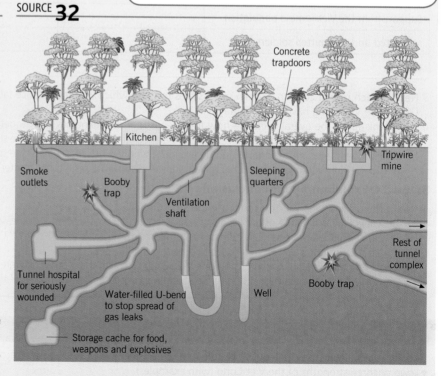

A Viet Cong tunnel complex. To avoid the worst effects of American air power, the Viet Cong built a vast network of underground tunnels, probably around 240 km of them.

US tactics

Bombing

The main US tactic was bombing. For seven years from 1965–72 the USA bombed military and industrial targets in North Vietnam; they bombed towns and cities in North and South Vietnam; they bombed the Ho Chi Minh trail; they bombed Vietnam's neighbours Laos and Cambodia (who were sympathetic to the Viet Cong).

To some extent bombing worked.
- It damaged North Vietnam's war effort and it disrupted supply routes.
- From 1970 to 1972, intense bombing of North Vietnam forced them to negotiate for peace.

However, air power could not defeat the Communists. It could only slow them down. Even after major air raids on North Vietnam in 1972, the Communists were still able to launch a major assault on the South. Even more important, civilian casualties helped turn the Vietnamese people against the Americans.

Search and destroy

To combat guerrilla warfare the US commander General Westmoreland developed a policy of search and destroy. He set up heavily defended US bases in South Vietnam near to the coasts. From here helicopters full of troops would descend on a village and search out and destroy any Viet Cong forces they found. Soldiers had to send back reports of body counts.

Search-and-destroy missions did kill Viet Cong soldiers, but there were problems.
- The raids were often based on inadequate information.
- Inexperienced US troops often walked into traps.
- Innocent villages were mistaken for Viet Cong strongholds. For every Viet Cong weapon captured by search and destroy, there was a body count of six. Many of these were innocent civilians.
- Search-and-destroy tactics made the US and South Vietnamese forces very unpopular with the peasants. It pushed them towards supporting the Viet Cong.

SOURCE 33

You would go out, you would secure a piece of terrain during the daylight hours, [but at night] you'd surrender that — and I mean literally surrender … you'd give it up, because … the helicopters would come in and pick you up at night and fly you back to the security of your base camp.

Lieutenant Colonel George Forrest, US Army.

Chemical weapons

The US also used chemical weapons to combat the Viet Cong.
- **Agent Orange** was a highly toxic 'weedkiller' sprayed from planes to destroy the jungle where the Viet Cong hid. The Americans used 82 million litres of Agent Orange to spray thousands of square kilometres of jungle.
- **Napalm** was another widely used chemical weapon. It destroyed jungles where guerrillas might hide. It also burned through skin to the bone.
- Many civilians and soldiers were also killed or harmed by these chemical weapons.

US troops

In the early stages of the war most US troops were professional soldiers. Morale was good and they performed well. However, as the war intensified the US needed more soldiers so they introduced the draft (conscription). As soon as young men left school or college they could be called up into the US army. So from 1967:
- Many soldiers were young men who had never been in the military before. The average age of US troops was only 19.
- In theory American troops came from all walks of life. In reality the majority of combat troops were from poor and immigrant backgrounds.
- The conscripts knew little about Vietnam — and some cared little about democracy or communism. They just wanted to get home alive. In contrast the Viet Cong were fighting for their own country, and a cause many of them believed in.
- Morale among the US conscripts was often very low. To tackle this problem the generals introduced a policy of giving troops just a one-year term of service. This backfired because as soon as the soldiers gained experience they were sent home.

SOURCE 34

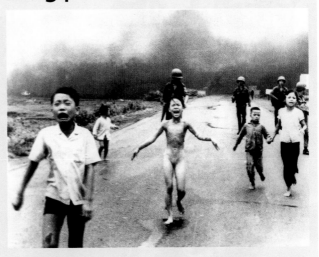

A ten-year-old Vietnamese girl, Phan Thi Kim, runs naked after tearing her burning clothes from her body following a napalm attack in 1972. This photograph became one of the most enduring images of the war.

SOURCE 35

In the end anybody who was still in that country was the enemy. The same village you'd gone in to give them medical treatment … you could go through that village later and get shot at by a sniper. Go back in and you would not find anybody. Nobody knew anything. We were trying to work with these people, they were basically doing a number on us. You didn't trust them anymore. You didn't trust anybody.

Fred Widmer, an American soldier, speaking in 1969.

The Tet Offensive

Despite these problems the official American view of the war from 1965 to 1967 was that it was going reasonably well. The US and South Vietnamese forces were killing large numbers of Viet Cong. Although they were struggling against guerrilla tactics they were confident that the enemy was being worn down. The press reports reflected this positive view.

This confidence was shattered early in 1968. During the New Year holiday, Viet Cong fighters attacked over 100 cities and other military targets. One Viet Cong commando unit tried to capture the US embassy in Saigon. US forces had to fight to regain control room by room. Around 4,500 Viet Cong fighters tied down a much larger US and South Vietnamese force in Saigon for two days.

In many ways the Tet Offensive was a disaster for the Communists. They had hoped that the people of South Vietnam would rise up and join them. They didn't. The Viet Cong lost around 10,000 experienced fighters and were badly weakened by it.

However, the Tet Offensive proved to be a turning point in the war because it raised hard questions in the USA about the war.

- There were nearly 500,000 troops in Vietnam and the USA was spending $20 billion a year on the war. So why had the Communists been able to launch a major offensive that took US forces completely by surprise?
- US and South Vietnamese forces quickly retook the towns captured in the offensive, but in the process they used enormous amounts of artillery and air power. Many civilians were killed. The ancient city of Hue was destroyed. Was this right?

SOURCE 36

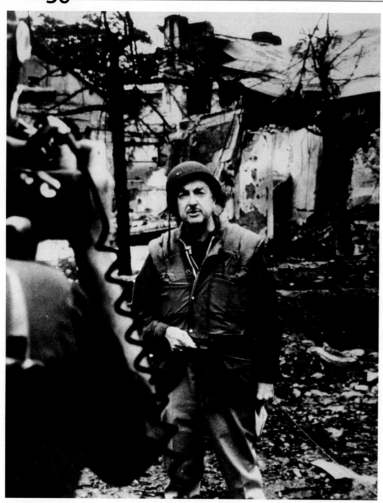

CBS News journalist Walter Cronkite reporting in Vietnam in February 1968. He was regarded as the most trusted man in America.

The media

Until this point media coverage of the war was generally positive, although some journalists were beginning to ask difficult questions in 1967. During the Tet Offensive the gloves came off. CBS journalist Walter Cronkite (see Source 36) asked 'What the hell is going on? I thought we were winning this war'. Don Oberdorfer of *The Washington Post* later wrote (in 1971) that as a result of the Tet Offensive 'the American people and most of their leaders reached the conclusion that the Vietnam War would require greater effort over a far longer period of time than it was worth'.

SOURCE 37

The Tet Offensive was the decisive battle of the Vietnam War because of its profound impact on American attitudes about involvement in Southeast Asia. In the aftermath of Tet, many Americans became disillusioned ... To the American public and even to members of the administration, the offensive demonstrated that US intervention ... had produced a negligible effect on the will and capability of the Viet Cong and North Vietnamese.

Extract from *The Tet Offensive: Intelligence Failure in War* by James Wirtz.

One does not use napalm on villages and hamlets sheltering civilians if one is attempting to persuade these people of the rightness of one's cause. One does not defoliate [destroy the vegetation of] the country and deform its people with chemicals if one is attempting to persuade them of the foe's evil nature.

An American comments on US policy failure in Vietnam.

The peace movement in the USA

For a war on such a scale the government had to have the support of the American people. With deaths and injuries to so many young Americans, public opinion had been turning against the war even before the Tet Offensive. After it the trickle of anti-war feeling became a flood.

- The war was draining money that could be used to better purposes at home (see Sources 39 and 40). Yet despite all that spending the USA did not seem to be any closer to winning the war.
- The draft exposed racial inequality in the USA: 30 per cent of African Americans were drafted compared to only 19 per cent of white Americans; 22 per cent of US casualties were black Americans, even though this group made up only 11 per cent of the total US force. World champion boxer Muhammad Ali refused to join the army on the grounds of his Muslim faith. He was stripped of his world title and his passport was removed. Ali was a follower of the radical Black Power group called Nation of Islam. They argued: How could they fight for a country which discriminated against them at home? As some of them pointed out, 'the Viet Cong never called us nigger'.
- Most damaging of all, an increasing number of Americans felt deeply uncomfortable about what was going on in Vietnam.

The Vietnam War was a media war. Thousands of television, radio and newspaper reporters, and a vast army of photographers sent back to the USA and Europe reports and pictures of the fighting. The newspapers showed crying children burned by American napalm bombs (see Source 34). Television showed prisoners being tortured or executed, or women and children watching with horror as their house was set on fire. To see such casual violence beamed into the living rooms of the USA was deeply shocking to the average American. Was this why 900,000 young Americans had been drafted? Instead of Vietnam being a symbol of a US crusade against Communism, Vietnam had become a symbol of defeat, confusion and moral corruption. The most powerful illustration of this was the My Lai massacre (see page 118).

The anti-war protests reached their height during 1968–70 led by students and civil rights campaigners.

- In the first half of 1968, there were over 100 demonstrations against the Vietnam War involving 40,000 students. Frequently, the protest would involve burning the American flag – a criminal offence in the USA and a powerful symbol of the students' rejection of American values. Students taunted the American President Lyndon B Johnson with the chant 'Hey, Hey LBJ; how many kids did you kill today?'
- In November 1969, almost 700,000 anti-war protesters demonstrated in Washington DC. It was the largest political protest in American history.

Source Analysis

1 Who or what is the cartoonist criticising in Source 39?
2 Which do you think is more effective as a criticism of the Vietnam War – Source 38, 39 or 40? Give reasons based on the source and your knowledge of the USA at this time.

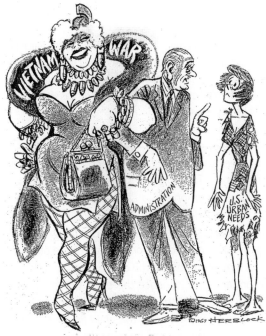

"There's Money Enough To Support Both Of You — Now, Doesn't That Make You Feel Better?"

---from <u>The Herblock Gallery</u> (Simon & Schuster, 1968)

An American cartoon from 1967.

This confused war has played havoc with our domestic destinies. The promises of the great society have been shot down on the battlefields of Vietnam. The pursuit of this widened war has narrowed the promised dimensions of the domestic welfare programs, making the poor – white and Negro – bear the heaviest burdens both at the front and at home.

The war has put us in the position of protecting a corrupt government that is stacked against the poor. We are spending $500,000 to kill every Viet Cong soldier while we spend only $53 for every person considered to be in poverty in the USA. It has put us in a position of appearing to the world as an arrogant nation. Here we are 10,000 miles away from home fighting for the so-called freedom of the Vietnamese people when we have so much to do in our own country.

Civil rights leader Martin Luther King speaking in the USA in April 1968.

SOURCE 41

Most of the soldiers had never been away from home before they went into service. And they end up in Vietnam going there many of them because they thought they were going to do something courageous on behalf of their country, something which they thought was in the American ideal.

But it didn't mean slaughtering whole villages of women and children. One of my friends, when he told me about it, said: 'You know it was a Nazi kind of thing.' We didn't go there to be Nazis. At least none of the people I knew went there to be Nazis.

Written by Ronald Ridenhour, a US soldier in Vietnam. He was not at My Lai, but interviewed many witnesses and started a campaign to pressure the US authorities to investigate properly.

SOURCE 42

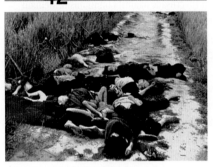

A photograph taken at My Lai on 16 March 1968 by Ron Haeberle (see Source 43).

Think!

1 Why do you think it took twelve months for anyone to do anything about the massacre?
2 Why was the massacre so shocking to the American public?

Source Analysis ▶

1 Source 43 was written by someone who worked for the US Army. Does that make it a trustworthy source?

The My Lai massacre

In March 1968, a unit of young American soldiers called Charlie Company started a search-and-destroy mission. They had been told that in the My Lai area there was a Viet Cong headquarters, and 200 Viet Cong guerrillas. They had been ordered to destroy all houses, dwellings and livestock. They had been told that all the villagers would have left for market because it was a Saturday. Most of them were under the impression that they had been ordered to kill everyone they found in the village.

Early in the morning of 16 March, Charlie Company arrived in My Lai. In the next four hours, between 300 and 400 civilians were killed. They were mostly women, children and old men. Some were killed while they worked in their fields. Many of them were mown down by machine-gun fire as they were herded into an irrigation ditch. Others were shot in their homes. No Viet Cong were found in the village. Only three weapons were recovered.

'Something dark and bloody'

At the time, the army treated the operation as a success. The commanding officer's report said that 20 non-combatants had been killed by accident in the attack, but the rest of the dead were recorded as being Viet Cong. The officers and men involved were praised.

However, twelve months later, a letter arrived in the offices of 30 leading politicians and government officials in Washington. It was written by Ronald Ridenhour, an American soldier who had served in Vietnam and who personally knew many of the soldiers who took part in the massacre. He had evidence, he said, of 'something rather dark and bloody' that had occurred in My Lai – or Pinkville as the American soldiers called it. He recounted in detail the stories he had been told about what had taken place and asked Congress to investigate.

Investigation

Soon after, *Life* magazine, one of the most influential magazines in the USA, published photographs of the massacre at My Lai (see Source 42) that had been taken by an official army photographer. This triggered an investigation that ended in the trial for mass murder of Lieutenant William Calley. He was an officer in Charlie Company. He had personally shot many of the people in the irrigation ditch at My Lai. In September 1969 he was formally charged with murdering 109 people. Ten other members of the company and the commanding officers were also charged.

Aftermath

The revelations were deeply shocking to the American people. The charges were also too much for the army. They placed responsibility on Calley. They denied that Calley was acting under orders. His senior officers were acquitted. After a long court case surrounded by massive media attention and publicity, Calley was found guilty of the murder of 22 civilians. In August 1971 he was sentenced to 20 years' hard labour. In November 1974 he was released.

SOURCE 43

I think I was in a kind of daze from seeing all these shootings and not seeing any returning fire. Yet the killing kept going on. The Americans were rounding up the people and shooting them, not taking any prisoners … I was part of it, everyone who was there was part of it and that includes the General and the Colonel flying above in their helicopters … Just as soon as I turned away I heard firing. I saw people drop. They started falling on top of each other, one on top of the other. I just kept on walking. I did not pay any attention to who did it. By that time I knew what the score was. It was an atrocity … I notice this one small boy had been shot in the foot … he was walking toward the group of bodies looking for his mother … then suddenly I heard a crack and … I saw this child flip on top of the pile of bodies. The GI just stood and walked away. No remorse. Nothing.

Ron Haeberle, the US Army official photographer. His black and white pictures for the Army and his colour photographs taken with his own private camera had a dramatic public impact.

Ending the war in Vietnam

After the Tet Offensive President Johnson concluded that the war could not be won militarily. He reduced the bombing campaign against North Vietnam and instructed his officials to begin negotiating for peace with the Communists.

Johnson also announced that he would not be seeking re-election as President. It was an admission of failure. In the election campaign both candidates campaigned to end US involvement in Vietnam. The anti-war feeling was so strong that if they had supported continuing the war they would have had no chance of being elected anyway. It was no longer a question of 'could the USA win the war?' but 'how can the USA get out of Vietnam without it looking like a defeat?'

A new President

In November 1968 Richard Nixon was elected President. From 1969 to 1973 he and his National Security Adviser Henry Kissinger worked to end US involvement in Vietnam. This was not easy because the bigger question of how to contain world Communism – the one that had got the USA into Vietnam in the first place – had not gone away. They did not want to appear simply to hand Vietnam to the Communists. They used a range of strategies.

Improved relations with USSR and China	Peace negotiations with North Vietnam
In 1969 the USSR and China fell out. It seemed possible that there would even be a war between these two powerful Communist countries. As a result, both the USSR and China tried to improve relations with the USA.	From early 1969, Kissinger had regular meetings with the chief Vietnamese peace negotiator, Le Duc Tho.
'Vietnamisation' of the war effort	**Increased bombing**
In Vietnam Nixon began handing responsibility for the war to South Vietnamese forces and withdrawing US troops. Between April 1969 and the end of 1971 almost 400,000 US troops left Vietnam.	At the same time Nixon increased bombing campaigns against North Vietnam to show he was not weak. US and South Vietnamese troops also invaded Viet Cong bases in Cambodia, causing outrage across the world, and even in the USA.

'Peace with honour'

In Paris in January 1973 all parties signed a peace agreement. Nixon described it as 'peace with honour'. Others disagreed (see Source 44), but the door was now open for Nixon to pull out all US troops. By 29 March 1973, the last American forces had left Vietnam.

It is not clear whether Nixon really believed he had secured a lasting peace settlement. But within two years, without the support of the USA, South Vietnam had fallen to the Communists. One of the bleakest symbols of American failure in Vietnam was the televised news images of desperate Vietnamese men, women and children trying to clamber aboard American helicopters taking off from the US embassy. All around them Communist forces swarmed through Saigon. After 30 years of constant conflict, the struggle for control of Vietnam had finally been settled and the Communists had won.

Source Analysis ▶

1 Describe the attitude of Source 44 to the agreement of January 1973.
2 Are you surprised by this source?

SOURCE **44**

FOR WHOM THE BELL TOLLS

... the nation began at last to extricate itself from a quicksandy war that had plagued four Presidents and driven one from office, that had sundered the country more deeply than any event since the Civil War, that in the end came to be seen by a great majority of Americans as having been a tragic mistake.

... but its more grievous toll was paid at home — a wound to the spirit so sore that news of peace stirred only the relief that comes with an end to pain. A war that produced no famous victories, no national heroes and no strong patriotic songs, produced no memorable armistice day celebrations either. America was too exhausted by the war and too chary of peace to celebrate.

Reaction to the agreement of January 1973 in the influential American news magazine *Newsweek*, 5 February 1973.

Why did US policy fail in Vietnam?

Despite all the money they spent and the effort they put in, the US failed to contain the spread of Communism to South Vietnam. You are now going to consider the reasons for this.

1 Make cards like these. On each card write an explanation or paste a source which shows the importance of the reason, i.e. how it damaged the policy of containment. Add other cards if you think there are reasons you should consider.

2 Lay your cards out on a large sheet of paper and add lines to show connections between the reasons. Write an explanation of the connection.

US military tactics in Vietnam	The unpopularity of the South Vietnamese regime	The experience of the Viet Cong and the inexperience of the American soldiers	Opposition in the USA	Other countries' support for the Viet Cong

Use these cards for your revision. Take a photo of your completed layout showing and annotating the connections. This will be a good essay plan if you have to write on this topic for an assignment. Make sure you can remember one piece of evidence to go with each point.

How did the Vietnam War affect the policy of containment?

The American policy of containment was in tatters.

- It had failed **militarily**. The war had shown that even the USA's vast military strength could not stem the spread of Communism.

- It had also failed **strategically**. Not only did the USA fail to stop South Vietnam going Communist, but the heavy bombing of Vietnam's neighbours, Laos and Cambodia, actually helped the Communist forces in those countries to win support. By 1975 both Laos and Cambodia had Communist governments. Instead of slowing down the domino effect in the region, American policies actually speeded it up.

- It was also a **propaganda disaster**. The Americans had always presented their campaign against Communism as a moral crusade. But atrocities committed by American soldiers and the use of chemical weapons damaged the USA's reputation. In terms of a crusade for 'democracy' the Americans were seen to be propping up a government that did not have the support of its own people.

Theses failures greatly affected the USA's future policies towards Communist states. After the war, the Americans tried to improve their relations with China. They ended their block on China's membership of the UN. The President made visits to China. The USA also entered into a period of greater understanding with the Soviet Union. In fact, during the 1970s both the Soviet Union and China got on better with the USA than they did with each other.

The Americans also became very suspicious of involving their troops in any other conflict that they could not easily and overwhelmingly win. This was an attitude that continued to affect American foreign policy into the twenty-first century.

How successful was the USA's policy of containment in Vietnam?

1 Look back at your chart from page 109. Complete it for the Vietnam War.

2 You have now looked at three very different case studies of the USA's attempts to contain Communism. Using the work you have done for the Focus Tasks on pages 99, 109 and this page, explain:
   ♦ how far did the policy of containment succeed
   ♦ what the main reasons for its success or failure were.

All these case studies (Korea, Cuba, Vietnam) are important because they each show different aspects of containment in action. Make sure you are equally confident about each one and can explain in your own words whether it was a success or failure for containment.

Keywords

Make sure you know what these terms mean and be able to define them confidently.

- Agent Orange
- Armistice
- Arms race
- Atomic bomb/H bomb
- Bay of Pigs
- Blockade
- Capitalism
- CENTO
- CIA
- Cold War
- Cominform
- Communism
- Containment
- Conventional weapons
- Democracy
- Dictator
- Diplomatic relations
- Domino theory
- Draft
- Guerrilla warfare
- Ho Chi Minh Trail
- ICBM
- Indochina
- Intelligence (as in CIA)
- Landlord/peasant
- MAD
- Missile gap
- Napalm
- Nuclear deterrent
- Operation Rolling Thunder
- Satellite state
- Search and destroy
- SEATO
- Surveillance
- Tet Offensive
- United Nations
- US sphere of influence
- Viet Cong
- Viet Minh
- Vietnamisation
- Warsaw Pact

Chapter Summary

Containment

1 The USA was anti-Communist and wanted to limit the spread of Communism around the world – this policy was called containment.

Korea

2 When a Communist government tried to take over in Korea in 1950 the USA sent troops to help prevent Korea falling to the Communists.

3 The result was a stalemate and in 1953 Korea was divided into a Communist north (friendly towards China) and a capitalist south (friendly towards the USA).

Cuba

4 Cuba turned Communist in 1959. Cuba is a large island very close to the USA.

5 In the 1960s there was a nuclear arms race between the USA and USSR with ever more dangerous nuclear weapons being developed and tested by both sides.

6 The Soviet leader Khrushchev sent nuclear weapons to Cuba. The USA and much of the world were worried that this might lead to the first nuclear war with dreadful consequences.

7 The US President Kennedy ordered a blockade of Cuba to prevent the weapons arriving and the crisis was averted. Better relations between the two leaders followed.

Vietnam

8 The next area of worry was South-east Asia where Communism was very strong. The USA believed in the domino theory – if one country turned Communist then the neighbouring countries would follow so they wanted to stop any country turning Communist.

9 In 1954 following a civil war Vietnam was divided into a Communist north and a capitalist south but the north, with the help of Communist China, tried to take over the south too.

10 The USA decided to help the south to resist the threat of the Communist north by first sending money and advisers then combat troops.

11 They got more and more involved, to the point where hundreds of thousands of US troops were fighting in Vietnam (the US introduced conscription to provide enough soldiers), and thousands were being killed each year.

12 Despite all this investment the US was not winning this war. The war lost support at home and the USA decided to withdraw from Vietnam and leave South Vietnam to its fate. It finally fell to the Communists in 1975.

Exam Practice

See pages 168–175 and pages 316–319 for advice on the different types of questions you might face.

1 (a) Describe the Domino Theory. [4]
  (b) Explain why the USA sent troops to Vietnam in the mid 1960s. [6]
  (c) 'The Americans failed in Vietnam because they used the wrong tactics.' How far do you agree with this statement? Explain your answer. [10]
2 Study Source 15 on page 103. How reliable is this source? Use the source and your knowledge to explain your answer. [7]
3 Study Sources 19 and 20 on page 106. How similar are these two sources? Use the source and your knowledge to explain your answer. [8]

Before

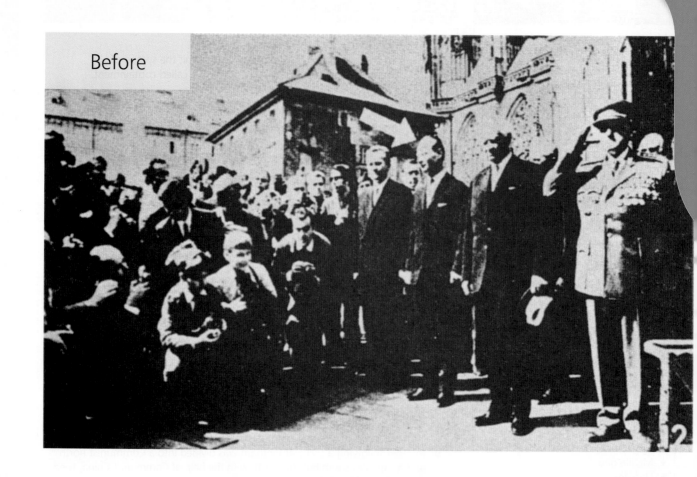

After

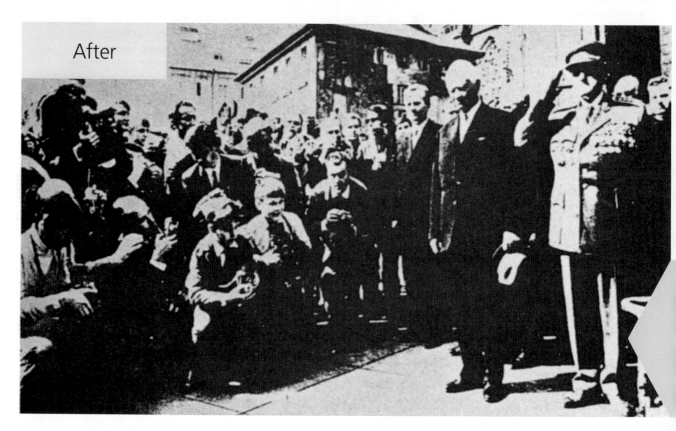

How secure was the USSR's control over eastern Europe, 1948–c.1989?

FOCUS POINTS

- Why was there opposition to Soviet control in Hungary in 1956 and Czechoslovakia in 1968, and how did the USSR react to this opposition?
- How similar were events in Hungary in 1956 and in Czechoslovakia in 1968?
- Why was the Berlin Wall built in 1961?
- What was the significance of 'Solidarity' in Poland for the decline of Soviet influence in eastern Europe?
- How far was Gorbachev personally responsible for the collapse of Soviet control over eastern Europe?

In Chapter 4 you saw how the Soviet Union took control of eastern Europe. You are now going to return to that story and see how far the Soviet Union was able to maintain that control.

You will investigate:

- how the Soviet Union took control in eastern Europe and how it tried to maintain control
- why and how some people challenged Soviet control and what happened to them when they did
- how, finally, changes in the Soviet Union led to the collapse of all the Communist regimes in eastern Europe and indeed the collapse of the Soviet Union.

The key question you will consider is 'how secure' was this control.

The Soviet Union almost certainly did not feel it was secure. It kept up constant pressure on the governments and people of eastern Europe. It was really only the threat of sending in the Red Army that propped up some of the Communist regimes in the region long after their people had lost faith in their government. In the end it was Mikhail Gorbachev's unwillingness to prop them up any longer with Soviet troops that signalled the end of Soviet domination.

So which of these graphs do you think is the best representation of Soviet control through this period?

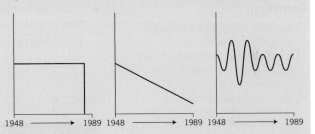

And remember...

This chapter overlaps with Chapter 5 (see timeline on pages 74–75). So you will get a more rounded view of the period if you remember that both chapters take their place within the tense Cold War environment. For example:

- while the USA was fighting the Korean War to push back Communism in the early 1950s, the USSR was sending troops to East Germany to keep Communism in place
- in 1968 when the USA was facing fierce criticism at home against its policy of containment and the Vietnam War in particular, the Soviet Union was trying to keep the lid on the anti-Soviet ideas that were developing in Czechoslovakia in the Prague Spring.

◀ Here are two version of the same photo. The first shows the leader of Czechoslovakia, Alexander Dubček. The second is the same photo used by the Communist-controlled media after Dubček had been ousted from power by Soviet troops in 1968.

1 How has the photo been changed?
2 Why might the photo have been changed?
3 What does this tell you about Communist control of Czechoslovakia in 1968?

Cominform

➤ Cominform stands for the Communist Information Bureau.

➤ Stalin set up the Cominform in 1947 as an organisation to co-ordinate the various Communist governments in eastern Europe.

➤ The office was originally based in Belgrade in Yugoslavia but moved to Bucharest in Romania in 1948 after Yugoslavia was expelled by Stalin because it would not do what the Soviet Union told it to do.

➤ Cominform ran meetings and sent out instructions to Communist governments about what the Soviet Union wanted them to do.

Comecon

➤ Comecon stands for the Council for Mutual Economic Assistance.

➤ It was set up in 1949 to co-ordinate the industries and trade of the eastern European countries.

➤ The idea was that members of Comecon traded mostly with one another rather than trading with the West.

➤ Comecon favoured the USSR far more than any of its other members. It provided the USSR with a market to sell its goods. It also guaranteed it a cheap supply of raw materials. For example, Poland was forced to sell its coal to the USSR at one-tenth of the price that it could have got selling it on the open market.

➤ It set up a bank for socialist countries in 1964.

Stalin used a 'carrot and stick' approach to control eastern Europe. Explain what this means and refer to the information on this page in your answer.

The cartoonist who drew Source 1 was a critic of Stalin. How is he criticising Stalin in this cartoon?

How did the Soviet Union seize control in eastern Europe?

As you saw in Chapter 4, after the Second World War the Communists quickly gained control of eastern Europe (see Source 17, page 84). The chaotic situation in many of the countries helped them.

● After the war there was a **political vacuum** in many countries in eastern Europe. The Soviet leader Stalin helped the Communist parties in them to win power. Through Cominform (see Factfile) he made sure that these eastern European countries followed the same policies as the Soviet Union. They became one-party states. The Communist Party was the only legal party. Secret police arrested the Communists' opponents.

● There was also a need to **restore law and order**. This provided a good excuse to station Soviet troops in each country.

● The **economies** of eastern Europe were shattered. To rebuild them, the governments followed the economic policies of the Soviet Union. They took over all industry. Workers and farmers were told what to produce. Through Comecon (see Factfile) Stalin made sure that the countries of eastern Europe traded with the USSR. He promised aid to countries that co-operated with the Soviet Union.

● Stalin's public reason for wanting to control eastern Europe was to defend the Soviet Union from invasion from the west. However his subsequent policies showed that he also wanted to benefit from the wealth and resources of eastern Europe.

SOURCE **1**

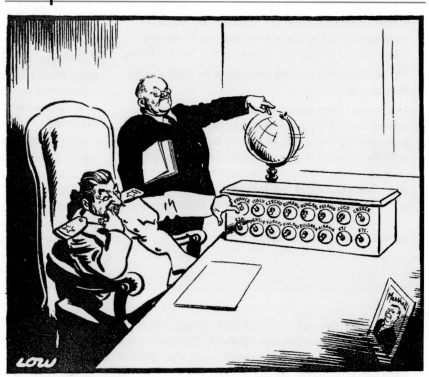

"WHO'S NEXT TO BE LIBERATED FROM FREEDOM, COMRADE?"

David Low comments on Stalin's control of eastern Europe, 2 March 1948. The person spinning the globe is Molotov, Stalin's foreign minister. On the desk is a photo of General Marshall (see page 86 to see what he proposed for Europe).

SOURCE 2

Twenty years ago we jumped head first into politics as though we were jumping into uncharted waters . . . There was a lot of enthusiasm . . . You're like this when you are young and we had an opportunity, which had long been denied, to be there while something new was being created.

Jiří Ruml, a Czech Communist, writing in 1968.

How did Soviet control affect the people of eastern Europe?

For some people of eastern Europe to start with the Communists brought hope. The Soviet Union had achieved amazing industrial growth before the Second World War. Maybe, by following Soviet methods, they could do the same. Soviet-style Communism also offered them stable government and security because they were backed by one of the world's superpowers. Faced by shortages and poverty after the war, many people hoped for great things from Communism (see Source 2).

However, the reality of Soviet control of eastern Europe was very different from what people had hoped for.

- **Freedom** Countries that had a long tradition of free speech and democratic government suddenly lost the right to criticise the government. Newspapers were censored. Non-Communists were put in prison for criticising the government. People were forbidden to travel to countries in western Europe.
- **Wealth** Such repression and loss of freedom might have been more accepted if Communism had made people better off. Between 1945 and 1955 eastern European economies did recover. Wages in eastern Europe fell behind the wages in other countries. They even fell behind the wages in the Soviet Union. Eastern Europe was forbidden by Stalin to apply for Marshall Aid from the USA (see page 87) which could have helped it in its economic recovery.
- **Consumer goods** Long after economic recovery had ended the wartime shortages in western Europe, people in eastern Europe were short of coal to heat their houses, short of milk and meat. Clothing and shoes were very expensive. People could not get consumer goods like radios, electric kettles or televisions which were becoming common in the West. Factories did not produce what ordinary people wanted. They actually produced what the Soviet Union wanted.

In addition, they had little chance to protest. In June 1953 there were huge demonstrations across East Germany protesting about Communist policies. Soviet tanks rolled in and Soviet troops killed 40 protesters and wounded over 400. Thousands were arrested and the protests were crushed. Similar protests in Czechoslovakia, Hungary and Romania were dealt with in the same way.

Think!

1 Study Source 3. Why do you think Tito wished to remain independent of the Soviet Union?
2 Why do you think the Soviet Union was worried about Tito's independence?
3 Look at Source 17 on page 84. Does this help to explain why the Soviet Union allowed Tito to remain independent?
4 On a scale of 0–10, how secure do you think Soviet control was in 1953?

Revision Tip

Make sure you can explain in your own words:
- the role of Cominform
- the role of the Red Army
in keeping control of eastern Europe.

SOURCE 3

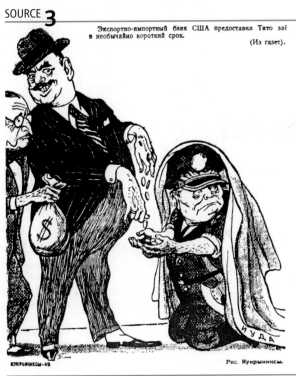

A 1949 Soviet cartoon. Marshal Tito, leader of Yugoslavia, is shown accepting money from the Americans. His cloak is labelled 'Judas' – 'the betrayer'. Yugoslavia was the only Communist state to resist domination by Stalin. The Soviet Union kept up a propaganda battle against Tito. Despite the Cold War, there were more cartoons in the official Communist newspapers attacking Tito than cartoons criticising the USA.

Profile

Nikita Khrushchev

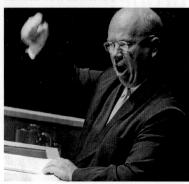

- ◆ Born 1894, the son of a coal miner.
- ◆ Fought in the Red Army during the Civil War, 1922–23.
- ◆ Afterwards worked for the Communist Party in Moscow. Was awarded the Order of Lenin for his work building the Moscow underground railway.
- ◆ In 1949 he was appointed by the Communist Party to run Soviet agriculture.
- ◆ There was a power struggle after Stalin's death over who would succeed him. Khrushchev had come out on top by 1955 and by 1956 he felt secure enough in his position to attack Stalin's reputation.
- ◆ Became Prime Minister in 1958.
- ◆ Took his country close to nuclear war with the USA during the Cuban missile crisis in 1962 (see pages 102–109).
- ◆ Was forced into retirement in 1964.
- ◆ Died in 1971.

Revision Tip

Khrushchev

Make sure you know two ways in which Khrushchev appeared to be different from Stalin in 1955.

De-Stalinisation

Write your own definition of 'de-Stalinisation'. Make sure you include:
- ◆ at least two examples
- ◆ an explanation of why it was radical.

The rise of Khrushchev

Stalin was a hero to millions of people in the USSR. He had defeated Hitler and given the USSR an empire in eastern Europe. He made the USSR a nuclear superpower. When he died in 1953, amid the grief and mourning, many minds turned to the question of who would succeed Stalin as Soviet leader. The man who emerged by 1955 was Nikita Khrushchev. Khruschev seemed very different from Stalin. He

- ● ended the USSR's long feuds with China and with Yugoslavia
- ● talked of peaceful co-existence with the West
- ● made plans to reduce expenditure on arms
- ● attended the first post-war summit between the USSR, the USA, France and Britain in July 1955
- ● said he wanted to improve the living standards of ordinary citizens.

De-Stalinisation

At the Communist Party International in 1956, Khruschev made an astonishing attack on Stalin. He dredged up the gory evidence of Stalin's purges (see page 220) and denounced him as a wicked tyrant who was an enemy of the people and kept all power to himself. Khruschev went on to say much worse things about Stalin and began a programme of de-Stalinisation.

- ● He closed down Cominform.
- ● He released thousands of political prisoners.
- ● He agreed to pull Soviet troops out of Austria (they had been posted there since the end of the Second World War).
- ● He invited Marshall Tito to Moscow.
- ● He dismissed Stalin's former Foreign Minister Molotov.
- ● He seemed to be signalling to the countries of eastern Europe that they would be allowed much greater independence to control their own affairs.

Those in eastern Europe who wanted greater freedom from the Soviet Union saw hopeful times ahead.

SOURCE 4

We must produce more grain. The more grain there is, the more meat, lard and fruit there will be. Our tables will be better covered. Marxist theory helped us win power and consolidate it. Having done this we must help the people eat well, dress well and live well. If after forty years of Communism, a person cannot have a glass of milk or a pair of shoes, he will not believe Communism is a good thing, whatever you tell him.

Nikita Khrushchev speaking in 1955.

SOURCE 5

Stalin used extreme methods and mass repressions at a time when the revolution was already victorious . . . Stalin showed in a whole series of cases his intolerance, his brutality and his abuse of power . . . He often chose the path of repression and physical annihilation, not only against actual enemies, but also against individuals who had not committed any crimes against the Party and the Soviet government.

Khrushchev denounces Stalin in 1956. For citizens of eastern Europe who had been bombarded with propaganda praising Stalin, this was a shocking change of direction.

Look at Source 6.
1 Make a list of the features of the cartoon that show Khrushchev as a new type of leader.
2 Design another cartoon that shows him relaxing the Soviet grip on eastern Europe. Think about:
♦ how you would show Khrushchev
♦ how you would represent the states of eastern Europe (as maps? as people?)
♦ hcw you would represent Soviet control (as a rope? getting looser? tighter?).
You could either draw the cartoon or write instructions for an artist to do so.

How secure was Soviet control?

On page 123 we showed you three graphs. At the end of this chapter you will decide which is the most accurate way to represent Soviet control 1945–90.

Through the rest of this chapter you are going to examine a number of different case studies of Soviet control. Each is to be studied in its own right but you are also going to use them to to build your understanding of the bigger picture. Here are some features of the Polish uprising of 1956:
♦ workers go on strike for more wages
♦ 53 rioters killed by Polish army
♦ Polish army loses control
♦ Khrushchev moves troops to the Polish border
♦ a new leader is appointed who is more acceptable to the Polish people
♦ Communists agreed to stop persecuting the Catholic Church.
For each feature decide whether it suggests that Soviet control was strong or weak. There may be some events that could be used to support either view. Make sure you can explain your decisions.

SOURCE 6

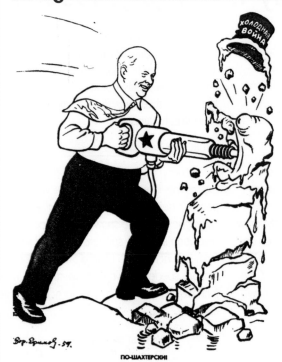

A 1959 Soviet cartoon. The writing on the snowman's hat reads 'cold war'. Khrushchev is drilling through the cold war using what the caption calls 'miners' methods'. The cartoon uses very strong visual images like Khrushchev's modern style of clothing to emphasise his new ideas. And of course he is breaking up the Cold War!

The Warsaw Pact

One aspect of Stalin's policy did not change, however. His aim in eastern Europe had always been to create a buffer against attack from the West. Khrushchev continued this policy. In 1955 he created the Warsaw Pact. This was a military alliance similar to NATO (see page 91). The members would defend each other if one was attacked. The Warsaw Pact included all the Communist countries of eastern Europe except Yugoslavia, but it was dominated by the Soviet Union (see Source 17, page 84).

Challenges to Soviet control in eastern Europe

Khrushchev's criticism of Stalin sent a strong signal to opposition groups in eastern Europe that they could now press for changes. The question was: how far would Khrushchev let them go? The first opposition Khrushchev had to deal with as leader was in Poland.

In the summer of 1956 demonstrators attacked the Polish police, protesting about the fact that the government had increased food prices but not wages. Fifty-three workers were killed by the Polish army in riots in Poznan. The Polish government itself was unable to control the demonstrators. Alarmed, Khrushchev moved troops to the Polish border.

By October 1956 Poland was becoming more stabilised. A new leader, Wladyslaw Gomulka, took charge on 20 October. During the Nazi occupation Gomulka had been a popular leader of Communist resistance. However, he was also a nationalist. He had not seen eye to eye with many Polish Communists, who were totally loyal to Stalin. Khrushchev accepted Gomulka's appointment – a popular move in Poland for the next couple of years.

There was also an agreement that the Communists would stop persecuting members of the Catholic Church. The Red Army moved away from the Polish border and left the Polish army and government to sort things out.

Khruschev was soon put to the test again in Hungary in October 1956.

Case study 1: Hungary, 1956

From 1949 to 1956 Hungary was led by a hard-line Communist called Mátyás Rákosi. Hungarians hated the restrictions which Rákosi's Communism imposed on them. Most Hungarians felt bitter about losing their freedom of speech. They lived in fear of the secret police. They resented the presence of thousands of Soviet troops and officials in their country. Some areas of Hungary even had Russian street signs, Russian schools and shops. Worst of all, Hungarians had to pay for Soviet forces to be in Hungary.

SOURCE **7**

Living standards were declining and yet the papers and radio kept saying that we had never had it so good. Why? Why these lies? Everybody knew the state was spending the money on armaments. Why could they not admit that we were worse off because of the war effort and the need to build new factories? . . . I finally arrived at the realisation that the system was wrong and stupid.

A Hungarian student describes the mood in 1953.

SOURCE **8**

. . . wearing clothes patterned after Western styles, showing interest in Jazz, expressing liberalism in the arts – was considered dangerous in the eyes of the people's democracy. To cite a small example, let us take the case of my university colleague, John. He showed up at lectures one day several weeks before the revolution in a new suit and a striped shirt and necktie, all of which he had received from an uncle in the United States through gift-parcel channels. His shoes were smooth suede and would have cost one month's wages in Hungary. After classes John was summoned by the party officer. He received a tongue-lashing and was expelled.

Written by László Beke, a student who helped lead the Hungarian uprising in 1956, in *A Student's Diary: Budapest October 16–November 1, 1956.*

What happened?

In June 1956 a group within the Communist Party in Hungary opposed Rákosi. He appealed to Moscow for help. He wanted to arrest 400 leading opponents. Moscow would not back him. The Kremlin ordered Rákosi to be retired 'for health reasons'.

The new leader, Ernö Gerö, was no more acceptable to the Hungarian people. Discontent came to a head with a huge student demonstration **on 23 October**, when the giant statue of Stalin in Budapest was pulled down.

The USSR allowed a new government to be formed under the well-respected Imre Nagy on 24 October. Soviet troops and tanks stationed in Hungary since the Second World War began to withdraw. Hungarians created thousands of local councils to replace Soviet power. Several thousand Hungarian soldiers defected from the army to the rebel cause, taking their weapons with them.

Nagy's government began to make plans. It would hold free elections, create impartial courts, restore farmland to private ownership. It wanted the total withdrawal of the Soviet army from Hungary. It also planned to leave the Warsaw Pact and declare Hungary neutral in the Cold War struggle between East and West. There was widespread optimism that the new American President Eisenhower, who had been the wartime supreme commander of all Allied Forces in western Europe, would support the new independent Hungary with armed troops if necessary.

How did the Soviet Union respond?

Khrushchev at first seemed ready to accept some of the reforms. However, he could not accept Hungary's leaving the Warsaw Pact. In November 1956 thousands of Soviet troops and tanks moved into Budapest. The Hungarians did not give in. Two weeks of bitter fighting followed. Some estimates put the number of Hungarians killed at 30,000. However, the latest research suggests about 3,000 Hungarians and up to 1,000 Russians were killed. Another 200,000 Hungarians fled across the border into Austria to escape the Communist forces.

Focus Task

Why was there opposition to Soviet control in Hungary?

1 Use the text and Sources 7 and 8 to list reasons why some Hungarians were opposed to Communist control – for example, they resented the presence of Soviet troops.
2 List the changes proposed by Nagy's government.
3 Which of these proposed changes do you think would be most threatening of the USSR? Give reasons.

Revision Tip

Test yourself to see if you can remember:
♦ two important reasons that the Hungarians rebelled against Soviet control in 1956
♦ two changes brought about by Nagy
♦ how Khrushchev reacted at first, then changed his mind, then changed it again.

SOURCE 9

In Hungary thousands of people have obtained arms by disarming soldiers and militia men . . . Soldiers have been making friends with the embittered and dissatisfied masses . . . The authorities are paralysed, unable to stop the bloody events.

From a report in a Yugoslav newspaper. Yugoslavia, although Communist, did not approve of Soviet policies.

SOURCE 10

We have almost no weapons, no heavy guns of any kind. People are running up to the tanks, throwing in hand grenades and closing the drivers' windows. The Hungarian people are not afraid of death. It is only a pity that we cannot last longer. Now the firing is starting again. The tanks are coming nearer and nearer. You can't let people attack tanks with their bare hands. What is the United Nations doing?

A telex message sent by the Hungarian rebels fighting the Communists. Quoted in George Mikes, *The Hungarian Revolution*, 1957.

SOURCE 11

October 27, 1956. On my way home I saw a little girl propped up against the doorway of a building with a machine gun clutched in her hands. When I tried to move her, I saw she was dead. She couldn't have been more than eleven or twelve years old. There was a neatly folded note in her pocket she had evidently meant to pass on through someone to her parents. In childish scrawl it read: 'Dear Mama, Brother is dead. He asked me to take care of his gun. I am all right, and I'm going with friends now. I kiss you. Kati.'

Written by László Beke, a Hungarian student.

SOURCE 12

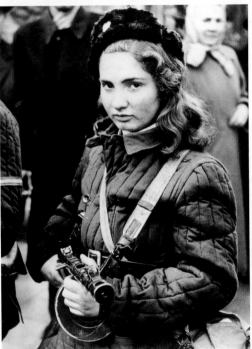

An armed fifteen-year-old girl in Budapest during the Hungarian rising of 1956.

Source Analysis

1 How do Sources 9 and 10 differ in the impression they give of the Hungarian uprising?
2 Why do you think they differ?
3 Does the photo in Source 12 give the same impression as either Source 9 or Source 10?
4 Work in pairs. Study Sources 9–12 and choose one source. Try to convince your partner that your source is the most useful source for studying events in Hungary in 1956.

Think!

1 Look back at Source 17 in Chapter 4. Why do you think Hungary's membership of the Warsaw Pact was so important to the Soviet Union?
2 Why do you think the Hungarians received no support from the West?
3 Explain which of these statements you most agree with:

> The speed at which the Red Army crushed resistance in Hungary shows how completely the Soviet Union controlled Hungary.

> The severity of the Red Army in dealing with Hungary in 1956 shows how fragile the Soviet hold on Hungary really was.

The Western powers protested to the USSR but sent no help; they were too preoccupied with a crisis of their own (the Suez crisis in the Middle East)!

Outcomes

Khrushchev put János Kádár in place as leader. Kádár took several months to crush all resistance. Around 35,000 anti-Communist activists were arrested and 300 were executed. Kádár cautiously introduced some of the reforms being demanded by the Hungarian people. However, he did not waver on the central issue – membership of the Warsaw Pact.

Case study 2: Czechoslovakia and the Prague Spring, 1968

SOURCE **13**

In Czechoslovakia the people who were trusted [by the Communist government] were the obedient ones, those who did not cause any trouble, who didn't ask questions. It was the mediocre man who came off best.

In twenty years not one human problem has been solved in our country, from primary needs like flats, schools, to the more subtle needs such as fulfilling oneself . . . the need for people to trust one another . . . development of education.

I feel that our Republic has lost its good reputation.

From a speech given by Ludvik Vaculik, a leading figure in the reform movement, in March 1968.

SOURCE **14**

The Director told them they would produce 400 locomotives a year. They are making seventy.

And go look at the scrapyard, at all the work that has been thrown out. They built a railway and then took it down again. Who's responsible for all this? The Communist Party set up the system.

We were robbed of our output, our wages . . . How can I believe that in five years' time it won't be worse?

Ludvik Vaculik quotes from an interview he had with the workers in a locomotive factory run by the Communists.

Focus Task

Why was there opposition to Soviet control in Czechoslovakia?

Use the text and Sources 13–15 to list the reasons for opposition to soviet control in Czechoslovakia.

Twelve years after the brutal suppression of the Hungarians, Czechoslovakia posed a similar challenge to Soviet domination of eastern Europe. Khrushchev had by now been ousted from power in the USSR. A new leader, Leonid Brezhnev, had replaced him.

What happened?

In the 1960s a new mood developed in Czechoslovakia. People examined what had been happening in twenty years of Communist control and they did not like what they saw. In 1967 the old Stalinist leader was replaced by Alexander Dubček. He proposed a policy of 'socialism with a human face': less censorship, more freedom of speech and a reduction in the activities of the secret police. Dubček was a committed Communist, but he believed that Communism did not have to be as restrictive as it had been before he came to power. He had learned the lessons of the Hungarian uprising and reassured Brezhnev that Czechoslovakia had no plans to pull out of the Warsaw Pact or Comecon.

The Czech opposition was led by intellectuals who felt that the Communists had failed to lead the country forward. As censorship had been eased, they were able to launch attacks on the Communist leadership, pointing out how corrupt and useless they were. Communist government ministers were 'grilled' on live television and radio about how they were running the country and about events before 1968. This period became known as 'The Prague Spring' because of all the new ideas that seemed to be appearing everywhere.

By the summer even more radical ideas were emerging. There was even talk of allowing another political party, the Social Democratic Party, to be set up as a rival to the Communist Party.

SOURCE **15**

All the different kinds of state in which the Communist Party has taken power have gone through rigged trials . . . There must be a fault other than just the wrong people were chosen. There must be a fault in the theory [of Communism] itself.

Written by Luboš Dubrovsky, a Czech writer, in May 1968.

How did the Soviet Union respond?

The Soviet Union was very suspicious of the changes taking place in Czechoslovakia. Czechoslovakia was one of the most important countries in the Warsaw Pact. It was centrally placed, and had the strongest industry. The Soviets were worried that the new ideas in Czechoslovakia might spread to other countries in eastern Europe. Brezhnev came under pressure from the East German leader, Walter Ulbricht, and the Polish leader, Gomulka, to restrain reform in Czechoslovakia.

The USSR tried various methods in response. To start with, it tried to slow Dubček down. It argued with him. Soviet, Polish and East German troops performed very public training exercises right on the Czech border. It thought about imposing economic sanctions – for example, cancelling wheat exports to Czechoslovakia – but didn't because it thought that the Czechs would ask for help from the West.

In July the USSR had a summit conference with the Czechs. Dubček agreed not to allow a new Social Democratic Party. However, he insisted on keeping most of his reforms. The tension seemed to ease. Early in August, a conference of all the other Warsaw Pact countries produced a vague declaration simply calling on Czechoslovakia to maintain political stability.

Then seventeen days later, on 20 August 1968, to the stunned amazement of the Czechs and the outside world, Soviet tanks moved into Czechoslovakia.

There was little violent resistance, although many Czechs refused to co-operate with the Soviet troops. Dubček was removed from power. His experiment in socialism with a human face had not failed; it had simply proved unacceptable to the other Communist countries.

SOURCE 16

Yesterday troops from the Soviet Union, Poland, East Germany, Hungary and Bulgaria crossed the frontier of Czechoslovakia . . . The Czechoslovak Communist Party Central Committee regard this act as contrary to the basic principles of good relations between socialist states.

A Prague radio report, 21 August 1968.

SOURCE 17

The party and government leaders of the Czechoslovak Socialist Republic have asked the Soviet Union and other allies to give the Czechoslovak people urgent assistance, including assistance with armed forces. This request was brought about . . . by the threat from counter revolutionary forces . . . working with foreign forces hostile to socialism.

A Soviet news agency report, 21 August 1968.

SOURCE 18

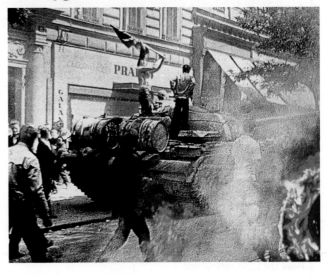

Czechs burning Soviet tanks in Prague, August 1968.

Source Analysis

1 Explain how and why Sources 16 and 17 differ in their interpretation of the Soviet intervention.
2 What is the message of Source 19?

SOURCE 19

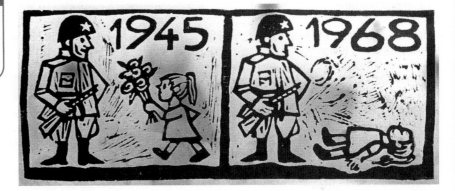

A street cartoon in Prague.

SOURCE 20

When internal and external forces hostile to socialism attempt to turn the development of any socialist country in the direction of the capitalist system, when a threat arises to the cause of socialism in that country, a threat to the socialist commonwealth as a whole – it becomes not only a problem for the people of that country but also a general problem, the concern of all socialist countries.

The Brezhnev Doctrine.

Outcomes

Unlike Nagy in Hungary, Dubček was not executed. But he was gradually downgraded. First he was sent to be ambassador to Turkey, then expelled from the Communist Party altogether. Photographs showing him as leader were 'censored' (see page 122).

Before the Soviet invasion, Czechoslovakia's mood had been one of optimism. After, it was despair. A country that had been pro-Soviet now became resentful of the Soviet connection. Ideas that could have reformed Communism were silenced.

Dubček always expressed loyalty to Communism and the Warsaw Pact, but Brezhnev was very worried that the new ideas coming out of Czechoslovakia would spread. He was under pressure from the leaders of other Communist countries in eastern Europe, particularly Ulbricht in East Germany. These leaders feared that their own people would demand the same freedom that Dubček had allowed in Czechoslovakia.

The Brezhnev Doctrine

The Czechoslovak episode gave rise to the Brezhnev Doctrine. The essentials of Communism were defined as:

● a one-party system
● to remain a member of the Warsaw Pact.

Focus Task A

How similar were the uprisings of 1956 and 1968?

One question which historians often consider is how similar the uprisings of 1956 in Hungary and 1968 in Czechoslovakia actually were. The table below gives you a number of ways to compare the two events. Work through pages 128–31, make your own copy then complete the table.

Issue	Hungary, 1956	Czechoslovakia, 1968	How similar? Give reasons
Aims of rebels			
Attitude towards Communism			
Attitude towards democracy			
Attitude towards the USSR			
Attitude towards the West			
Why the USSR intervened			
How the USSR intervened			
Response of the rebels			
Casualties			
Eventual outcome			

Here are a few points to help you get the table started, but you will have to decide where they fit and add your own as well.

♦ Abolish secret police
♦ Around 200,000 fled the country
♦ Because of the threat to leave Warsaw Pact
♦ Dubček downgraded
♦ Fear that other states would demand the same freedoms
♦ Less censorship
♦ Pitched battles in the streets
♦ Wanted a more human form of Communism
♦ Wanted free elections with more than one party
♦ Withdraw Soviet troops

Revision Tip

You don't need to learn this whole table but be sure you can explain:
♦ two ways in which the Hungarian and Czech uprisings were similar
♦ two ways in which they were different.

Focus Task B

How secure was Soviet control of Hungary and Czechoslovakia?

Here are various events from the two invasions. For each event decide where it should go on this line. Does it suggest that Soviet control was weak, strong or somewhere in between?

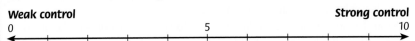

Weak control   **Strong control**
0   5   10

There may be some events that you think could be used to support either view. Whatever you decide you must include notes to explain your decision.

Hungary

♦ Imre Nagy forms new government
♦ Khruschev sends in troops
♦ Nagy imprisoned and executed
♦ Nagy's plans
♦ Opposition to Rákosi
♦ Rákosi not supported by Moscow
♦ Rákosi removed
♦ Rebellion
♦ Soviet tanks move in and then withdraw
♦ Two weeks of fierce street fighting

Czechoslovakia

♦ Censorship eased in Czechoslovakia
♦ Czech Communist leaders were heavily criticised for corrupt and incompetent rule
♦ Plans to set up Social Democratic Party
♦ USSR argued with Dubček to slow down the pace of reform
♦ Troops carried out training exercises on the border of Czechoslovakia
♦ The USSR considered sanctions against Czechoslovakia but feared they would not work
♦ Tanks moved into Prague on 20 August 1968
♦ There was little violent resistance in Czechoslovakia
♦ Dubček was removed
♦ The Brezhnev Doctrine

Case study 3: The Berlin Wall

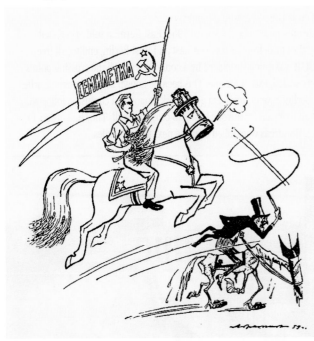

A 1959 Soviet cartoon – the caption was: 'The socialist stallion far outclasses the capitalist donkey'.

You have already seen how Berlin was a battleground of the Cold War (see Source 22). In 1961 it also became the focus of the Soviet Union's latest attempt to maintain control of its east European satellites.

The problem

The crushing of the Hungarian uprising (see page 128) had confirmed for many people in eastern Europe that it was impossible to fight the Communists. For many, it seemed that the only way of escaping the repression was to leave altogether. Some wished to leave eastern Europe for political reasons – they hated the Communists – while many more wished to leave for economic reasons. As standards of living in eastern Europe fell further and further behind the West, the attraction of going to live in a capitalist state was very great.

The contrast was particularly great in the divided city of Berlin. Living standards were tolerable in the East, but just a few hundred metres away in West Berlin, East Germans could see some of the prize exhibits of capitalist West Germany – shops full of goods, great freedom, great wealth and great variety. This had been deliberately done by the Western powers. They had poured massive investment into Berlin. East Germans could also watch West German television.

In the 1950s East Germans were still able to travel freely into West Berlin. From there they could travel on into West Germany. It was very tempting to leave East Germany, with its harsh Communist regime and its hardline leader, Walter Ulbricht. By the late 1950s thousands were leaving and never coming back (see Source 23).

Source Analysis

1 Look at Source 21. What is the aim of this cartoon?
2 How might someone living in a Communist country react to it?

West Berlin . . . has many roles. It is more than a showcase of liberty, an island of freedom in a Communist sea. It is more than a link with the free world, a beacon of hope behind the iron curtain, an escape hatch for refugees. Above all, it has become the resting place of Western courage and will . . . We cannot and will not permit the Communists to drive us out of Berlin.

President Kennedy speaking in 1960, before he became President.

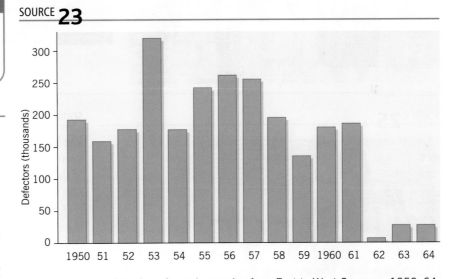

Number of people crossing from East to West Germany, 1950–64.

Those who were defecting were very often highly skilled workers or well-qualified managers. The Communist government could not afford to lose these high-quality people. More importantly, from Khrushchev's point of view, the sight of thousands of Germans fleeing Communist rule for a better life under capitalism undermined Communism generally.

The solution

In 1961 the USA had a new President, the young and inexperienced John F Kennedy. Khrushchev thought he could bully Kennedy and chose to pick a fight over Berlin. He insisted that Kennedy withdraw US troops from the city. He was certain that Kennedy would back down. Kennedy refused. However, all eyes were now on Berlin. What would happen next?

At two o'clock in the morning on Sunday 13 August 1961, East German soldiers erected a barbed-wire barrier along the entire frontier between East and West Berlin, ending all free movement from East to West. It was quickly replaced by a concrete wall. All the crossing points from East to West Berlin were sealed, except for one. This became known as Checkpoint Charlie.

Families were divided. Berliners were unable to go to work; chaos and confusion followed. Border guards kept a constant look-out for anyone trying to cross the wall. They had orders to shoot people trying to defect. Hundreds were killed over the next three decades.

SOURCE 24

A

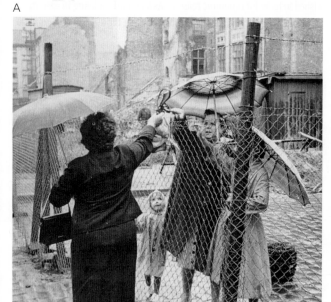

B

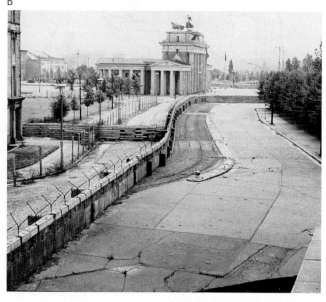

Stages in the building of the Berlin Wall.

SOURCE 25

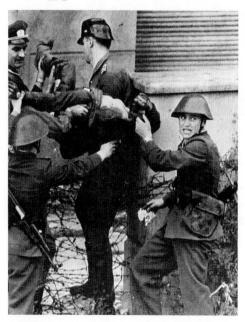

East German security guards recover the body of a man shot attempting to cross the wall in 1962.

SOURCE 26

The Western powers in Berlin use it as a centre of subversive activity against the GDR [the initial letters of the German name for East Germany]. In no other part of the world are so many espionage centres to be found. These centres smuggle their agents into the GDR for all kinds of subversion: recruiting spies; sabotage; provoking disturbances.

The government presents all working people of the GDR with a proposal that will securely block subversive activity so that reliable safeguards and effective control will be established around West Berlin, including its border with democratic Berlin.

A Soviet explanation for the building of the wall, 1961.

Outcomes

For a while, the wall created a major crisis. Access to East Berlin had been guaranteed to the Allies since 1945. In October 1961 US diplomats and troops crossed regularly into East Berlin to find out how the Soviets would react.

On 27 October Soviet tanks pulled up to Checkpoint Charlie and refused to allow any further access to the East. All day, US and Soviet tanks, fully armed, faced each other in a tense stand-off. Then, after eighteen hours, one by one, five metres at a time, the tanks pulled back. Another crisis, another retreat.

The international reaction was relief. Khrushchev ordered Ulbricht to avoid any actions that would increase tension. Kennedy said, 'It's not a very nice solution, but a wall is a hell of a lot better than a war.' So the wall stayed, and over the following years became the symbol of division – the division of Germany, the division of Europe, the division of Communist East and democratic West. The Communists presented the wall as a protective shell around East Berlin. The West presented it as a prison wall.

SOURCE 27

There are some who say, in Europe and elsewhere, we can work with the Communists. Let them come to Berlin.

President Kennedy speaking in 1963 after the building of the Berlin Wall.

SOURCE 28

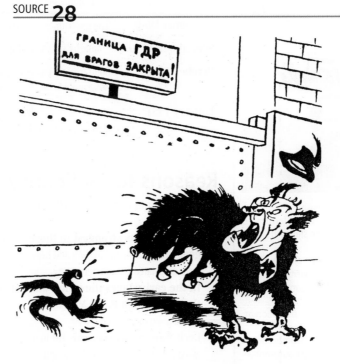

A Soviet cartoon from the 1960s. The sign reads: 'The border of the GDR (East Germany) is closed to all enemies.' Notice the shape of the dog's tail.

Revision Tip

You need to be able to give:
♦ two reasons that the Soviet Union built the Berlin Wall
♦ a full explanation of each reason.

Focus Task

Why was the Berlin Wall built in 1961?

Stage 1

Work in pairs.

Make a poster or notice to be stuck on the Berlin Wall explaining the purpose of the wall. One of you do a poster for the East German side and the other do a poster for the West German side. You can use pictures and quotations from the sources in this chapter or use your own research.

Make sure you explain in your poster the reasons why the wall was built and what the results of building the wall will be.

Stage 2

Discuss with your partner: Do you think the building of the Berlin Wall shows that Communist control of East Germany was weak or that it was strong?

Choose pieces of evidence from the past three pages that could be used to support either viewpoint and explain how it could be used that way.

Case study 4: Solidarity in Poland, 1980–81

SOURCE **29**

- *More pay*
- *End to censorship*
- *Same welfare benefits as police and party workers*
- *Broadcasting of Catholic church services*
- *Election of factory managers*

Some of Solidarity's 21 demands.

Profile

Lech Walesa

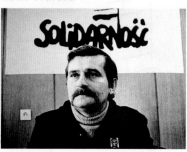

- ➤ Pronounced Lek Fowensa.
- ➤ Born 1943. His father was a farmer.
- ➤ He went to work in the shipyards at Gdansk.
- ➤ In 1976 he was sacked from the shipyard for making 'malicious' statements about the organisation and working climate.
- ➤ In 1978 he helped organise a union at another factory. He was dismissed.
- ➤ In 1979 he worked for Eltromontage. He was said to be the best automotive electrician. He was sacked.
- ➤ With others, he set up Solidarity in August 1980 and became its leader.
- ➤ He was a committed Catholic.
- ➤ In 1989 he became the leader of Poland's first non-Communist government since the Second World War.

Revision Tip

Make sure you know:
- ◆ two demands made by Solidarity in 1980
- ◆ one reason why Solidarity was crushed in 1981
- ◆ one reason why you think the rise and fall of Solidarity is a significant event in history.

Throughout the years of Communist control of Poland there were regular protests. However, they were generally more about living standards and prices than attempts to overthrow Communist government.

During the first half of the 1970s Polish industry performed well so the country was relatively calm. But in the late 1970s the Polish economy hit a crisis and 1979 was the worst year for Polish industry since Communism had been introduced. This is what happened next.

July 1980	The government announced increases in the price of meat.
August 1980	Workers at the Gdansk shipyard, led by Lech Walesa, put forward 21 demands to the government, including free trade unions and the right to strike (see Source 29). They also started a free trade union called Solidarity. Poland had trade unions but they were ineffective in challenging goverment policies.
30 August 1980	The government agreed to all 21 of Solidarity's demands.
September 1980	Solidarity's membership grew to 3.5 million.
October 1980	Solidarity's membership was 7 million. Solidarity was officially recognised by the government.
January 1981	Membership of Solidarity reached its peak at 9.4 million – more than a third of all the workers in Poland.

Reasons for Solidarity's success

You might be surprised that the government gave in to Solidarity in 1980. There are many different reasons for this.

- **The union was strongest in those industries that were most important to the government** – shipbuilding and heavy industry. A general strike in these industries would have devastated Poland's economy.
- **In the early stages the union was not seen by its members as an alternative to the Communist Party.** More than 1 million members (30 per cent) of the Communist Party joined Solidarity.
- **Lech Walesa was very careful** in his negotiations with the government and worked to avoid provoking a dispute that might bring in the Soviet Union.
- **The union was immensely popular.** Almost half of all workers belonged. Lech Walesa was a kind of folk hero.
- **Solidarity had the support of the Catholic Church** which was still very strong in Poland.
- **The government was playing for time.** It hoped Solidarity would break into rival factions. The government also drew up plans for martial law (rule by the army).
- **Finally, the Soviet Union had half an eye on the West.** Solidarity had gained support in the West in a way that neither the Hungarian nor the Czech rising had. Walesa was well known on Western media and people in the West bought Solidarity badges to show their support. The scale of the movement ensured that the Soviet Union treated the Polish crisis cautiously.

Following this success membership of Solidarity increased quickly.

Think!

Between August 1980 and December 1981, Solidarity went through some rapid changes. Choose two moments in this period that you think were particularly important in the rise and fall of Solidarity and explain why they were important.

SOURCE **31**

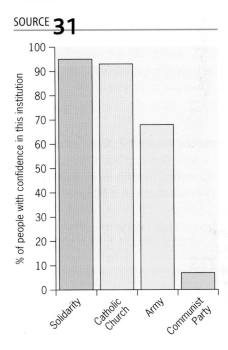

The results of an opinion poll in Poland, November 1981. The people polled were asked whether they had confidence in key institutions in Poland. It is known that 11 per cent of those polled were Communist Party members.

In February 1981 the civilian Prime Minister 'resigned' and the leader of the army, General Jaruzelski, took over. From the moment he took office, people in Poland, and observers outside Poland, expected the Soviet Union to 'send in the tanks' at any time, especially when the Solidarity Congress produced an 'open letter' saying that they were campaigning not only for their own rights but for the rights of workers throughout the Communist bloc. It proclaimed that the Poles were fighting 'For Your Freedom and For Ours'.

Jaruzelski and Walesa negotiated to form a government of national understanding but when that broke down in December, after nine months of tense relationships, the Communist government acted. Brezhnev ordered the Red Army to carry out 'training manoeuvres' on the Polish border. Jaruzelski introduced martial law. He put Walesa and almost 10,000 other Solidarity leaders in prison. He suspended Solidarity.

Reasons for the crushing of Solidarity

Military dictators are not required to give reasons for their actions. But if they did what might Jaruzelski have to say?

- **Solidarity was acting as a political party.** The government declared that it had secret tapes of a Solidarity meeting setting up a new provisional government – without the Communist Party.
- **Poland was sinking into chaos.** Almost all Poles felt the impact of food shortages. Rationing had been introduced in April 1981. Wages had increased by less than inflation. Unemployment was rising.
- **Solidarity itself was also tumbling into chaos.** There were many different factions. Some felt that the only way to make progress was to push the Communists harder until they cracked under the pressure. Strikes were continuing long after the Solidarity leadership had ordered them to stop.

The Soviet Union had seen enough. It thought the situation in Poland had gone too far. If Poland's leaders would not restore Communist control in Poland, then it would. This was something the Polish leaders wanted to avoid.

The Communist government had regained control of Poland but in December 1981, looking back on the past eighteen months, two things were obvious:

- The Polish people no longer trusted the Communists leadership.
- The only thing that kept the Communists in power was force or the threat of force backed by the USSR. When Jaruzelski finally decided to use force, Solidarity was easily crushed. The lesson was clear. If military force was not used, then Communist control seemed very shaky indeed.

The significance of Solidarity

In the story of Soviet control of eastern Europe Solidarity was significant for a number of reasons:

- It highlighted the failure of Communism to provide good living standards and this undermined Communism's claim to be a system which benefited ordinary people.
- It highlighted inefficiency and corruption (see Source 30 for example).
- It showed that there were organisations which were capable of resisting a Communist government.
- It showed that Communist governments could be threatened by 'people power'.

If Soviet policy were to change Communist control would not survive.

What do you expect to happen next?

Focus Task

What was the significance of Solidarity for the decline of Soviet influence in eastern Europe?

'Solidarity died as quickly as it started, having achieved nothing.'
How far do you agree with this statement? Support your answer with evidence from pages 136 and 137.

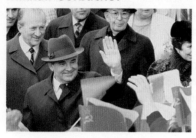
Enter Mikhail Gorbachev

Gorbachev became leader of the Soviet Union in 1985. He was an unusual mix of idealist, optimist and realist.

- The realist in him could see that the USSR was in a terrible state. Its economy was very weak. It was spending far too much money on the arms race. It was locked into an unwinnable war in Afghanistan.
- The idealist in Gorbachev believed that Communist rule should make life better for the people of the USSR and other Communist states. As a loyal Communist and a proud Russian, he was offended by the fact that goods made in Soviet factories were shoddy, living standards were higher in the West and that many Soviet citizens had no loyalty to the government.
- The optimist in Gorbachev believed that a reformed Communist system of government could give people pride and belief in their country. He definitely did not intend to dismantle Communism in the USSR and eastern Europe, but he did want to reform it radically.

Gorbachev's policies in eastern Europe

Gorbachev also had a very different attitude to eastern Europe from Brezhnev. In March he called the leaders of the Warsaw Pact countries together. This meeting should have been a turning point in the history of eastern Europe. He had two messages.

'We won't intervene'

SOURCE **32**

The time is ripe for abandoning views on foreign policy which are influenced by an imperial standpoint. Neither the Soviet Union nor the USA is able to force its will on others. It is possible to suppress, compel, bribe, break or blast, but only for a certain period. From the point of view of long-term big time politics, no one will be able to subordinate others. That is why only one thing – relations of equality – remains. All of us must realise this . . .

Gorbachev speaking in 1987.

Gorbachev made it very clear to the countries of eastern Europe that they were responsible for their own fates. However, most of the Warsaw Pact leaders were old style, hardline Communists. To them, Gorbachev's ideas were insane and they simply did not believe he meant what he said.

'You have to reform'

Gorbachev also made it clear that they needed to reform their own countries. He did not think Communism was doomed. In fact he felt the opposite was true. Gorbachev believed the Communist system could provide better healthcare, education and transport. The task in the USSR and eastern Europe was to renew Communism so as to match capitalism in other areas of public life. However, they did not believe him on this count either.

In the next few year these leaders would realise they had made a serious error of judgement.

Gorbachev's reforms

He had to be cautious, because he faced great opposition from hardliners in his own government, but gradually he declared his policies. The two key ideas were glasnost (openness) and perestroika (restructuring).

- **Glasnost:** He called for open debate on government policy and honesty in facing up to problems. It was not a detailed set of policies but it did mean radical change.
- In 1987 his **perestroika** programme allowed market forces to be introduced into the Soviet economy. For the first time in 60 years it was no longer illegal to buy and sell for profit.

SOURCE 33

A

Polish, Hungarian and Romanian dogs get to talking. 'What's life like in your country?' the Polish dog asks the Hungarian dog.

'Well, we have meat to eat but we can't bark. What are things like where you are from?' says the Hungarian dog to the Polish dog.

'With us, there's no meat, but at least we can bark,' says the Polish dog.

'What's meat? What's barking?' asks the Romanian dog.

B

East German leader Erich Honecker is touring East German towns. He is shown a run-down kindergarten. The staff ask for funds to renovate the institution. Honecker refuses. Next he visits a hospital, where the doctors petition him for a grant to buy new surgical equipment. Honecker refuses. The third place on Honecker's itinerary is a prison. This is pretty dilapidated, and here too the governor asks for money to refurbish. This time Honecker immediately pulls out his cheque book and insists that not only should the cells be repainted but that they should be fitted with new mattresses, colour televisions and sofas. Afterwards an aide asks him why he said no to a school and a hospital, but yes to a prison. Honecker says, 'Where do you think we will be living in a few months' time?'

Examples of anti-Communist jokes collected by researchers in eastern Europe in the 1980s.

Source Analysis

1 Why do you think President Reagan was so fond of jokes like those in Source 34A and B?
2 Do you think it is strange that Gorbachev was upset by these jokes? Explain your answer.
3 Can jokes really be useful historical sources? Explain your answer.
4 If you think jokes are useful sources, do you think the jokes in Source 33 are more or less useful than the jokes in Source 34? Explain your answer.

Defence spending

He also began to cut spending on defence. The nuclear arms race was an enormous drain on the Soviet economy at a time when it was in trouble anyway.

After almost 50 years on a constant war footing, the **Red Army** began to shrink.

International relations

At the same time, Gorbachev brought a new attitude to the USSR's relations with the wider world.
- He withdrew Soviet troops from Afghanistan, which had become such a costly yet unwinnable war.
- In speech after speech, he talked about international trust and co-operation as the way forward for the USSR, rather than confrontation.

Gorbachev and President Reagan

Ronald Reagan became US President in January 1981. He was President until 1988. He had only one policy towards the USSR – get tough. He criticised its control over eastern Europe and increased US military spending.

In a way, Reagan's toughness helped Gorbachev.
- It was clear by the late 1980s that the USSR could not compete with American military spending. This helped Gorbachev to push through his military spending cuts.
- Reagan got on quite well with Gorbachev himself. As superpower relations improved, the USSR felt less threatened by the USA. This meant there was less need for the USSR to control eastern Europe.

SOURCE 34

A

The Soviet Union would remain a one party state even if the Communists allowed an opposition party to exist. Everyone would join the opposition party.

B

When American college students are asked what they want to do after graduation, they reply: 'I don't know, I haven't decided'. Russian students answer the same question by saying: 'I don't know, they haven't told me'.

Anti-Communist jokes told by US President Reagan to Mikhail Gorbachev at their summit meetings in the late 1980s.

Implications for eastern Europe

As Gorbachev introduced his reforms in the USSR the demand rose for similar reforms in eastern European states as well. Most people in these states were sick of the poor economic conditions and the harsh restrictions that Communism imposed. Gorbachev's policies gave people some hope for reform.

'Listen to your people'

In July 1988 Gorbachev made a speech to the leaders of the Warsaw Pact countries. He planned to withdraw large numbers of troops, tanks and aircraft from eastern Europe. Hungary was particularly eager to get rid of Soviet troops and, when pressed, Gorbachev seemed to accept this. In March 1989 he made clear again that the Red Army would not intervene to prop up Communist regimes in eastern Europe. What followed was staggering.

The collapse of Communism in eastern Europe

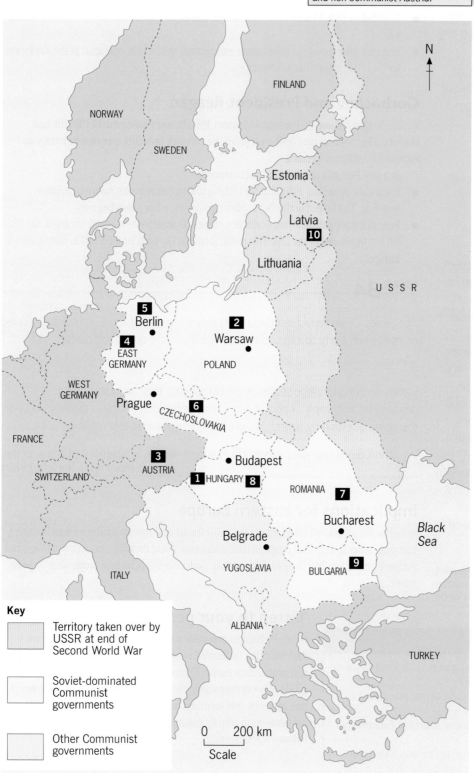

2
June
In Poland, free elections are held for the first time since the Second World War. Solidarity wins almost all the seats it contests. Eastern Europe gets its first non-Communist leader, President Lech Walesa.

3
September
Thousands of East Germans on holiday in Hungary and Czechoslovakia refuse to go home. They escape through Austria into West Germany.

4
October
There are enormous demonstrations in East German cities when Gorbachev visits the country. He tells the East German leader Erich Honecker to reform. Honecker orders troops to fire on demonstrators but they refuse.

Gorbachev makes it clear that Soviet tanks will not move in to 'restore order'.

5
November
East Germans march in their thousands to the checkpoints at the Berlin Wall. The guards throw down their weapons and join the crowds. The Berlin Wall is dismantled.

6
November
There are huge demonstrations in Czechoslovakia. The Czech government opens its borders with the West, and allows the formation of other parties.

7
December
In Romania there is a short but very bloody revolution that ends with the execution of the Communist dictator Nicolae Ceausescu.

8
The Communist Party in Hungary renames itself the Socialist Party and declares that free elections will be held in 1990.

9
In Bulgaria, there are huge demonstrations against the Communist government.

10
March 1990
Latvia leads the Baltic republics in declaring independence from the USSR.

Key

Territory taken over by USSR at end of Second World War

Soviet-dominated Communist governments

Other Communist governments

0   200 km

Scale

People power

The western media came up with a phrase to explain these events – people power. Communist control was toppled because ordinary people were not prepared to accept it any longer. They took control of events. It was not political leaders guiding the future of eastern Europe in 1989 but ordinary people.

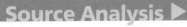
SOURCE **35**

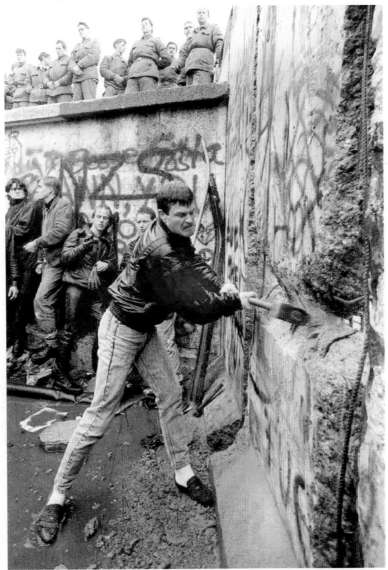

A demonstrator pounds away at the Berlin Wall as East German border guards look on from above, 4 November 1989. The wall was dismantled five days later.

SOURCE **36**

For most west Europeans now alive, the world has always ended at the East German border and the Wall; beyond lay darkness . . . The opening of the frontiers declares that the world has no edge any more. Europe is becoming once more round and whole.

The Independent, November 1989.

Reunification of Germany

With the Berlin Wall down, West German Chancellor Helmut Kohl proposed a speedy reunification of Germany. Germans in both countries embraced the idea enthusiastically.

Despite his idealism, Gorbachev was less enthusiastic. He expected that a new united Germany would be more friendly to the West than to the East. But after many months of hard negotiations, not all of them friendly, Gorbachev accepted German reunification and even accepted that the new Germany could become a member of NATO. This was no small thing for Gorbachev to accept. Like all Russians, he lived with the memory that it was German aggression in the Second World War that had cost the lives of 20 million Soviet citizens.

On 3 October 1990, Germany became a united country once again.

The collapse of the USSR

Even more dramatic events were to follow in the Soviet Union itself.

1990	
MARCH	Gorbachev visited the Baltic state of **Lithuania** – part of the Soviet Union. Its leaders put their views to him. They were very clear. They wanted independence. They did not want to be part of the USSR. Gorbachev was for once uncompromising. He would not allow this. But in March they did it anyway.
	Almost as soon as he returned to Moscow from Lithuania, Gorbachev received a similar demand from the Muslim Soviet Republic of **Azerbaijan**. What should Gorbachev do now? He sent troops to Azerbaijan to end rioting there. He sent troops to Lithuania. But as the summer approached, the crisis situation got worse.
MAY	The **Russian Republic**, the largest within the USSR, elected Boris Yeltsin as its President. Yeltsin made it clear that he saw no future in a Soviet Union. He said that the many republics that made up the USSR should become independent states.
JULY	**Ukraine** declared its independence. Other republics followed.
	By the end of 1990 nobody was quite sure what the USSR meant any longer. Meanwhile Gorbachev was an international superstar. In October 1990 Gorbachev received the **Nobel Peace Prize** for his contribution to ending the Cold War.
1991	
APRIL	The Republic of **Georgia** declared its independence.
AUGUST	The USSR was disintegrating. Reformers within the USSR itself demanded an end to the Communist Party's domination of government. Gorbachev was struggling to hold it together, but members of the Communist elite had had enough.
	Hardline Communist Party members and leading military officers attempted a **coup** to take over the USSR. The plotters included Gorbachev's Prime Minister, Pavlov, and the head of the armed forces, Dimitry Yazov. They held Gorbachev prisoner in his holiday home in the Crimea. They sent tanks and troops on to the streets of Moscow. This was the old Soviet way to keep control. Would it work this time?
	Huge crowds gathered in Moscow. They strongly opposed this military coup. The Russian President, Boris Yeltsin, emerged as the leader of the popular opposition. Faced by this resistance, the conspirators lost faith in themselves and the coup collapsed.
	This last-ditch attempt by the Communist Party to save the USSR had failed. A few days later, Gorbachev returned to Moscow.
DECEMBER	Gorbachev might have survived the coup, but it had not strengthened his position as Soviet leader. He had to admit that the USSR was finished and he with it.
	In a televised speech on 25 December 1991, Gorbachev announced his own resignation and the end of the Soviet Union (see Source 37).

Think!

Think of a suitable headline for each of the six episodes in the collapse of the USSR summarised in the table.

The end of the Cold War

Read Source 37 carefully. Three statements are in bold.

Do you agree or disagree with each statement? For each statement, write a short paragraph to:
a) explain what it means, and
b) express your own view on it.

SOURCE 37

A sense of failure and regret came through his [Gorbachev's] Christmas Day abdication speech – especially in his sorrow over his people 'ceasing to be citizens of a great power'. Certainly, if man-in-the-street interviews can be believed, **the former Soviet peoples consider him a failure**.

History will be kinder. *The Nobel Prize he received for ending the Cold War was well deserved. Every man, woman and child in this country should be eternally grateful.*

His statue should stand in the centre of every east European capital; *for it was Gorbachev who allowed them their independence. The same is true for the newly independent countries further east and in Central Asia. No Russian has done more to free his people from bondage since Alexander II who freed the serfs.*

From a report on Gorbachev's abdication speech, 25 December 1991, in the US newspaper the *Boston Globe*.

SOURCE 38

He had no grand plan and no predetermined policies; but if Gorbachev had not been Party General Secretary, the decisions of the late 1980s would have been different. The USSR's long-lasting order would have endured for many more years, and almost certainly the eventual collapse of the order would have been much bloodier than it was to be in 1991. The irony was that Gorbachev, in trying to prevent the descent of the system into general crisis, proved instrumental in bringing forward that crisis and destroying the USSR.

Extract from *History of Modern Russia* by historian Robert Service, published 2003. In this extract he is commenting on the meeting in March 1985.

SOURCE 39

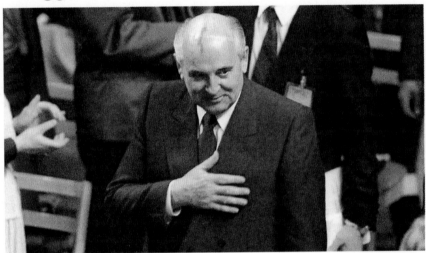

Mikhail Gorbachev after receiving the Nobel Peace Prize, 15 October 1990.

SOURCE 40

Doonesbury   BY GARRY TRUDEAU

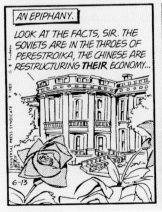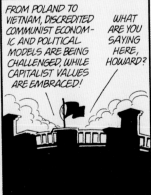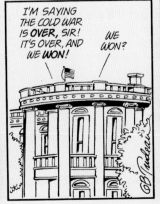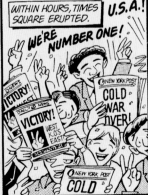

A cartoon by Doonesbury which appeared in the *Guardian* on 13 June 1988.

Focus Task A

How far was Gorbachev personally responsible for the collapse of control over eastern Europe?

You are making a documentary film called 'The Collapse of the Red Empire' to explain the how and why of Soviet control of eastern Europe. The film will be 60 minutes long.

1 Decide what proportion of this time should concentrate on:
   a) people power
   b) problems in the USSR
   c) Actions by Western leaders such as Reagan
   d) Actions of political leaders in eastern Europe
   e) Mikhail Gorbachev.

2 Choose one of these aspects and summarise the important points, stories, pictures or sources that your film should cover under that heading.

Focus Task B

How secure was Soviet control of eastern Europe?

You now know a lot about Soviet control of eastern Europe:
♦ how and why Communists seized control of each country in the 1940s (Chapter 4)
♦ how the Soviet Union successfully crushed opposition and threats to control from the 1950s to the 1980s
♦ how the Communist regimes of eastern Europe and the USSR collapsed so suddenly in 1989–90.
Here are the three graphs from page 123. Which do you think best represents the story of Soviet control of eastern Europe?

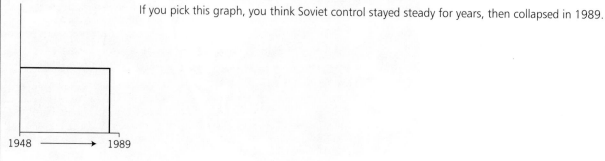
If you pick this graph, you think Soviet control stayed steady for years, then collapsed in 1989.

1948 ⟶ 1989

If you pick this graph, you think Soviet control gradually decreased over time.

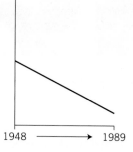

1948 ⟶ 1989

If you pick this graph, you think Soviet control fluctuated in response to various crises.

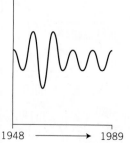

1948 ⟶ 1989

If you think none of them is right then draw your own. Explain your graph using evidence from this chapter. You could refer back to your work for the Focus Tasks on pages 127, 132 and 137.

Keywords

Make sure you know what these terms mean and are able to define them confidently.

- Berlin Wall
- Brezhnev Doctrine
- Censorship
- Checkpoint Charlie
- Co-existence
- Comecon
- Cominform
- Communism
- Communist bloc
- De-Stalinisation
- Freedom of speech
- Glasnost
- Iron curtain
- Martial law
- NATO
- Nobel Peace Prize
- One-party state
- People power
- Perestroika
- Politburo
- Red Army
- Reunification
- Secret police
- Socialism
- Solidarity
- Soviet republics
- Summit meeting
- Superpower
- The Prague Spring
- Trade union
- Warsaw Pact

Chapter Summary

The USSR and eastern Europe

1 After the Second World War, Communist governments were elected or forced on most countries of eastern Europe.

2 They were not directly ruled by the USSR but their Communist governments did what the USSR wanted and when they did not the USSR sent troops and tanks (the Red Army) to force them to follow the USSR's wishes.

3 Life in these countries was tightly controlled with censorship, a secret police and all industry directed to meeting the needs of the Soviet Union rather than making goods for ordinary people.

4 The countries formed a military alliance called the Warsaw Pact – the members would defend each other if any member was attacked.

5 In Hungary in 1956 the Communist government was very unpopular and the people resented the lack of freedom. There were demonstrations and protests. A new leader was chosen (with Soviet approval) who promised greater freedom but when he also decided to leave the Warsaw Pact the USSR changed and sent the Red Army to crush the rising.

6 In 1961 an increasing number of people in Communist East Germany were leaving by crossing into capitalist West Germany. The USSR responded by building the Berlin Wall – and stopping all movement from East to West Berlin. It stayed in place for 28 years and became a symbol of Cold War tension.

7 In Czechoslovakia in 1968 after mass protests the Communist government tried to introduce more freedom for its people. Again, the Soviet Union sent the Red Army to crush the protests.

8 In 1980 a trade union in Poland called Solidarity led a protest movement against Communist control that was tolerated to start with until the army took over in Poland and Solidarity was crushed.

9 In 1985 Gorbachev became leader of the USSR. He believed the USSR needed to change and he introduced two key ideas: glasnost (openness) and perestroika (restructuring).

10 He also told the Communist governments of eastern Europe that the USSR was no longer going to intervene to prop them up. They were on their own. In 1988 he began to withdraw Soviet troops from eastern Europe.

11 The impact of this was not immediately clear but by 1989 people in eastern Europe began to test what this meant in practice. First of all Hungarians began to dismantle the barbed-wire fence between Hungary and the west. Over the rest of the summer of 1989 people acted similarly throughout eastern Europe, culminating with the dismantling of the Berlin Wall (while troops looked on) in November.

12 Gorbachev was awarded the Nobel Peace Price for helping to end the Cold War between the USA and the USSR but he was not popular in the USSR. The USSR fragmented and he resigned as leader on Christmas Day 1991.

Exam Practice

See pages 168–175 and pages 316–319 for advice on the different types of questions you might face.

1(a) What were glasnost and perestroika? **[4]**

(b) Explain why Mikhail Gorbachev changed Soviet policy towards eastern Europe. **[6]**

(c) 'Gorbachev almost singlehandedly ended Communist control of eastern Europe.' How far do you agree with this statement? Explain your answer. **[10]**

2 Study Source 26 on page 134. How far do you think Source 26 is a reliable source? Explain your answer using the source and your own knowledge. **[7]**

3 Study Source 28 on page 135. Why was this source published at this time? Explain your answer using details of the source and your knowledge. **[7]**

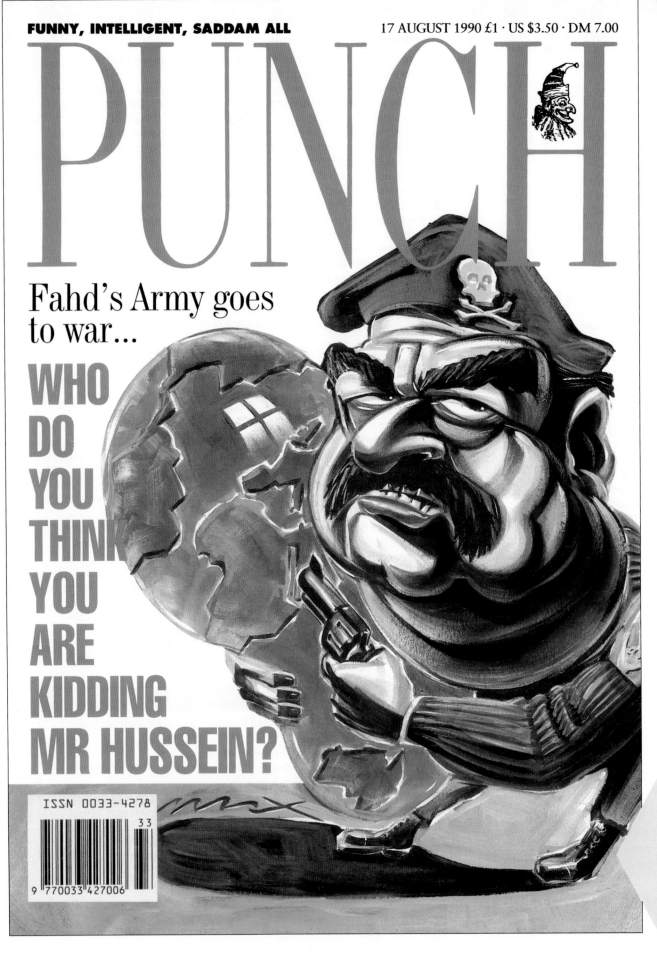

17 AUGUST 1990 £1 · US $3.50 · DM 7.00

PUNCH

Fahd's Army goes
to war...

WHO DO YOU THINK YOU ARE KIDDING MR HUSSEIN?

ISSN 0033-4278

9 770033 427006

33

7 Why did events in the Gulf matter, c. 1970–2000?

FOCUS POINTS

- Why was Saddam Hussein able to come to power in Iraq?
- What was the nature of Saddam Hussein's rule in Iraq?
- Why was there a revolution in Iran in 1979?
- What were the causes and consequences of the Iran–Iraq War, 1980–88?
- Why did the First Gulf War take place?

In Chapters 4–6 you have been studying the development of the Cold War and the impact of the superpowers on countries and events around the world. This chapter shifts the focus away from the superpowers onto the oil-rich states around the Persian Gulf (see map on page 148).

The region has seen rapid change over the past 40 years. There is a lot of political tension within and between the Gulf states that has caused some costly and ferocious wars, especially the Iran–Iraq War of 1980–88. It has also drawn into the conflict many outside nations: the First Gulf War of 1991 saw a multinational force of 35 different countries at war with Saddam Hussein's Iraq.

Your first task in this chapter will be to understand why the Gulf has been the source of such tension. It would easy to focus it all on individuals such as Saddam Hussein (pictured opposite) or on the importance of oil. As you will see those are both very important but there are also factors at work.

Your second task is to think about why these events matter so much to so many people. It should be obvious that they matter to people living in the region, but they have also mattered a lot to people living far away from the Gulf states. Western powers have got involved in wars much more readily than they have in conflicts in other parts of the world. Why did events in the Gulf matter to them?

Timeline

The timeline on the right gives you an overview of the main events you will be studying in this chapter. You will be focusing on two countries in particular, Iran and Iraq.

◀ This is the front cover of Punch magazine in August 1990. Punch was a satirical news magazine published in Britain from the nineteenth century through into the 1990s. This shows Saddam Hussein, leader of Iraq.

1 What impression does this give you of Saddam Hussein?
2 What is the message of this illustration?

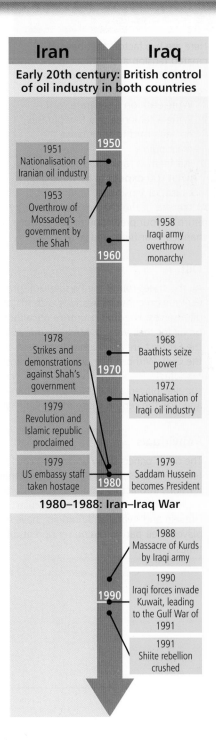

Iran | **Iraq**

Early 20th century: British control of oil industry in both countries

1950

1951 Nationalisation of Iranian oil industry

1953 Overthrow of Mossadeq's government by the Shah

1958 Iraqi army overthrow monarchy

1960

1978 Strikes and demonstrations against Shah's government

1968 Baathists seize power

1970

1972 Nationalisation of Iraqi oil industry

1979 Revolution and Islamic republic proclaimed

1979 US embassy staff taken hostage

1979 Saddam Hussein becomes President

1980

1980–1988: Iran–Iraq War

1988 Massacre of Kurds by Iraqi army

1990 Iraqi forces invade Kuwait, leading to the Gulf War of 1991

1990

1991 Shiite rebellion crushed

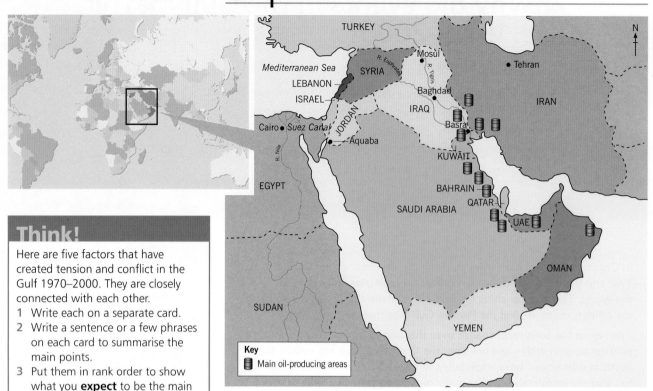

Map showing the main countries and key features of the Gulf region. All the states named are Arab except Iran and Turkey.

Think!

Here are five factors that have created tension and conflict in the Gulf 1970–2000. They are closely connected with each other.

1 Write each on a separate card.
2 Write a sentence or a few phrases on each card to summarise the main points.
3 Put them in rank order to show what you **expect** to be the main causes of tension.

At the end of the chapter you can return to your prediction to see if you changed your mind and why.

Oil!

All the states round the Persian Gulf produce oil; in fact, the Gulf region contains nearly two-thirds of the world's known oil reserves. The Gulf countries are almost entirely dependent on oil for their wealth. Many countries in the West and in the Far East are also highly dependent on imports of oil from the Gulf. Without it, much of their transport systems and manufacturing industry would break down. Control of oil supplies played a major part in the Iran–Iraq War of 1980–88 and was the central cause of the Gulf War of 1991.

Individuals

The other panels show underlying causes of tension. It is usually people who turn these tensions into actual conflicts. The different leaders of the Gulf states, in particular Saddam Hussein and Ayatollah Khomeini, have each played their part in raising tension at different times.

Reasons for tension in the Gulf

Israel

Not far from the Gulf is the state of Israel – the Jewish state created in 1948 and carved out of land inhabited by Arabs. The creation of the state of Israel was opposed by all Arab states, including those in the Gulf, and Israel has been a source of tension ever since.

Religion

The vast majority of the people in this area are Muslims. However there is a huge split between Sunni and Shia Muslims. The origins of this split are explained in the Factfile on the opposite page. Disagreement between these two branches of Islam has been a major cause of conflict throughout this period.

National identity

The two countries you will be focussing on most of all are Iran and Iraq. One is Arab while the other is not. They are both ancient civilisations dating back thousands of years. Their people are independent and proud of who they are and where they have come from. Yet for much of their history the area has been controlled by foreign empires. While outsiders might care most about oil, many Iranians and Iraqis care more about their country, their identity and their religion than they do about money or oil. This has sometimes brought them into conflict with foreign powers or with rulers who co-operate with them.

Why was Saddam Hussein able to come to power in Iraq?

Factfile

Baath Party

➤ The Baath Party had originally been established in Syria in the 1950s but its influence extended to several Arab countries, including Iraq.

➤ Baath means 'Renaissance' or rebirth of Arab power.

➤ The Baathists called for unity among Arabs throughout the Middle East. This was known as Arab Nationalism.

➤ In Iraq, they were mainly supported because they demanded a strong stand against foreign interference in the affairs of Iraq.

Factfile

Sunni and Shiite Muslims

➤ All Muslims, whose religion is Islam, believe in Allah (God). They believe that Muhammad, born in Mecca (in today's Saudi Arabia in AD 572), is the messenger and prophet of Allah.

➤ The Sunni–Shiite difference originated with a major disagreement over who should succeed Muhammad as the Caliph, or leader (in Arabic, it literally means deputy or successor) of the Muslim world.

➤ Ali, the cousin and son-in-law of Muhammad, believed he should be leader and he was recognised as Caliph in Iraq and Persia (modern Iran). But the Muslim rulers in Syria chose another successor.

➤ This led to division and warfare amongst Muslims with the creation of two groups: the Shia, or Shiite, Muslims who followed Ali, and the Sunni Muslims.

➤ Most Arabs became Sunni Muslims while the Arabs of southern Iraq and the (non-Arab) Persians became Shiite Muslims.

Ancient Iraq

Iraq lies in the ancient land of Mesopotamia, one of the world's oldest civilisations. The first cities were built here, the most famous of which was Baghdad. The Hanging Gardens of Babylon became one of the Seven Wonders of the Ancient World.

Many centuries later, in the seventh century AD, the land of Iraq was invaded by the Arabs and its people adopted the language, Arabic, and the religion, Islam, of the invaders.

The British mandate

By 1900, the area that we now think of as Iraq was actually three provinces of the Turkish Empire. At the end of the First World War the Turkish Empire was broken up. Under the Treaty of Sevres (see page 19) the three provinces were combined as a League of Nations mandate (see page 31) run by the British. The main reason the British were keen to do this was oil.

This was a bitter blow to Iraqi nationalists who wanted (and, in some cases, had fought for) complete independence for Iraq. The British soon had a rebellion on their hands. By October 1920, they had 100,000 troops in Iraq. They crushed the uprising but, in doing so, they aroused even more opposition. Today Iraqi schoolchildren all learn about the 'Revolution of 1920' and how their nationalist heroes stood up to foreign, imperialist armies.

King Faisal

The British soon realised they could not run the country on their own. They needed collaborators: Iraqis who were willing to run the country in partnership with them. So in 1921, they invited Faisal, member of a leading Arab family in the Middle East, to become King of Iraq and head of a new government. However, the country was far from independent. The British:

● kept control of Iraq's foreign policy and kept two airbases (near Basra and Baghdad)
● controlled the oil: they did this through the British-owned Iraqi Petroleum Company which owned, drilled and sold all of Iraq's oil.

Discontent

The monarchy lasted 35 years. During this time Iraq saw considerable economic development. Education was improved and more people learned to read and write. However there was much discontent:

● Inequality: the country was dominated by a small number of big landowners while the vast majority of the population was very poor.
● Israel: Britain supported the new Jewish state of Israel in 1948 against the opposition of the Arab states.
● Control of oil: in 1952, the Iraqi government agreed with the Iraqi Petroleum Company that profits from Iraqi oil would be shared equally between the Iraqi government and the British-dominated company. However the company still controlled production and prices.

Republic

In 1958 the monarchy was overthrown and Iraq became a republic. After another coup by army officers in 1968 the republic was ruled by the Baath Party. Most Baathists were Sunni Muslims. The Sunnis had been the dominant group in Iraq ever since the state of Iraq was set up in 1921, although the Shiites formed the majority of the population. Many Shiites were now brought into the new government in a show of unity.

Saddam Hussein

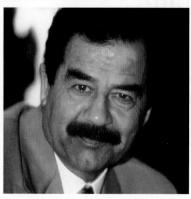

- Born in 1937 into a poor peasant family in Takrit, near Baghdad.
- He was named Saddam and is always referred to by this name.
- He never knew his father, who disappeared before he was born, and he was brought up by his uncle.
- He failed to gain admission to the military academy and, at the age of 20, he became a Baath Party activist.
- In 1963 he became head of the Iraqi Intelligence Services.
- He was Vice-President from 1968 to 1979 when he became President.
- As President, he was ruthless in eliminating his rivals.
- Many of his closest advisers came from the same Takrit clan as he did and several members of his close family, including his two sons, held important posts in government.
- In 1980, he went to war with neighbouring Iran. The war was to last for eight years yet, two years after it ended, his forces invaded Kuwait.
- In 2003, his government was overthrown by invading US forces and, in 2006, he was executed, after trial by an Iraqi court, for crimes against humanity.

SOURCE 2

In July 1969 another eighty prominent Iraqis were on trial for espionage. They were merely the prelude to thousands of hangings, almost all for 'espionage' and 'spying'. Eleven years later, when Saddam Hussein was confirmed in power, Iraqi hangmen were dispatching victims to the gallows at the rate of a hundred every six weeks.

From *The Great War for Civilisation; The Conquest of the Middle East* by Robert Fisk, who has lived in, and reported from, the Middle East for over 30 years.

The rise of Saddam Hussein

One of the Baathists who had played a key role in the 1968 coup/takeover was Saddam Hussein. As a young man, Saddam had been immersed in the anti-British, anti-Western atmosphere of the Arab world in the late 1950s and the 1960s. He had been involved in the overthrow of the pro-British monarchy in 1958 and played a key role in the coup of 1968. He was made Vice-President, serving under a much older President. However, it was Saddam who emerged as the strong man of the regime. How was he able to do this?

A strong power base

You may have read about Stalin if your chosen Depth Study is Russia 1905–41. Stalin came to power there by building up support within the Communist Party. By the time he was challenging for power there was a wide network of people in the USSR who owed their jobs to Stalin and thought they might be promoted if they stayed loyal to him. We know Saddam was an admirer of Stalin, and he used similar methods to build up his own power.

To begin with, he made sure that he had control of key positions within the ruling Baath Party and he also controlled the most important departments in the government and the army. You can see how he did this in the Factfile. In Iraq, family and tribal connections were (and still are) a very important source of power. Saddam placed family and friends in positions of power.

The other main source of power in Iraq was the army. Saddam placed friends and allies in important positions here, too. He also kept the military commanders happy by spending on defence.

Popularity

In 1972, the government nationalised, and took complete control of, the Iraqi oil industry, despite the opposition of the British. This was a daring and popular move. Saddam oversaw the process of nationalisation and used Iraq's oil wealth to build up education, health and welfare services that were among the best in the Arab world. He was recognised with an award from the United Nations for creating the most modern public health system in the Middle East.

Then, in 1973, the Iraqis joined other Arab oil-producing states in reducing oil production and sales to Western countries. This was done to punish the West, for supporting Israel in a war against the Arab states of Egypt and Syria. However, it also had the effect of driving up oil prices by 400 per cent. Iraq's income from oil was to rise from $575 million in 1972 to $26,500 million in 1980.

As the country became richer, Saddam improved the national economy: electricity was extended to the countryside; agriculture was increasingly mechanised; and roads, bridges, hospitals, schools and dams were built. The Iraqis became more educated and healthcare improved. An urban middle class of lawyers, businessmen and government officials emerged.

Control

Saddam and the Baathists became much more powerful, extending their control over Iraqi government and society. Trade unions, schools and even sports clubs came under state control and membership of the Baath Party determined who was appointed to positions in the government. The main aim of education was to immunise the young against foreign culture and promote Arab unity and 'love of order'. Saddam Hussein said that the ideal student was one who could 'stand in the sun holding his weapon day and night without flinching'.

Repression

In 1976, Saddam was made a general in the army. By now he was the effective leader of Iraq as the President became increasingly frail. Saddam extended government control over the army and the secret police. High military spending kept the armed forces happy, but they were also kept under control by regular indoctrination, by rotating the officers (so that none could build up opposition) and by the imprisonment and execution of those suspected of disloyalty.

Repression was extended throughout Iraqi society. There were increasing reports of torture and rape of those held in prison. The secret police, under Saddam's control, came to dominate both the army and the Baath Party. Most of its recruits came from rural, tribal areas in the Sunni-dominated region to the north and west of Baghdad and many were from Saddam's own tribe. In 1979, Saddam Hussein forced the ailing President to resign and he formally became President of Iraq.

Focus Task

Why was Saddam Hussein able to come to power in Iraq?

1 Work in pairs or groups. Create cards which set out the key factors which brought Saddam to power: power base; popularity; control; repression. Write each one on a separate card.
2 On the back of each card, note down as briefly as you can how Saddam made use of each factor.
3 Look for connections between the factors on your cards.
4 Now use your cards to help you write an essay (of 150–300 words) in answer to the question. It could consist of four main paragraphs, beginning like this:
   a) He built up a strong power base.
   b) He pursued policies which made him popular.
   c) He shaped and controlled Iraqi life.
   d) He used indoctrination and terror to control people.
5 Finally, in a conclusion, decide which of the reason(s) are most important and explain why.

What was the nature of Saddam Hussein's rule in Iraq?

Once he took power, Saddam held on to it for another 25 years, despite several plots against him and defeats in two wars. Becoming President in 1979 did not mark any change in policy. In many ways he continued to rule Iraq in similar ways to those he had used before 1979. He combined the 'stick' of terror, and indoctrination, with the 'carrot' of social and infrastructure improvements. But the big change was that each aspect was taken to a new level. He was very skilful in exploiting rivalries between different groups in Iraq to divide his enemies. When he came to power in 1979 he carried out a brutal purge of anyone who might be a threat to him. Around 500 members of his own party were executed. Many more were arrested or fled the country.

'Show trials'

Saddam was an admirer of Stalin's use of terror to enforce submission. Saddam's presidency started with the televised trial of a number of opponents; 21 were later executed. There had always been repression, but Saddam raised the level, terrorising his own party as well as opponents. Baath party members faced the death penalty for joining another party. There were many attempts to overthrow Saddam and they were met with overwhelming violence. After an attempt to assassinate him in the village of Dujail to the north of Baghdad in 1982, he ordered his security forces to kill nearly 150 villagers in retaliation.

The cult of leadership

Saddam became more aggressive towards Israel. He condemned Egypt for making a peace treaty with Israel in 1979. At home Saddam was glorified by the media, who portrayed him as the leader and protector of the Arab world as well as his own people. There were statues of him everywhere, his portraits hung in all public buildings and his birthday was made a national holiday. When a referendum was held on his presidency, 99 per cent of Iraqis voted in support.

SOURCE 3

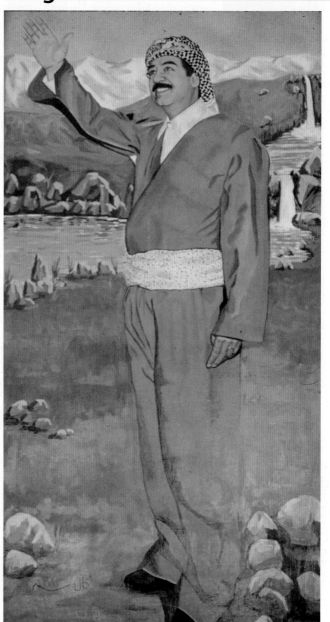

A poster of Saddam Hussein published in Iraq in 1989.

The Kurds

Iraq's population was made up of three main groups: Shia Muslims (the majority), Sunni Muslims and Kurds. Ever since the state of Iraq was created in 1921, the Kurds had enjoyed a certain amount of self-rule, but many of their leaders were determined to achieve a separate homeland, Kurdistan. However, Saddam wanted the opposite. He was determined to extend *his* government's control over the Kurdish north.

In 1974–75, his forces attacked the Kurds. Many of their leaders were executed or driven into exile and the Kurds lost much of their self-government. The Kurds stood little chance but they did get help from Iran. Iranian help increased when Iran and Iraq went to war in 1980 (see page 158). As a result the Kurds gained greater control of Kurdish northern Iraq. Saddam saw this as a betrayal. In March 1988 Saddam's planes bombarded the Kurdish town of Halabja using chemical weapons (see Source 4). This was one of the episodes for which Saddam Hussein was later put on trial, found guilty and executed.

Factfile

The Kurds

➤ The Kurds form about 20 per cent of the population of Iraq.
➤ They are mostly situated in the north, especially along the borders with Syria, Turkey and Iran (see Source 1 on page 148).
➤ There are millions of Kurds inside these neighbouring countries as well as in Iraq itself. However, the Iraqi Kurds were probably the most organised.
➤ The Kurds are Muslim but not Arab and they speak a different language.
➤ There had been almost constant conflict between Iraqi troops and Kurdish nationalist fighters from the time the state of Iraq was created in 1921.
➤ Since the end of the monarchy in 1958, some Kurds and many Shiites had done well and become better off in Iraq as long as they proved loyal. But, under Saddam, there were mass expulsions.

Dead bodies – human and animal – littered the streets, huddled in doorways, slumped over the steering wheels of their cars. Survivors stumbled around, laughing hysterically, before collapsing. Those who had been directly exposed to the gas found that their symptoms worsened as the night wore on. Many children died along the way and were abandoned where they fell.

An eyewitness account quoted in T. McDowall, *A Modern History of the Kurds*, p. 358.

Source Analysis

1 How far do Sources 4, 5 and 6 agree about the treatment of the Kurds by Iraqi forces?
2 Which of Sources 4, 5 and 6 are more useful for the historian studying the massacre at Halabja in northern Iraq?

SOURCE **6**

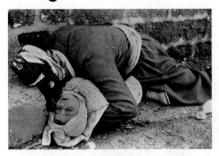

A scene from the Kurdish town of Halabja, in northern Iraq, in March 1988. The Iraqi air force had attacked the town with chemical weapons, including mustard gas and cyanide.

Revision Tip

Saddam Hussein maintained his hold on power by use of terror and indoctrination and by crushing the opposition. Make sure you can remember examples of how:
♦ he crushed opposition
♦ he used the cult of personality
♦ some Iraqis benefited from Saddam's rule
♦ Shiites suffered.

Saddam's solution to the 'Kurdish problem'

When the war with Iran ended in July 1988, Saddam decided to solve the 'Kurdish problem' once and for all. He set out to depopulate much of the Kurdish north and destroy the Kurdish nationalist movement. His cousin, later nicknamed 'Chemical Ali' by the Kurds, was put in charge. Saddam's forces used chemical weapons and carried out mass executions as well as bulldozing villages. About 180,000 Kurds were killed and at least another 100,000 refugees fled into neighbouring Turkey. It was not until the first Gulf War that the situation of the Kurds improved (see page 164).

SOURCE **5**

Some groups of prisoners were lined up, shot from the front, and dragged into pre-dug mass graves; others were made to lie down in pairs, sardine-style, next to mounds of fresh corpses, before being killed; still others were tied together, made to stand on the tip of the pit, and shot in the back so that they would fall forward into it. Bulldozers then pushed earth or sand loosely over the heaps of corpses.

From a report gathered by the pressure group Human Rights Watch, and based on the testimonies of several eyewitnesses.

Repression of the Shiite Iraqis

Shiites, who form the majority of the population in the south and centre of Iraq, continued to suffer persecution under Saddam Hussein's rule. In the early days of Baath rule, some had prospered. Many of the rank-and-file Baath party members were Shiite. Most Shiites wanted greater *inclusion* in Iraqi government and society, not the *separatism* that many Kurds wanted. However, after the Islamic revolution in neighbouring Shiite Iran in 1979 (see page 155), Saddam became increasingly suspicious of the Shiite majority in Iraq. In 1980–81, 200,000 Shiites were deported to Iran as their 'loyalty was not proven'. Many of them were successful businessmen whose businesses were then handed over to the government's supporters.

Infrastructure

At the same time Saddam continued to use Iraq's immense oil revenue to improve the health, education and other services for the people of Iraq. As you have already read, he brought electricity and similar improvements to rural villages. Daily life for many ordinary Iraqis improved due to improved road transport and water supplies. Access to university education and high quality health care was free. Painters, musicians and other artists, helped by government subsidies, flourished. Saddam even introduced penalties for avoiding literacy classes and bullied his own ministers to lose weight to set an example to the people. There was freedom of religious worship and government in Iraq was relatively free from corruption. However, all of these benefits depended on people not getting on the wrong side of the regime.

Focus Task

What was the nature of Saddam Hussein's rule in Iraq?

Divide into groups. Each group should take one of the following themes and build up a detailed picture of this aspect of Saddam's rule.
♦ **Use of terror**, especially in his treatment of non-Sunni peoples in Iraq.
♦ **Indoctrination and the cult of leadership**, for example, his control of education and his portrayal as a national and Arab hero.
♦ **Development of Iraq's infrastructure**, i.e. the facilities, services and communications needed for the country to function properly.
You might also think of things which do not fit easily into any of these categories (such as Saddam giving preferential treatment to people from his own clan or region), or which would be appropriate in more than one category.
Now write an essay of 200–400 words to answer the question: 'Terror, and terror alone, explains Saddam Hussein's success in holding on to power.' How far do you agree with this interpretation?

Why was there a revolution in Iran in 1979?

You are now going to leave Iraq for a while, to study what was going on in Iraq's neighbour Iran. The events overlap with those you have already studied.

Iran and the British

At the start of the twentieth century, Iran was ruled by a Shah. Iran was an independent country (not part of anyone's empire) but its oil fields were controlled by a British company (Anglo-Iranian Oil) that paid the Shah's government for the right to operate them.

After the Second World War, an increasing number of Iranians demanded that their government take control of the oil fields. They insisted that Iranians should receive at least half of the oil profits. The leading Iranian nationalist Mohammed Mossadeq, said: 'The oil resources of Iran, like its soil, its rivers and mountains, are the property of the people of Iran.'

He gained huge popular support and, in 1951, the Shah made him Prime Minister. The Iranian Parliament then passed a law to nationalise the oil industry. This defiant move thrilled the Iranians. Many in the Arab world also applauded and Mossadeq became a hero to millions, both in and beyond Iran.

In retaliation, the British company withdrew its workforce and refused to allow any of its technicians to work with the new Iranian National Oil Company. The British also persuaded other Western oil companies not to buy Iran's oil and the British navy imposed a blockade of Iran's ports, refusing to allow any ships to enter or leave.

Source Analysis ▼

1 What impression does the cartoon in Source 7 give of Mossadeq and of Britain?
2 What is the message of this cartoon?

SOURCE **7**

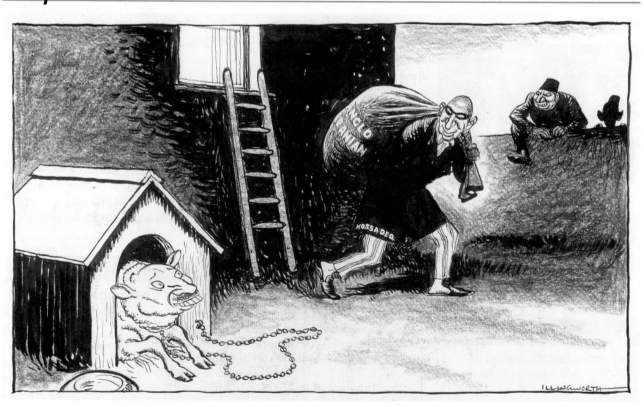

A British cartoon from October 1951. The animal in the kennel represents the British Prime Minister, Clement Attlee. The bag is marked Anglo-Iranian and the man is marked Mossadeq.

The overthrow of Mossadeq's government, 1953

Iran's income from oil sales dwindled but Mossadeq remained hugely popular for standing up to the West and asserting Iran's independence. The British persuaded the USA to join them in overthrowing Mossadeq. They played on America's fear of Communism. This was at the height of the Cold War and Iran had a long border with Soviet Russia. What might happen if the Soviet Union extended its influence into Iran and even got its hands on Iran's oil!

So under pressure from the Americans and the British the Shah dismissed Mossadeq and replaced him with a more pro-Western Prime Minister. Mossadeq was put on trial and imprisoned and the Iranian Parliament was closed down.

Following this coup:

● A group of Western oil companies agreed with the Shah to restart production in return for a 40 per cent share in Iran's oil profits.
● The Shah's new government signed a treaty with the USA in 1955 and, a year later, joined Britain, Turkey and Iraq in an anti-Soviet alliance. For the West, the Shah was a useful ally in the Middle East: reliably anti-Soviet and guardian of much of the West's oil supplies.
● Iran grew rich on income from the oil industry, which the National Iranian Oil Company now controlled. The Shah made some reforms – he transferred some of Iran's land from the biggest landowners to poorer farmers; he gave women the vote; he increased the number of schools and raised literacy rates, but there was still a vast contrast between the rich elite and the poor masses.

Opposition to the Shah

In the 1970s the Shah faced increasing opposition. With the parliament suppressed, the opposition was led by was led by the mullahs (Muslim religious leaders). In the mosques, especially at the weekly, Friday prayers, the mullahs criticised the wealth, luxury and corruption of the Shah and his supporters. In 1971, the Shah held a huge celebration of what he claimed was the 2500th anniversary of the Persian monarchy. Very few believed the claim. Worse still, for most Iranians, it was seen as far too extravagant at a cost of $330 million, especially in a country where millions struggled to feed themselves.

They also criticised the Shah's close relations with the non-Muslim West. Many saw the Shah as a pawn in the hands of the USA, being exploited for American gain. He even supported the existence of the state of Israel. The mullahs encouraged street demonstrations which targeted banks, because of their close ties to Western companies, or cinemas which showed mostly foreign, often sexual, films. These were felt to be unIslamic.

In response, the Shah's secret police arrested, exiled, imprisoned and tortured thousands of the government's critics, including mullahs. The outstanding leader of the opposition was Ayatollah Khomeini, a leading Muslim scholar. Like many other Muslim religious leaders, he had been forced into exile by the Shah's government. At first, in 1964, he went to Turkey, later Iraq and, finally, Paris. From here, his writings and speeches were smuggled into Iran, often in the form of cassette tapes.

The Islamic Revolution 1979

In 1978, there were huge strikes and demonstrations calling on the Shah to abdicate. Every time the Shah's army and police killed people in these protests, there followed even bigger demonstrations, often a million-strong in the capital, Tehran. In September 1978, the government introduced military rule and, the next day, troops killed over 500 people in a massive demonstration. In October, there was a wave of strikes which brought most industry, including oil production, to a halt.

By the end of 1978 some soldiers were refusing to fire on crowds. Many of them, especially conscripts, sympathised with the protestors. Meanwhile, the Shah's advisers assured him that he was still popular and that it was only a minority of agitators who were misleading people and causing the protests.

In January 1979, the Shah left Iran in order to receive treatment for cancer. He never returned. Instead, the 76-year-old Khomeini returned in triumph amid huge celebrations, and declared an Islamic Revolution. The Shah's last prime minister fled the country and most of the army declared support for the revolution. A national referendum produced a large majority in favour of abolishing the monarchy and establishing an Islamic republic.

Source Analysis

Study Sources 8 and 9.
1 Do they prove that ordinary Iranians supported the revolution?
2 Is one source more convincing as evidence than the other? Explain your answers.

SOURCE 9

Numerous eyewitnesses have commented on the almost universal enthusiasm, discipline, mutual cooperation and the organisation which added to the spirit and extent of the last months of the revolution and distributed supplies and heating oil during the revolutionary strikes.

Written in 2003 by historian Nikki Keddie, an expert on Iranian history who has written several books, over 40 years, on the subject.

SOURCE 8

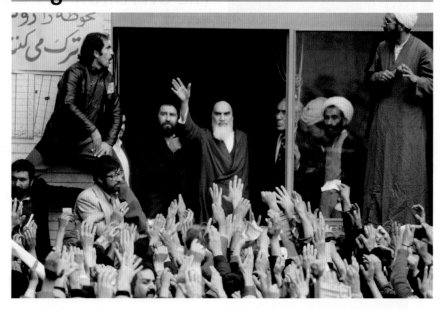

Ayatollah Khomeini waving to a crowd of enthusiastic supporters on his return to Tehran, February 1979.

Focus Task

Extravagance in a country where many are poor	Role of Khomeini
Foreign films	Hatred of the secret police
Pro-Western foreign policy	Importance of mullahs and mosques
Strikes and demonstrations	Huge Western profits from oil
Banks closely tied to the West	Killing of protestors led to bigger demonstrations and more strikes

Why was there a revolution in Iran in 1979?

1 Here are some factors which help to explain the 1979 revolution. Work in groups to decide how the factors could be grouped, and also how some factors are connected to each other. Possible groups might be:
 ♦ dislike of Western influence
 ♦ religious leaders' opposition to Shah
 ♦ the Shah's attitude towards opponents.
 You can probably think of other groupings – and remember some factors may be relevant to more than one group.

2 Use the results of your sorting exercise to write an essay to answer this question: 'The main reason for the revolution in Iran in 1979 was the Shah's close relations with the West.' To what extent do you agree with this view?
 ♦ It is probably best to start by selecting reasons which support this view and explain why they are important.
 ♦ Then select other reasons, some of which may also be connected to the Shah's close relations with the West. This second part of your answer will contain more short-term reasons such as the growing opposition in the late 1970s.
 ♦ Finally, you need to make a judgement about the extent to which the Shah's overthrow was a result of his closeness to the West.

Revision Tip

The Shah's government was overthrown because of its unpopular, pro-Western policies and replaced by an Islamic republic. Make sure you can remember the role of the following in overthrowing the Shah:
♦ Ayatollah Khomeini
♦ anti-Western feeling/opinion
♦ injustices and inequalities in Iran.

Ayatollah Khomeini

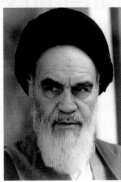

➤ Born in 1902, he was brought up by his mother following the murder of his father in 1903. He had a traditional religious education.

➤ He spent much of his life in studying, writing and teaching Islamic law, philosophy and ethics.

➤ Became an ayatollah in the early 1920s. The term 'ayatollah' is used by Shia Muslims to refer to the most senior religious scholars.

➤ From 1964 to 1979 Khomeini lived in exile.

➤ He was popular in Iran for his opposition to the Shah and the Shah's dependence on the USA, for his simple lifestyle and language, and his religious beliefs.

➤ He reminded people that Muhammad, the founder of Islam, had established and ruled over an Islamic state in Arabia in the seventh century AD. In other words, Muhammad had been a political as well as a religious leader. As Khomeini said: 'Islam is politics or it is nothing.'

The establishment of an Islamic state

Despite the huge support for the Ayatollah, there were other groups competing for power in Iran. For instance, there was the Communist Party and there were middle-class liberals who wanted a Western-style democracy. However, it was Ayatollah Khomeini's supporters, organised in the Islamic Republican Party, who came to dominate Parliament and hold key positions in the government. Although Khomeini was not president or prime minister, he held ultimate power as the 'supreme leader' of Shiite Iran. He had the final say in government and law-making. New laws, based on the Koran, the Muslim holy book, were passed: education was purged of unIslamic influences; women had to cover their heads in public; and alcohol, Western pop music and most Western films were banned. There were also mass trials of the Shah's former supporters and many were executed.

Khomeini and his government were keen to spread the Islamic revolution to what they saw as the corrupt, unIslamic regimes in other parts of the Muslim world. Above all, they denounced the ties which bound other states to the West.

The storming of the US embassy, November 1979

The USA, the former ally of the Shah, was seen as the main enemy in Iran and came to be known as 'the Great Satan'. When the US government allowed the Shah into America to receive medical treatment in November 1979, Iranian students stormed the US embassy in Tehran, and took 50 of the American staff as hostages. The US government declared Iran to be an international 'outlaw'. Yet millions in the Muslim world, both Arab and non-Arab, admired Khomeini for standing up to the West.

Meanwhile neighbouring Iraq was a prime target for the export of the Islamic revolution. It had a completely secular, non-religious government and a growing religious opposition. It also had a large Shiite population, who were excluded from top positions in government. Khomeini accused the Iraq government of being 'atheist' and 'corrupt' and, in one of his broadcasts to the people of Iraq, he called on them to: 'Wake up and topple this corrupt regime in your Islamic country before it is too late.'

Think!

It is December 1979. You are a Western journalist who has been asked to review the first twelve months of the Islamic republic for people who know very little about it. You should explain:

1 Why was an Islamic government established?
2 What form it takes e.g. is it democratic or a one-party state? Is there a parliament?
3 What is the role of Khomeini?
4 What reforms have been passed?
5 What are its policies towards:
  a) other Muslim countries?
  b) the USA?

Revision Tip

Make sure you can:
♦ describe two aims of the Khomeini regime
♦ explain one reason why it was hostile to the USA
♦ give an example of one other country in the region which might be concerned about the new regime.

What were the causes and consequences of the Iran–Iraq War 1980–88?

In 1980 Saddam Hussein decided to invade Iran. Why did he do this?

- The Iranian leader, Ayatollah Khomeini, had called on Iraqis to rise up and overthrow Saddam Hussein. The majority of Iraq's population were Shi'ite Muslims whereas Saddam and his allies were Sunni Muslims. Saddam saw Khomeini's influence as a potentially very serious threat.
- Saddam had evidence that Iran was involved in the assassination of leading members of the Baathist Party in Iraq. He feared they were now plotting to overthrow him as well.
- Saddam saw an opportunity to gain valuable territory.
  - As you can see from Source 1 Iraq's access to the sea was very narrow while Iran had a long coastline and several ports through which to export its oil (see map in Source 13). Iraq wanted to gain complete control of the Shatt al-Arab waterway to gain a secure outlet to the sea.
  - At the same time Saddam thought he might be able to seize parts of oil-rich, south-west Iran.
- Iran was weak so now seemed the ideal time to attack.
  - It's economy was in chaos following the fall of the Shah's regime.
  - The country was facing a western boycott of its trade because of the capture of the US embassy.
  - The Iranian armed forces were demoralised.

Saddam saw an opportunity to exploit Iran's weak position. He planned a short, limited war which would force Iran to make concessions, but more importantly would warn Iran that Iraq would not be intimidated or undermined. He hoped war would not only strengthen his regime but also would make Iraq the leading power in the oil-rich Gulf.

Revision Tip

Make sure you can explain:
- one way in which oil was an important cause of the war
- one other factor which caused the war.

Focus Task

Why did Iraq invade Iran in 1980?

The text gives various reasons for the invasion. Which of them are examples of:
- concern for the security of Saddam's Iraq
- opportunism
- a desire to enrich Iraq
- territorial ambition (to gain more land)?

Some will be examples of more than one of these. Explain which one you think figured most prominently in Saddam's mind.

The war reaches stalemate

When Iraqi forces invaded Iran in September 1980, there was little resistance and most observers felt that Iraq would soon win. Saddam himself predicted a 'whirlwind war', confident that a swift, heavy blow would dislodge Khomeini's government. He was soon proved wrong.

Within a month Iraqi forces were halted in the Iranian desert. They now resorted to firing missiles at Iran's cities in order to terrorise the civilian population. So began the so-called 'War of the Cities' in which both sides bombed and killed hundreds of thousands of civilians.

Iraq had superior firepower but Iran, with its much bigger population, sent in hundreds of thousands of new recruits, in 'human waves', many of them fired up with revolutionary enthusiasm, willing to become martyrs – to sacrifice their lives for the Islamic revolution. A message left by one young Iranian soldier for his parents was typical: 'Don't cry mother, because I am happy. I am not dead. Dear father, don't cry because you will be proud when you realise I am a martyr.' Most Iranians believed they were fighting for good against evil.

Source Analysis

1 How far do Sources 10, 11 and 12 agree about the importance of religion in this war?

SOURCE **10**

The Iranian front lines tend to be scenes of chaos and dedication, with turbaned mullahs, rifles slung on their backs, rushing about on brightly coloured motorcycles encouraging the troops. Religious slogans are posted everywhere, and sometimes reinforcements arrive cheerfully carrying their own coffins as a sign of willingness to be 'martyred'.

A description by a reporter of what he observed on the Iranian battle front.

SOURCE **11**

My involvement in the war was a reflection of the nature of our Islamic revolution. It was based on a new interpretation of religion – getting involved in the war was a sacred duty. We were led by a prophet-like statesman Khomeini so this is how we perceived the war. This was the reason for our overwhelming commitment. The war could not be separated from our religion.

An Iranian man tells the British journalist, Robert Fisk, what had motivated him when he went to the war front in 1984.

SOURCE **12**

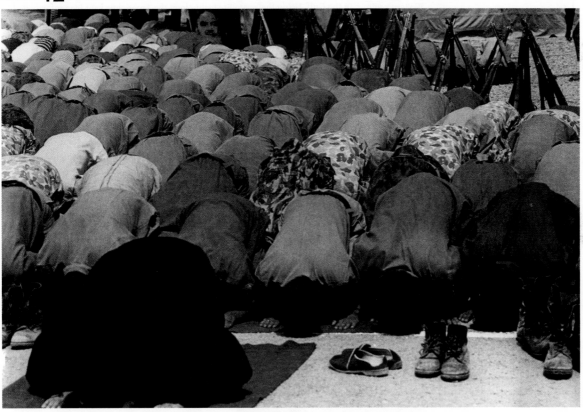

Members of the Iranian Basiji (mobilized volunteer forces) pray behind a cleric, their weapons stacked to one side, during military training in Tehran, Iran, during the Iran-Iraq War, 6th November 1981.

Within two years, Iran had recaptured all of its land and had cut off Iraq from its only sea ports. There were calls for a ceasefire but these came to nothing because Iran said it would not settle for anything less than the overthrow of Saddam's regime.

When Iran stated that its target was to seize Baghdad, the Iraqi capital, the Iraqi forces became more united in their determination to defend their country. By 1984, the two sides were bogged down in trench warfare along the 1,000-mile border. It was similar, in this way, to the fighting in the trenches on the western front in the First World War except that sand, not mud, was what bogged the soldiers down.

Foreign involvement

Most of the Arab states supported Iraq. In particular the Sunni rulers of the Gulf states (see Source 1) had little support for Iran's Islamic revolution. They were opposed to the spread of Iran's revolutionary, Shiite version of an Islamic state. They feared that if it won the war Iran might liberate the Iraqi Shiites and establish an Iraqi state loyal to Khomeini. They feared Iran would stir up the Shiite minorities in their own countries. They also believed Iran posed a threat to their oil fields. So:

● Saudi Arabia and the smaller oil-rich Gulf states, together with Egypt and Jordan, supplied money and arms to Iraq

● Jordan also provided a route for Iraq's imports and exports through the port of Aqaba (see Source 1). This was vital for Iraq when her access to the Gulf was cut off by Iranian forces.

Syria, however, supported Iran because of intense rivalry with its neighbour, Iraq. The Syrians shut the Iraqi pipelines which passed through its territory to the Mediterranean. In return, Syria received free Iranian oil.

France, Germany and the Soviet Union also sided with Iraq, as did the USA. They were all bitterly opposed to the new regime in Iran. France became the main non-Arab supplier of arms to Iraq. America's support became more active when the Iranians counter-attacked and talked of advancing on Baghdad. The thought of the revolutionary Iranians controlling so much of the oil in the Gulf terrified the Americans as well as most of the Arab states. Khomeini might then be able to control world oil prices! Furthermore, an Iranian victory might lead to the collapse of pro-Western regimes in the Gulf. Using their satellite technology, the Americans kept Iraq informed of Iranian troop movements. They also provided Iraq with equipment which was later used to make chemical weapons and, like the Arab states, they turned a blind eye when these were used against the Iranians.

From 1986 the fighting was focused on the Gulf, the vital route through which both Iraq and Iran exported their oil. Each side attacked the enemy's oil installations and tankers. The Iraqi air force controlled the skies but the Iranian navy was stronger. When the Iranians began to attack Kuwaiti ships in retaliation for Kuwait's support for Iraq, the Soviet Union offered to help the Kuwaitis. The USA swiftly stepped in to provide protection for Kuwaiti ships, both to pre-empt further Soviet aid and to maintain its influence with the oil-rich Gulf states. When the Iranians cut off Iraq's access to the Gulf through the Shatt al-Arab waterway (see Source 13), the US provided protection for Iraqi shipping and destroyed much of the Iranian navy.

SOURCE **13**

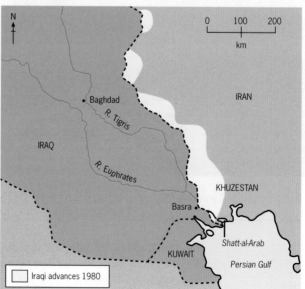

This map shows some of the main areas of fighting in the Iran–Iraq War.

Revision Tip

Make sure you can:
♦ describe how one other state became involved in the war
♦ explain one reason why other states became involved in the war.

Ceasefire, 1988

In July 1988, the Iranians finally accepted a ceasefire. Their economy was in ruins, the stream of 'martyrs' had subsided and they faced the prospect of a direct war with the USA. There was no peace treaty, only a truce, and both sides continued to re-arm.

It had been one of the longest and most destructive wars since the Second World War. No one knows the exact casualties but it is estimated that nearly a million Iranians and half a million Iraqis had died. Although there had been a stalemate between the two sides for much of the war, the 'War of the Cities' had killed many civilians and caused massive destruction. There was brutality, on a huge scale, by both sides.

Both sides had hoped that minority ethnic groups within the enemy country would rise up and welcome the invaders. That did not happen. National feelings proved stronger in both cases. No doubt terror played a part too: they feared what might happen to their families if they went over to the other side.

Consequences for Iran

Khomeini said that he found agreeing to a ceasefire 'more deadly than poison'. He died a year later, in 1989. Despite eight years of warfare, in which hundreds of thousands had died, he was still revered by millions of Iranians for his proud, defiant stand after years of humiliation by stronger powers. Twelve million people filled the streets of Tehran for his funeral, lining the streets leading to the cemetery. The Islamic Republic continued to attract wide support in Iran.

Although Iran suffered widespread destruction and huge loss of life, it had a population of 55 million and was still a major power. However, it had not succeeded in exporting its revolutionary, Shiite brand of Islam.

Consequences for Iraq

Iraq's economy and society had also suffered extensive damage. Not only had half a million people been killed, but the health and education of the entire population suffered. During the war, more and more was spent on weapons (accounting for 93 per cent of all imports by 1984) so that less and less was spent on hospitals and schools. Life expectancy fell and infant mortality increased.

When the war ended, the Iraqi government promised its people peace and prosperity. What they got instead was further hardship and more terror. Iraq faced debts of $80 billion yet instead of rebuilding the country, Saddam kept a million men in arms and poured money into developing the most advanced weapons. He had the fourth largest army in the world and, by 1990, he had more aircraft and tanks than Britain and France combined.

The economy was in tatters and there was no post-war recovery: the value of Iraq's oil exports had declined because of war damage and a fall in the oil prices on the world market. Many people in the oil industry lost their jobs and, to make matters worse, thousands of soldiers were demobilised, thus adding to mounting unemployment.

Despite the terror exercised by Saddam's police and army, there were riots and strikes. Some opposition was co-ordinated in the mosques, which were beyond the control of Saddam's police and army. The army would not dare to attack the mosques, the most holy places, because it would intensify the opposition of all Muslims. But the main threat to Saddam came from his army. Many officers felt cheated of victory over Iran and some privately blamed Saddam for the failure to defeat their neighbour. There were several attempts to overthrow him between 1988 and 1990 and many officers were executed for conspiracy. Saddam needed to divert attention away from a growing military crisis in Baghdad. This may have been one of the reasons for the invasion of Kuwait.

Focus Task

What were the consequences of the Iran-Iraq War?

1 From the text above, list the consequences of the war for Iran, for Iraq and for the West.
2 'A war with no winners!' How far do you agree with this description of the Iran–Iraq War? Use your list to support your judgement.

What was Saddam thinking?

I have the most powerful army in the region. I have chemical and biological weapons stockpiled and a nuclear weapons programme underway. Nobody will dare to stand up to me.

Those Kuwaitis have had it coming.

Invading Kuwait will show that I am a serious player in this region.

I will get the concessions I want on oil production and then pull out of Kuwait.

Why did Saddam invade Kuwait in 1990?

Background to the invasion

Kuwait is a small and oil rich state on the southern border of Iraq. Both had been run by Britain after World War 1 but Britain did not leave Kuwait until 1961. When the British left, Iraq had laid claim to Kuwait but other Arab states had sent troops to keep the Iraqis out and Iraq reluctantly recognised Kuwait's independence in 1963.

In 1990 Iraq was again threatening Kuwait. The Iran–Iraq war left Saddam with rising discontent among his own population and even among his military commanders. He also had $80 billion debt to pay off. The only way he could do this was to increase oil production in Iraq. The problem with this was that Iraq was a member of OPEC (Oil Producing and Exporting Countries). OPEC controlled oil production in order to keep prices high — too much production meant the price dropped. Some leading states in OPEC, particularly Kuwait and Saudi Arabia, refused Saddam's request. Worse still, they demanded repayment of funds given to Iraq during the war. Saddam claimed this was an insult as Iraqi lives had defended Kuwait. He also accused Kuwait of drilling under Iraq's borders and taking oil which belonged to Iraq.

Saddam's invasion of Kuwait, August 1990

Facing an increase in discontent at home and a military crisis on his hands, Saddam decided to invade Kuwait. On 2 August 1990, a huge force of 300,000 crossed into Kuwait and overran the country. It took just three days and the rest of the world was taken completely by surprise. However, the international reaction was almost unanimous. Nearly all Arab states condemned Saddam's action while the United Nations Security Council agreed to impose complete trade sanctions against Iraq: no country was to have any trade with Iraq until their forces had withdrawn from Kuwait. These were the most complete and effective sanctions ever imposed by the UN.

Saddam's response to UN sanctions

Saddam, however, was defiant. He declared Kuwait a province of Iraq. He tried to win Arab support by saying that he would withdraw Iraqi forces only when the Israelis withdrew *their* forces from Palestinian lands that had been occupied since 1967. The Palestinians were thrilled but most Arab states still condemned Iraq.

News soon emerged of atrocities committed by Iraqi troops against Kuwaiti citizens: thousands of Kuwaiti protestors were arrested and hundreds were gunned down, often and deliberately in front of their families. Then came news that Saddam had ordered the detention of hundreds of foreigners as hostages, most of whom were Westerners caught in Iraq or Kuwait. This caused outrage. Some of the hostages were used as human shields by being kept near to military targets. Although the women and children, the sick and the old were soon released, there was still widespread condemnation of Iraqi behaviour.

Revision Tip

Make sure you can remember:
♦ one long-term reason and
♦ one short-term reason why Saddam invaded Kuwait in August 1990.

Think!

How do you think the invasion would be reported in a newspaper in your own country? Write a headline and a brief article explaining why Saddam Hussein ordered his forces to invade Kuwait. Your word limit is 200 words.

SOURCE **14**

Our jobs, our way of life, our own freedom and the freedom of friendly countries around the world would all suffer if control of the world's great oil reserves fell into the hands of Saddam Hussein.

US President Bush speaking a fortnight after the Iraqi invasion of Kuwait.

The American reaction

No one was more horrified at the Iraqi invasion of Kuwait than the Americans. Iraqi forces were now massed on Kuwait's border with Saudi Arabia. Many feared that Iraq might also seize the Saudi oil fields, the biggest in the world, and thus gain control of more than half of the world's oil fields.

As long ago as 1957, US President Eisenhower had written to one of his advisers: 'Should a crisis arise threatening to cut the Western world off from the Mid East oil, we would *have* to use force.' When the King of Saudi Arabia requested the USA to send military forces to defend his country in case of attack, the Americans were quick to oblige. Over the next few months, they built up large naval, land and air forces.

Multi-national force

Although some Arab states, like Jordan, preferred an 'Arab' solution to the problem, the majority fully supported the deadline which the UN delivered to Iraq at the end of November: withdraw from Kuwait by 15 January 1991 or face military force.

Saddam predicted the 'mother of all battles'. Over 700,000 troops had been assembled in the deserts of Saudi Arabia. Most were American but Britain and France also sent large forces. Most significant of all was that many Arab countries such as Egypt and Syria sent troops, as did other Muslim countries like Pakistan and Bangladesh. Saudi Arabia itself contributed 100,000 soldiers. In all, 34 countries joined the coalition. It was the broadest coalition ever assembled for a UN operation. Saddam would not be able to claim that this was a Western crusade against the Arabs and Islam.

SOURCE **15**

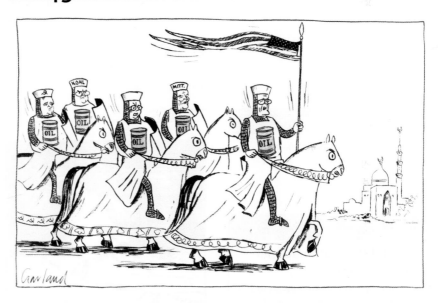

A cartoon by Nicholas Garland, in the British newspaper, the *Independent*, 10 August 1990, six days after Iraqi forces invaded Kuwait. The leading figure represents the US President George Bush, followed in order by the French President, the British Foreign Secretary, the German Chancellor and the Russian Foreign Minister.

Source Analysis ▶

1 To what extent do you think the cartoonist in Source 15 approves the actions of the United Nations?

2 How useful is it for the historian studying the role of the UN in the Kuwait crisis?

3 Nicholas Garland created many cartoons commenting on the Gulf War. Sources 15 and 16 are two examples. You can look up more of his work at www.cartoons.ac.uk.

In 1966, Garland became the first political cartoonist for the *Daily Telegraph*, a paper that is usually seen as right wing whereas Garland came from a left-wing background (both of his parents were Communists). In 1986 he became one of the founders of the *Independent* newspaper. He had freedom to draw what he liked, noting in 1988 that political cartoonists derive most of their impact from their ability to express contrasting views to the rest of the paper.

Do these cartoons tell us more about the cartoonist or the events he portrays? Explain your view.

Think!

There have been many acts of aggression by one country against another since the Second World War, but rarely have so many countries joined together to use military force in order to repel the aggressor. So why did so many countries agree to join the force this time?

Make a table listing the different reasons countries had for joining the multi-national force. Look through the text and sources on pages 162–63 and gather evidence of these reasons. You could work in pairs or small groups.

♦ To punish Iraq
♦ To protect the world's oil supplies
♦ Fear of what Saddam might do next
♦ Motives of USA and other Western countries
♦ Motives of Saudi Arabia and other Arab states
♦ Other reasons

Factfile

Gulf War ceasefire

Peace terms were imposed on Iraq by the UN. These included:

➤ Iraq had to recognise Kuwait's sovereignty

➤ Iraq had to pay reparations (war damages)

➤ Iraqi aircraft could not enter the 'no-fly zones' in the Kurdish north and the south

➤ Iraq had to comply with weapons inspections from the UN to uncover and destroy all weapons of mass destruction (WMD). WMD are biological, chemical or nuclear weapons that could be used to kill as many people as possible

➤ Until all WMD were destroyed the UN imposed wide-ranging trade sanctions (which virtually cut off Iraq from the rest of the world).

The Gulf War, January–March 1991

The war to liberate Kuwait became known as the Gulf War (and later 'The First Gulf War'). It began with a five-week air assault on military targets but also on airports, bridges, factories and roads. The coalition forces had complete air superiority and the most powerful air force in the world armed with the most up-to-date weapons. Saddam hoped world opinion would turn against the coalition but his hopes came to nothing. He tried to involve Israel by firing missiles in the hope that this would cause a split between the West and their Arab allies. The US persuaded the Israelis not to retaliate and the Arab members of the US-led coalition stayed firm.

In February, the ground attack began. The Iraqi forces were no match for the coalition and were quickly defeated with heavy casualties. US and coalition troops were better trained, better equipped and more motivated than many of the reluctant conscripts in the Iraqi army. They were also backed by fearsome air power including helicopter gunships. As they retreated, Iraqi forces tried to wreck Kuwait by pouring oil into the Gulf and setting fire to the oilfields. With the Iraqis driven out of Kuwait the US-led forces continued into Iraq itself. The US President called on the Kurds in the north and the Shiites in the south to rise up and overthrow Saddam. They both responded, but they lacked arms and received no support from US troops. In the Shia south, about 50,000 were killed by Saddam's forces and similar reprisals were expected in the Kurdish north. With a humanitarian catastrophe looming, media coverage rallied world opinion and forced the USA and Britain to act. The Americans and British established 'no-fly zones', which prevented Saddam regaining control of the north. A 'safe haven' was created for the Kurds who have been effectively in control of their areas ever since.

The coalition forces stopped short of Baghdad. There were strong voices in the US government that wanted to go further and get rid of Saddam Hussein altogether. However their UN mission had been restricted to the liberation of Kuwait and America's Arab allies would not have supported an American overthrow of Saddam. The coalition would have split if the Americans had attacked Baghdad. Many Arab commentators believed that the United States used the war to establish its military presence in the Gulf and to dominate the world's oil resources. On 28 February, a ceasefire was called (see Factfile).

Source Analysis ▶

Using the information on pages 164–165 explain the message of Source 16.

Focus Task

Why did the multi-national force succeed?

'The attempt to liberate Kuwait was a very risky operation because Saddam had 300,000 troops in Kuwait and a further 700,000 in Iraq. He had huge numbers of tanks and aircraft and a stockpile of chemical weapons. It is therefore surprising that the coalition forces even tried to liberate Kuwait and even more surprising that they succeeded.'

Build an argument against this statement and use the sources and information on pages 162–166 as evidence to support your view. Try to keep your argument under 150 words long.

SOURCE 16

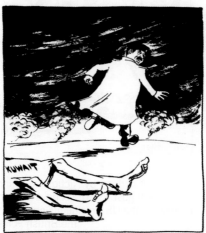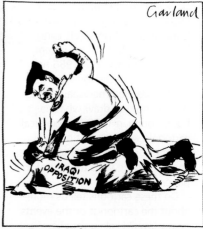

A cartoon by Nicholas Garland, from the British newspaper, the *Daily Telegraph*, 8 March 1991, a week after the ceasefire.

SOURCE **17**

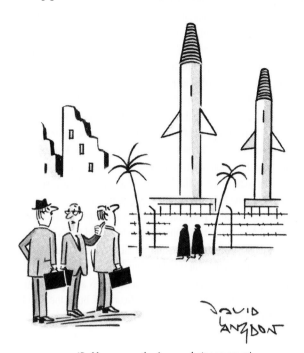

'Saddam swears they're new design mosques'

A Punch cartoon by David Langdon published in 1991

Weapons inspections

A month after the ceasefire, the United Nations Special Committee (UNSCOM) started to search for and destroy Iraq's weapons of mass destruction. Because of the serious effect of sanctions Iraq co-operated. It admitted that it had stockpiled nerve gas and chemical warheads. The UN inspectors uncovered a nuclear programme with several kilograms of highly enriched uranium, necessary for the production of nuclear weapons.

After a year, UNSCOM declared that it had destroyed all medium- and long-range missiles. Three years later, it said it had destroyed all the material for making nuclear and chemical weapons. However, it had not been able to eliminate all of Iraq's biological weapons programme. Nevertheless, by 1995, the Iraqi government was confident that sanctions would soon be lifted and confessed to the production of some anthrax and nerve gas whilst claiming that the stockpiles had been destroyed during the Gulf War. UNSCOM demanded proof but this was not forthcoming.

At this time, Saddam's son-in-law, who had fallen out of favour with Saddam because of a family feud, defected to Jordan. He told those who questioned him in Jordan that, after the Gulf War, Saddam's second son had been given the job of hiding Iraq's weapons of mass destruction. (He was later promised a pardon by Saddam and returned to Baghdad, only to be shot three days later.) The Americans were now increasingly suspicious and distrustful of the Iraqi government and they began to demand 'regime change' (i.e. the removal of Saddam) before they would agree to lift sanctions.

> **Source Analysis** ▲
>
> 1 What is the message of the cartoon in Source 17?
> 2 What does it reveal about people's views on whether Saddam had WMD?

The impact of sanctions on Iraq

Within a short period of time the living conditions of the Iraqi people became increasingly hard:

- A blockade prevented any imports of machinery, fertilisers, most medicines and even books.
- At first Iraq was not allowed to sell oil. After some months sales were allowed but they were strictly limited.
- As Iraq imported much of its food, this had disastrous consequences. A UN survey in the mid-1990s claimed that, in the Baghdad area, a quarter of those under the age of five were 'severely malnourished'. By 1997, 7,000 children were dying each month of hunger and disease.
- Iraq was not allowed to import chlorine to purify water in case it was used in making chemical weapons. The contamination of water led to widespread outbreaks of dysentery. It is reckoned that between a quarter and half a million children died during this period.
- As the humanitarian crisis worsened, the UN came up with a plan in 1996 to allow Iraq to sell its oil in order to buy food. This 'Oil for Food' programme was to be run by the UN. It brought much-needed relief to a desperate people.

Yet sanctions did not increase the opposition to Saddam's regime in Iraq, let alone lead to rebellion. Saddam used violence and terror, as ever, to control resources and reward his most loyal supporters. Disloyal elements in the army were purged, sometimes executed. A special army unit was created to protect the President and nearly all the top jobs in government and the armed forces went to Sunnis, particularly to members of Saddam's own family and tribe.

The roads, bridges and electricity systems in Baghdad and the Sunni areas were largely rebuilt and, although Iraq's WMD programme was depleted, the army was still the biggest in the Arab world. Meanwhile Saddam allowed the filming of mass suffering, especially for Arab television networks, so that the image of Iraq as the victim of the greedy, uncaring West would be propagated. International opinion began to turn against the policy of sanctions.

Focus Task A

How successful were UN sanctions?

Create a table to show your analysis of the following measures of success:

♦ Did they eliminate WMD?
♦ Effects on lives of Iraqis
♦ Effects on the USA's image in the Arab world

For your overall judgement, give a score out of ten and explain it using specific examples.

Iraq emerges from isolation

Saddam did not want to give up all his secret weapons and had always tried to disrupt the UN weapons inspectors. Besides, he knew that the inspection teams were working closely with the US Central Intelligence Agency (CIA) and other Western intelligence agencies. He no doubt suspected that they were planning to overthrow him. When the UN inspection team demanded access to the headquarters of the Iraqi special security services and to the presidential palaces, Saddam refused and, in 1997, the inspectors were forced to leave Iraq. A year later, in 1998, American (and British) planes started bombing Iraqi military sites, despite the commonly-held view that Iraq had no more WMD.

Most Arab states had been happy to see Iraq taught a lesson in 1991 but now the bombing campaign turned many of them against the USA. When the US Secretary of State, Madeleine Albright, was asked on television if the starvation of half a million people was justified, she said it had been 'worth it'. This caused widespread anger in the Arab world and several states started to trade with Iraq again. Iraq was re-emerging from international isolation.

Even the USA seemed to accept the revival of Iraq's oil industry. A growing global economy was pushing up oil prices and several American firms won contracts to rebuild Iraq's oil wells. By 1999 the UN had approved unlimited oil exports from Iraq and Saddam's regime had restored diplomatic relations with all its neighbours. It had got rid of the hated UN inspectors and still had the most feared army in the Arab world. Saddam had challenged both the UN and the USA (now the world's one and only superpower), and he had survived. When George W. Bush, the son of the previous President, was elected President of the USA in 2000, there was renewed talk in Washington of the need to 'remove Saddam'.

Focus Task B

To what extent was Saddam Hussein responsible for conflict in the Gulf region, 1970–2000?

The two most obvious examples of conflict in the Gulf in this period are, of course, the Iran–Iraq War and the Gulf War of 1990–91, but you should also make *some* reference to conflict within states. Some examples are listed in the table below.

1 Copy out and complete this table using what you have found out from your study of this chapter. Some cells have been started for you.

Conflict	Saddam Hussein responsible?	Other states, UN or Western powers responsible?
1970s: conflict and revolution in Iran		
1980: Invasion of Iran	*Saddam ordered the invasion, confident of a quick victory.*	
1980s: The Iran–Iraq war		*Iran said it would not agree to a ceasefire until Saddam's government was overthrown.*
1980s (and especially in 1988): conflict with Kurds and Shiites		
1990: invasion of Kuwait		*Saddam accused the Kuwaitis of producing too much oil so that the price would go down and the Iraqi economy be weakened.*
1990–91: and subsequent war		
1990s Saddam Hussein and UN sanctions		*After the UN inspectors were forced to leave Iraq in 1997, US and British planes bombed Iraqi military sites.*

2 Look back to your prediction on page 148. Do you now think that you got these factors in the right order?

3 Now write an essay in answer to this question. In your conclusion you should make a judgement about the *extent* of Saddam Hussein's role. Do you think he was wholly responsible? Mostly responsible? No more responsible than others? Use the table above to support your answer.

Keywords

Make sure you know what these terms mean and be able to define them confidently.

♦ Arab nationalism
♦ Ayatollah
♦ Baath Party
♦ Chemical weapons
♦ Coup
♦ Martyr
♦ Mullah
♦ Multi-national force
♦ Nationalism
♦ Sanctions
♦ Shia
♦ Shiite
♦ Sunni
♦ Superpowers
♦ WMD (Weapons of Mass Destruction)

Chapter Summary

Why did events in the Gulf matter, c.1970–2000?

Iraq

1 Iraq was ruled by a pro-British monarchy until 1958. Saddam Hussein came to power after the Baathist Party took control in 1968. Saddam nationalised the oil industry and built up Iraq's economy.

2 He held on to power by the use of terror, propaganda and a Sunni-dominated government, and he crushed Kurdish and Shiite opposition.

Iran

3 Iran was ruled by the Shah although the British controlled the oil fields. Prime Minister Mossadeq nationalised the oil industry in 1951 but was overthrown under Anglo–US pressure two years later.

4 Growing opposition led to the downfall of the pro-Western Shah and the establishment of an Islamic republic led by Ayatollah Khomeini in 1979.

Iran–Iraq War, 1980–88

5 Saddam took advantage of Iran's post-revolutionary weakness and invaded his neighbour in 1980. Iraq scored early victories but the Iranians sent in human waves, many of them willing to be martyrs. The 'War of the Cities' led to widespread destruction and a huge death toll.

6 Foreign intervention also intensified the fighting. The Sunni-dominated, Arab Gulf states feared a victory for Shiite revolutionary Iran and supported Iraq, as did the Soviet Union and Western powers. In the oil tanker war that developed after 1986, the US actively supported Iraq.

The Gulf War, 1990–91

7 Iraqi forces invaded Kuwait to gain control of its oil fields and the UN imposed trade sanctions on Iraq.

8 To liberate Kuwait and also prevent a possible Iraqi attack on Saudi oil fields, the US led a huge multi-national force against Iraq. This was supported by most of the Arab states.

9 The Iraqis were driven out of Kuwait and forced to agree to harsh peace terms. UN sanctions were imposed to force Iraq to destroy all its Weapons of Mass Destruction (WMD).

10 Most WMD were destroyed while sanctions hurt the Iraqi population but Saddam remained in power.

Exam Practice

See pages 168–175 and pages 316–319 for advice on the different types of questions you might face.

1 (a) Describe the methods used by Saddam Hussein to consolidate his power in Iraq. **[4]**

(b) Why did Iraq and Iran go to war in 1980? **[6]**

(c) 'Saddam Hussein brought nothing but misery to the Iraqi people.' Explain how far you agree with this statement. **[10]**

2 Study Source 8 on page 156. Why did the revolutionary government of Iran publish this photograph in 1979?

Paper 1: Core Content – Introduction

Structure of the paper

Paper 1 is split into two parts:

Section A: Core content

Section B: Depth studies.

This Exam Focus deals with the core content. See page 316 for advice on the Depth Studies.

- The core content has two options. In this book we have only covered Option B: The 20th Century.
- The exam paper will have four questions on Option B and you have to answer two, so make sure you revise at least two of the seven chapters in Section 1.

Structure of the questions

All core content questions on Paper 1 are similar:

There is a **source** or a **simple statement** to read or look at – however there are no questions on this; it is just to help you to focus your thinking on the topic. Then there are three parts:

a) a **knowledge** question worth 4 marks. This will often begin 'describe' or 'what'

b) an **explanation** question worth 6 marks. This will often begin with 'explain' or 'why'

c) an **evaluation** question worth 10 marks. One common type of question gives you a statement to agree or disagree with. You need to make a judgement and back up your judgement with evidence and argument.

Four key steps

1 Choose questions carefully: Read all the questions carefully before you decide which to answer. You should have revised enough to give you a choice of questions, but don't just immediately opt for your favourite topic – sometimes your less favoured topic might have a question which suits you better.

2 Plan your time: Timing is important – running out of time is NOT unlucky, it is a mistake!

- The core content is worth two-thirds of the marks so you should spend two-thirds of the time on it – i.e. 80 minutes.
- The marks for each question give you a guide as to how long to spend as well.

3 Read the question carefully: This might sound obvious but there is a skill to it.

- Make sure you understand what the question asks you to do: write a description? Write an explanation? Write a comparison?
- Make sure you focus on the right topic and the right sub-topic. Selecting the right material is critical. Think of your knowledge like a wardrobe. You do not wear all of your clothes every day, you select the different clothes for school, going out, sport, cold weather, warm weather, etc. So, if you see a question on the League of Nations it could be on the structure of the League, the League in the 1920s, or one crisis like Abyssinia. Make sure you focus on the right area.
- Make sure you focus on the right time period. For example, if you are facing a question on the Vietnam War make sure whether it is asking about the early stages or the later stages. Focusing on the wrong period could be very costly.

4 Plan your answer: Are you fed up with teachers telling you to plan your answer before you start writing? Well, you are going to be fed up with us as well then because your teachers are right! Just remember this simple advice:

- If you think through your answer first, then writing it is easy. Start by stating your case and then support it.
- If you try to skip the thinking and planning and just start writing, you will make a mess of it because it will not be clear what points you are trying to make. You will also run the danger of running out of time.

1919–39 example questions

These first examples are based on the content of Chapters 1 to 3.

Part (a) questions

These are usually questions which ask you to describe. So, an example of a part (a) question would be:

> What were Germany's main losses under the Treaty of Versailles? **[4]**

Advice on how to answer

These questions are usually straightforward but there are two key things to bear in mind:

- Show that you can select material which is relevant to the question – this is a vital skill for a historian (and in the exam). This question asks about Germany's territorial losses, so do not write about restrictions on the German army!
- Be precise. Many students waste time by over-answering this question – writing far more than is needed. A part (a) question is only 4 marks so make 4 points! You would normally get one mark for each relevant point you make.

It is better to write a paragraph rather than just a list of points. Here is an example we have written of a good answer which would be likely to get full marks. Read it all through and ignore the fact that some of it is crossed out.

> None of the answers on pages 169–179 is a real student answer. We have written them to help show the features.

> Under the Treaty of Versailles Germany lost 10 per cent of its land, ~~so many Germans ended up living in other countries. Some German land was given to its European neighbours.~~ Alsace-Lorraine was given to France and West Prussia was given to Poland ~~to ensure that Poland had a sea port.~~ Germany also lost all its overseas colonies ~~including Togoland and Cameroon and German East Africa which were given to Britain and France.~~

Now read just the parts which have not been crossed out. Just these parts would have been likely to gain full marks!

Part (b) questions

These are usually questions which ask for an explanation. An explanation is hard to define, but one way to think of it is to say what you think and then say why you think it. So, a typical part (b) question might be:

> Explain why Clemenceau and Lloyd George disagreed at the Paris Peace Conference about how to treat Germany. **[6]**

Advice on how to answer

The best answers usually get straight to the point – no background information about the leaders or the Conference. For a question like this you should say what Lloyd George and Clemenceau disagreed about and then explain why they held these different views. One word of warning – a common error which students make is to simply describe the disagreements and not explain them.

> This paragraph would be likely to get a good mark because it explains one reason for their disagreement. So would the next paragraph.

> Lloyd George and Clemenceau disagreed over what to do about Germany because Clemenceau saw Germany as a bigger threat than Lloyd George did. During the war France suffered massive damage to its industries, towns and agriculture. Over two-thirds of French troops were killed or injured in the war. Germany's population was still much greater than France's (75 million compared to 40 million) and Germany had invaded France in 1870 and 1914. Lloyd George did not see Germany as a threat in the same way. In fact he wanted to rebuild Germany so that British industries could start trading with Germany.

> This paragraph explains that Clemenceau felt that the best way to get future peace was to cripple Germany, but Lloyd George felt this would not work and would make Germany vengeful.

> Lloyd George and Clemenceau also disagreed about what measures would work. Clemenceau wanted to cripple Germany by breaking it up into separate states, reducing its army and forcing it to pay huge fines. Lloyd George felt that this would simply make Germany want revenge in the future so although he favoured fines and some limits on German arms he did not think Germany should be treated as harshly as Clemenceau.

Part (c) questions

These are usually questions which ask you to think like a historian and make a judgement. They can come in many different forms but they usually want you to show whether you think one or more factors are more important than others in historical situations. They might ask you how far you agree or disagree with a statement or they might state some important factors and ask you how far you think one was more important than another. So a (c) question might look something like this:

> 'The Treaty of Versailles was a fair settlement.' How far do you agree with this statement? Explain your answer. **[10]**

Advice on how to answer

Step 1: You have to understand the statement.
Step 2: List the key points which support or oppose the statement.
Step 3: Decide on your argument (the one you are best able to support) and support it with evidence.
Step 4: You are ready to write your answer.

Planning your answer to this question is important to prevent rambling. There are many different ways to structure your answer but the safest is to explain why you might agree with the statement; then reasons why you might not; then finally express your judgement as to how far you agree, for example:

> There are many arguments to support the view that the Treaty of Versailles was a fair settlement. To begin with, it was strongly believed that Germany had started the war and was therefore responsible for it. It was certainly true that Germany invaded neutral Belgium in 1914, which broke international treaties. Another argument was that most of the fighting on the western front took place in Belgium and France. France lost around 1.6 million troops and civilians as well as suffering huge damage to industry, towns and agriculture. There was no fighting on German soil and so there was a strong case that Germany should pay compensation.

> A second argument was that the Treaty was not as harsh as its critics claimed. Germany certainly lost territory in the Versailles settlement — 10 per cent of its land, all colonies, 12.5 per cent of its population. However, it could have been a lot harsher. Clemenceau wanted Germany to be broken up into small states. And when we look at the Treaty of Brest-Litovsk, which Germany forced Russia to sign in 1918, we can see that Germany was much harsher in its terms with Russia than the Allies were with Germany at Versailles.

> Of course, there were terms that were seen as unfair. Germans regarded the Treaty as a diktat because they were not consulted about it. They also believed that the Allies operated double standards. For example, the German army was limited to 100,000 men but France and Britain and most other countries did not reduce their armed forces to the same levels. Another term that could be seen as unfair was the fact that many Germans were left outside Germany as a result of the Treaty.

> Overall, I agree with the statement. Obviously no treaty will be seen as fair by all sides but the Treaty of Versailles was as fair as it possibly could have been, and was a lot fairer on Germany than it might have been. The arguments against the Treaty were mainly complaints from the German point of view at the time. But most historians, such as Margaret Macmillan, with the benefit of hindsight, believe that the Treaty could have been a lot harsher. I put more faith in the historians and therefore this convinces me that the Treaty was not unfair.

Reasons why historians or people at the time would argue the Treaty was fair.

Reasons why historians or people at the time would argue the Treaty was unfair.

Which side you think is the stronger, and why. It is really strong to end with a clear statement.

Practice

Before you turn the page have a go at these three practice questions. Then you can judge your answers against our comments on page 172.

(a) Describe how the Treaty of Versailles punished Germany. **[4]**
(b) Explain what Wilson wanted to achieve from the peace settlement at Versailles. **[6]**
(c) 'Clemenceau did not get what he wanted out of the Paris Peace Conference.' How far do you agree with this statement? Explain your answer. **[10]**

1945–2000 example questions

These examples are based on the content of Chapters 4 to 7.

Part (a) questions   These are usually questions which ask you to describe. So, an example of a part (a) question might be:

> Describe Saddam Hussein's rise to power in Iraq. **[4]**

Advice on how to answer   These questions are usually straightforward but there are two key things to bear in mind:

- Show that you can select material which is relevant to the question – this is a vital skill for a historian (and for any written answers). This question asks about Saddam's rise to power. So don't get bogged down into details about where he was from, or who he was related to, unless you think it helps describe his rise to power.
- Be precise. Many students waste time by over-answering this question – writing far more than is needed. If a question is only worth 4 marks try to make 4 points!

And remember, it is better to write a paragraph rather than just a list of points. It reads better.

Part (b) questions   These are usually questions which ask for an explanation. An explanation is hard to define, but one way to think of it is to say what you think and then say why you think it. So, a possible part (b) question might be:

> Why was the Truman Doctrine important? **[6]**

Advice on how to answer   The best answers usually get straight to the point – no background information about the Cold War. For a question like this you should say what the Truman Doctrine was and then explain why it was important. One word of warning – do not just describe the Truman Doctrine. You need to describe what Truman did **and** explain why this had an impact on US policy and Soviet policy in the years that followed.

Part (c) questions   These are usually questions which ask you to think like a historian and make a judgement. They can come in many different forms but they usually want you to show whether you think one or more factors are more important than others in historical situations. They might ask you how far you agree or disagree with a statement or they might state some important factors and ask you how far you think one was more important than another. So a (c) question might look something like this:

> 'The USA was more responsible than the USSR in causing the Cold War in the late 1940s.' How far do you agree with this statement? Explain your answer. **[10]**

Advice on how to answer   Planning your answer to this question is important to prevent rambling. There are many different ways to do this but the safest is to explain first of all why you might agree with the statement; then reasons why you might not; then finally express your judgement as to how far you agree. So think along these lines:

- set out two to three events or developments and use them as evidence which points to the USA being to blame
- set out two to three events or developments and use them as evidence which points to the USSR being to blame
- come off the fence and give your view.

Before you turn the page have a go at these three practice questions. Then you can judge your answers against the answers and comments on page 173.

> **(a)** Describe the Bay of Pigs incident of 1961. **[4]**
> **(b)** Explain the reasons that Khrushchev put nuclear missiles on Cuba in 1962. **[6]**
> **(c)** 'The Cuban Missile Crisis was a victory for the USA.' How far do you agree with this statement? Explain your answer. **[10]**

1919–39 worked examples

Here are some example answers that we have written to show you how to tackle the questions you might face.

(a) Describe how the Treaty of Versailles punished Germany **[4]**

The Treaty punished Germany by limiting the size of its army to 100,000 men and banning conscription. It also had to pay reparations of £6,600 million to the Allies. All of its overseas empire was taken away from it.

(b) Explain what Wilson wanted to achieve from the peace settlement at Versailles. **[6]**

Wilson hoped to achieve several things. Firstly, he wanted to set up an international body called the League of Nations. He wanted this because he felt that nations had to work together in order to achieve world peace.

He also wanted to make sure that the different people in eastern Europe, like the Poles, would no longer be part of Austria–Hungary's empire. This was because he believed in self-determination – the idea that nations should rule themselves.

(c) 'Clemenceau did not get what he wanted out of the Paris Peace Conference.' How far do you agree with this statement? Explain your answer. **[10]**

Clemenceau was dissatisfied with the Treaty of Versailles although there were many terms that did please him.

He was happy that the threat from Germany was reduced with their armed forces being limited.

Clemenceau was also pleased with some of the territorial terms of the Treaty, such as claiming Alsace-Lorraine back from Germany, which had taken it in 1870.

However, Clemenceau was not satisfied that the Treaty reduced the threat from Germany enough. He was dissatisfied with the reparations settlement, thinking it was too low. He wanted Germany broken up into smaller states. He wanted Germany to be permanently economically and militarily crippled so as not to pose a future threat.

Overall, I do not agree with the statement that Clemenceau got what he wanted. I think Clemenceau got a lot of what he wanted out of the Treaty, such as reparations and Alsace-Lorraine, but he did not get the one thing he wanted most, which was guaranteed security from a German attack in the future, either through alliances or by crippling Germany. This is what he wanted above all, and he did not get it.

1945–2000 worked examples

Here are some example answers that we have written to show you how to tackle the questions you might face.

(a) Describe the Bay of Pigs incident of 1961. **[4]**

> This response is excellent – clear and straight to the point. The question is only worth 4 marks, so it would not be worthwhile here explaining lots of background about the run up to the invasion.

The Bay of Pigs invasion was not a direct invasion of Cuba by the US. Kennedy sent arms and equipment for 1400 anti-Castro exiles to invade Cuba and overthrow him. They landed at the Bay of Pigs but were met by 20,000 Cuban troops who had tanks and modern weapons. The invasion failed because Castro had killed or captured all of them within a matter of days.

(b) Explain the reasons that Khrushchev put nuclear missiles on Cuba in 1962. **[6]**

> This is a very good start because the answer **fully explains** how placing missiles on Cuba was a good defensive tactic for the USSR.

Khrushchev was concerned about the missile gap between the USSR and the US. The US had more long-range missiles than the USSR. He could put medium-range missiles on Cuba and still reach most of the US. So with missiles on Cuba it was less likely that the USA would ever launch a 'first strike' against the USSR.

> Unfortunately, the answer has drifted off and has lost focus on the question: in this case, **why** the missiles were placed in Cuba. You wouldn't get marks for giving lots of detail about things which you haven't been asked about. Possible other reasons could have included Khrushchev's wish to defend Cuba and how the missiles would give him bargaining power.

So in October 1962 a US spy plane flew over Cuba and found the nuclear missile sites. They took detailed pictures which showed that the sites would be ready to launch the missiles within a week. The Americans also found that there were Soviet ships on their way to Cuba with more missiles.

(c) 'The Cuban Missile Crisis was a victory for the USA.' How far do you agree with this statement? Explain your answer. **[10]**

In some ways the crisis was a victory for the US. Kennedy had secured the removal of the missiles and Khrushchev had been forced to back down after the naval blockade. The Soviet military was particularly unhappy with this and felt humiliated. In 1964 Khrushchev was removed from power; his enemies certainly thought he had failed.

> It's excellent that this answer has managed to demonstrate two different ways that the US came off as the victor.

However, Khrushchev had managed to avoid a US invasion of Cuba, a major achievement. Cuba was able to keep Soviet aid and protection despite the loss of the missiles. Also, Kennedy did have to remove the US missiles from Turkey, which was an uncomfortable position as it should have been NATO's decision and his NATO colleagues were unhappy.

> A **balanced argument** is key to earning a high mark in this question. This fully explains the evidence which **challenges** the statement.

In practical terms, the USSR gained overall because the crisis made it clear that even though they couldn't match the numbers of US weapons, their nuclear capacity alone was enough of a threat to make them respected. However, it was Kennedy, and therefore the US, who won the propaganda battle. He came off as the hero who had held firm against Communism and his reputation was enhanced. Khrushchev, meanwhile, was ousted from office, unable to use the Turkish withdrawal for propaganda as it was all done in secret.

> This answer attempts a balanced conclusion rather than a clinching argument. It argues that the USA won in some respects while the USSR won in others. This can be a good way of tackling a conclusion if you do not feel confident enough to decide one way or the other.

Paper 2: Introduction

Paper 2 will also be based on your study of the core content in Chapters 1 to 7. The difference between Paper 1 and Paper 2 is that Paper 2 is source-based – it is testing your ability to use your knowledge and skill to interrogate and compare a range of sources.

It is essentially a source-based investigation into one historical question drawn from the core content. You will already know the general area that this investigation will be based on (for example, in June 2015 it will be the causes of the First World War and why international peace collapsed in 1939, and in November 2015 it will be the causes of the Cold War).

Structure
- There is no choice of questions – you have to answer them all. The questions will be designed to test how well you can use historical sources but you will also need to use your historical knowledge as well.
- There will be up to eight sources, some pictures and some written, some from the time, some written by historians.
- There are no trick sources designed to catch you out, but there will usually be some sources which agree with each other and some which disagree, and some which do a bit of both!
- The questions take you step-by-step through the sources and are carefully designed to allow you to show that you can think like a historian. This means doing more than extracting basic information from a source. It means looking at sources to see what they reveal about:
  - why the source was produced
  - the audience for the source and the methods used in the source to convince its audience
  - what it reveals about the people who produced it, e.g. attitudes, values, concerns, anger (sources will often involve a person or organisation who is denying; criticising; mocking; praising; accusing; threatening; warning; afraid; unhappy; campaigning; outraged .... and much more!)
- It can be helpful to use your contextual knowledge, comment on the tone of a source, and point out its purpose .... **but only if these things are supporting your answer to the question being asked**. So if the question gives you a source in which a politician claims a particular policy was successful and asks whether that source can be trusted, there is no need to use your knowledge to give more detail about the policy or the politician unless that knowledge supports what you are saying about why the source can or cannot be trusted.

Question types
The exam could include any type of question about any type of source so what you are about to read is not foolproof! It is also important to remember that answers to the different types of questions should vary depending on the actual source – there is no 'one size fits all' formula. However, it is still worth thinking about question types and how you might answer them.

Type 1: Analysing the message of a source

This type of question uses a source where the author or artist is trying to make a particular point. The source could be part of a speech, or a cartoon, or possibly a poster. With a cartoon, you might be asked: 'What is the message of the cartoonist?'. With a question like this, remember these key points:

- For or against? What is the cartoonist for or against? Cartoonists do not draw cartoons simply to tell the public something is happening. Usually cartoons criticise or disapprove of something or maybe mock.
- How do you know? What details in the cartoon tell you what the cartoonist's view is?
- Why now? Why is the cartoon being drawn at this point in time?
- For message questions, you do not need to consider reliability.

Type 2: Similarity/difference

These questions are designed to get you think on two levels:

- Similarities and/or differences of in the content of the sources.
- Similarities and/or differences at a more subtle level e.g. the attitudes shown in each source, or the purpose of each source. For example, you might face two text sources where the two sources agree about events or details (e.g. that the USSR did place missiles in Cuba) but differ in purpose or attitudes (e.g. one might be critical of the USSR whereas the other is supportive).

If you do spot the higher level points, don't forget to state clearly whether the two sources are similar or different – this is an easy mistake to make when you are thinking hard!

Type 3: How useful?

A good way to think of these questions is not 'How useful is this source …?' but 'How is this source useful …?' Even a biased source is useful. The really important thing to think about is '**useful for what?**'
All sources are useful in telling you something about the attitudes or concerns of the person or organisation who created them. An American poster accusing Communists of crimes is not reliable about Communists but it is useful in showing that Americans were worried about Communism.

Type 4: Purpose

To tackle this type of question you need to work out the message of the source and then think about what the author of the source would want to achieve by getting that message across. Usually this would involve:

● changing people's attitudes (e.g. voting for a particular party)
● changing people's behaviour (e.g. getting them to join a movement or contribute funds to a particular cause).

Type 5: Surprise

The aim of these questions is for you to show you understand the period being studied and how historians use sources. So for example:

● whether or not the events described in the source are surprising in the context of the time (e.g. a speech by US President Richard Nixon attempting to build friendly relations with Communist China in the 1970s when the USA was traditionally very anti-Communist)
● whether or not it is surprising that the creator of the source was saying what they were saying in this place at this time (e.g. Nixon's speech is less surprising when we know that he was trying to get US troops out of the war in Vietnam and part of his plan involved better relations with China).

Type 6: Reliability

It's a good idea to explain in what way you think the sources are reliable or unreliable about particular people, issues or events. In other words, if you say the source is reliable or unreliable, make sure you explain what it is reliable or unreliable about! For example:

● If you know or can work out something about the author, explain why you think he/she is reliable or unreliable about particular people, issues or events.
● If there is any emotive language or a biased tone, explain why you think this shows the author has a particular point of view or purpose which makes the source reliable or unreliable about particular people, issues or events.
● If you think the source is reliable or unreliable because the content of the source fits with or contradicts your own knowledge about particular people, issues or events.
● Whether any other sources in the paper support or contradict the source – just because you are comparing two does not mean you can't use the other sources to help you evaluate those two.
You might conclude sources are equally trustworthy or untrustworthy.

Type 7: Conclusion

This usually starts with a statement and then asks you to explain whether you think the sources show that the statement is true or not.

● Address both sides of the statement – the yes/no or agree/disagree sides.
● You can approach this in two ways:
   – Either use two paragraphs, one for each side of the argument. Start each paragraph clearly. Group the yes/agree sources together and explain how they support the statement. Then group the no/disagree sources together and explain how they oppose the statement.
   – Work through source by source.
● When you make use of a source in your answer, don't just refer to it by letter. Explain how the content of the source supports or challenges the statement.
● Show awareness that some sources might be more reliable than others.

On pages 176–179 are some practice questions. We have provided possible answers and comments. When you have read these, you can test yourself out on a mock exam paper we have put together!

Paper 2: 1919–39 example answers with comments

SOURCE **A**

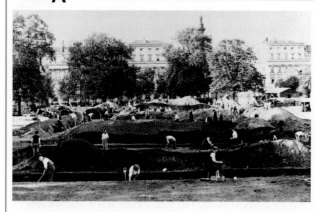

Digging air raid defences in London, September 1938.

Good use of **contextual knowledge** to show that the events in the source are not surprising. Another way of explaining this would have been to point out that people in Britain thought war was close (see Source C).

1 Study Source A. Are you surprised by this source? **[8]**

I am not surprised that they were digging air raid shelters. Even though war had not broken out, the whole of the summer of 1938 was full of tension in Europe. In May, Hitler had laid claim to the Sudetenland area and said he would fight Czechoslovakia for it if necessary. This news put the whole of Europe on full war alert. The photo of the building of air raid defences is therefore in keeping with air raid shelters being built and people buying gas masks.

SOURCE **B**

The Sudetenland is the last problem that must be solved and it will be solved. It is the last territorial claim which I have to make in Europe.

The aims of our foreign policy are not unlimited … They are grounded on the determination to save the German people alone … Ten million Germans found themselves beyond the frontiers of the Reich … Germans who wished to return to the Reich as their homeland.

Hitler speaking in Berlin, September 1938.

Recognises that biased and untrustworthy sources are useful! In this case, we may not be able to **trust** what Hitler is saying, but it is still **useful** in revealing how Hitler manipulated the situation.

2 Study Source B. How useful is this source to an historian? **[8]**

The source is definitely useful because it tells us how Hitler was publicly portraying the issue of the Sudetenland to the German people and the rest of the world. He says that it is the 'last problem' and the 'last territorial claim' Germany has in Europe. Even though this, of course, turned out not to be the case, it is still useful in showing us the methods Hitler employed to get what he wanted. It also gives us an insight into why some people may have supported Appeasement.

This is not a real exam paper. We have written the questions for you to practise and provided some example answers.

SOURCE C

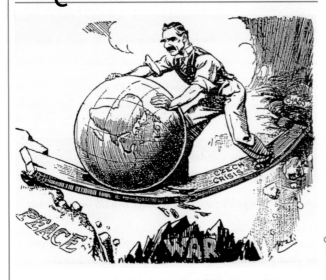

A British cartoon published in the *News of the World*, shortly after the Munich Agreement.

3 Study Source C. What is the message of the cartoonist? **[6]**

Good idea to start your answer in this way. It gets you straight to the point. This answer has carefully correctly identified that the source is **supportive** of the Munich Agreement.

The message that the cartoonist was trying to put across is that Chamberlain has done a good job by signing the Munich Agreement, avoiding a crisis and taking the world to war, and moving it towards peace.

You can see this because he's shown as tough and strong with his sleeves rolled up, successfully rolling the globe across the sheer drop to war below.

The cartoonist clearly thinks that giving Hitler the Sudetenland in 1938 was the right decision.

The answer has not simply described the cartoon but has actually **used** the details to **support** the point made above.

Understands the **context** in which this cartoon was drawn, and gets this across, without too much unnecessary detail.

SOURCE D

People of Britain, your children are safe. Your husbands and your sons will not march to war. Peace is a victory for all mankind. If we must have a victor, let us choose Chamberlain, for the Prime Minister's conquests are mighty and enduring – millions of happy homes and hearts relieved of their burden.

The *Daily Express* comments on the Munich Agreement, 30 September 1938.

SOURCE E

We have suffered a total defeat ... I think you will find that in a period of time Czechoslovakia will be engulfed in the Nazi regime. We have passed an awful milestone in our history. This is only the beginning of the reckoning.

Winston Churchill speaking in October 1938. He felt that Britain should resist the demands of Hitler. However, he was an isolated figure in the 1930s.

Uses the **content** of the sources to show how they **disagree**. This is a useful starting point – it is saying that Source E says Source D is wrong about people's attitudes to the Munich Agreement. It is important to explain 'wrong about what?'.

4 Study Sources D and E. How far does Source E prove Source D wrong? **[9]**

In some ways Source E does prove Source D wrong. The newspaper says that the Munich Agreement will bring peace – 'your husbands and sons will not march to war'. This is contradicted by Churchill when he says 'This is only the beginning of the reckoning'. The overall impression given by Source D is that people are relieved by the Munich Agreement, whereas Churchill seems to prove this wrong by being very critical of it.

However, Source E cannot prove Source D wrong about people's reactions to the Munich Agreement. Lots of people in Britain were relieved that it had averted war, or at least delayed it in the short term. This can be seen by looking at Source C, where the cartoonist seems to support Chamberlain's actions, showing how he has dealt well with a tricky situation.

Improves the answer because it looks at the issue of 'proof' in a different way. By **cross-referencing** Source D with another source on the paper, it can be shown that whilst Churchill may be right about the Munich Agreement in general, he cannot prove Source D wrong about people's **reactions to it**.

Paper 2: 1945–2000 example answers with comments

SOURCE A

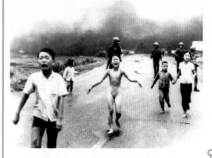

A ten-year-old Vietnamese girl, Phan Thi Kim, runs naked after tearing her burning clothes from her body following a napalm attack in 1972. This photograph became one of the most enduring images of the war.

1 Study Source A. Why was this published in 1972? **[7]**

> An excellent start because it is entirely focused on the question; it identifies a specific **outcome** of the picture's publication.

The source was published to turn public opinion against the US involvement in Vietnam.

We can see this because the picture will immediately make the viewer feel huge sympathy for the young children who have been burned by napalm.

By 1967 the media had started to ask difficult questions about American involvement in Vietnam and the media coverage was no longer generally positive.

> Here, the answer **uses** the detail from the photograph to show how it supports the point made above.

> The answer correctly places the photograph into its context.

SOURCE B

We were not in My Lai to kill human beings. We were there to kill ideology that is carried by – I don't know – pawns. Blobs. Pieces of flesh. And I wasn't in My Lai to destroy intelligent men. I was there to destroy an intangible idea … To destroy Communism.

From Lieutenant Calley's account of the event, *Body Count*, published in 1970.

SOURCE C

This was a time for us to get even. A time for us to settle the score. A time for revenge – when we can get revenge for our fallen comrades. The order we were given was to kill and destroy everything that was in the village. It was to kill the pigs, drop them in the wells; pollute the water supply … burn the village, burn the hootches as we went through it. It was clearly explained that there were to be no prisoners. The order that was given was to kill everyone in the village. Someone asked if this meant the women and children. And the order was: everyone in the village, because those people that were in the village – the women, the kids, the old men – were VC … or they were sympathetic to the Viet Cong.

Sergeant Hodge of Charlie Company.

2 Study Sources B and C. Why do they differ in their accounts of what happened at My Lai in 1968? **[9]**

> Even though this response has not yet tackled the question of **why** the sources differ, it is a good approach because we can see the sources are being **compared to each other**, and not dealt with in isolation.

In Source B, Lieutenant Calley gives the impression that the massacre at My Lai was not really a massacre or a revenge operation: 'We were not in My Lai to kill human beings.' But in Source C, Sergeant Hodge says it was revenge – the operation was 'a time for us to get even'.

I think the sources say different things because at the time they were produced, Calley and other officers in Charlie Company had been charged with murder for what happened at My Lai. So Hodge is trying to put the blame for what happened on his senior officers, placing all the responsibility on them, whilst Calley is trying to justify his actions. He's trying to appeal to people's fear of Communism.

> This part now successfully tackles the question of **why** the sources differ and uses the **context** and **purpose** of the sources to fully explain this.

SOURCE D

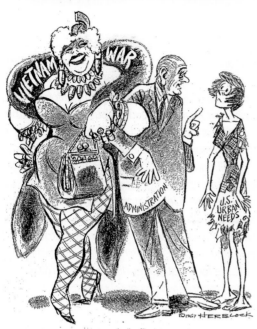

"There's Money Enough To Support Both Of You —
Now, Doesn't That Make You Feel Better?"

VIETNAM WAR

ADMINISTRATION

U.S. URBAN NEEDS

—from The Herblock Gallery (Simon & Schuster, 1968)

An American cartoon from 1967.

3 Study Source D. What is the message of the cartoonist? **[7]**

The cartoonist is criticising President Lyndon Johnson for lying to the American people when he says there is enough money to fight the Vietnam War and help poorer areas of the USA (shown by the ragged woman labelled US Urban Needs). The cartoonist clearly thinks that the Vietnam War is getting all the money and poor Americans are being ignored.

This was published in 1967 and by this time a lot of the US media were starting to question American involvement.

> This answer correctly identifies that this cartoonist is **critical** of America's sustained involvement.

SOURCE E

The American military was not defeated in Vietnam –

The American military did not lose a battle of any consequence. From a military standpoint, it was almost an unprecedented performance. This included Tet 68, which was a major military defeat for the VC and NVA.

The United States did not lose the war in Vietnam, the South Vietnamese did –

The fall of Saigon happened 30 April 1975, two years AFTER the American military left Vietnam. The last American troops departed in their entirety 29 March 1973. How could we lose a war we had already stopped fighting? We fought to an agreed stalemate.

The Fall of Saigon –

The 140,000 evacuees in April 1975 during the fall of Saigon consisted almost entirely of civilians and Vietnamese military, NOT American military running for their lives.

There were almost twice as many casualties in Southeast Asia (primarily Cambodia) the first two years after the fall of Saigon in 1975 than there were during the ten years the US was involved in Vietnam.

An extract from a website, www.slideshare.net, 'Vietnam War Statistics', by an American ex-serviceman.

4 Study Source E. How reliable is this source about the Vietnam War? **[8]**

I don't think Source E is very reliable at all about the Vietnam War. I think the source's whole purpose seems to be to convince people that America shouldn't be embarrassed about its actions in Vietnam and that it could have won the war had it chosen to stay because the author is very selective in the evidence put forward, such as the fact that Saigon did not technically fall to North Vietnam until after the Americans left. He neglects evidence such as the fact America spent $110 billion on the war and had been there over ten years without securing victory.

> This is a very good response which tackles the question of reliability in different ways. Firstly, the answer uses **contextual knowledge** to challenge details in the source, and secondly, the answer examines the purpose of the source and uses that to question its reliability.

Paper 2: Sample Paper A: League of Nations in the 1920s

SOURCE **A**

The League was created, first and foremost, as a security organisation. But in this respect it fell badly short of its original aims. There was no way to guarantee that members would carry out their obligations to enforce sanctions or undertake military force where it might be needed. But it was not without its achievements. For most countries attendance at League meetings in the 1920s was seen as essential, because the foreign ministers of the major powers were almost always present. The small and middle sized states found the League was a vital platform for them to talk about their interests and concerns. Even those outside the League, including the United States, found it useful to attend League-sponsored Conferences and similar events. Without exaggerating its importance the League developed useful ways of handling inter-state disputes. For the most part the League handled the 'small change' of international diplomacy. It was not a substitute for great power diplomacy as Wilson had hoped, but it was an additional resource which contributed to the handling of international politics.

An American historian writing in 2005.

SOURCE **B**

Despite its poor historical reputation, the League of Nations should not be dismissed as a complete failure. Of sixty-six international disputes it had to deal with (four of which had led to open hostilities), it successfully resolved thirty-five important disputes and quite legitimately passed back twenty to the traditional channels of diplomacy where major powers negotiated settlements outside the League. It failed to resolve eleven conflicts. Like its successor the United Nations, it was capable of being effective.

A British historian writing in 2009.

SOURCE **C**

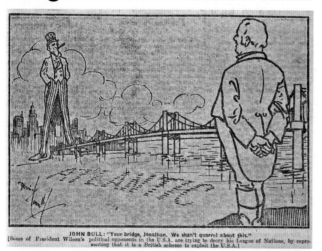

JOHN BULL: "Your bridge, Jonathan. We shan't quarrel about this."
[Some of President Wilson's political opponents in the U.S.A. are trying to decry his League of Nations, by representing that it is a British scheme to exploit the U.S.A.]

A cartoon published in the USA in 1919.

SOURCE **D**

The League Council felt that our role under the League Covenant was to do everything we could to promote a settlement, and since the two parties had willingly agreed to accept the decision of the Conference of Ambassadors our job from this point was to do everything we could to help the Ambassadors make decisions which were in line with the opinions expressed in the Assembly in Geneva. In this I believe we acted rightly and properly.

British government minister Lord Robert Cecil writing in October 1923 about the Corfu Crisis. Cecil was the British minister responsible for League of Nations matters.

SOURCE **E**

In response to the successive menaces of Mussolini we muzzled the League, we imposed the fine on Greece without evidence of her guilt and without reference to the International Court of Justice, and we disbanded the Commission of Enquiry. A settlement was thus achieved. At the time I felt that British public opinion will wonder how it came about that we entered into the dispute upon a firm moral basis and that in the end we forced Greece to accept a settlement that was unjust. Corfu was evacuated by the Italians, but the League of Nations had suffered a defeat from which its prestige has never recovered.

British government official Sir Harold Nicolson writing in 1929, soon after he resigned from the British diplomatic service after criticising one of his ministers.

SOURCE F

Greek forces have invaded our sovereign territory. Make only slight resistance. Protect the refugees. Prevent the spread of panic. Do not expose the troops to unnecessary losses in view of the fact that the incident has been laid before the Council of the League of Nations, which is expected to stop the invasion.

A telegram from the Bulgarian Ministry of War in Sofia to its army commanders, 22 October 1925.

SOURCE G

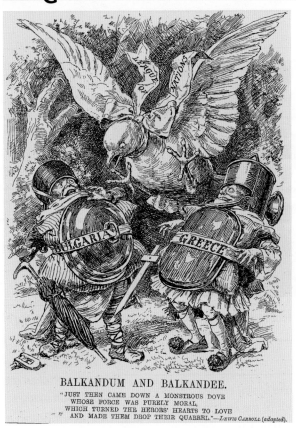

A British cartoon about the conflict between Greece and Bulgaria, published in December 1925.

Study Sources A and B.
1   How far do Sources A and B agree about the League of Nations? Explain your answer using details from the sources. **[8]**

Study Source C.
2   Was Source C produced by a supporter or an opponent of America joining the League? Explain your answer using details from the source and your own knowledge. **[7]**

Study Sources D and E.
3   Why do these sources give such different accounts of the League's actions over Corfu? Explain your answer using details from the sources and your own knowledge. **[8]**

Study Source F.
4   Are you surprised by Source F? Explain your answer using details from the source and your own knowledge. **[8]**

Study Source G.
5   What is the message of the cartoonist? Explain your answer using details from the source and your own knowledge. **[7]**

Study Sources A–G.
6   'The League of Nations was very successful in the 1920s.' How far do these sources support this statement? Use the sources to explain your answer. **[12]**

Paper 2: Sample Paper B: The beginnings of the Cold War

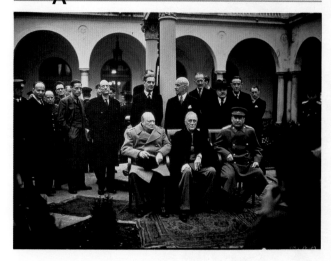

A publicity photograph of the Big Three taken at the Yalta Conference in 1945.

SOURCE **B**

We (Roosevelt, Churchill and Stalin) argued freely and frankly across the table. But at the end on every point unanimous agreement was reached … We know, of course, that it was Hitler's hope and the German war lords' hope that we would not agree – that some slight crack might appear in the solid wall of allied unity … But Hitler has failed. Never before have the major allies been more closely united – not only in their war aims but also in their peace aims.

Extract from President Roosevelt's report to the US Congress on the Yalta Conference, April 1945.

SOURCE **C**

I have always worked for friendship with Russia but, like you, I feel deep anxiety because of their misinterpretation of the Yalta decisions, their attitude towards Poland, their overwhelming influence in the Balkans excepting Greece, the difficulties they make about Vienna, the combination of Russian power and the territories under their control or occupied, coupled with the Communist technique in so many other countries, and above all their power to maintain very large Armies in the field for a long time. What will be the position in a year or two?

Extract from a telegram sent by Prime Minister Churchill to President Roosevelt in May 1945.

SOURCE **D**

OPERATION UNTHINKABLE

REPORT BY THE JOINT PLANNING STAFF

We have examined Operation Unthinkable. As instructed, we have taken the following assumptions on which to base our examination:

Great Britain and the United States have full assistance from the Polish armed forces and can count upon the use of German manpower and what remains of German industrial capacity . . .

Owing to the special need for secrecy, the normal staffs in Service Ministries have not been consulted.

OBJECT

The overall or political object is to impose upon Russia the will of the United States and British Empire. The only way we can achieve our object with certainty and lasting results is by victory in a total war.

Extract from a top secret document called Operation Unthinkable. It was presented by the Army Chiefs to Churchill in May 1945 but the research and planning had begun in February 1945.

This is not a real exam paper. We have written the questions for you to practise.

SOURCE E

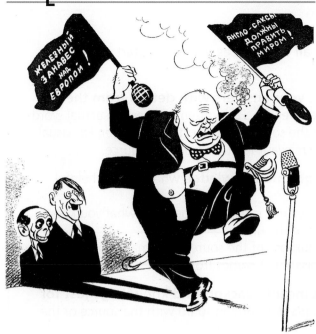

A Soviet cartoon published in 1946.

SOURCE F

A shadow has fallen upon the scenes so lately lighted by the Allied victory. From Stettin on the Baltic to Trieste on the Adriatic, an iron curtain has descended. Behind that line lie all the states of central and eastern Europe. The Communist parties have been raised to power far beyond their numbers and are seeking everywhere to obtain totalitarian control. This is certainly not the liberated Europe we fought to build. Nor is it one which allows permanent peace.

A speech by Winston Churchill in 1946. It was given in the USA and was broadcast widely. At the time Churchill was no longer British Prime Minister.

SOURCE G

The following circumstances should not be forgotten. The Germans made their invasion of the USSR through Finland, Poland and Romania. The Germans were able to make their invasion through these countries because, at the time, governments hostile to the Soviet Union existed in these countries. What can there be surprising about the fact that the Soviet Union, anxious for its future safety, is trying to see to it that governments loyal in their attitude to the Soviet Union should exist in these countries?

A speech by Soviet leader Stalin given in 1946. It was broadcast in the USSR and reported in Britain and the USA.

Study Source A.
1   What can you learn from this source? Explain your answer using details from the sources. **[7]**

Study Sources B and C.
2   How far do Sources A and B agree? Explain your answer using details from the sources. **[8]**

Study Source D.
3   Are you surprised by Source D? Explain your answer using details from the source and your own knowledge. **[7]**

Study Source E.
4   What is the cartoonist's message? Explain your answer using details from the sources and your own knowledge. **[8]**

Study Sources F and G.
5   How far do you think Source F influenced Source G? Explain your answer using details from the source and your own knowledge. **[8]**

Study Sources A–G.
6   'The Cold War began because Churchill had such a poor relationship with Stalin.' How far do these sources support this statement? Use the sources to explain your answer. **[12]**

TOP TIPS for Paper 2

1 Read through all the **sources** before you start writing anything.

2 Always **support your answers with details from the sources** and **be specific**. For written sources use actual words or phrases from the source to support your answer. For visual sources describe relevant features from the source.

3 Use your background knowledge whenever it's helpful, particularly to:
- work out if a source is reliable (does it fit what you know about events of the time)
- explain the purpose of the source (you may know the author or the organisation it comes from).

4 However, **don't include background knowledge just for its own sake** if it's got nothing to do with the source or the question.

5 When you use your own knowledge avoid saying 'my knowledge tells me …'. Just **state what you know**.

6 Avoid speculation – so avoid using words like 'might' and 'could' (such as 'The author might be a supporter so he could be biased …').

7 Avoid phrases such as 'we don't know what else …' or 'she could have forgotten ….'. Examiners call this 'stock evaluation' because it could be applied to any source. You will not get any credit for this type of answer.

8 Cross-referencing is essential but it is not easy to do this well. When you cross-reference you should argue that Source X is strong or weak evidence because it is supported by what is said in Source Y – and then quote from or summarise what it says in Source Y which proves your point.

9 Don't include your own personal views which are not historical (such as, 'I think it was awful the way the USA used chemical weapons in Vietnam …').

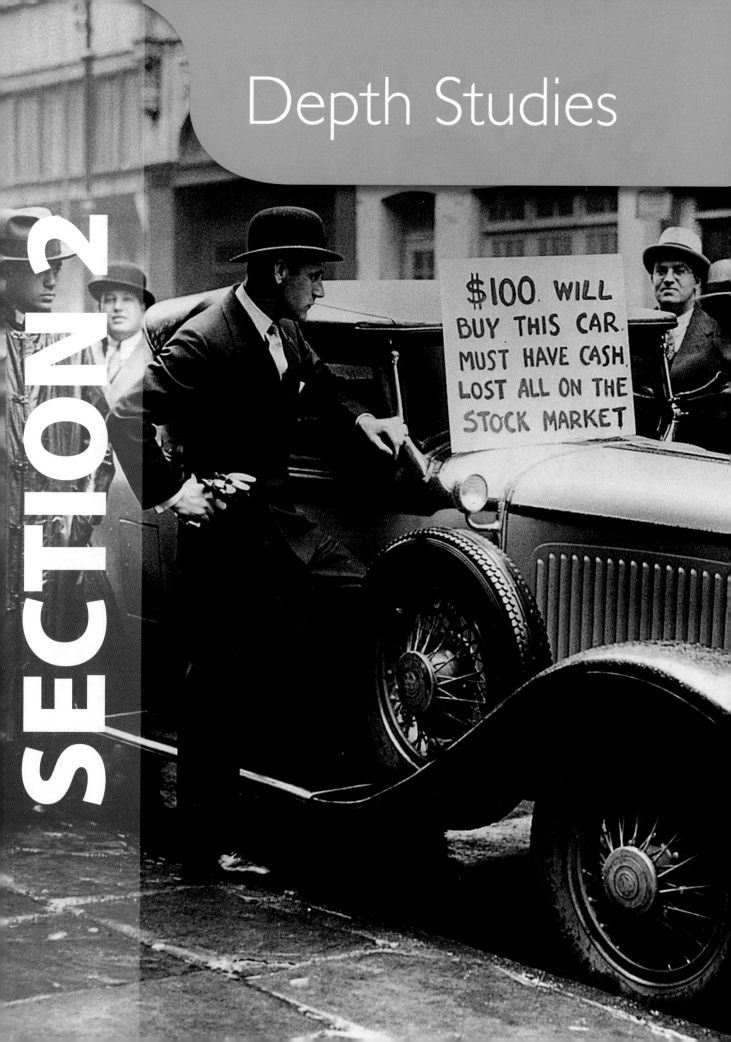

Depth Studies

SECTION 2

$100. WILL BUY THIS CAR. MUST HAVE CASH. LOST ALL ON THE STOCK MARKET

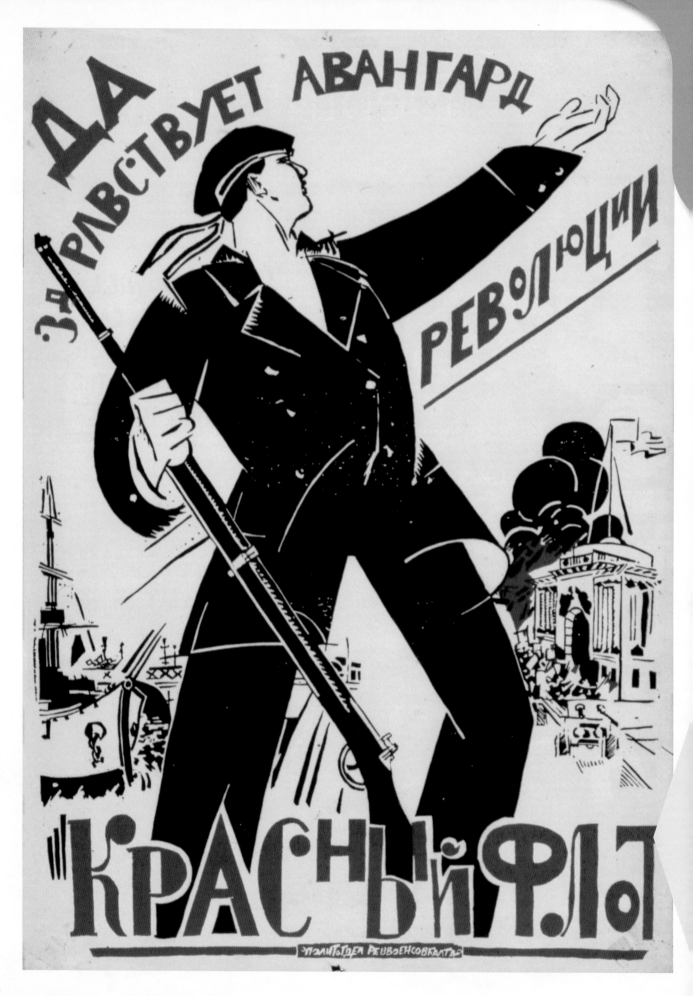

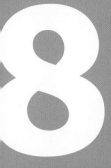

8 Russia, 1905–41

KEY QUESTIONS

8.1 Why did the Tsarist regime collapse in 1917?

8.2 How did the Bolsheviks gain and hold on to power?

8.3 How did Stalin gain and hold on to power? What was the impact of Stalin's economic policies?

In 1905 Russia was a vast but backward agricultural country. Its industry was underdeveloped, its people mainly poor and uneducated. It was ruled by a Tsar who had complete power. In March 1917 the Tsar was overthrown and in November of the same year the Bolsheviks took over the running of Russia. Over the next 30 years the country was transformed by Stalin into a modern industrial state which became a world superpower.

In 8.1 you will investigate why the Tsar's regime survived one revolution in 1905 but then collapsed in 1917. What changed?

In 8.2 you will explore how the Bolsheviks (Communists) under Lenin seized power in 1917 and, against all the odds, held on to power.

In 8.3 you will look at how Stalin became the new leader of Russia (by this time the USSR) after Lenin, how he changed the Soviet Union, and the consequences of his rule for his people.

Timeline

This timeline shows the period you will be covering in this chapter. Some of the key dates are filled in already. To help you get a complete picture of the period make your own much larger version of the timeline and add other details to it as you work through the chapter.

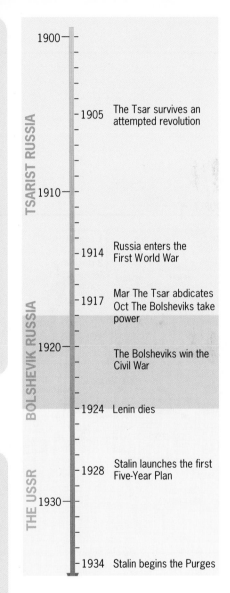

1900	
1905	The Tsar survives an attempted revolution
1910	
1914	Russia enters the First World War
1917	Mar The Tsar abdicates Oct The Bolsheviks take power
1920	The Bolsheviks win the Civil War
1924	Lenin dies
1928	Stalin launches the first Five-Year Plan
1930	
1934	Stalin begins the Purges

TSARIST RUSSIA · BOLSHEVIK RUSSIA · THE USSR

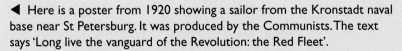

◄ Here is a poster from 1920 showing a sailor from the Kronstadt naval base near St Petersburg. It was produced by the Communists. The text says 'Long live the vanguard of the Revolution: the Red Fleet'.

On pages 205–209 you will be looking at the period from which this poster comes. Try to answer the following questions (you will have to guess intelligently) and then keep your answers and check whether you were right.

1 How would you describe the poster's view of the sailor – for example, cowardly, weak, brave?

2 Does this mean the sailors support the Communists or the other way around?

3 Do you get the impression that Russia is a peaceful place at this time?

4 Would you expect the relationship between the Communists and the sailors to change in the next few months?

8.1 Why did the Tsarist regime collapse in 1917?

Focus

When Nicholas II was crowned Tsar of Russia in 1894, the crowds flocked to St Petersburg to cheer. There were so many people that a police report said 1,200 people were crushed to death as the crowd surged forward to see the new Tsar, whom they called 'the Little Father of Russia'.

Twenty-three years later, he had been removed from power and he and his family were prisoners. They were held under armed guard in a lonely house at Ekaterinburg, far from the Tsar's luxurious palaces. Perhaps the Tsar might have asked himself how this had happened, but commentators were predicting collapse long before 1917. In fact some people think the surprise is that the Tsar had actually survived so long. How could one man rule such a vast and troubled empire? So your focus in 8.1 is why, having survived for 23 years, did the Tsar's regime finally collapse *in 1917*?

Focus Points

♦ How well did the Tsarist regime deal with the difficulties of ruling Russia up to 1914?
♦ How did the Tsar survive the 1905 Revolution?
♦ How far was the Tsar weakened by the First World War?
♦ Why was the revolution of March 1917 successful?

SOURCE **1**

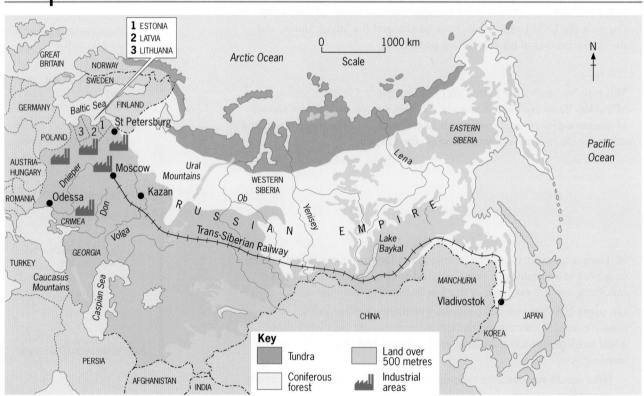

The Russian empire in 1900.

Tsar Nicholas II

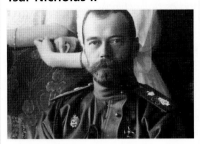

> Born 1868.
> Crowned as Tsar in 1896.
> Married to Alexandra of Hesse (a granddaughter of Queen Victoria).
> Both the Tsar and his wife were totally committed to the idea of the Tsar as autocrat – absolute ruler of Russia.
> Nicholas regularly rejected requests for reform.
> He was interested in the Far East. This got him into a disastrous war with Japan in 1905.
> He was not very effective as a ruler, unable to concentrate on the business of being Tsar.
> He was a kind, loving family man but did not really understand the changes Russia was going through.
> By 1917 he had lost control of Russia and abdicated.
> In 1918 he and his family were shot by Bolsheviks during the Russian Civil War.

The Russian empire

Russia was a vast empire of many nationalities rather than a single country, and the Tsar was its supreme ruler.

Nationalities

Only 40 per cent of the Tsar's subjects spoke Russian as their first language. Some subjects, for example the Cossacks, were loyal to the Tsar. Others, for example the Poles and Finns, hated Russian rule. Jews often suffered racial prejudice and even attacks called pogroms, sponsored by the government.

Peasants and the countryside

Around 80 per cent of Russia's population were peasants who lived in communes. There were some prosperous peasant farmers called kulaks, but living and working conditions for most peasants were dreadful. Farming was backward and primitive. There was no education. Hunger and disease were common. Life expectancy was only 40 in some areas. Worse still, a rising population meant there was a shortage of good quality land. Despite this, mainly because of the teachings of the Church, most peasants were loyal to the Tsar although some peasants did support the opposition Social Revolutionaries who wanted to take the good farming land from the aristocrats and the Church and give it to the peasants.

New industries, cities and the working class

From the later nineteenth century, the Tsars had been keen to see Russia become an industrial power. The senior minister Sergei Witte introduced policies that led to rapid industrial growth. Oil and coal production trebled, while iron production quadrupled. Some peasants left the land to work in these newly developing industries. However, their living conditions hardly improved. They were jammed into slum housing in the cities, especially St Petersburg and Moscow. Within a short distance of the Tsar's glittering palaces workers suffered from illnesses, alcoholism, appalling working conditions and low pay. Trade unions were illegal so there was no way to protest. Most workers were probably no better off than the peasants.

SOURCE **2**

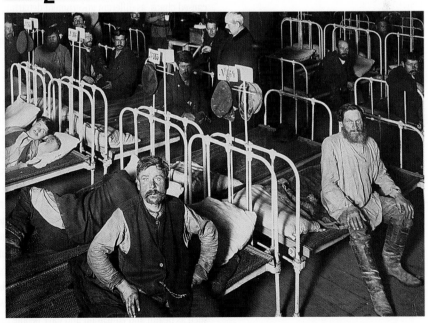

Workers' living conditions: a dormitory in Moscow. Urban workers made up about 4 per cent of the population in 1900.

SOURCE 3

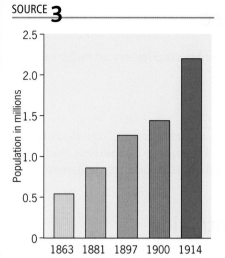

Graph showing the growth of St Petersburg.

SOURCE 4

Let all know that I, devoting all my strength to the welfare of the people, will uphold the principle of autocracy as firmly and as unflinchingly as my late unforgettable father.

Part of Tsar Nicholas II's coronation speech in 1894.

The middle classes

As a result of industrialisation, a new class began to emerge in Russia – the capitalists. They were landowners, industrialists, bankers, traders and businessmen. Until this time, Russia had had only a small middle class which included people such as shopkeepers, lawyers and university lecturers. The capitalists increased the size of Russia's middle class, particularly in the towns. Their main concerns were the management of the economy, although the capitalists were also concerned about controlling their workforce. Clashes between workers and capitalists were to play an important role in Russia's history in the years up to 1917.

The Tsar and his government

The huge and diverse empire was ruled by an autocracy. One man, the Tsar, had absolute power. By the early twentieth century most of the great powers had given their people at least some say in how they were run, but Nicholas was utterly committed to the idea of autocracy. He had many good qualities such as his willingness to work hard and his attention to detail. However, Nicholas tended to avoid making important decisions and wasted time by getting involved in the tiniest details of government.

Nicholas tended to avoid making important decisions. He did not delegate day-to-day tasks. In a country as vast as Russia, where tasks had to be delegated to officials, this was a major problem. He insisted on getting involved in the tiniest details of government. He personally answered letters from peasants and appointed provincial midwives. He even wrote out the instructions for the royal car to be brought round!

Nicholas also managed his officials poorly. He felt threatened by able and talented ministers, such as Count Witte and Peter Stolypin. He dismissed Witte in 1906 and was about to sack Stolypin (see page 195) when Stolypin was murdered in 1911. Nicholas refused to chair the Council of Ministers because he disliked confrontation. He encouraged rivalry between ministers. This caused chaos, as different government departments refused to co-operate with each other. He also appointed family members and friends from the court to important positions. Many of them were incompetent or even corrupt, making huge fortunes from bribes.

Control

The Tsar's regime exercised strong control over the people. Newspapers were censored and political parties banned. The police had a special force with 10,000 officers whose job was to concentrate on dealing with political opponents of the regime. The Tsar's secret police force, the Okhrana, was very effective, sending thousands to prison and exile in Siberia. Backing them up was the army which could be counted to put down any disturbances, particularly those of the terrifying Cossack regiments. A loyal army was crucial to the Tsar's regime.

In the countryside the peasants belonged to a *mir* or village commune which controlled different aspects of daily life. There were also land captains, local nobility who dealt with crimes and disputes; they were hated by the peasants. Larger regions were controlled by governors, aristocrats appointed by the Tsar. They had all sorts of powers to arrest people, put down trouble, censor newspapers and so on. Some of these were petty tyrants running their own little police states.

There were elected town and district councils called *zemstva*, but these were dominated by the nobility and professional classes (doctors, lawyers). The *zemstva* did some good work in areas such as health and education and gave people useful experienced in running local government. Some people wanted a national *zemstvo* through which elected representatives could play a part in running the country.

Think!

1. Draw up your own chart to summarise the Tsarist system of government.
2. Describe and explain at least two ways in which Nicholas II made Russia's government weak.

Opposition to the Tsar

The Tsarist government faced opposition from three particular groups. Many middle-class people wanted greater democracy in Russia and pointed out that Britain still had a king but also a powerful parliament. These people were called liberals.

Two other groups were more violently opposed to the Tsar. They believed that revolution was the answer to the people's troubles. The Socialist Revolutionaries (SRs) were a radical movement. Their main aim was to carve up the huge estates of the nobility and hand them over to the peasants. They believed in a violent struggle and were responsible for the assassination of two government officials, as well as the murder of a large number of Okhrana (police) agents and spies. They had support in the towns and the countryside.

The Social Democratic Party was a smaller but more disciplined party which followed the ideas of Karl Marx. In 1903 the party split itself into Bolsheviks and Mensheviks. The Bolsheviks (led by Lenin) believed it was the job of the party to create a revolution whereas the Mensheviks believed Russia was not ready for revolution. Both of these organisations were illegal and many of their members had been executed or sent in exile to Siberia. Many of the leading Social Democrat leaders were forced to live abroad.

Factfile

Marxist theory

➤ Karl Marx was a German writer and political thinker. He believed that history was dominated by class struggle and revolution.

➤ In Marxist theory the first change brought about by the class struggle would be the middle classes taking control from the monarchy and aristocracy.

➤ There would then be a revolution in which the workers (the proletariat) would overthrow the middle classes.

➤ For a short while the Communist Party would rule on behalf of the people, but as selfish desires disappeared there would be no need for any government.

➤ All would live in a peaceful, Communist society.

Source Analysis ▶

Look carefully at Source 5. It was drawn by opponents of the Tsar's regime who had been forced to live in Switzerland to avoid the Tsar's secret police. It is a representation of life in Russia under the rule of the Tsar. Discuss how far you think it is an accurate view of Russian society. Think about:

♦ ways in which its claims are supported by the information and sources in the text

♦ ways in which its claims are not supported by the information and sources in the text

♦ aspects of life in Russia that are not covered by the drawing.

Think!

You are a minister of the Tsar in 1903. Write a report for him, informing him truthfully of the situation in Russia.

Your report should mention:

♦ inefficient and corrupt government

♦ the condition of the peasants

♦ the contrast between rich and poor in Russia

♦ conditions for the workers in the towns

♦ the activities of opposition groups.

SOURCE 5

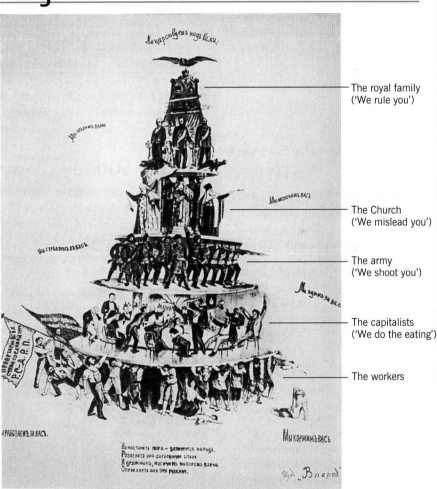

- The royal family ('We rule you')
- The Church ('We mislead you')
- The army ('We shoot you')
- The capitalists ('We do the eating')
- The workers

Cartoon showing the Tsarist system. This was published in Switzerland by exiled opponents of the Tsar.

SOURCE 6

Lord, we workers, our children, our wives and our old, helpless parents have come, Lord, to seek truth, justice and protection from you.

We are impoverished and oppressed, unbearable work is imposed on us, we are despised and not recognised as human beings. We are treated as slaves, who must bear their fate and be silent. We have suffered terrible things, but we are pressed ever deeper into the abyss of poverty, ignorance and lack of rights.

We ask but little: to reduce the working day to eight hours and to provide a minimum wage of a rouble a day.

Officials have taken the country into a shameful war. We working men have no say in how the taxes we pay are spent.

Do not refuse to help your people. Destroy the wall between yourself and your people.

From the Petition to the Tsar presented by Father Gapon, 1905.

Source Analysis

1 Read Source 6. Make two lists:
   a) the petitioners' complaints
   b) their demands.
2 Are these demands revolutionary demands? Explain your answer.
3 Choose two words to sum up the attitude of the petitioners to the Tsar in Source 6.
4 Look carefully at Source 7. Would you interpret the contents of this source as:
   a) evidence of the strength of the Tsar's regime
   b) evidence of the weakness of the regime?
   Explain your answer and refer to the information in the text as well.
5 a) Describe in detail what you can see in Source 8.
   b) What do you think the artist is trying to show?
   c) How might this event change the attitude of the petitioners (see your answer to Q.3)?

The 1905 revolution

At the beginning of the new century Russia was a fast-changing society as industry and cities grew rapidly. This was causing lots of stresses and strains as people flooded into towns and cities, often living and working in appalling conditions. After 1900 Russia was hit by economic depression – wages fell, factories and mines closed and people were thrown out of work. This led to strikes and unrest. When the police set up 'approved' trade unions to try to control the workers, this only led to more strikes. To make matters worse, a poor harvest in 1901 led to hunger and peasant revolt. The only answer the government could come up with to this growing discontent was force and suppression (see Source 7).

SOURCE 7

A third of Russia lives under emergency legislation. The numbers of the regular police and of the secret police are continually growing. The prisons are overcrowded with convicts and political prisoners. At no time have religious persecutions [of Jews] been so cruel as they are today. In all cities and industrial centres soldiers are employed and equipped with live ammunition to be sent out against the people. Autocracy is an outdated form of government that may suit the needs of a central African tribe but not those of the Russian people who are increasingly aware of the culture of the rest of the world.

Part of a letter from the landowner and writer Leo Tolstoy to the Tsar in 1902. The letter was an open letter – it was published openly as well as being sent to the Tsar.

On top of this, the Tsar decided to go to war with Japan. This may have been an attempt by the Tsar to unite the Russian people against an outside enemy. But the Russians suffered a serious of humiliating defeats which made the government appear unfit and incompetent.

Bloody Sunday

These tensions all came together on Sunday, 22 January 1905, when a crowd of 200,000 protesters, led by the priest Father Gapon, came to the Winter Palace to give a petition to the Tsar. Many of the marchers carried pictures of the Tsar to show their respect for him.

The Tsar was not in the Winter Palace. He had left St Petersburg when the first signs of trouble appeared. The protesters were met by a regiment of soldiers and mounted Cossacks. Without warning, the soldiers opened fire and the Cossacks charged. It was a decisive day. The Tsar finally lost the respect of the ordinary people of Russia.

SOURCE 8

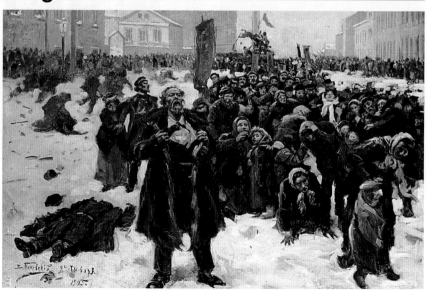

Bloody Sunday – as painted in around 1910.

A clear, frosty day. Went for a long walk. Since yesterday all the factories and workshops in St Petersburg have been on strike. Troops have been brought in to strengthen the garrison. The workers have conducted themselves calmly hitherto. At the head of the workers is some socialist priest: Gapon.

Sunday 22 January

A painful day. There have been serious disorders in St Petersburg because workmen wanted to come up to the Winter Palace. Troops had to open fire in several places in the city; there were many killed and wounded. God, how painful and sad! Mama arrived from town, straight to church. I lunched with all the others. Went for a walk with Misha. Mama stayed overnight.

From the Tsar's diary, recording the events of Bloody Sunday.

Bloody Sunday sparked a wave of strikes which spread to other cities. Barricades appeared in the streets accompanied by riots and violence. The Tsar's uncle was assassinated and it seemed the Tsar might well lose control of Russia. All sorts of groups joined the workers demanding change. These included the liberals and middle classes who wanted civil rights and a say in government, students who wanted freedom in the universities, and the nationalities demanding independence. However they did not combine to form a united opposition.

In June the sailors on Battleship Potemkin mutinied. This was dangerous for the Tsar who needed the armed forces to remain loyal. In the countryside, peasants attacked landlords and seized land. Workers' councils (or soviets) were formed, becoming particularly strong in St Petersburg and Moscow, and revolutionaries like Trotsky returned from exile to join in. In September a general strike began and paralysed Russian industry.

How did the Tsar survive?

Things were so bad at the end of September that the Tsar was persuaded, unwillingly, to issue the October Manifesto. This offered the people an elected parliament called the Duma, the right to free speech and the right to form political parties. This divided the Tsar's opponents. The liberals were delighted, feeling this had achieved their main aim, and the middle classes, desperate to end the violence and disorder, now supported moves to end the revolution.

The Tsar made peace with Japan and brought his troops back to help put down the trouble. To ensure their loyalty he promised them better pay and conditions. Now the government moved to restore order. In December 1905 the leaders of the St Petersburg and Moscow soviets were arrested. This led to fighting in Moscow and other cities but the workers were no match for the army and their resistance was crushed. In the countryside it took much of 1906 to bring peasant unrest under control. The Tsar promised financial help in setting up a peasants' bank to help them buy land but it was force that won the day. Troops were sent out in huge numbers to crush the peasants and the nationalities. Thousands were executed or imprisoned. Beatings and rape were used to terrify peasants into submission. It was clear that no revolution would succeed if the army stayed loyal to the Tsar.

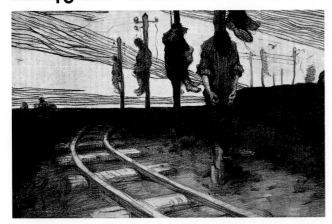

Nightmare: the aftermath of a Cossack punishment expedition: an illustration from the Russian magazine *Leshii*, 1906.

Source Analysis ▲

1 Read Source 9. Do you agree that it suggests the Tsar was out of touch? Explain your answer.
2 Do you think 'Nightmare' is a good title for Source 10?

Focus Task

How did the Tsar survive the 1905 revolution?

Copy and complete the diagram. Describe how each of the factors helped the Tsar survive and bring Russia back under control. We have started one branch for you.

THE TSAR SURVIVES

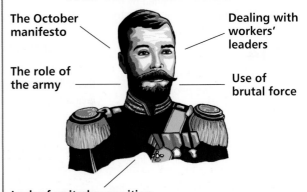

The October manifesto

Dealing with workers' leaders

The role of the army

Use of brutal force

Lack of united opposition

All the different groups — workers, peasants, liberals etc. — had different aims and never united together to bring down the Tsar's government.

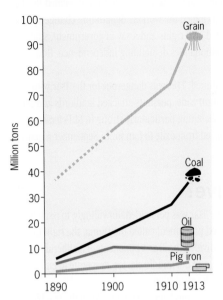

Agricultural and industrial production, 1890–1913.

SOURCE 13

Year	Strikes	Strikers
1905	13,995	2,863,173
1906	6,114	1,108,406
1907	3,573	740,074
1908	892	176,101
1909	340	64,166
1910	222	46,623
1911	466	105,110
1912	2,032	725,491
1913	2,404	887,096
1914	3,534	1,337,458

These figures were compiled by the Tsar's Ministry of Trade and Industry.

SOURCE 14

Let those in power make no mistake about the mood of the people . . . never were the Russian people . . . so profoundly revolutionised by the actions of the government, for day by day, faith in the government is steadily waning . . .

Guchkov, a Russian conservative in the Duma, 1913. By 1913, even staunch supporters of the Tsar were beginning to want change.

The troubled years, 1905–14

The Tsar survived the 1905 revolution, but some serious questions remained. Nicholas needed to reform Russia and satisfy at least some of the discontented groups that had joined the revolution in 1905. The Duma deputies who gathered for its first meeting in 1906 were hopeful that they could help to steer Russia on a new course. They were soon disappointed (see Source 12). The Tsar continued to rule without taking any serious notice of them. The first and second Dumas were very critical of the Tsar. They lasted less than a year before Nicholas sent them home. In 1907 Tsar Nicholas changed the voting rules so that his opponents were not elected to the Duma. This third Duma lasted until 1912, mainly because it was much less critical of the Tsar than the previous two. But by 1912 even this 'loyal' Duma was becoming critical of the Tsar's ministers and policies.

SOURCE 12

The two hostile sides stood confronting each other. The old and grey court dignitaries, keepers of etiquette and tradition, looked across in a haughty manner, though not without fear and confusion, at 'the people of the street', whom the revolution had swept into the palace, and quietly whispered to one another. The other side looked across at them with no less disdain or contempt.

The court side of the hall resounded with orchestrated cheers as the Tsar approached the throne. But the Duma deputies remained completely silent. It was a natural expression of our feelings towards the monarch, who in the twelve years of his reign had managed to destroy all the prestige of his predecessors. The feeling was mutual: not once did the Tsar glance towards the Duma side of the hall. Sitting on the throne he delivered a short, perfunctory speech in which he promised to uphold the principles of autocracy . . . .

From the memoirs of Duma deputy Obolensky, published in 1925. He is describing the first session of the Duma in April 1906.

Stolypin

In 1906 the Tsar appointed a tough new Prime Minister – Peter Stolypin. Stolypin used a 'carrot and stick' approach to the problems of Russia.

The stick: He came down hard on strikers, protesters and revolutionaries. Over 20,000 were exiled and over 1,000 hanged (the noose came to be known as 'Stolypin's necktie'). This brutal suppression effectively killed off opposition to the regime in the countryside until after 1914.

The carrot: Stolypin also tried to win over the peasants with the 'carrot' they had always wanted – land. He allowed wealthier peasants, the kulaks, to opt out of the mir communes and buy up land. These kulaks prospered and in the process created larger and more efficient farms. Production did increase significantly (see Source 11). On the other hand, 90 per cent of land in the fertile west of Russia was still run by inefficient communes in 1916. Farm sizes remained small even in Ukraine, Russia's best farmland. Most peasants still lived in the conditions and remained discontented.

Stolypin also tried to boost Russia's industries. There was impressive economic growth between 1908 and 1911. But Russia was still far behind modern industrial powers such as Britain, Germany and the USA.

Think!

1 What does Source 12 suggest about the attitude of the Tsar and the members of his court to the idea of the 'people' being more involved in running the country?

2 What does Source 13 suggest about working people's attitudes to the Tsar's regime?

The profits being made by industry were going to the capitalists, or they were being paid back to banks in France which had loaned the money to pay for much of Russia's industrial growth. Very little of this new wealth found its way back to the urban workers whose wages remained low while the cost of food and housing was rising. Living and working conditions had not really improved – they were still appalling.

Stolypin was assassinated in 1911, but the Tsar was about to sack him anyway. He worried that Stolypin was trying to change Russia too much. Nicholas had already blocked some of Stolypin's plans for basic education for the people and regulations to protect factory workers. The Tsar was influenced by the landlords and members of the court. They saw Stolypin's reforms as a threat to the traditional Russian society in which everyone knew their place.

Relations between the Tsar and his people became steadily worse. The year 1913 saw huge celebrations for the three hundredth anniversary of the Romanovs' rule in Russia. The celebrations were meant to bring the country together, but enthusiasm was limited.

Discontent grew, especially among the growing industrial working class in the cities. Strikes were on the rise (see Source 13), including the highly publicised Lena gold field strike where troops opened fire on striking miners. However, the army and police dealt with these problems and so, to its opponents, the government must have seemed firmly in control.

Strangely, some of the government's supporters were less sure about the government (see Source 14). Industrialists were concerned by the way in which the Tsar preferred to appoint loyal but unimaginative and sometimes incompetent ministers.

SOURCE 15

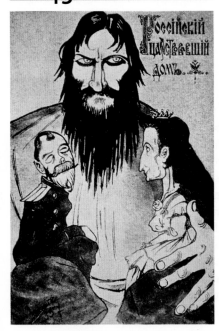

Russian cartoon. The caption reads: 'The Russian Tsars at home.'

Rasputin

Some of the Tsar's supporters were particularly alarmed about the influence of a strange and dangerous figure – Gregory Yefimovich, generally known as Rasputin. The Tsar's son Alexis was very ill with a blood disease called haemophilia. Through hypnosis, it appeared that Rasputin could control the disease. He was greeted as a miracle worker by the Tsarina (the Tsar's wife). Before long, Rasputin was also giving her and the Tsar advice on how to run the country. People in Russia were very suspicious of Rasputin. He was said to be a drinker and a womaniser. His name means 'disreputable'. The Tsar's opponents seized on Rasputin as a sign of the Tsar's weakness and unfitness to rule Russia. The fact that the Tsar either didn't notice their concern or, worse still, didn't care showed just how out of touch he was.

How far was the Tsar weakened by the First World War?

The First World War had a massive impact on Russia. Your task is to use the material on pages 196–197 to present an overview of how the war affected four different groups of people in Russian society. The groups are:

♦ the army
♦ the workers
♦ the middle classes
♦ the aristocracy.

As you read through pages 196–197 you will find out about the impact of the war on each group. Write a paragraph or series of notes summarising the impact of war on each group.

SOURCE 16

The army had neither wagons nor horses nor first aid supplies . . . We visited the Warsaw station where there were about 17,000 men wounded in battle. At the station we found a terrible scene: on the platform in dirt, filth and cold, on the ground, even without straw, wounded men, who filled the air with heart-rending cries, dolefully asked: 'For God's sake order them to dress our wounds. For five days we have not been attended to.'

From a report by Michael Rodzianko, President of the Duma.

SOURCE 17

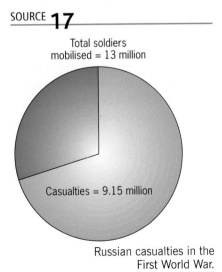

Total soldiers mobilised = 13 million

Casualties = 9.15 million

Russian casualties in the First World War.

War and revolution

In August 1914 Russia entered the First World War. Tensions in the country seemed to disappear. The Tsar seemed genuinely popular with his people and there was an instant display of patriotism. The Tsar's action was applauded. Workers, peasants and aristocrats all joined in the patriotic enthusiasm. Anti-government strikes and demonstrations were abandoned. The good feeling, however, was very short-lived. As the war continued, the Tsar began to lose the support of key sectors of Russian society.

The army

The Russian army was a huge army of conscripts. At first, the soldiers were enthusiastic, as was the rest of society. Even so, many peasants felt that they were fighting to defend their country against the Germans rather than showing any loyalty to the Tsar. Russian soldiers fought bravely, but they stood little chance against the German army. They were badly led and treated appallingly by their aristocrat officers. They were also poorly supported by the industries at home. They were short of rifles, ammunition, artillery and shells. Many did not even have boots.

The Tsar took personal command of the armed forces in September 1915. This made little difference to the war, since Nicholas was not a particularly able commander. However, it did mean that people held Nicholas personally responsible for the defeats and the blunders. The defeats and huge losses continued throughout 1916. It is not surprising that by 1917 there was deep discontent in the army.

Peasants and workers

It did not take long for the strain of war to alienate the peasants and the workers. The huge casualty figures took their toll. In August 1916, the local governor of the village of Grushevka reported that the war had killed 13 per cent of the population of the village. This left many widows and orphans needing state war pensions which they did not always receive.

Despite the losses, food production remained high until 1916. By then, the government could not always be relied on to pay for the food produced. The government planned to take food by force but abandoned the idea because it feared it might spark a widespread revolt.

By 1916 there was much discontent in the cities. War contracts created an extra 3.5 million industrial jobs between 1914 and 1916. The workers got little in the way of extra wages. They also had to cope with even worse overcrowding than before the war. There were fuel and food shortages. What made it worse was that there was enough food and fuel, but it could not be transported to the cities. The rail network could not cope with the needs of the army, industry and the populations of the cities. The prices of almost everything got higher and higher. As 1916 turned into 1917, many working men and women stood and shivered in bread queues and cursed the Tsar.

The middle classes

The middle classes did not suffer in the same way as the peasants and workers, but they too were unhappy with the Tsar by the end of 1916. Many middle-class activists in the zemstva were appalled by reports such as Source 16. They set up their own medical organisations along the lines of the modern Red Cross, or joined war committees to send other supplies to the troops. These organisations were generally far more effective than the government agencies. By 1916 many industrialists were complaining that they could not fulfil their war contracts because of a shortage of raw materials (especially metals) and fuel. In 1915 an alliance of Duma politicians, the Progressive Bloc, had urged the Tsar to work with them in a more representative style of government that would unite the people. The Tsar dismissed the Duma a month later.

SOURCE 18

The average worker's wage in 1917 was 5 roubles a day. This would buy you:

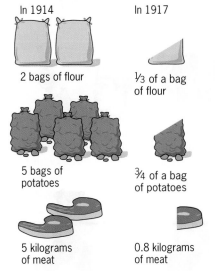

In 1914 — 2 bags of flour   In 1917 — ⅓ of a bag of flour

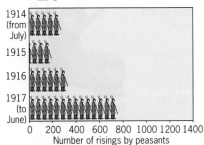

5 bags of potatoes   ¾ of a bag of potatoes

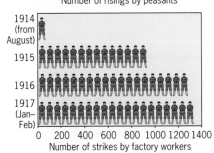

5 kilograms of meat   0.8 kilograms of meat

Prices in Russia, 1914–17.

SOURCE 20

1914 (from July)
1915
1916
1917 (to June)
0 200 400 600 800 1000 1200 1400
Number of risings by peasants

1914 (from August)
1915
1916
1917 (Jan–Feb)
0 200 400 600 800 1000 1200 1400
Number of strikes by factory workers

Peasant risings and strikes, 1914–17.

Think!

Imagine you are an adviser to the Tsar in 1916. Which of the sources on pages 196–197 would give you most concern? Explain your answer.

The aristocracy

The situation was so bad by late 1916 that the Council of the United Nobility was calling for the Tsar to step down. The junior officers in the army had suffered devastating losses in the war. Many of these officers were the future of the aristocrat class. The conscription of 13 million peasants also threatened aristocrats' livelihoods, because they had no workers for their estates. Most of all, many of the leading aristocrats were appalled by the influence of Rasputin over the government of Russia. When the Tsar left Petrograd (the new Russian version of the Germanic name St Petersburg) to take charge of the army, he left his wife in control of the country. The fact that she was German started rumours flying in the capital. There were also rumours of an affair between her and Rasputin. Ministers were dismissed and then replaced. The concerns were so serious that a group of leading aristocrats murdered Rasputin in December 1916.

SOURCE 19

I asked for an audience and was received by him [the Tsar] on March 8th. 'I must tell Your Majesty that this cannot continue much longer. No one opens your eyes to the true role which this man is playing. His presence in Your Majesty's court undermines confidence in the Supreme Power and may have an evil effect on the fate of the dynasty and turn the hearts of the people from their Emperor' . . . My report did some good. On March 11th an order was issued sending Rasputin to Tobolsk; but a few days later, at the demand of the Empress, this order was cancelled.

M Rodzianko, President of the Duma, March 1916.

The March 1917 revolution

As 1917 dawned, few people had great hopes for the survival of the Tsar's regime. In January strikes broke out all over Russia. In February the strikes spread. They were supported and even joined by members of the army. The Tsar's best troops lay dead on the battlefields. These soldiers were recent conscripts and had more in common with the strikers than their officers. On 7 March workers at the Putilov steelworks in Petrograd went on strike. They joined with thousands of women – it was International Women's Day – and other discontented workers demanding that the government provide bread. From 7 to 10 March the number of striking workers rose to 250,000. Industry came to a standstill. The Duma set up a Provisional Committee to take over the government. The Tsar ordered them to disband. They refused. On 12 March the Tsar ordered his army to put down the revolt by force. They refused. This was the decisive moment. Some soldiers even shot their own officers and joined the demonstrators. They marched to the Duma demanding that they take over the government. Reluctantly, the Duma leaders accepted – they had always wanted reform rather than revolution, but now there seemed no choice.

On the same day, revolutionaries set up the Petrograd Soviet again, and began taking control of food supplies to the city. They set up soldiers' committees, undermining the authority of the officers. It was not clear who was in charge of Russia, but it was obvious that the Tsar was not! On 15 March he issued a statement that he was abdicating. There was an initial plan for his brother Michael to take over, but Michael refused: Russia had finished with Tsars.

SOURCE 21

One company of the Pavlovsky Regiment's reserve battalion had declared on 26 February that it would not fire on people . . . We have just received a telegram from the Minister of War stating that the rebels have seized the most important buildings in all parts of the city. Due to fatigue and propaganda the troops have laid down their arms, passed to the side of the rebels or become neutral . . .

General Alekseyev, February 1917.

Focus Task A

How important was the war in the collapse of the Tsarist regime?

Historians have furiously debated this question since the revolution took place. There are two main views:

View 1

The Tsar's regime was basically stable up to 1914, even if it had some important problems to deal with. It was making steady progress towards becoming a modern state, but this progress was destroyed by the coming of war. Don't forget that this war was so severe that it also brought Germany, Austria–Hungary and Turkey to their knees as well.

View 2

The regime in Russia was cursed with a weak Tsar, a backward economy and a class of aristocrats who were not prepared to share their power and privileges with the millions of ordinary Russians. Revolution was only a matter of time. The war did not cause it, although it may have speeded up the process.

Divide the class into two groups.

One group has to find evidence and arguments to support View 1, the other to support View 2.

You could compare notes in a class discussion or organise a formal debate. You may even be able to compare your views with students in other schools using email conferencing.

Focus Task B

Why was the March 1917 revolution successful?

The Tsar faced a major revolution in 1905 but he survived. Why was 1917 different? Why was he not able to survive in 1917?

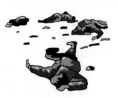

The military failures of the war
(Questioned deaths, competence of Tsar and government)

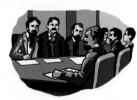

Duma formed provisional government
(Alternatives to Tsar's government)

The workers
(Strikes, unrest)

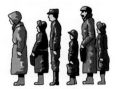

Shortages at home
(Food, fuel, rising prices)

Tsarina and Rasputin
(Damaged reputations)

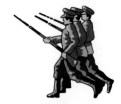

Mutiny of the army

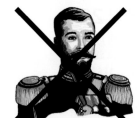

Tsar's supporters
(Aristocrats, middle classes, army officers had lost faith in Tsar as leader)

Stage 1

1 Copy the headings in this diagram. They show seven reasons why the Tsar was forced to abdicate in March 1917.
2 For each of the factors, write one or two sentences explaining how it contributed to the fall of the Tsar.
3 Draw lines between any of the factors that seem to be connected. Label your line explaining what the link is.

Stage 2

4 In pairs or small groups, discuss the following points:
   a) Which factors were present in 1905?
   b) Were these same factors more or less serious than in 1905?
   c) Which factors were not present in 1905?
   d) Were the new factors decisive in making the March 1917 revolution successful?

Key Question Summary

Why did the Tsarist regime collapse in 1917?

1 The Tsar was a weak, indecisive leader whose government did not run the country well.
2 The regime had lost the support and loyalty of the people.
   a) The workers were deeply resentful because their living and working conditions had improved little despite the wealth produced by a rapidly developing industry.
   b) The peasants would only be satisfied when they owned the land. Some improvements had been made by the land reforms but most peasants lived very poor lives.
3 The middle classes wanted a say in government. The Tsar refused to respond to this demand and would not work with the Duma, even during the war.
4 The Russian army had done badly in the war, losing many lives, and the Tsar was held responsible for this.
5 The Tsarina and Rasputin had damaged the reputation of the royal family and made a terrible mess of running the country when the Tsar went to the warfront. Even top aristocrats and army generals thought the Tsar was unfit to run Russia.
6 The war had caused extreme shortages in St Petersburg leaving an angry strike-prone, discontented population which exploded in March 1917.
7 The crucial factor was when the soldiers mutinied and went over to the side of the people. Support for the Tsarist regime had crumbled.

8.2 How did the Bolsheviks gain and hold on to power?

The Provisional Government should do nothing now which would break our ties with the allies. The worst thing that could happen to us would be separate peace. It would be ruinous for the Russian revolution, ruinous for international democracy . . .

As to the land question, we regard it as our duty at the present to prepare the ground for a just solution of the problem by the Constituent Assembly.

A Provisional Government Minister explains why Russia should stay in the war, 1917.

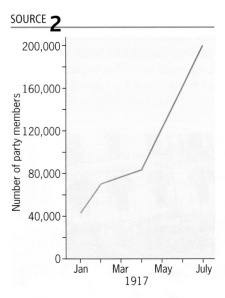

Growth of Bolshevik support, 1917.

Think!

Read Source 1. How popular do you think the Provisional Government's policies on the war and land would be with the peasants and the soldiers?

Focus

If you had asked Russians in Petrograd in March 1917 what they thought of the Bolsheviks, most would probably have said, 'Who are the Bolsheviks?' Yet this small party quite dramatically seized control of Russia just six months later in November 1917.

Once in power most people thought the Bolsheviks would survive only a few weeks. They had a formidable set of enemies lined up against them. In the first few days they could not even get into the central bank to get money to run the government. Yet, against all the odds, they did survive.

So your focus in pages 199–210 is all about how they did it. It all begins with the problems facing the Provisional Government of Russia in March 1917.

Focus Points

♦ How effectively did the Provisional Government rule Russia in 1917?
♦ Why were the Bolsheviks able to seize power in November 1917?
♦ Why did the Bolsheviks win the Civil War?
♦ How far was the New Economic Policy a success?

The Provisional Government (Mar–Oct 1917)

Russia's problems were not solved by the abdication of the Tsar. The Duma's Provisional Committee took over government. It faced three overwhelmingly urgent decisions:

● to continue the war or make peace
● to distribute land to the peasants (who had already started taking it) or ask them to wait until elections had been held
● how best to get food to the starving workers in the cities.

The Provisional Government was dominated by middle-class liberals, particularly the Cadets, although some revolutionary leaders joined them later. It included men such as the lawyer Alexander Kerensky – Justice Minister in the Provisional Government but also a respected member of the Petrograd Soviet – it also included angry revolutionaries who had no experience of government at all. The Provisional Government promised Russia's allies that it would continue the war, while trying to settle the situation in Russia. It also urged the peasants to be restrained and wait for elections before taking any land. The idea was that the Provisional Government could then stand down and allow free elections to take place to elect a new Constituent Assembly that would fairly and democratically represent the people of Russia. It was a very cautious message for a people who had just gone through a revolution.

However, the Provisional Government was not the only possible government. The newly formed Petrograd Soviet held the real power in St Petersburg. It had the support of the workers, e.g. railway men, and, crucially, the soldiers in St Petersburg. It could control what went on in the city. However, the Soviet decided to work with the Provisional Government in the spring and summer of 1917.

One man was determined to push the revolution further. He was Lenin, leader of the Bolsheviks (see page 202). When he heard of the March revolution he immediately returned to Russia from exile in Europe. The Germans even provided him with a special train, hoping that he might cause more chaos in Russia!

When Lenin arrived at Petrograd station, he set out the Bolshevik programme in his April Theses. He urged the people to support the Bolsheviks in a second revolution. Lenin's slogans 'Peace, Land and Bread' and 'All power to the soviets' contrasted sharply with the cautious message of the Provisional Government. Support for the Bolsheviks increased quickly (see Sources 2 and 4), particularly in the soviets and in the army.

SOURCE 3

A sudden and disastrous change has occurred in the attitude of the troops . . . Authority and obedience no longer exist . . . for hundreds of miles one can see deserters, armed and unarmed, in good health and in high spirits, certain they will not be punished.

A Russian officer reporting back to the Provisional Government, 1917.

SOURCE 4

The Bolshevik speaker would ask the crowd 'Do you need more land?'

Do you have as much land as the landlords do?'

'But will the Kerensky government give you land? No, never. It protects the interests of the landlords. Only our party, the Bolsheviks, will immediately give you land . . .'

Several times I tried to take the floor and explain that the Bolsheviks make promises which they can never fulfil. I used figures from farming statistics to prove my point; but I saw that the crowded square was unsuitable for this kind of discussion.

A Menshevik writer, summer 1917.

Source Analysis

How useful is Source 4 to a historian studying Russia at this time? Use the source and your own knowledge to explain your answer.

In the second half of 1917, the Provisional Government's authority steadily collapsed.

- The war effort was failing. Soldiers had been deserting in thousands from the army. Kerensky became Minister for War and rallied the army for a great offensive in June. It was a disaster. The army began to fall apart in the face of a German counter-attack (see Source 3). The deserters decided to come home.

- Desertions were made worse because another element of the Provisional Government's policy had failed. The peasants ignored the orders of the government to wait. They were simply taking control of the countryside. The soldiers, who were mostly peasants, did not want to miss their turn when the land was shared out.

The Provisional Government's problems got worse in the summer. In July (the 'July Days'), Bolshevik-led protests against the war turned into a rebellion. However, when Kerensky produced evidence that Lenin had been helped by the Germans, support for the rebellion fell. Lenin, in disguise, fled to Finland. Kerensky used troops to crush the rebellion and took over the government.

SOURCE 5

The Provisional Government possesses no real power and its orders are executed only in so far as this is permitted by the Soviet of Workers' and Soldiers' Deputies, which holds in its hands the most important elements of actual power, such as troops, railroads, postal and telegraph service . . .

A letter from Guchkov, Minister for War in the Provisional Government, to General Alekseyev, 22 March 1917.

SOURCE 6

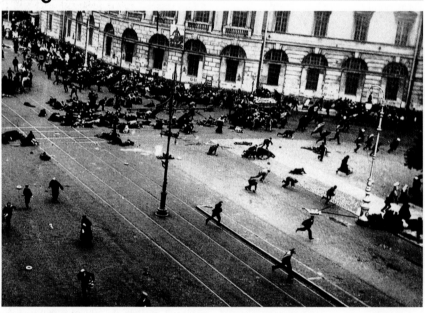

Troops loyal to the Provisional Government fire on Bolshevik demonstrators during the July Days.

Kerensky was in a very difficult situation. In the cities strikes, lawlessness and violence were rife. The upper and middle classes expected him to restore order. Kerensky seemed unable to do anything about this or the deteriorating economic situation.

There was little reason for the ordinary people of Russia to be grateful to the Provisional Government (see Sources 7 and 8).

SOURCE 7

Cabs and horse-drawn carriages began to disappear. Street-car service was erratic. The railway stations filled with tramps and deserting soldiers, often drunk, sometimes threatening. The police force had vanished in the first days of the Revolution. Now 'revolutionary order' was over. Hold-ups and robberies became the order of the day. Politically, signs of chaos were everywhere.

HE Salisbury, *Russia in Revolution*.

Source Analysis

How far do you think Source 8 is a reliable source about the situation in Russia under the Provisional Government? Use the source, your knowledge and the other sources in this section to explain your answer.

SOURCE 8

Week by week food became scarcer . . . one had to queue for long hours in the chill rain . . . Think of the poorly clad people standing on the streets of Petrograd for whole days in the Russian winter! I have listened in the bread-lines, hearing the bitter discontent which from time to time burst through the miraculous good nature of the Russian crowd.

John Reed, an American writer who lived in Petrograd in 1917.

Others were also fed up with the Provisional Government. In September 1917, the army leader Kornilov marched his troops towards Moscow, intending to get rid of the Bolsheviks and the Provisional Government, and restore order. Kerensky was in an impossible situation. He had some troops who supported him but they were no match for Kornilov's. Kerensky turned to the only group which could save him: his Bolshevik opponents. The Bolsheviks organised themselves into an army which they called the Red Guards. Kornilov's troops refused to fight members of the Soviet so his plans collapsed.

But it was hardly a victory for Kerensky. In fact, by October Kerensky's government was doomed. It had tried to carry on the war and failed. It had therefore lost the army's support. It had tried to stop the peasants from taking over the land and so lost their support too. Without peasant support it had failed to bring food into the towns and food prices had spiralled upwards. This had lost the government any support it had from the urban workers.

In contrast, the Bolsheviks were promising what the people wanted most (bread, peace, land). It was the Bolsheviks who had removed the threat of Kornilov. By the end of September 1917, the Bolsheviks had control of the Petrograd Soviet and Leon Trotsky was its chairman. They also controlled the soviets in Moscow and other major cities.

What do you think happened next?

Focus Task

How effectively did the Provisional Government rule Russia in 1917?

Step 1

1 Here is a list of some decisions that faced the Provisional Government when it took over in March 1917:
   a) what to do about the war
   b) what to do about land
   c) what to do about food.
   For each one, say how the government dealt with it, and what the result of the action was.
2 Based on your answers to question 1, how effective do you think the Provisional Government was? Give it a mark out of ten.

Step 2

3 Read through pages 199–201 again. Think about how effectively the Provisional Government dealt with their opponents:
   ♦ Petrograd Soviet
   ♦ Bolsheviks
   ♦ Kornilov's attempted coup..
4 Based on your answers to question 3, would you revise the score you gave the government in question 2?

Step 3

5 Now reach an overview score. Out of 10, how effective was the Provisional Government? Write a paragraph to explain your score.

SOURCE 9

The Provisional Government has been overthrown. The cause for which the people have fought has been made safe: the immediate proposal of a democratic peace, the end of land owners' rights, workers' control over production, the creation of a Soviet government. Long live the revolution of workers, soldiers and peasants.

Proclamation of the Petrograd Soviet, 8 November 1917.

The Bolshevik Revolution

By the end of October 1917, Lenin was convinced that the time was right for the Bolsheviks to seize power. They had the support of many workers and control of the Soviet. Lenin convinced the other Bolsheviks to act swiftly. It was not easy — leading Bolsheviks like Kamenev felt that Russia was not ready, but neither he nor any other Bolshevik could match Lenin in an argument.

During the night of 6 November, the Red Guards led by Leon Trotsky took control of post offices, bridges and the State Bank. On 7 November, Kerensky awoke to find the Bolsheviks were in control of most of Petrograd. Through the day, with almost no opposition, the Red Guards continued to take over railway stations and other important targets. On the evening of 7 November, they stormed the Winter Palace (again, without much opposition) and arrested the ministers of the Provisional Government. Kerensky managed to escape and tried to rally loyal troops. When this failed, he fled into exile. On 8 November an announcement was made to the Russian people (see Source 9).

Why did the Bolsheviks succeed?

Despite what they claimed, the Bolsheviks did not have the support of the majority of the Russian people. So how were they able to carry out their takeover in November 1917?

- The unpopularity of the Provisional Government was a critical factor — there were no massive demonstrations demanding the return of Kerensky!
- A second factor was that the Bolsheviks were a disciplined party dedicated to revolution, even though not all the Bolshevik leaders believed this was the right way to change Russia.
- The Bolsheviks had some 800,000 members, and their supporters were also in the right places, including substantial numbers of soldiers and sailors. (The Bolsheviks were still the only party demanding that Russia should pull out of the war.)
- The major industrial centres, and the Petrograd and Moscow Soviets especially, were also pro-Bolshevik.
- The Bolsheviks also had some outstanding personalities in their ranks, particularly Trotsky and their leader Lenin.

Profile

Vladimir Ilich Lenin

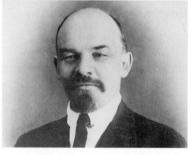

- Born 1870 into a respectable Russian family.
- Brother hanged in 1887 for plotting against the Tsar.
- Graduated from St Petersburg University after being thrown out of Kazan University for his political beliefs.
- One of the largest Okhrana files was about him!
- Exiled to Siberia 1897–1900.
- 1900–03 lived in various countries writing the revolutionary newspaper 'Iskra' ('The Spark').
- Became leader of the Bolsheviks in 1903.
- Was exiled in European countries, 1905–17.
- Returned to Russia after the first revolution in 1917.
- Led the Bolsheviks to power in November 1917.

Think!

Work in pairs, taking either Lenin or Trotsky.
1. Using Sources 10–14 add extra bullet points to the profiles of Lenin (this page) and Trotsky (page 203):
   - why he appealed to people
   - his personal qualities
   - his strengths as a leader.
2. Finally, write a short report on the contribution of your individual to the Bolsheviks' success in 1917.

SOURCE 10

This extraordinary figure [Lenin] was first and foremost a professional revolutionary. He had no other occupation. A man of iron will and inflexible ambition, he was absolutely ruthless and used human beings as mere material for his purpose. Short and sturdy with a bald head, small beard and deep set eyes, Lenin looked like a small tradesman. When he spoke at meetings his ill-fitting suit, his crooked tie, his ordinary appearance disposed the crowd in his favour. 'He is not one of the gentlefolk, he is one of us', they would say.

The Times, writing about Lenin after his death, 1924.

Profile

Leon Trotsky

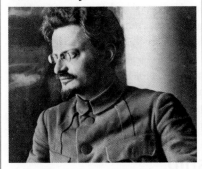

- Born 1879 into a respectable and prosperous Jewish farming family.
- Exceptionally bright at school and brilliant at university.
- Politically active – arrested in 1900 and deported to Siberia.
- Escaped to London in 1902 and met Lenin there.
- Joined the Social Democratic Party, but supported the Menshevik wing rather than the Bolsheviks.
- Played an important role in the 1905 revolution – imprisoned for his activities.
- Escaped in 1907 and worked as a writer and journalist in Europe, especially in Vienna, Austria. Edited *Pravda*, the newspaper of the Social Democratic Party.
- In 1917 he returned to Russia and played a key role in the Bolshevik Revolution.
- In 1918 he became the Commissar for War and led the Bolsheviks to victory in the Civil War which broke out in 1918.

SOURCE 15

The [November] Revolution has often and widely been held to have been mainly Lenin's revolution. But was it? Certainly Lenin had a heavier impact on the course [of events] than anyone else. The point is, however, that great historical changes are brought about not only by individuals. There were other mighty factors at work as well in Russia in 1917 . . . Lenin simply could not have done or even co-ordinated everything.

Historian Robert Service, writing in 1990.

SOURCE 11

Lenin . . . was the overall planner of the revolution: he also dealt with internal divisions within the party and provided tight control, and a degree of discipline and unity which the other parties lacked.

SJ Lee, *The European Dictatorships*, 1987.

SOURCE 12

The struggle was headed by Lenin who guided the Party's Central Committee, the editorial board of Pravda, and who kept in touch with the Party organisations in the provinces . . . He frequently addressed mass rallies and meetings. Lenin's appearance on the platform inevitably triggered off the cheers of the audience. Lenin's brilliant speeches inspired the workers and soldiers to a determined struggle.

Soviet historian Y Kukushkin, *History of the USSR*, 1981

SOURCE 13

Now that the great revolution has come, one feels that however intelligent Lenin may be he begins to fade beside the genius of Trotsky.

Mikhail Uritsky, 1917. Uritsky was a Bolshevik activist and went on to play an important role in Bolshevik governments after 1917.

SOURCE 14

Under the influence of his [Trotsky's] tremendous activity and blinding success, certain people close to Trotsky were even inclined to see in him the real leader of the Russian revolution . . . It is true that during that period, after the thunderous success of his arrival in Russia and before the July days, Lenin did keep rather in the background, not speaking often, not writing much, but largely engaged in directing organisational work in the Bolshevik camp, whilst Trotsky thundered forth at meetings in Petrograd. Trotsky's most obvious gifts were his talents as an orator and as a writer. I regard Trotsky as probably the greatest orator of our age. In my time I have heard all the greatest parliamentarians and popular tribunes of socialism and very many famous orators of the bourgeois world and I would find it difficult to name any of them whom I could put in the same class as Trotsky.

From *Revolutionary Silhouettes*, by Anatoly Lunacharsky, published in 1918. The book was a series of portraits of leading revolutionaries. The author was a Bolshevik activist and knew Lenin and Trotsky well.

Focus Task

Why were the Bolsheviks able to seize power in November 1917?

1 Using your answers in this section, sum up how **Bolshevik organisation** and **leadership** contributed to their success.
2 Read Source 15.
3 Here are some of the 'other mighty factors at work'. Write some notes to explain how each one helped the Bolsheviks. The first has been done for you:
   - Collapse of the Tsar's regime – *This had left a power vacuum. It was difficult to set up a new democratic regime which everybody would support.*
   - War (people war weary, disruption)
   - Army disintegrating (officers and soldiers in St Petersburg)
   - Peasants (had already begun to seize land)
   - Desperate economic situation (desperate people)

Bolshevik decrees, 1917

8 November
➤ Land belonging to Tsar, Church and nobles handed over to peasants.
➤ Russia asked for peace with Germany.
12 November
➤ Working day limited to eight hours; 48-hour week; rules made about overtime and holidays.
14 November
➤ Workers to be insured against illness or accident.
1 December
➤ All non-Bolshevik newspapers banned.
11 December
➤ The opposition Constitutional Democratic Party (Cadets) banned; its leaders arrested.
20 December
➤ Cheka (secret police) set up to deal with 'spies and counter-revolutionaries'.
27 December
➤ Factories put under control of workers' committees.
➤ Banks put under Bolshevik government control.
31 December
➤ Marriages could take place without a priest if desired.
➤ Divorce made easier.

Think!

Study the Factfile. Which of the Bolshevik decrees would you say aimed to:
a) keep the peasants happy
b) keep the workers happy
c) increase Bolshevik control
d) improve personal freedom in Russia?

Lenin in power

Lenin and the Bolsheviks had promised the people bread, peace and land. Lenin knew that if he failed to deliver, the Bolsheviks would suffer the same fate as the Provisional Government.

Lenin immediately set up the Council of People's Commissars (the Sovnarkom). It issued its first decree on 8 November, announcing that Russia was asking for peace with Germany. There followed an enormous number of decrees from the new government that aimed to strengthen the Bolsheviks' hold on power (see Factfile). The peasants were given the nobles' lands. The factories and industries were put into the hands of the workers. The Bolsheviks were given power to deal ruthlessly with their opponents – and they did (see page 205).

The Bolshevik dictatorship

Lenin had also promised free elections to the new Constituent Assembly. Elections were held in late 1917. As Lenin had feared, the Bolsheviks did not gain a majority (see Source 16). Their rivals, the peasant-based Socialist Revolutionaries, were the biggest party when the Assembly opened on 18 January 1918.

Lenin solved this problem in his typically direct style. He sent the Red Guards to close down the Assembly. After brief protests (again put down by the Red Guards) the Assembly was forgotten. Lenin instead used the Congress of Soviets to pass his laws as it did contain a Bolshevik majority.

Russia's democratic experiment therefore lasted less than 24 hours, but this did not trouble Lenin's conscience. He believed he was establishing a dictatorship of the proletariat which in time would give way to true Communism.

SOURCE **16**

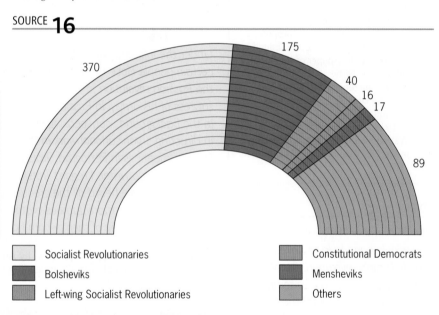

Socialist Revolutionaries		Constitutional Democrats
Bolsheviks		Mensheviks
Left-wing Socialist Revolutionaries		Others

The results of the Constituent Assembly elections, 1917.

Making peace

The next promise that Lenin had to make good was for peace. He put Trotsky in charge of negotiating a peace treaty. He told Trotsky to try to spin out the peace negotiations as long as possible. He hoped that very soon a socialist revolution would break out in Germany as it had in Russia. By February of 1918, however, there was no revolution and the Germans began to advance again. Lenin had to accept their terms in the Treaty of Brest–Litovsk in March 1918.

The Treaty was a severe blow to Russia. You can see how much land was lost in Source 17, but this was not the whole story. Russia's losses included 34 per cent of its population, 32 per cent of its agricultural land, 54 per cent of its industry, 26 per cent of its railways and 89 per cent of its coalmines. A final blow was the imposition of a fine of 300 million gold roubles. It was another example of Lenin's single-minded leadership. If this much had to be sacrificed to safeguard his revolution, then so be it. Many Russians, including revolutionaries, were opposed to the signing of the treaty.

SOURCE **17**

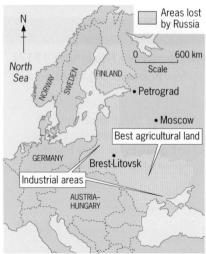

The Treaty of Brest-Litovsk, 1918.

Opposition and Civil War

Lenin's activities in 1917–18 were bound to make him enemies. He survived an attempted assassination in August 1918 (he was hit three times). In December he set up a secret police force called the Cheka to crush his opponents.

By the end of 1918 an unlikely collection of anti-Bolshevik elements had united against the Bolsheviks. They became known as the Whites (in contrast to the Bolshevik Reds) and consisted of enemies of the Bolsheviks from inside and outside Russia (see Factfile). By the spring of 1918 three separate White armies were marching on Bolshevik-controlled western Russia. Generals Yudenich and Denikin marched towards Petrograd and Moscow, while Admiral Kolchak marched on Moscow from central southern Russia.

Factfile

The Whites

'Whites' was a very broad term and was applied to any anti-Bolshevik group(s). Whites were made up of:

➤ Socialist Revolutionaries
➤ Mensheviks
➤ supporters of the Tsar
➤ landlords and capitalists who had lost land or money in the revolution
➤ the Czech Legion (former prisoners of war).

The Whites were also supported for part of the Civil War by foreign troops from the USA, Japan, France and Britain. They were sent by their governments to force Russia back into war against Germany.

SOURCE 19

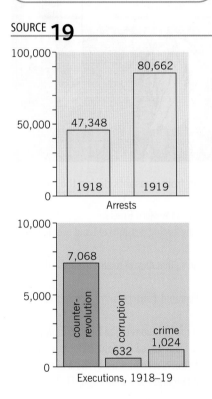

The Red Terror.

SOURCE 18

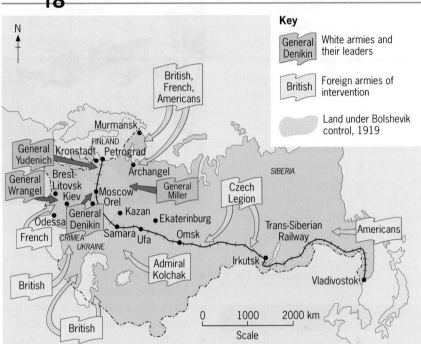

The main developments of the Civil War.

The reaction of the Bolsheviks was ruthless and determined. In an amazingly short time, Leon Trotsky created a new Red Army of over 300,000 men. They were led by former Tsarist officers. Trotsky made sure of their loyalty by holding their families hostage and by appointing political commissars to watch over them. The Cheka (secret police) terrorised the populations of Bolshevik territories so that nobody co-operated. In July 1918, White forces were approaching Ekaterinburg where the Tsar was being held. The Bolshevik commander ordered the execution of the Tsar and his family. Lenin could not risk the Tsar being rescued and returned as leader of the Whites. The fighting was savage with both sides committing terrible acts of cruelty.

Through harsh discipline and brilliant leadership, Trotsky's Red Army began to turn back the White forces. Kolchak's forces were destroyed towards the end of 1919 and at the same time the foreign 'armies of intervention' withdrew. The Whites were not really a strong alliance, and their armies were unable to work together. Trotsky defeated them one by one. The last major White army was defeated in the Crimea in November 1920.

Why did the Bolsheviks win the Civil War?

The Red Army was no match for the armies that were still fighting on the Western Front in 1918. However, compared to the Whites, the Red Army was united and disciplined. It was also brilliantly led by Trotsky.

SOURCE 20

In the villages the peasant will not give grain to the Bolsheviks because he hates them. Armed companies are sent to take grain from the peasant and every day, all over Russia, fights for grain are fought to a finish.

In the Red Army, for any military offence, there is only one punishment, death. If a regiment retreats against orders, machine guns are turned on them. The position of the bourgeoisie [middle class] defies all description. Payments by the banks have been stopped. It is forbidden to sell furniture. All owners and managers of works, offices and shops have been called up for compulsory labour. In Petrograd hundreds of people are dying from hunger. People are arrested daily and kept in prison for months without trial.

The Red Terror, observed by a British businessman in Russia in 1918.

Source Analysis

1 Use Sources 20 and 21 to describe how the Civil War affected ordinary people.
2 Do you think Source 21 was painted by opponents or supporters of the Bolsheviks?
3 Look at Source 24. Who is controlling the White forces?
4 Who do you think Source 23 is talking to?

SOURCE 21

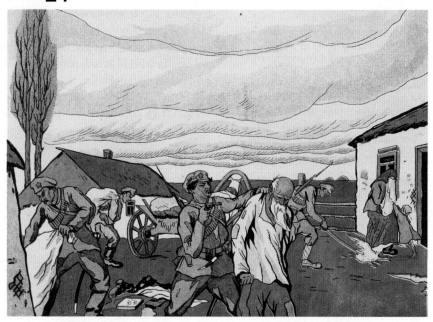

Members of the Red Guard requisition grain from peasants during the Civil War.

The Bolsheviks also kept strict control over their heartlands in western Russia.

- They made sure that the towns and armies were fed, by forcing peasants to hand over food and by rationing supplies (see Source 22).
- They took over the factories of Moscow and Petrograd so that they were able to supply their armies with equipment and ammunition.
- The Red Terror made sure that the population was kept under strict control (see Sources 19 and 20).
- The Bolsheviks used propaganda to raise fears about the intentions of the foreign armies in league with the Whites (Source 24). A propaganda train spread Communist ideas across Russia. Effective propaganda also made good use of atrocities committed by the Whites and raised fears about the possible return of the Tsar and landlords (see Sources 20, 21, 23 and 24).

SOURCE 22

Having surrounded the village [the Whites] fired a couple of volleys in the direction of the village and everyone took cover. Then the mounted soldiers entered the village, met the Bolshevik committee and put the members to death . . . After the execution the houses of the culprits were burned and the male population under forty-five whipped . . . Then the population was ordered to deliver without pay the best cattle, pigs, fowl, forage and bread for the soldiers as well as the best horses.

Diary of Colonel Drozdovsky, from his memoirs written in 1923. He was a White commander during the Civil War.

SOURCE 23

For the first time in history the working people have got control of their country. The workers of all countries are striving to achieve this objective. We in Russia have succeeded. We have thrown off the rule of the Tsar, of landlords and of capitalists. But we still have tremendous difficulties to overcome. We cannot build a new society in a day. We ask you, are you going to crush us? To help give Russia back to the landlords, the capitalists and the Tsar?

Red propaganda leaflet, *Why Have You Come to Murmansk?*

SOURCE 24

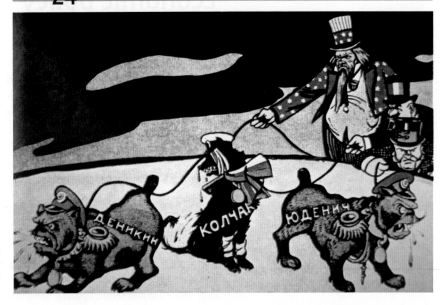

Bolshevik propaganda cartoon, 1919. The dogs represent the White generals Denikin, Kolchak and Yudenich.

SOURCE 25

The Civil War, 1918–1920, was a time of great chaos and estimates of Cheka executions vary from twelve to fifty thousands. But even the highest figure does not compare to the ferocity of the White Terror . . . for instance, in Finland alone, the number of workers executed by the Whites approaches 100,000.

R Appignanesi, *Lenin for Beginners*, 1977.

Finally, the Reds had important territorial advantages. Their enemies were spread around the edge of Russia while they controlled the centre and also the all-important railway system. This enabled them to move troops and supplies quickly and effectively by rail, while their enemies used less efficient methods.

The Whites, in contrast with the Bolsheviks, were not united.

● They were made up of many different groups, all with different aims.

● They were also widely spread so they were unable to co-ordinate their campaigns against the Reds. Trotsky was able to defeat them one by one.

● They had limited support from the Russian population. Russian peasants did not especially like the Bolsheviks, but they preferred them to the Whites. If the Whites won, the peasants knew the landlords would return. Both sides were guilty of atrocities, but the Whites in general caused more suffering to the peasants than the Reds.

Source Analysis

'Most Russians saw the Bolsheviks as the lesser of two evils.' Explain how Sources 20, 22, 23 and 25 support this statement or not.

Focus Task

Why did the Bolsheviks win the Civil War?

1 Draw a table and use the text to make notes about how each of these factors helped the Bolsheviks win.

♦ Unity
♦ Leadership
♦ Communications, e.g. railways
♦ Geography
♦ Support of the workers
♦ Support of the peasants
♦ The Red Army
♦ Foreign intervention
♦ Propaganda

2 Now write some paragraphs to show how some of these factors were connected. Two examples are shown below.

Linking Geography and Communications:

In such a vast country communications were a key to success. The Bolsheviks held the central industrial area which included all the main railway lines out of Moscow and Petrograd. This meant that they could get soldiers and military supplies to the different fronts much more easily that the Whites who found it very difficult to communicate with each other and move troops around the edges of the centre.

Linking Foreign intervention and Propaganda:

The foreign intervention was a gift to the Reds. They could use it in their propaganda to show that the Red Army was fighting foreign invaders.

Economic policy

War Communism

War Communism was the name given to the harsh economic measures the Bolsheviks adopted during the Civil War in order to survive. It had two main aims. The first aim was to put Communist theories into practice by redistributing (sharing out) wealth among the Russian people. The second aim was to help with the Civil War by keeping the towns and the Red Army supplied with food and weapons.

- All large factories were taken over by the government.
- Production was planned and organised by the government.
- Discipline for workers was strict and strikers could be shot.
- Peasants had to hand over surplus food to the government. If they didn't, they could be shot.
- Food was rationed.
- Free enterprise became illegal – all production and trade was controlled by the state.

War Communism achieved its aim of winning the war, but in doing so it caused terrible hardship. Peasants refused to co-operate in producing more food because the government simply took it away. This led to food shortages which, along with the bad weather in 1920 and 1921, caused a terrible famine. Some estimates suggest that 7 million Russian people died in this famine. There were even reports of cannibalism.

SOURCE 26

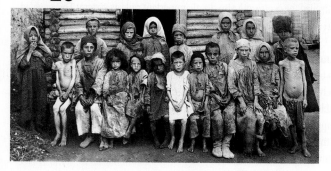

Starving children photographed during the Russian famine of 1921.

SOURCE 27

After carrying out the October Revolution, the working classes hoped for freedom. But the result has been greater slavery. The bayonets, bullets and harsh commands of the Cheka – these are what the working man of Soviet Russia has won. The glorious emblem of the workers' state – the hammer and sickle – has been replaced by the Communist authorities with the bayonet and the barred window. Here in Kronstadt we are making a third revolution which will free the workers and the Soviets from the Communists.

Official statement from the Kronstadt sailors.

Kronstadt mutiny

As you saw on page 186 the sailors from the Kronstadt naval base were strong supporters of the Bolsheviks during the revolution and the Civil War. Many of them were Bolshevik Party members. However, they were concerned at the impact that Bolshevik policies were having on ordinary Russians. In February 1921 a delegation of sailors visited Petrograd and learned first hand of the hardships people were suffering and the repressive policies being used by the Bolsheviks against their own people. Sailors from two of the battleships at Kronstadt passed a resolution calling on the Bolsheviks to change their policies. The made 15 demands, including new elections, freedom of speech, equal rations and the scrapping of the militia units which were taking peasants' grain.

This was a potentially serious threat to Lenin and the Bolsheviks. The Kronstadt sailors had been loyal supporters and losing their support was serious. More importantly, they were well armed and well organised and could potentially threaten the Bolshevik war effort. Lenin issued a statement claiming the rebellion was a plot by the White force. He demanded the rebels surrender. They refused, so in early March Trotsky's forces stormed the Kronstadt base. There was heavy fighting and although there are no reliable figures about casualties the death toll was probably in the thousands. Thousands more of the rebels were executed or imprisoned in labour camps. Nevertheless the rebellion had affected Lenin. Soon afterwards he abandoned the emergency policies of War Communism. Considering the chaos of the Civil War years, it may seem strange that this particular revolt had such a startling effect on Lenin. It did so because the Kronstadt sailors had been among the strongest supporters of Lenin and Bolshevism in 1917–20. Lenin began to think that he had to make some concessions.

Think!

1 Read Source 27. What aspects of War Communism are the sailors most angry about?
2 Would you expect peasants in Russia to feel the same?
3 Why do you think Lenin was more worried about the revolt of the sailors than about starvation among the peasants?

Source Analysis

Why do you think the photograph in Source 26 was taken and published in 1921? Use the source and your knowledge to explain your answer.

Source Analysis

Does the evidence of Source 32 prove that the NEP was a success? Explain your answer with reference to Sources 28, 30 and 31.

The New Economic Policy

Many thousands of the Kronstadt sailors were killed. The mutiny was crushed. But Lenin recognised that changes were necessary. In March 1921, at the Party Congress, Lenin announced some startling new policies which he called the New Economic Policy (NEP). The NEP effectively brought back capitalism for some sections of Russian society. Peasants were allowed to sell surplus grain for profit and would pay tax on what they produced rather than giving some of it up to the government.

SOURCE **29**

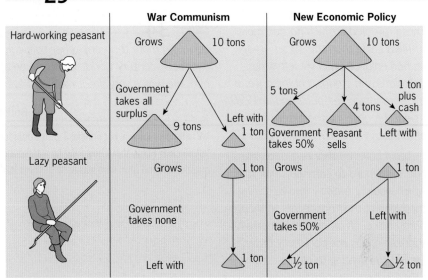

How the NEP differed from War Communism.

In the towns, small factories were handed back into private ownership and private trading of small goods was allowed.

Lenin made it clear that the NEP was temporary and that the vital heavy industries (coal, oil, iron and steel) would remain in state hands. Nevertheless, many Bolsheviks were horrified when the NEP was announced, seeing it as a betrayal of Communism. As always, Lenin won the argument and the NEP went into operation from 1921 onwards. By 1925 there seemed to be strong evidence that it was working, as food production in particular rose steeply. However, as Source 31 suggests, increases in production did not necessarily improve the situation of industrial workers.

SOURCE **32**

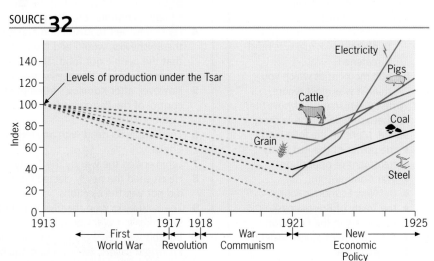

Production under the New Economic Policy, 1921–25.

Source Analysis

From all you have found out about Lenin, do you agree with Source 34? (Don't forget to look at Source 33.)

SOURCE 33

In the late 1980s and 1990s, Soviet archives were opened up as the Communist regime came to an end. These revealed a much harder, more ruthless Lenin than the 'softer' image he had enjoyed amongst left-wing historians and groups. For instance, a memorandum, first published in 1990, reveals his ordering the extermination of the clergy in a place called Shuya …

Lenin believed that revolutionaries had to be hard to carry out their role, which would inevitably involve spilling the blood of their opponents. Although hard and tough on others, it seems that Lenin was not personally brave. He left the fighting to others.

An extract from *Communist Russia under Lenin and Stalin*. This was an A level History textbook published in 2002.

Focus Task

How did the Bolsheviks consolidate their rule?

1 Draw a timeline from 1917 to 1924, and mark on it the events of that period mentioned in the text.
2 Mark on the timeline:
  a) one moment at which you think Bolshevik rule was most threatened
  b) one moment at which you think it was most secure.
3 Write an explanation of how the Bolsheviks made their rule more secure. Mention the following:
  ♦ the power of the Red Army
  ♦ treatment of opposition
  ♦ War Communism
  ♦ the New Economic Policy
  ♦ the Treaty of Brest-Litovsk
  ♦ the victory in the Civil War
  ♦ the promise of a new society
  ♦ propaganda.
4 Is any one of these factors more important than any of the others? Explain your answer.

The death of Lenin and the creation of the USSR

Lenin did not live to see the recovery of the Russian economy. He suffered several strokes in 1922 and 1923 which left him paralysed and which led to his death in January 1924. He was a remarkable man by any standards. He led Russia through revolution and civil war and even in 1923 he supervised the drawing up of a new constitution that turned the Russian Empire into the Union of Soviet Socialist Republics. Source 34 gives the opinion of a British historian.

SOURCE 34

Lenin did more than any other political leader to change the face of the twentieth-century world. The creation of Soviet Russia and its survival were due to him. He was a very great man and even, despite his faults, a very good man.

The British historian AJP Taylor writing in the 1960s.

We will never know what policies Lenin would have pursued if he had lived longer – he certainly left no clear plans about how long he wanted the NEP to last. He also left another big unanswered question behind him: who was to be the next leader of the USSR?

Key Question Summary

How did the Bolsheviks gain power and how did they hold on to power?

1 After the Tsar's abdication, a Provisional Government was set up to run Russia until elections could be held to choose a new government.
2 The Petrograd Soviet had the real power in the capital because it controlled the army and the workers in the factories.
3 The Provisional Government was weak and failed to deal with the problems of the war and the land to the satisfaction of the people. The economic situation continued to deteriorate throughout 1917.
4 Lenin returned to Russia and announced, in the April Theses, that his party, the Bolsheviks, would end the war, give the land to the peasants and ensure that the people got food. This brought them popular support although an attempt by some Bolsheviks to stage a rising in the July Days was a failure.
5 However, after Kornilov's attempted coup, they had enough support to take control of the Petrograd Soviet. On Lenin's urging, they seized power in October 1917.
6 The Bolsheviks dealt with any internal opposition ruthlessly by using the Cheka.
7 Lenin ended the war by the Treaty of Brest-Litovsk.
8 He crushed the newly elected Constituent Assembly because the Bolsheviks did not win the elections.
9 The Bolsheviks won the Civil War and kept the economy going through a system called War Communism.
10 But this was very harsh and people, including former supporters like the Kronstadt sailors, were turning against the Communists. So Lenin introduced a compromise – the New Economic Policy – which allowed the economy to recover and bring the people respite and some prosperity. So by 1924 the Bolsheviks were still firmly in power and had consolidated their position.

8.3 Stalin's Russia

Focus

Most people thought Trotsky was the person most likely to succeed Lenin. Yet not only did Stalin become the new leader of the USSR, but over the next 40 years he changed it radically. He created a modern industrial state that became a superpower but he also created a totalitarian state where opposition was not tolerated and where the government imprisoned or murdered millions of its own citizens.

How did Stalin gain and hold on to power?

Focus Points

- Why did Stalin, and not Trotsky, emerge as Lenin's successor?
- Why did Stalin launch the Purges?
- What methods did Stalin use to control the Soviet Union?
- How complete was Stalin's control over the Soviet Union by 1941?

What was the impact of Stalin's economic policies?

Focus Points

- Why did Stalin introduce the Five-Year Plans?
- Why did Stalin introduce collectivisation?
- How successful were Stalin's economic changes?
- How were the Soviet people affected by these changes?

In this section you will look at two overlapping themes: how Stalin modernised the USSR and how he controlled it.

Source Analysis

1 Study Source 1. What achievements is Stalin pointing out?
2 Which figure can you see top left? Why do you think he has been placed in this position?
3 Why do you think this poster was produced at the end of the 1930s?

SOURCE **1**

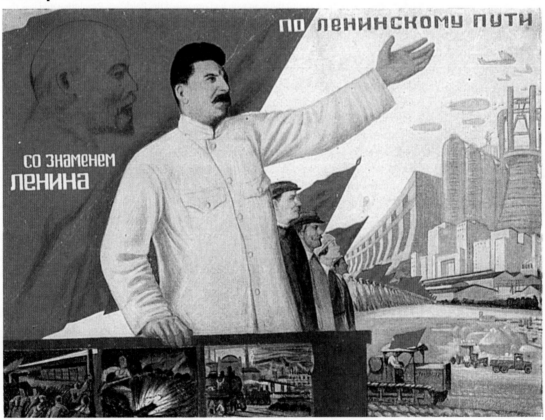

An official poster from the mid to late 1930s showing Stalin pointing out the achievements of the USSR and its people.

211

Stalin's steps to power

- **1923** Lenin calls for Stalin to be replaced. Trotsky calls him 'the party's most eminent mediocrity'.
- **1924** Lenin's death. Stalin attends funeral as chief mourner. Trotsky does not turn up (tricked by Stalin).
- **1924** Stalin, Kamenev and Zinoviev form the triumvirate that dominates the Politburo, the policy-making committee of the Communist Party. Working together, these three cut off their opponents (Trotsky and Bukharin) because between them they control the important posts in the party.
- **1925** Trotsky sacked as War Commissar. Stalin introduces his idea of Socialism in One Country.
- **1926** Stalin turns against Kamenev and Zinoviev and allies himself with Bukharin.
- **1927** Kamenev, Zinoviev and Trotsky all expelled from the Communist Party.
- **1928** Trotsky exiled to Siberia. Stalin begins attacking Bukharin.
- **1929** Trotsky expelled from USSR and Bukharin expelled from the Communist Party.

Stalin or Trotsky?

When Lenin died in 1924 there were several leading Communists who were possible candidates to take his place. Among the contenders were Kamenev and Zinoviev, leading Bolsheviks who had played important parts in the Bolshevik Revolution of 1917, and Bukharin was a more moderate member of the party who favoured the NEP and wanted to introduce Communism gradually to the USSR. However, the real struggle to succeed Lenin was between two bitter rivals, Joseph Stalin and Leon Trotsky. The power struggle went on for some time and it was not until 1929 that Stalin made himself completely secure as the supreme leader of the USSR. Stalin achieved this through a combination of political scheming, the mistakes of his opponents and the clever way in which he built up his power base in the Communist Party.

Lenin's Testament

SOURCE 2

Comrade Stalin, having become Secretary General, has unlimited authority in his hands and I am not sure whether he will always be capable of using that authority with sufficient caution.

Comrade Trotsky, on the other hand, is distinguished not only by his outstanding ability. He is personally probably the most capable man in the present Central Committee, but he has displayed excessive self-assurance and preoccupation with the purely administrative side of the work.

Lenin's Testament. This is often used as evidence that Stalin was an outsider. However, the document contained many remarks critical of other leading Communists as well. It was never published in Russia, although, if it had been, it would certainly have damaged Stalin.

Source 2 shows Lenin's opinions of Trotsky and Stalin. As Lenin lay dying in late 1923 Trotsky seemed most likely to win. He was a brilliant speaker and writer, as well as the party's best political thinker, after Lenin. He was also the man who had organised the Bolshevik Revolution and was the hero of the Civil War as leader of the Red Army (see page 206).

Trotsky's mistakes

So how did Trotsky lose this contest? Much of the blame lies with Trotsky himself. He was brilliant, but also arrogant and high-handed. He often offended other senior party members. More importantly, he failed to take the opposition seriously. He made little effort to build up any support in the ranks of the party. And he seriously underestimated Stalin, as did the other contenders. No one saw Stalin as a threat. They were all more concerned with each other. Stalin kept in the shadows, not taking a clear position and seeming to be the friend and ally of different groups. This allowed him to become steadily more powerful without the others realising it.

Trotsky also frightened many people in the USSR. They were worried he might become a dictator, especially because he had a great deal of support in the army. Trotsky argued that the future security of the USSR lay in trying to spread permanent revolution across the globe until the whole world was Communist. Many people were worried that Trotsky would involve the USSR in new conflicts and that his radical policies might split the party.

SOURCE 3

Trotsky refrained from attacking Stalin because he felt secure. No contemporary, and he least of all, saw in the Stalin of 1923 the menacing and towering figure he was to become. It seemed to Trotsky almost a joke that Stalin, the wilful and sly but shabby and inarticulate man in the background, should be his rival.

Historian I Deutscher in *The Prophet Unarmed, Trotsky 1921–1929*, published in 1959.

Luck

As it often does in history, chance also played a part. Trotsky was unfortunate in falling ill late in 1923 with a malaria-like infection – just when Lenin was dying, and Trotsky needed to be at his most active.

Stalin's cunning

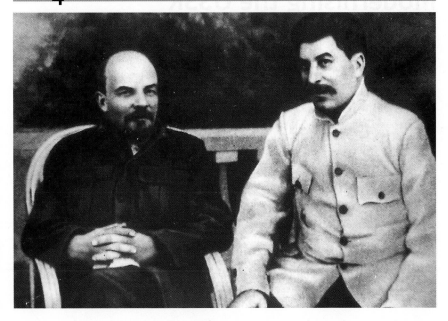

Lenin and Stalin. Stalin made the most of any opportunity to appear close to Lenin. This photograph is a suspected fake.

We have already seen that Stalin was a clever politician and he planned his bid for power carefully. He made great efforts to associate himself with Lenin wherever possible and got off to an excellent start at Lenin's funeral. He played a trick on Trotsky. Stalin cabled Trotsky to tell him that Lenin's funeral was to be on 26 January, when it was in fact going to be on the 27th. Trotsky was away in the south of Russia and would not have had time to get back for the 26th, although he could have got back for the 27th. As a result, Trotsky did not appear at the funeral whereas Stalin appeared as chief mourner and Lenin's closest comrade and follower.

He was also extremely clever in using his power within the Communist Party. He took on many boring but important jobs including the post of General Secretary. He used these positions to put his own supporters into important posts and remove people likely to support his opponents from the Party. He was also very good at political manoeuvring. First of all he allied himself with Zinoviev and Kamanev to push out Trotsky. Then he allied himself with Bukharin in the debate about the NEP (see page 209) to defeat Zinoviev and Kamanev and later get them, along with Trotsky, expelled from the Party. All the time he was building his own power base, bringing in his supporters to the Party Congress and Central Committee to make sure he was chosen as leader. Finally he turned on Bukharin and his supporters, removing them from powerful positions. By 1929 he was the unchallenged leader.

Stalin's policies also met with greater favour than Trotsky's. Stalin proposed that in future the party should try to establish 'Socialism in One Country' rather than try to spread revolution worldwide. The idea that they could achieve socialism on their own appealed to the Russian sense of nationalism. Finally, Stalin appeared to be a straightforward Georgian peasant – much more a man of the people than his intellectual rivals. To a Soviet people weary of years of war and revolution, Stalin seemed to be the man who understood their feelings.

Profile

Joseph Stalin

➤ Born 1879 in Georgia. His father was a shoemaker and an alcoholic.
➤ Original name was Iosif Dzhugashvili but changed his name to Stalin (man of steel).
➤ Twice exiled to Siberia by the Tsarist secret police, he escaped each time.
➤ Made his name in violent bank raids to raise party funds.
➤ He was slow and steady, but very hardworking.
➤ He also held grudges and generally made his enemies suffer.
➤ Became a leading Communist after playing an important role in defending the Bolshevik city of Tsaritsyn (later Stalingrad) during the Civil War.
➤ Had become undisputed party leader by 1929.

Think!

In groups, look at the following statements and decide on a scale of 1–5 how far you agree with them.
♦ Stalin was a dull and unimaginative politician.
♦ Stalin appeared to be a dull and unimaginative politician.
♦ Trotsky lost the contest because of his mistakes.
♦ Stalin trusted to luck rather than careful planning.
♦ Stalin was ruthless and devious.
Try to find evidence on these two pages to back up your judgements.

Focus Task

Why did Stalin and not Trotsky emerge as Lenin's successor?

Write notes under the following headings to explain why Stalin rather than Trotsky emerged as the new leader of Russia.
♦ Trotsky's strengths and weaknesses in the leadership contest
♦ Why other contenders underestimated Stalin
♦ How Stalin outmanoeuvred other contenders
♦ Why Stalin's policies were attractive to Party members
Then combine your notes to write your own account in answer to the question: 'Why did Stalin and not Trotsky emerge as Lenin's successor?'

SOURCE 5

Throughout history Russia has been beaten again and again because she was backward . . . All have beaten her because of her military, industrial and agricultural backwardness. She was beaten because people have been able to get away with it. If you are backward and weak, then you are in the wrong and may be beaten and enslaved. But if you are powerful, people must beware of you.

It is sometimes asked whether it is not possible to slow down industrialisation a bit. No, comrades, it is not possible . . . To slacken would mean falling behind. And those who fall behind get beaten . . . That is why Lenin said during the October Revolution: 'Either perish, or overtake and outstrip the advanced capitalist countries.' We are 50 to 100 years behind the advanced countries. Either we make good the difference in ten years or they crush us.

Stalin speaking in 1931.

SOURCE 6

Key
🏭 New industry

0   500 km
Scale

Locations of the new industrial centres.

Modernising the USSR

Once in power, Stalin was determined to modernise the USSR quickly. He had many reasons.

- **To increase the USSR's military strength:** The First World War had shown that a country could only fight a modern war if it had the industries to produce the weapons and other equipment which were needed (see Source 5).
- **To rival the economies of the USA and other capitalist countries:** When Stalin took power, much of Russia's industrial equipment had to be imported. Stalin wanted to make the USSR self-sufficient so that it could make everything it needed for itself. He also wanted to improve standards of living in Russia so that people would value Communist rule.
- **To increase food supplies:** Stalin wanted more workers in industries, towns and cities. He also wanted to sell grain abroad to raise cash to buy industrial equipment. This meant fewer peasants had to produce more food which meant that farming would have to be reorganised.
- **To create a Communist society:** Communist theory said that most people had to be workers for Communism to work. In 1928 only about one in five Russians were industrial workers.
- **To establish his reputation:** Lenin had made big changes to the USSR. Stalin wanted to prove himself as a great leader by bringing about even greater changes.

Modernising industry: the Five-Year Plans

Stalin ended Lenin's NEP and set about achieving modernisation through a series of Five-Year Plans. These plans were drawn up by GOSPLAN, the state planning organisation that Lenin had set up in 1921. It set ambitious targets for production in the vital heavy industries (coal, iron, oil, electricity). The plans were very complex but they were set out in such a way that by 1929 every worker knew what he or she had to achieve.

| GOSPLAN set overall targets for an industry. | ▶ | Each region was told its targets. | ▶ | The region set targets for each mine, factory, etc. | ▶ | The manager of each mine, factory, etc. set targets for each foreman. | ▶ | The foremen set targets for each shift and even for individual workers. |

The first Five-Year Plan focused on the major industries and although most targets were not met, the achievements were still staggering. The USSR increased production and created a foundation on which to build the next Five-Year Plans. The USSR was rich in natural resources, but many of them were in remote places such as Siberia. So whole cities were built from nothing and workers taken out to the new industrial centres. Foreign observers marvelled as huge new steel mills appeared at Magnitogorsk in the Urals and Sverdlovsk in central Siberia. New dams and hydro-electric power fed industry's energy requirements. Russian 'experts' flooded into the Muslim republics of central Asia such as Uzbekistan and Kazakhstan, creating industry from scratch in previously undeveloped areas.

The second Five-Year Plan (1933–37) built on the achievements of the first. Heavy industry was still a priority, but other areas were also developed. Mining for lead, tin, zinc and other minerals intensified as Stalin further exploited Siberia's rich mineral resources. Transport and communications were also boosted, and new railways and canals were built. The most spectacular showpiece project was the Moscow underground railway.

Stalin also wanted industrialisation to help improve Russia's agriculture. The production of tractors and other farm machinery increased dramatically. In the third Five-Year Plan, which was begun in 1938, some factories were to switch to the production of consumer goods. However, this plan was disrupted by the Second World War.

Think!

1 How does Source 5 help explain why Stalin introduced the Five-Year Plan with such ambitious targets?
2 What were the other key reasons why he introduced them?

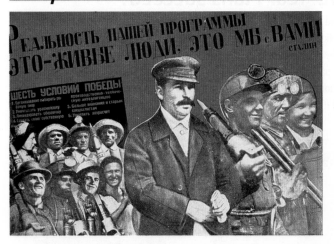

Propaganda poster showing Stalin as a comrade side by side with Soviet workers. The text means 'It is our workers who make our programme achievable.'

How was industrialisation achieved?

Any programme as extreme as Stalin's Five-Year Plans was bound to carry a cost. In the USSR this cost was paid by the workers. Many foreign experts and engineers were called in by Stalin to supervise the work and in their letters and reports they marvel at the toughness of the Russian people. The workers were constantly bombarded with propaganda, posters, slogans and radio broadcasts. They all had strict targets to meet and were fined if they did not meet them.

The most famous worker was Alexei Stakhanov. In 1935 with two helpers and an easy coal seam to work on, he managed to cut an amazing 102 tons of coal in one shift. This was fourteen times the average for a shift. Stakhanov became a 'Hero of Socialist Labour' and the propaganda machine encouraged all Soviet workers to be Stakhanovites.

The first Five-Year Plan revealed a shortage of workers, so from 1930 the government concentrated on drafting more women into industry. It set up thousands of new crèches and day-care centres so that mothers could work. By 1937 women were 40 per cent of industrial workers (compared to 28 per cent in 1927), 21 per cent of building workers and 72 per cent of health workers. Four out of five new workers recruited between 1932 and 1937 were women.

By the late 1930s many Soviet workers had improved their conditions by acquiring well-paid skilled jobs and earning bonuses for meeting targets. Unemployment was almost non-existent. In 1940 the USSR had more doctors per head of population than Britain. Education became free and compulsory for all and Stalin invested huge sums in training schemes based in colleges and in the work place.

But, on the other hand, life was very harsh under Stalin. Factory discipline was strict and punishments were severe. Lateness or absences were punished by sacking, and that often meant losing your flat or house as well. In the headlong rush to fulfil targets, many of the products were of poor quality. Some factories overproduced in massive amounts while others had to shut down for short periods because they could not get parts and raw materials. However things did improve in the second and third Five-Year Plans.

On the great engineering projects, such as dams and canals, many of the workers were prisoners who had been sentenced to hard labour for being political opponents, or suspected opponents, of Stalin, or for being kulaks (rich peasants) or Jews. Many other prisoners were simply unfortunate workers who had had accidents or made mistakes in their work but had been found guilty of 'sabotage'.

On these major projects conditions were appalling and there were many deaths and accidents. It is estimated that 100,000 workers died in the construction of the Belomor Canal.

At the same time, the concentration on heavy industry meant that there were few consumer goods (such as clothes or radios) which ordinary people wanted to buy. In the towns and cities, most housing was provided by the state, but overcrowding was a problem. Most families lived in flats and were crowded into two rooms which were used for living, sleeping and eating. What's more, wages actually fell between 1928 and 1937. In 1932 a husband and wife who both worked earned only as much as one man or woman had in 1928.

Stalin was also quite prepared to destroy the way of life of the Soviet people to help industrialisation. For example, in the republics of central Asia the influence of Islam was thought to hold back industrialisation, so between 1928 and 1932 it was repressed. Many Muslim leaders were imprisoned or deported, mosques were closed and pilgrimages to Mecca were forbidden.

We got so dirty and we were such young things, small, slender, fragile. But we had our orders to build the metro and we wanted to do it more than anything else. We wore our miners' overalls with such style. My feet were size four and the boots were elevens. But there was such enthusiasm.

Tatyana Fyodorova, interviewed as an old lady in 1990, remembers building the Moscow underground.

Half a billion cubic feet of excavation work . . . 25,000 tons of structural steel . . . without sufficient labour, without necessary quantities of the most rudimentary materials. Brigades of young enthusiasts arrived in the summer of 1930 and did the groundwork of railroad and dam . . . Later groups of peasants came . . . Many were completely unfamiliar with industrial tools and processes . . .

J Scott, *Behind the Urals*, 1943.

SOURCE 10

What are the results of the Five-Year Plan in four years?

- *We did not have an iron and steel industry. Now we have one.*
- *We did not have a machine tool industry. Now we have one.*
- *We did not have a modern chemicals industry. Now we have one.*
- *We did not have a big industry for producing agricultural machinery. Now we have one.*

Stalin speaking about the first Five-Year Plan in 1932.

SOURCE 12

	1913	1928	1940
Gas (billion m³)	0.02	0.3	3.4
Fertilisers (million tons)	0.07	0.1	3.2
Plastics (million tons)	–	–	10.9
Tractors (thousand)	–	1.3	31.6

The growth in the output of the USSR, 1913–40.

SOURCE 13

Graph showing share of world manufacturing output, 1929–38.

Did the Five-Year Plans succeed?

There is much that could be and was criticised in the Five-Year Plans. Certainly there was a great deal of inefficiency, duplication of effort and waste. One feature of the plans was spectacular building projects, e.g. the Dnieprostroi Dam, which were used as a showcase of Soviet achievement. The Moscow Metro was particularly impressive with vast stations and stunning architectural design. There was an enormous human cost to these. But the fact remains that by 1937 the USSR was a modern state and it was this that saved it from defeat when Hitler invaded in 1941.

SOURCE 11

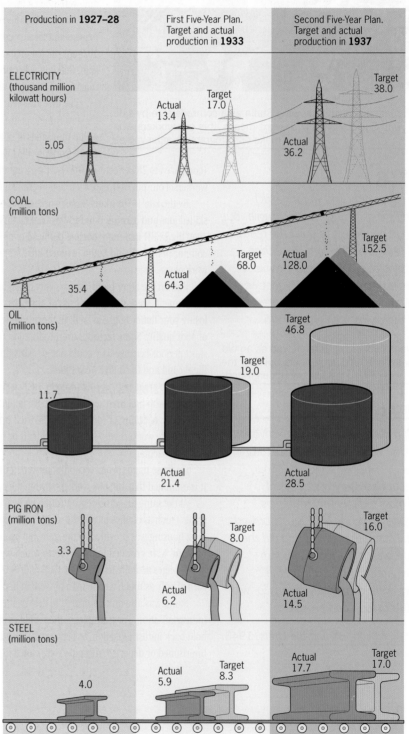

The achievements of the Five-Year Plans.

The Five-Year Plans were used very effectively for propaganda purposes. Stalin had wanted the Soviet Union to be a beacon of socialism and his publicity machine used the successes of industrialisation to further that objective. Blaming the workers was a good way of excusing mistakes made by management. However, many of the workers were unskilled ex-peasants and they did cause damage to machinery and equipment. To escape punishments and harsh conditions, or to try to get better wages and bonuses, workers moved jobs frequently (in some industries three times a year). This did not help industry or society to stabilise. To try to prevent this, internal passports were introduced to prevent the movement of workers inside the USSR.

SOURCE 14

There is evidence that he [Stalin] exaggerated Russia's industrial deficiency in 1929. The Tsars had developed a considerable industrial capacity . . . in a sense the spadework had already been done and it is not altogether surprising that Stalin should have achieved such rapid results.

Historian SJ Lee, *The European Dictatorships, 1918–1945*, published in 1987.

Source Analysis

1 What is the message of Source 15?
2 How could Stalin use Sources 12 and 13 to support the claims of Source 15?
3 Compare Sources 10 and 14. Do they agree or disagree about the Five-Year Plans? Explain your answer.
4 Which of Sources 10 or 14 do Sources 11, 12 and 13 most support?

SOURCE 15

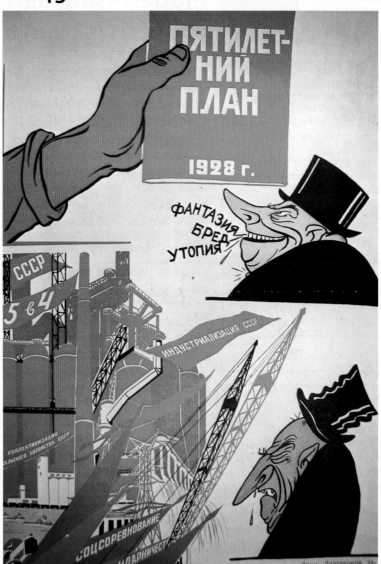

Soviet propaganda poster, 1933. In the top half, the hand is holding the first Five-Year Plan. The capitalist is saying (in 1928), 'Fantasy, Lies, Utopia.' The bottom half shows 1933.

Focus Task

How successful were Stalin's economic policies?

Step 1: The Five-Year Plans

Use all the information and sources in this section to assess the Five-Year Plans for industry. Copy and complete a table like this. Fill out column 2. You will come back to column 3 on page 219.

Policy	The Five-Year Plans	Collectivisation
Aims		
Key features		
Successes		
Failures		
Human cost		

Think!

1 Explain why Stalin needed to change farming in the USSR.
2 Why did the peasants resist?

SOURCE 16

In order to turn a peasant society into an industrialised country, countless material and human sacrifices were necessary. The people had to accept this, but it would not be achieved by enthusiasm alone . . . If a few million people had to perish in the process, history would forgive Comrade Stalin . . . The great aim demanded great energy that could be drawn from a backward people only by great harshness.

Anatoli Rybakov, *Children of the Arbat*, 1988. A Russian writer presents Stalin's viewpoint on the modernisation of Russia.

Modernising agriculture: collectivisation

For the enormous changes of the Five-Year Plan to be successful, Stalin needed to modernise the USSR's agriculture. This was vital because the population of the industrial centres was growing rapidly and yet as early as 1928 the country was already 2 million tons short of the grain it needed to feed its workers. Stalin also wanted to try to raise money for his industrialisation programme by selling exports of surplus food abroad.

His answer was collectivisation – forcing the farmers to combine their lands and cattle and farm them together (collectively) – see Factfile.

Most peasants were still working on small plots of land using backward methods. Making the peasants work on larger farms meant that it would be easier to make efficient use of tractors, fertilisers and other modern methods of farming. This would produce more food. Mechanised farming would require fewer peasants and release large numbers to work in growing industries. Moreover it would be easier to collect grain and taxes from larger farms. It would also be a more socialist way of farming as they would be co-operating rather than selling their own food for a profit.

There was one big problem with collectivisation. The peasants did not want to hand over their animals and tools and be ordered around by farm managers. All they wanted was to farm their own piece of land without interference from the government. This applied particularly to kulaks – richer peasants who owned larger farms and employed agricultural labourers.

The government sent out activists, backed up by the secret police, to 'persuade' them and a massive propaganda campaign was organised to inform peasants of the advantages of joining a collective farm. Some did join, but many resisted bitterly. They slaughtered and ate their animals rather than allow them to be taken, burnt crops and even their houses. In some areas there was armed resistance. The government blamed the kulaks for all the trouble and Stalin announced that 'We must liquidate the kulaks as a class'. In practice anybody who resisted became a kulak. Peasants were rounded up and deported in huge numbers to remote areas in Siberia, or to labour camps. Others fled to the cities.

This process in 1930–32 caused huge disruption in the countryside and there were severe food shortages. This, combined with a poor harvest in 1932, led to a famine on an unimaginable scale, particularly in the Ukraine, in the years 1932–33. The government would not acknowledge the famine and still sent out requisitioning gangs to collect grain for the workers and to export to other countries. Millions starved, perhaps as many as 13 million people. It was a man-made human tragedy of immense proportions. The way of life of millions of peasants had been destroyed.

After this traumatic period, the countryside did settle down and gradually more grain was produced, although the numbers of animals did not reach pre-collectivisation levels until 1940. Stalin had achieved his aim (see Source 17): he had established control of the grain supply and collectivised the peasants. Moreover he had a ready supply of labour for the factories.

SOURCE 17

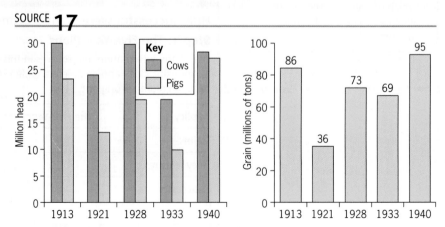

Agricultural production in the USSR 1913–40 based on figures produced by the Soviet government.

Source Analysis ▶

Read Source 18. Why do you think the only reports of the famine came from Western journalists?

SOURCE 18

'How are things with you?' I asked one old man. He looked around anxiously to see that no soldiers were about. 'We have nothing, absolutely nothing. They have taken everything away.' It was true. The famine is an organised one. Some of the food that has been taken away from them is being exported to foreign countries. It is literally true that whole villages have been exiled. I saw myself a group of some twenty peasants being marched off under escort. This is so common a sight that it no longer arouses even curiosity.

The *Manchester Guardian*, 1933.

Despite the famine, Stalin did not ease off. By 1934 there were no kulaks left. By 1941 almost all agricultural land was organised under the collective system. Stalin had achieved his aim of collectivisation.

SOURCE 19

Stalin, ignoring the great cost in human life and misery, claimed that collectivisation was a success; for, after the great famines caused at the time . . . no more famines came to haunt the Russian people. The collective farms, despite their inefficiencies, did grow more food than the tiny, privately owned holdings had done. For example, 30 to 40 million tons of grain were produced every year. Collectivisation also meant the introduction of machines into the countryside. Now 2 million previously backward peasants learned how to drive a tractor. New methods of farming were taught by agricultural experts. The countryside was transformed.

Historian E Roberts, *Stalin, Man of Steel*, published in 1986.

Focus Task

How successful were Stalin's economic policies?

Step 2: Collectivisation

1 You started a chart on page 217. Now complete column 3 to assess the policy of collectivisation.
2 Which policy do you think was more effective: the Five-Year Plans or collectivisation? Support your answer with evidence from pages 214–19.

Key Question Summary

What was the impact of Stalin's economic policies?

1 From 1928, Stalin embarked on a radical programme of change to modernise the USSR to increase its military power, rival Western economies and create a Communist society.

2 He initiated Five-Year Plans for industry in which production targets were set for every industry right down to individual factories.

3 The first two Five-Year Plans concentrated mainly on heavy industry – iron, coal and steel – and to a lesser extent on mining, chemicals and transport.

4 A feature of the plans was gigantic spectacular projects like the Moscow Underground.

5 The plans were very successful – the production of heavy industries rose dramatically, huge new industrial plants were built, new cities appeared and a modern industrial state was created. However, the quality of goods was often poor and there were inefficiencies.

6 Stalin needed to make farming more modern – using tractors and fertilisers – to produce the food he needed for the workers. He used collectivisation to do this – making peasants put their land and animals into collective farms under state control.

7 Many peasants resisted and were shot, sent to labour camps or exiled. Millions fled to the new cities to become workers.

8 As a result of this disruption, food production fell and there was a famine in parts of the USSR, especially the Ukraine, in 1932–33. However, Stalin had got what he wanted from collectivisation: food for the workers, food to export abroad, more industrial workers and control of the peasants and the food supply.

9 The cost to the Russian people of Stalin's economic plans was high. The peasants suffered immensely. But the workers also had to make sacrifices. Very few consumer goods were produced, the quality of housing was poor and the standard of living low. Factory discipline was harsh and workers who made mistakes could be punished severely or accused of sabotage and sent to labour camps.

SOURCE 20

A tribute to Comrade Stalin was called for. Of course, everyone stood up . . . for three minutes, four minutes, the 'stormy applause, rising to an ovation' continued . . . Who would dare to be the first to stop? After all, NKVD men were standing in the hall waiting to see who quit first! After 11 minutes the director [of the factory] . . . sat down . . . To a man, everyone else stopped dead and sat down. They had been saved!

. . . That, however, was how they discovered who the independent people were. And that was how they eliminated them. The same night the factory director was arrested.

Alexander Solzhenitsyn, *Gulag Archipelago*, published in 1973. Solzhenitsyn lost his Soviet citizenship as a result of this book.

Think!

According to Source 20, what sort of people did Stalin want in the USSR?

SOURCE 21

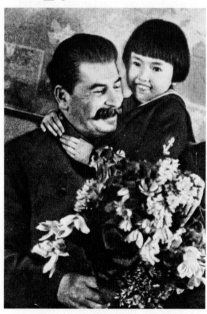

Stalin shown holding a young child, Gelya Markizova, in 1936. Stalin had both of her parents killed. This did not stop him using this image on propaganda leaflets to show him as a kind, fatherly figure.

How did Stalin control Russia?

You have already seen on pages 215–19 how Stalin was utterly ruthless in his crushing of any opposition to his industrial or agricultural policies.

The use of fear and terror to control Russians had been a feature of the Tsar's regime. It had also been a feature of the Communist state under Lenin, but Stalin took it to new heights. He was determined to stay in power and crush any opposition whether it came from inside or outside the Communist Party. Sitting behind him was the secret police, first called the OGPU and then the NKVD. In addition, there was an extensive system of labour camps, called the 'Gulag' – dreadful places which many did not survive.

The Purges

By 1934, some leading Communists wanted to slacken the breakneck pace of industrialisation and make life more bearable for ordinary Russians. When Sergei Kirov, virtually second to Stalin, suggested this at a Party conference, he was widely supported and there was talk of him replacing Stalin as leader.

Then Kirov was mysteriously murdered (probably on Stalin's orders) and Stalin used this as an excuse to 'purge' the Communist Party of his opponents suggesting there were spies and conspirators to be unmasked. He arranged for a series of show trials in which leading Bolsheviks confessed to their crimes, probably because of torture or threats to their families. Kamenev and Zinoviev were tried in the first big trial in 1936 along with fourteen others; Bukharin was tried in 1938. But these purges were not restricted to leading party members. Around 500,000 Communist Party members were arrested and either executed or sent to labour camps. Those left would carry out Stalin's orders to the letter.

It did not stop at the Communist Party. Anybody suspected of being disloyal to Stalin was arrested. Many people were denounced by neighbours trying to prove they were loyal. University lecturers and teachers, miners and engineers, factory managers and ordinary workers all disappeared. It is said that every family in the USSR lost someone in the Purges.

Stalin also purged the army, removing 25,000 officers – around one in five – including its supreme commander, Marshal Tukhachevsky, who had disagreed with Stalin in the past. This nearly proved fatal when Hitler invaded the USSR in 1941 since the Red Army suffered from a lack of good quality experienced officers.

By 1937 an estimated 18 million people had been transported to labour camps. Ten million died. Stalin seriously weakened the USSR by removing so many able individuals. Stalin had also succeeded in destroying any sense of independent thinking. Everyone who was spared knew that their lives depended on thinking exactly as Stalin did.

SOURCE 22

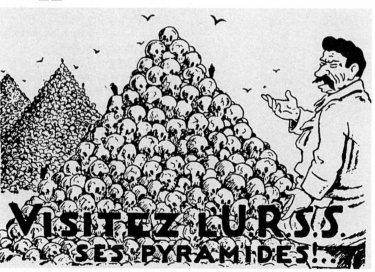

Russian exiles in France made this mock travel poster in the late 1930s. The text says: 'Visit the USSR's pyramids!'

Source Analysis

Choose either Source 22 or 24.
1 Summarise the message of the cartoon in your own words.
2 Do you think either of these cartoons could have been published in the USSR?

The new constitution

In 1936 Stalin created a new constitution for the USSR. It gave freedom of speech and free elections to the Russian people. This was, of course, a cosmetic measure. Only Communist Party candidates were allowed to stand in elections, and only approved newspapers and magazines could be published.

SOURCE **23**

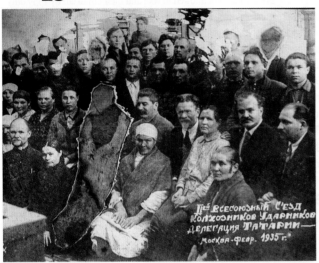

One of Stalin's opponents deleted from a photograph, 1935. Techniques of doctoring pictures became far more sophisticated in the 1930s. This allowed Stalin to create the impression that his enemies had never existed.

SOURCE **24**

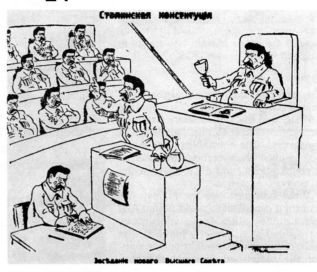

A cartoon published by Russian exiles in Paris in 1936. The title of the cartoon is 'The Stalinist Constitution' and the text at the bottom reads 'New seating arrangements in the Supreme Soviet'.

Revision Tip

You should have a view on whether terror or propaganda was more important in securing Stalin's rule. You need to:
♦ know at least two events which show how the terror regime worked.
♦ be able to describe at least two examples of propaganda.
♦ practise explaining which you think was more important – it does not matter which you decide as long as you can explain your reasoning.

The cult of personality

If you had visited the Soviet Union in the 1930s, you would probably have found that most Soviet citizens admired, even loved, Stalin and thought he was a great leader driving them forward to a great future. This is partly because of the deliberately created cult of the personality. The Soviet propaganda machine pushed Stalin into every aspect of their daily lives. Portraits (most homes had one), photographs and statues were everywhere. Regular processions were held in towns and cities praising Stalin. He was a super-being, almost godlike. Some historians argue that the Communist leaders thought that it was useful to have a figure like this to guide people through difficult times and make them willing to endure hardship. Of course, Stalin enjoyed the adulation he received. Moreover, he was determined to make himself an important historical figure. He had history books rewritten making Lenin and Stalin the only real heroes of the Revolution. Others, like Trotsky, were airbrushed out of history, their names and photos removed from books or given scant mention.

SOURCE **25**

These men lifted their villainous hands against Comrade Stalin. By lifting their hands against Comrade Stalin, they lifted them against all of us, against the working class . . . against the teaching of Marx, Engels, Lenin . . . Stalin is our hope, Stalin is the beacon which guides all progressive mankind. Stalin is our banner. Stalin is our will. Stalin is our victory.

From a speech made by Communist leader Nikita Khrushchev in 1937, at the height of the Purges. (Khrushchev later became leader of the USSR and in 1956 announced a 'de-Stalinisation' programme – see page 128).

Focus Task

Why did Stalin launch the Purges?

Some say that Stalin launched the Purges because he was power-mad and paranoid. Do you agree with this? Can you suggest other reasons? Use these headings to help you:
♦ Opposition to Stalin
♦ Why Stalin was determined to remain leader
♦ Controlling the Communist Party
♦ Controlling the people in an unstable society
♦ Getting rid of disruptive elements in the population
♦ Making sure the army stayed loyal.

Society and culture under Stalin

Stalin understood the power of ideas and the media. Newspapers were censored or run by government agencies. The radio was under state control. The state used propaganda extensively in posters, information leaflets and through public events like organised street theatre and processions. Soviet citizens could get very little information from the world outside apart from through state-controlled media. Stalin also controlled other areas that influenced the way people thought.

Religion came under sustained attack in the 1930s. Many churches were closed, priests deported and church buildings pulled down. Priests were not allowed to vote and their children. By 1939 only one in 40 churches were holding regular services in the USSR. Muslim worship was also attacked. Muslims were banned from practising Islamic law and women encouraged to abandon the veil. In 1917 there were 26,000 mosques in Russia but by 1939 there were only 1,300. Despite this aggressive action, in the 1937 census, around 60 per cent of Russians said that they were Christians.

All music and other arts in the USSR were carefully monitored by the NKVD. Poets and playwrights praised Stalin either directly or indirectly. Composers such as Shostakovich wrote music praising him and lived in dread of Stalin's disapproval. Artists and writers were forced to adopt a style called Soviet Realism. This meant that paintings and novels had to glorify ordinary workers, inspire people with socialism, and help build the future. Paintings showed happy collective farm workers in the fields or workers striving in the factories. It was a similar situation with literature (see Source 26).

Education and youth organisations

By the early 1930s Stalin set about reforming the Soviet education system. The discipline of teachers and parents was emphasised. Strict programmes of work were set out for key subjects like mathematics, physics and chemistry. History textbooks presented Stalin's view of history. There were compulsory lessons in socialist values and how a Soviet citizen should behave.

Children under fifteen joined the Pioneers where they were indoctrinated with Communist views, encouraged to be loyal to the state and to behave like a good citizens. It was like the Boy Scouts with activities stressing co-operation and teamwork.

Women in Stalin's USSR

Life under Stalin for women was a mixed picture. In many respects, women gained much more freedom and opportunity under Stalin's rule than they had had under the Tsar. Women were given the same educational and employment opportunities as men. Women entered the workforce in increasing numbers. By 1935 some 42 per cent of all industrial workers were women. The historian Wendy Goldman argues that the Second Five Year Plan in particular would have struggled to achieve what it did if it had not been for the huge influx of women workers. There is also some evidence that women were enrolled into technical training programs and management positions, although the vast majority of women remained in relatively low paid industrial jobs or traditional roles. There is also evidence of women facing resentment from male colleagues and relatively few women were able to achieve promotion.

The Communists also tried to challenge traditional views about women and the family. Communists thought that women should be free and not tied down to men by marriage. Children would be looked after in crèches and kindergarten. So divorce was made very easy and there was abortion on demand. The reality did not live up to the dream. In the cities many men abandoned and divorced women as soon as they became pregnant. In 1927 two-thirds of marriages in Moscow ended in divorce. The promised state-provided kindergartens did not materialise and thousands of women were left to manage as best they could with jobs and children. This situation was compounded by the upheavals in 1928–33, especially by collectivisation, which resulted in huge numbers of families being split. The result was millions of homeless children who roamed the streets in gangs, begging or taking part in petty crime.

The Great Retreat

By the mid 1930s there was a movement to return to traditional family values and discipline, often called 'The Great Retreat'.

- Abortion was made illegal except to protect the health of the mother.
- Divorce was made more difficult. Divorcing couples had to go to court and pay a fee.
- Divorced fathers had to pay maintenance for their children.

SOURCE 26

Whoever said that Soviet literature contains only real images is profoundly mistaken. The themes are dictated by the Party. The Party deals harshly with anybody who tries to depict the real state of affairs in their literature.

Is it not a fact that all of you now reading these lines saw people dying in the streets in 1932? People, swollen with hunger and foaming at the mouth, lying in their death throes in the streets. Is it not a fact that whole villages full of people perished in 1932? Does our literature show any of these horrors, which make your hair stand on end? No. Where will you find such appalling things depicted in Soviet literature? You call it realism?

A protest note pinned on the walls of a college by students in November 1935.

SOURCE 27

I, a Young Pioneer of the Soviet Union, in the presence of my comrades, solemnly promise to love my Soviet motherland passionately, and to live, learn and struggle as the great Lenin bade us and the Communist Party teaches us.

The promise made by each member of the Young Pioneers.

SOURCE 28

Interviews with Soviet citizens who fled the USSR in the Second World War showed that support for welfare policies, support for strong government and patriotic pride were all robust – and this was from a sample of persons who had shown their hatred of Stalin by leaving the country.

An extract from *A History of Modern Russia* by Robert Conquest, published in 2003. Conquest is a well-known historian in this field.

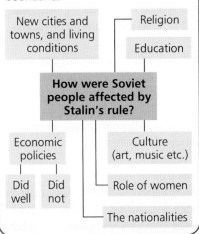

- Mothers received cash payments of 2,000 roubles per year for each child up to age five.
- A new law in 1935 allowed the NKVD to deal harshly with youth crime. There was even a death sentence introduced for young criminals, although there are no records of it being used.
- Parents could be fined if their children caused trouble. Their children could be taken to orphanages and their parents forced to pay for their upkeep.

It is very hard to judge the impact of these measures although they tended to have a much greater impact on women than men as they restricted many of the new opportunities which had opened up. Divorce rates did not fall and absent fathers meant women took the major role in holding family life together and became breadwinners as well. Overall, it seems that family life did not decline further in the 1930s and interviews with survivors of the period seem to suggest that most people supported the Great Retreat policies.

Equal society?

One of the main aims of Communist policies was to make life more equal and fair for all members of society. Critics of Communism have usually pointed out that it made life equally bad for everyone in society. There is some evidence to support this.

- The buying power of a worker's wages fell by over 50 per cent during the first Five Year Plan.
- The average worker in 1930s Moscow ate only 20 per cent of the meat and fish he ate in 1900.
- Housing was hard to find and expensive.
- It was difficult to get clothing, shoes and boots. Queuing to buy goods became part of life.

On the other hand, there were some positives. Health care improved enormously. Education improved and public libraries became available as literacy became a high priority. Sports facilities were good in most towns and cities.

Despite the ideology a divide in society began to open up. For some, if you were ambitious, you could become part of the new 'class' of skilled workers or a foreman, supervisor or technician. There was an army of managers and bureaucrats, and they created jobs for the secretaries who handled their paperwork. One manager employed a servant on eighteen roubles a week, while his wife earned 30 roubles a week as a typist. The manager could also get items like clothing and luxuries in the official Party shops. At the very top was a new ruling class – the nomenclatura. This was the special group loyal to Stalin who took all the top jobs in the Communist Party, the government and regional government. They and their families enjoyed many privileges such as better housing, food, clothes and schools for their children.

The groups mentioned above had done well out of the new industrial society and their support for Stalin was vital in helping him control Soviet society.

The nationalities

People often think of Russia and the USSR as the same thing, but this is wrong. Russia was the largest republic in a large collection of republics. As a Georgian, you might think Stalin would sympathise with people who did not want to be part of a Soviet Union dominated by Russia. In fact, Stalin had little time for nationalist feelings. He was much more concerned with control and obedience and he regarded the nationalities with suspicion. You have already read on page 222 how Communism attacked Islam, which was an attack on religion and nationality in the sense that the national identities of many nationalities (such as the Crimean Tatars, Kazhaks, Balkars and Azerbaijanis) were bound up with their religion.

In 1932 a new regulation was brought in that required Soviet citizens to carry identity booklets and these documents included a section in which they had to specify their nationality, another form of control. Many nationalities found that their homelands were dramatically changed by the arrival of large numbers of Russian immigrant workers who were sent there to develop new industrial projects. In some areas whole populations were deported from their homes because Stalin did not trust them. Between 1935 and 1938 Stalin carried out deportations against at least nine different ethnic groups. For example, when Japan began to expand in the Far East Stalin deported 142 000 Koreans away from his easternmost borders. This became a large-scale, systematic process once war broke out with Germany in 1941 as Stalin feared they would co-operate with the invading German forces and groups deported included Chechens in the south of the USSR and Poles, Lithuanians and other peoples of the Baltic territories.

Other groups were persecuted because of long-standing prejudices. For example, Jews still suffered discrimination and the Finnish population in the region around Leningrad fell by one-third during the 1930s.

SOURCE **29**

There are abominations in the supply of metal for the Stalingrad Tractor Plant and the Moscow and Gorky auto plants. It is disgraceful that the windbags at the People's Commissariat of Heavy Industry have still not gotten around to straightening out the supply system. Let the Central Committee place under its continuous supervision, without delay, the plants that are supplying them and make up for this disruption.

Stalin writing in 1932 to his deputy, Kaganovich.

Keywords

Make sure you know what these terms mean and are able to define them confidently.

- Bolshevik
- Capitalist
- Civil War
- Collectivisation
- Communist
- Cossack
- Duma
- Five-Year Plan
- Kerensky
- Lenin
- Marxist
- Mensheviks
- Nationalities
- New Economic Policy
- NKVD
- Okhrana
- Peasants
- Provisional Government
- Purges
- Show trials
- Social Democratic Party
- Socialist Revolutionaries
- Soviet Union
- Soviets
- Stalin
- Stolypin
- Trotsky
- Tsar
- Tsarina
- USSR
- War Communism
- Zemstva

How complete was Stalin's control over the Soviet Union by 1941?

By 1941 Stalin was the supreme unchallenged leader of Soviet Russia but how far was he in complete control?

On the one hand...

In the Purges which had mainly ended in 1938, Stalin had:

- removed all the old Bolsheviks capable of forming an alternative government and replacing him as leader
- removed the main officers in the army likely to cause him any trouble
- cowed intellectuals in education, sciences and the arts, making them unlikely to voice criticisms of his policies
- terrified the population at large who did not know where accusations of disloyalty might come from and feared being picked up by the secret police
- got rid of many of the unruly and disruptive elements in society by sending them to the Gulag where they might prove more useful as slave labour.

The vast organisation of the secret police, the NKVD, stood behind Stalin and behind the NKVD lay the terror of the Gulag concentration camps.

Stalin's position was cemented by the cult of the personality, which led many Russians to regard him as an almost superhuman leader whom they revered and even loved. Those who did not go along with the hype were very reluctant to voice their views in public. Stalin had complete control of the media and propaganda, which repeated the message that Stalin was great and the only person who could lead Russia to a bright future.

But on the other hand...

Soviet Russia was a still a difficult country to rule.

- Stalin found it difficult to control regions away from Moscow. People, including Communist officials, ran their own areas to suit themselves and would not always carry out instructions from the centre.
- There was a lot of bribery and corruption, especially as everybody had to reach unrealistic production targets in industry. Nobody, even Communist Party officials, wanted to be accused of not fulfilling targets, so they fiddled the figures, produced sub-standard goods or simply did not tell the centre what was going on.
- Even those higher up cheated and manipulated the system so they could escape any blame. The whole central planning system was rough and unwieldy despite the fact that it achieved its broad aims.

Soviet Russia in the 1930s was never very stable. Millions of people moved around as industrialisation created vast new centres and peasants were thrown off the land. People came and went seeking jobs and accommodation or trying to escape the authorities. Thousands changed jobs regularly so they could not be tracked down and subjected to the harsh labour laws, or to get better wages, especially if they were skilled workers. In all this fluid mix there were embittered, rebellious and criminal elements as well as young people who would not conform to Soviet laws, rules and regulations. Some historians think the Purges were in part an attempt to control this moving mass and weed out the troublemakers. But Stalin could never really bring this 'quicksand society' under control.

In the countryside, Stalin had subdued the peasants through collectivisation but most were still aggrieved by the loss of their land and independence. They adapted to the Stalinist system but resisted where they could. They made life difficult for farm managers, were insubordinate, neglected jobs, were apathetic and generally did not work hard. Agriculture never performed as well as it should have done.

What methods did Stalin use to control the USSR?

1 Draw up and complete a table to make notes and record examples for the methods of control listed. You can add more/different methods if you wish.

♦ Fear and terror (NKVD, Gulag)
♦ Purges
♦ Force and compulsion (e.g. collectivisation)
♦ Propaganda
♦ Cult of the personality
♦ Education and youth groups
♦ Control of mass media and the arts
♦ Improving living conditions for some

How complete was Stalin's control over the Soviet Union by 1941?

2 Now use your notes to write an answer to this question:
'By 1941 Stalin had complete control of the Soviet Union because he had crushed all opposition.' How far do you agree with this statement? Explain your answer.
You should structure this in three sections or paragraphs:

1 The argument that Stalin was in control. Here you should include:
♦ examples of the methods he used
♦ evidence that these methods actually worked (e.g. source extracts).

2 The argument that Stalin was not in control or that his control was not as great as it appeared. Here you should include:
♦ examples of resistance to Stalin and his methods
♦ an explanation of how serious this resistance was.

3 Your overall judgement as to how complete his control really was (e.g. that his control was not complete but the resistance was limited).

We know that Stalin tried to control things personally as far as he could. He sent out a constant stream of notes and letters giving very specific instructions about what should be done, even down to particular industrial plants. In letters to his henchmen Stalin talks frequently about fulfilling targets 'with unrelenting firmness and ruthlessness'. These could be used as evidence of Stalin's control but the frustration expressed in the letters can also be seen as evidence that Stalin was not able to get them to do what he wanted (see Source 29 for example).

Key Question Summary

How did Stalin gain and hold on to power?

1 Stalin emerged as the new leader of Russia through a mixture of political cunning, ruthlessness and the mistakes of the other contenders.
2 He gained control of the party machine and could appoint his supporters to key positions. He outmanoeuvred his opponents by playing them off against each other.
3 His main rival Trotsky, ill at the time, would not get involved in the power struggle. He was disliked by many Bolsheviks for being too aloof and they feared he would become a dictator.
4 Stalin's policy of 'Socialism in one country' was popular and appealed to Russian nationalism.
5 Stalin established a system of fear and terror to control the USSR, backed by an effective secret police force and the Gulag labour camps.
6 From 1936 he used the Purges to make sure he remained leader. He set up show trials to get rid of the old Bolsheviks who might form an alternative government and to frighten others.
7 He purged the Communist Party to make sure it would carry out his orders without question.
8 He purged the army to get rid of any officers who might be disloyal to him.
9 He undertook a general purge of the population to instil fear so that they would do as they were told. He got rid of leading members of the intelligentsia in education and the arts. He also got rid of troublesome individuals on the fringes of society who did not fit into the Stalinist system.
10 A cult of the personality saw Stalin promoted as a god-like leader who could guide the USSR to a great future.
11 Stalin tried to control what people thought through the mass media, education, the arts and culture in general. He tried to suppress religion but was not successful.

Exam Practice

See pages 168–175 and pages 316–319 for advice on the different types of questions you might face.

1 (a) What were the Five-Year Plans? **[4]**
   (b) Explain why Stalin was so committed to modernising industry in the USSR. **[6]**
   (c) 'The Five-Year Plans brought glory to Stalin but misery to his people.' How far do you agree with this statement? Explain your answer **[10]**

Component 3 or 4 questions

2 How important was the disunity of the Whites in the Bolshevik victory in the Civil War in Russia?
3 How significant was the role of terror and repression in maintaining Stalin's control of the USSR?

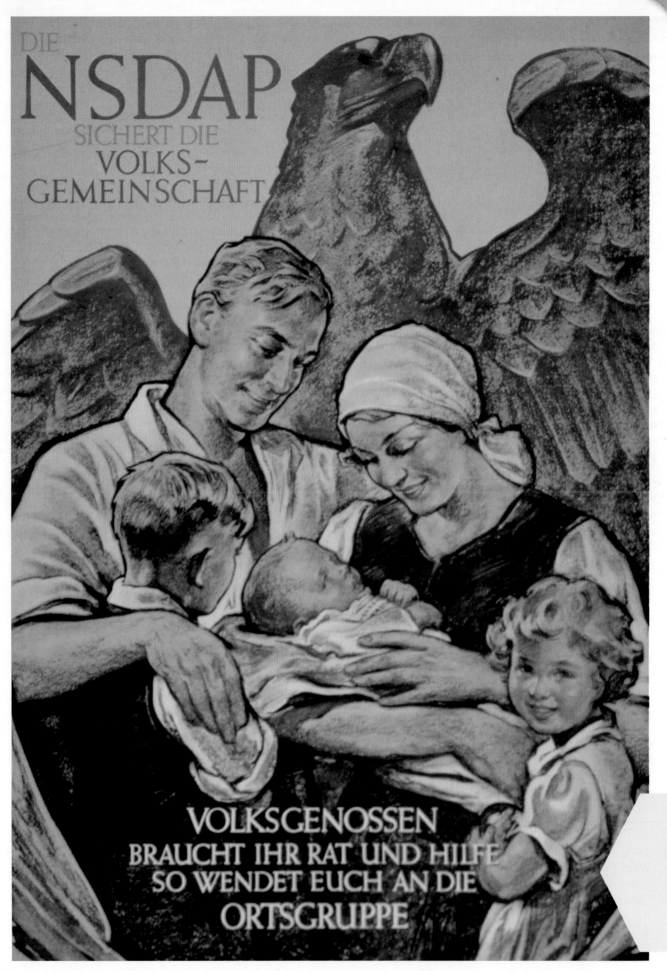

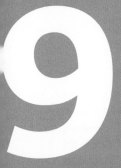

Germany, 1918–45

KEY QUESTIONS

9.1 Was the Weimar Republic doomed from the start?

9.2 Why was Hitler able to dominate Germany by 1934?

9.3 How effectively did the Nazis control Germany, 1933–45?

9.4 What was it like to live in Nazi Germany?

Germany emerged from the First World War in a state of chaos. The new Weimar government struggled from crisis to crisis. Out of this confusion Adolf Hitler and the Nazis emerged as the most powerful group in Germany and led Germany into a period of dictatorship ending in an international war and the deaths of tens of millions of people.

How could this happen in a modern, democratic European state?

In 9.1 you will investigate how the Weimar Republic was created out of post-war chaos and how its leaders tried to solve the problems left over from the war.

In 9.2 you will focus on the same period but view it through a different lens and examine the reasons for the birth and growth of the Nazi Party. You will see how its early failures turned into a runaway success after the economic Depression hit Germany in the early 1930s.

The Nazis had a very specific vision of what Germany should be like and they did not tolerate opposition. In 9.3 you will examine how they imposed their will on the German people through a combination of terror and propaganda.

In 9.4 you will see how specific groups of people were affected by Nazi rule – young people, women, workers and farmers – and how the lives of Germans began to change again as a result of the Second World War.

Timeline

This timeline shows the period you will be covering in this chapter. Some of the key dates are filled in already. To help you get a complete picture of the period make your own much larger version and add other details to it as you work through the chapter.

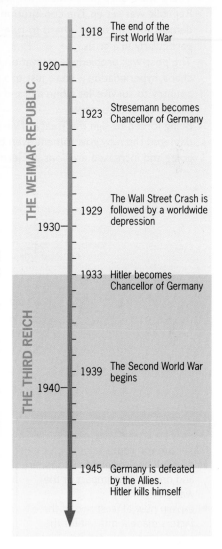

THE WEIMAR REPUBLIC

- 1918 — The end of the First World War
- 1920
- 1923 — Stresemann becomes Chancellor of Germany
- 1929 — The Wall Street Crash is followed by a worldwide depression
- 1930

THE THIRD REICH

- 1933 — Hitler becomes Chancellor of Germany
- 1939 — The Second World War begins
- 1940
- 1945 — Germany is defeated by the Allies. Hitler kills himself

◀ This Nazi poster from the 1930s encouraged people to turn to Nazi-led community groups for help and advice.

1 Using this source, describe the Nazis' ideal family.

2 What are the Nazis offering this ideal family and how is it represented in the poster?

3 Does this poster give the impression that people were afraid of the Nazis?

4 What message is the poster trying to convey to Germans?

9.1 Was the Weimar Republic doomed from the start?

Focus

The democratic Weimar government collapsed in 1933 and was replaced by a Nazi dictatorship. Some people suggest that this was inevitable: Germany had long been an authoritarian state so its fourteen-year experiment with democracy was doomed to fail – particularly given the problems that Germany faced after the war. Some would say:

♦ There were deep problems in the way the Weimar Republic was set up. The constitution was too democratic and made it hard to rule Germany, particularly in a crisis.
♦ The post-war problems – starvation, debt, political chaos, hyperinflation – were just too great for any country to survive, let alone a brand new one in a deeply divided country.
♦ Being forced to sign the Treaty of Versailles fatally damaged the new government even before it had got going and increased divisions in German society.

Others would disagree with these points and point to the recovery and successes of the 1920s. They would say that the successes of the 1920s were significant – the underlying problems had been solved and Germany's government was doing well.

There is plenty of evidence on both sides of the debate. As you study these events you can reach your own conclusions on these issues and arrive at your own judgement about whether the Weimar Republic was doomed to fail.

Focus Points

♦ How did Germany emerge from defeat at the end of the First World War?
♦ What was the impact of the Treaty of Versailles on the Republic?
♦ To what extent did the Republic recover after 1923?
♦ What were the achievements of the Weimar period?

The impact of the First World War

In 1914 the Germans were a proud people. Their Kaiser – virtually a dictator – was celebrated for his achievements. Their army was probably the finest in the world. A journey through the streets of Berlin in 1914 would have revealed prospering businesses and a well-educated and well-fed workforce. There was great optimism about the power and strength of Germany.

Four years later a similar journey would have revealed a very different picture. Although little fighting had taken place in Germany itself, the war had still destroyed much of the old Germany. The proud German army was defeated. The German people were surviving on turnips and bread, and even the flour for the bread was mixed with sawdust to make it go further. A flu epidemic was sweeping the country, killing thousands of people already weakened by lack of food.

Revision Tip

Make sure you can:
♦ describe one social, one economic and one political impact of the war on Germany.
♦ explain how at least two of these factors made it difficult for the new German government.

Focus Task

How did Germany emerge from defeat in the First World War?

1 Use the information on these two pages to make a list of all the challenges facing Ebert when he took over in Germany in 1918. You could organise the list into sections:
   ♦ Political challenges
   ♦ Social challenges
   ♦ Economic challenges.
2 Imagine you are advising Ebert. Explain what you think are the three most serious challenges that need tackling urgently.
3 Take a class vote and see if you can all agree on which are the most serious challenges.

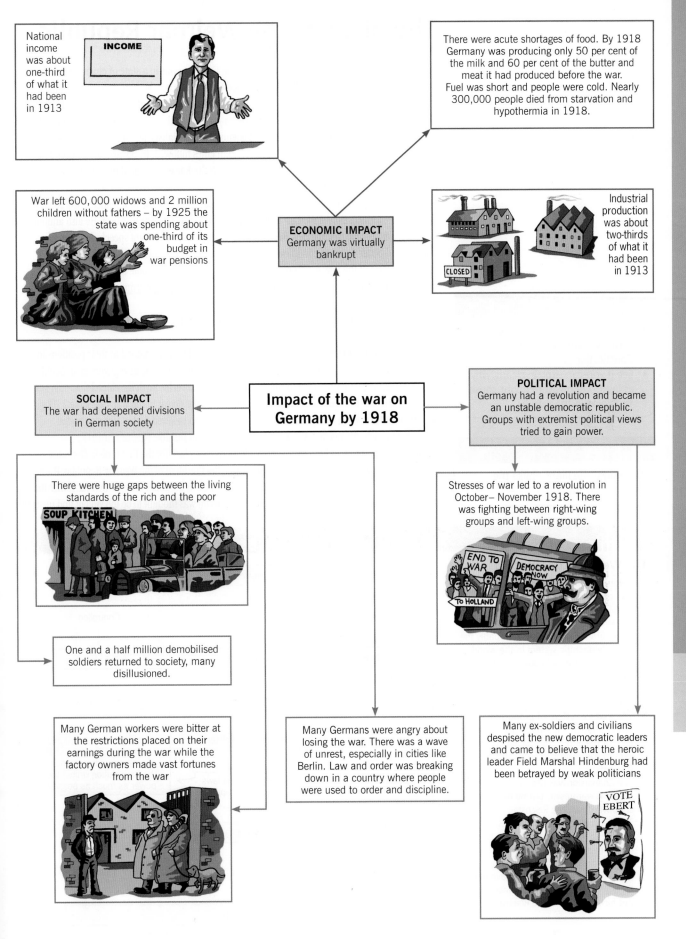

National income was about one-third of what it had been in 1913

INCOME

There were acute shortages of food. By 1918 Germany was producing only 50 per cent of the milk and 60 per cent of the butter and meat it had produced before the war. Fuel was short and people were cold. Nearly 300,000 people died from starvation and hypothermia in 1918.

War left 600,000 widows and 2 million children without fathers – by 1925 the state was spending about one-third of its budget in war pensions

ECONOMIC IMPACT
Germany was virtually bankrupt

Industrial production was about two-thirds of what it had been in 1913

CLOSED

SOCIAL IMPACT
The war had deepened divisions in German society

Impact of the war on Germany by 1918

POLITICAL IMPACT
Germany had a revolution and became an unstable democratic republic. Groups with extremist political views tried to gain power.

There were huge gaps between the living standards of the rich and the poor

SOUP KITCHEN

Stresses of war led to a revolution in October–November 1918. There was fighting between right-wing groups and left-wing groups.

END TO WAR
DEMOCRACY NOW
TO HOLLAND

One and a half million demobilised soldiers returned to society, many disillusioned.

Many German workers were bitter at the restrictions placed on their earnings during the war while the factory owners made vast fortunes from the war

Many Germans were angry about losing the war. There was a wave of unrest, especially in cities like Berlin. Law and order was breaking down in a country where people were used to order and discipline.

Many ex-soldiers and civilians despised the new democratic leaders and came to believe that the heroic leader Field Marshal Hindenburg had been betrayed by weak politicians

VOTE EBERT

The birth of the Weimar Republic

In autumn 1918 the Allies had clearly won the war. Germany was in a state of chaos, as you can see from the diagram on page 229,. The Allies offered Germany peace, but under strict conditions. One condition was that Germany should become more democratic and that the Kaiser should abdicate. When the Kaiser refused, sailors in northern Germany mutinied and took over the town of Kiel. This triggered other revolts. The Kaiser's old enemies, the Socialists, led uprisings of workers and soldiers in other German ports. Soon, other German cities followed. In Bavaria an independent Socialist Republic was declared. On 9 November 1918 the Kaiser abdicated his throne and left Germany for the Netherlands.

The following day, the Socialist leader Friedrich Ebert became the new leader of the Republic of Germany. He immediately signed an armistice with the Allies. The war was over. He also announced to the German people that the new Republic was giving them freedom of speech, freedom of worship and better working conditions. A new constitution was drawn up (see Factfile).

The success of the new government depended on the German people accepting an almost instant change from the traditional, autocratic German system of government to this new democratic system. The prospects for this did not look good.

The reaction of politicians in Germany was unenthusiastic. Ebert had opposition from both right and left.

- **On the right wing**, nearly all the Kaiser's former advisers remained in their positions in the army, judiciary, civil service and industry. They restricted what the new government could do. Many still hoped for a return to rule by the Kaiser. A powerful myth developed that men such as Ebert had stabbed Germany in the back and caused the defeat in the war (see page 231).
- **On the left wing** there were many Communists who believed that at this stage what Germany actually needed was a Communist revolution just like Russia's in 1917.

Despite this opposition, in January 1919 free elections took place for the first time in Germany's history. Ebert's party won a majority and he became the President of the Weimar Republic. It was called this because, to start with, the new government met in the small town of Weimar rather than in the German capital, Berlin. Even in February 1919, Berlin was thought to be too violent and unstable.

Revision Tip

- ◆ Make sure you can describe at least two features of the Weimar Constitution.
- ◆ See if you can explain clearly why at least one measure might cause problems in the future.

Think!

Why might the Right dislike the Weimar Constitution?

Factfile

The Weimar Constitution

- ➤ Before the war Germany had no real democracy. The Kaiser was virtually a dictator.
- ➤ The Weimar Constitution, on the other hand, attempted to set up probably the most democratic system in the world where no individual could gain too much power.
- ➤ All Germans over the age of 20 could vote.
- ➤ There was a system of proportional representation – if a party gained 20 per cent of the votes, they gained 20 per cent of the seats in the Parliament (Reichstag).
- ➤ The Chancellor was responsible for day-to-day government, but he needed the support of half the Reichstag.
- ➤ The Head of State was the President. The President stayed out of day-to-day government. In a crisis he could rule the country directly through Article 48 of the Constitution. This gave him emergency powers, which meant he did not have to consult the Reichstag.

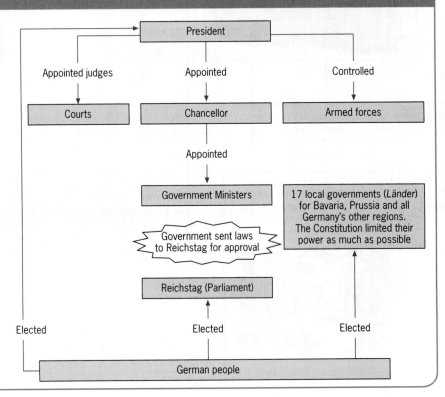

Think!

1 Draw up a table to compare the various threats from Left and Right described on this page. Include:
   ◆ Name of group
   ◆ Leadership
   ◆ Demands/Aims
   ◆ Supported by
   ◆ Methods
   ◆ How defeated
   ◆ Consequences
2 What differences can you see between the treatment of left-wing and right-wing extremists? Can you explain this?

Revision Tip

◆ Make sure you can describe at least one example of Left wing and one example of Right wing revolts.
◆ Practise explaining how the government defeated Left and Right wing threats.

The Republic in danger, 1919–24

From the start, Ebert's government faced violent opposition from both left-wing and right-wing opponents.

The threat from the Left

One left-wing group was known as the Spartacists. They were Communists led by Karl Liebknecht and Rosa Luxemburg. Their party was much like Lenin's Bolsheviks, who had just taken power in Russia. They argued strongly against Ebert's plans for a democratic Germany (see Factfile). They wanted a Germany ruled by workers' councils or soviets.

Early in 1919 the Spartacists launched their bid for power. Joined by rebel soldiers and sailors, they set up soviets in many towns. Not all soldiers were on the side of the Spartacists, however. Some anti-Communist ex-soldiers had formed themselves into vigilante groups called Freikorps. Ebert made an agreement with the commanders of the army and the Freikorps to put down the rebellion. Bitter street fighting followed between the Spartacists and Freikorps. Both sides were heavily armed. Casualties were high. The Freikorps won. Liebknecht and Luxemburg were murdered and this Communist revolution had failed. However, another one was soon to follow.

It emerged in Bavaria in the south of Germany. Bavaria was still an independent Socialist state led by Kurt Eisner, who was Ebert's ally. In February 1919 he was murdered by political opponents. The Communists in Bavaria seized the opportunity to declare a soviet republic in Bavaria. Ebert used the same tactics as he had against the Spartacists. The Freikorps moved in to crush the revolt in May 1919. Around 600 Communists were killed.

In 1920 there was more Communist agitation in the Ruhr industrial area. Again police, army and Freikorps clashed with Communists. There were 2,000 casualties.

Ebert's ruthless measures against the Communists created lasting bitterness between them and his Socialist Party. However, it gained approval from many in Germany. Ebert was terrified that Germany might go the same way as Russia (at that time rocked by bloody civil war). Many Germans shared his fears. Even so, despite these defeats, the Communists remained a powerful anti-government force in Germany throughout the 1920s.

The threat from the Right

At the same time Ebert's government faced violent opposition from the Right. His right-wing opponents were largely people who had grown up in the successful days of the Kaiser's Germany. They had liked the Kaiser's dictatorial style of government. They liked Germany having a strong army. They wanted Germany to expand its territory, and to have an empire. They had been proud of Germany's powerful industry. They deeply resented the treaty of Versailles and the restrictions placed on Germany's army and the losses of territory and industry (see page 232).

In March 1920 Dr Wolfgang Kapp led 5,000 Freikorps into Berlin in a rebellion known as the Kapp Putsch (Putsch means rebellion). The army refused to fire on the Freikorps and it looked as if Ebert's government was doomed. However, it was saved by the German people, especially the industrial workers of Berlin. They declared a general strike which brought the capital to a halt with no transport, power or water. After a few days Kapp realised he could not succeed and left the country. He was hunted down and died while awaiting trial. It seemed that Weimar had support and power after all. Even so, the rest of the rebels went unpunished by the courts and judges.

Ebert's government struggled to deal with the political violence in Germany. Political assassinations were frequent. In the summer of 1922 Ebert's foreign minister Walther Rathenau was murdered by extremists. Then in November 1923 Adolf Hitler led an attempted rebellion in Munich, known as the Munich Putsch (see page 239). Both Hitler and the murderers of Rathenau received short prison sentences. Strangely, Hitler's judge at the trial was the same judge who had tried him two years earlier for disorder. Both times he got off very lightly. It seemed that Weimar's right-wing opponents had friends in high places.

Focus Task

What was the impact of the Treaty of Versailles on the Republic?

1 **Research:** Using all the information and sources on pages 232–34 and pages 14–15 in Chapter 1, find out the impact of the treaty on:
   a) German territory
   b) the armed forces
   c) German attitudes and national pride
   d) the economy
   e) political stability.
2 **Reach a judgement:** Which of these do you think was most damaging to the Weimar republic in:
   ♦ the short term (in 1920)
   ♦ the long term (by 1923)?
   Support your answer with evidence from your research.

The Treaty of Versailles

The biggest crisis for the new republic came in May 1919 when the terms of the Treaty of Versailles were announced. You can read more about this in Chapter 1. Most people in Germany were appalled, but the right-wing opponents of Ebert's government were particularly angry. They blamed Ebert's government for betraying Germany. Germany lost:

- 10 per cent of its land
- all of its overseas colonies
- 12.5 per cent of its population
- 16 per cent of its coal and 48 per cent of its iron industry.

In addition:

- its army was reduced to 100,000; it was not allowed to have an air force; its navy was reduced
- Germany had to accept blame for starting the war and was forced to pay reparations.

Most Germans were appalled. Supporters of the Weimar government felt betrayed by the Allies. The Kaiser was gone — why should they be punished for his war and aggression? Opponents of the regime turned their fury on Ebert.

Ebert himself was very reluctant to sign the Treaty, but he had no choice. Germany could not go back to war. However, in the minds of many Germans, Ebert and his Weimar Republic were forever to blame for the Treaty. The injustice of the Treaty became a rallying point for all Ebert's opponents. They believed that the German army had been 'stabbed in the back' by the Socialist and Liberal politicians who agreed an armistice in November 1918. They believed that Germany had not been beaten on the battlefield, but that it had been betrayed by its civilian politicians who didn't dare continue the war. The Treaty was still a source of bitterness in Germany when Hitler came to power in 1933.

Revision Tip

♦ Make sure you can describe at least two ways the Treaty affected Germany.
♦ Try to explain at least two ways in which the Treaty caused economic problems in Germany.
♦ Practise explaining two reasons why the Treaty caused political problems.

SOURCE 2

The text reads: 'The Mammoth Military superiority of our neighbours'.

The chains = military treaties;
F = peace time strength;
R = reserve soldiers.

The German Reich is surrounded by Belgium, Czechoslovakia, Poland and France (clockwise from top left).

Nazi cartoon commenting on the military terms of the Versailles treaty.

Source Analysis

1 Study Source 2 carefully. What point is the cartoonist trying to make about Germany's position?
2 What point is the cartoonist making about France in relation to Germany?
3 What point is the cartoonist making about France in relation to the other countries in the cartoon?

SOURCE 3

There was a lot of official harassment. There was widespread hunger, squalor and poverty and – what really affected us – there was humiliation. The French ruled with an iron hand. If they disliked you walking on the pavement, for instance, they'd come along with their riding crops and you'd have to walk in the road.

The memories of Jutta Rudiger, a German woman living in the Ruhr during the French occupation.

Think!

1 Work in pairs. One of you study Source 4 and the other Source 5. Explain the message of each source to the other person in your pair. Remember to make a valid inference (for example, the cartoonist is saying …). Then remember to support the inference with a detail from the cartoon (for example this is shown in the cartoon by …).

Economic disaster

The Treaty of Versailles destabilised Germany politically, but Germans also blamed it for another problem – economic chaos. See if you agree that the Treaty of Versailles was responsible for economic problems in Germany.

The Treaty of Versailles forced Germany to pay reparations to the Allies. The reparations bill was announced in April 1921. It was set at £6,600 million, to be paid in annual instalments of 2 per cent of Germany's annual output. The Germans protested that this was an intolerable strain on the economy which they were struggling to rebuild after the war, but their protests were ignored.

The Ruhr

The first instalment of £50 million was paid in 1921, but in 1922 nothing was paid. Ebert did his best to play for time and to negotiate concessions from the Allies, but the French in particular ran out of patience. They too had war debts to pay to the USA. So in January 1923 French and Belgian troops entered the Ruhr (quite legally under the Treaty of Versailles) and began to take what was owed to them in the form of raw materials and goods.

The results of the occupation of the Ruhr were disastrous for Germany. The government ordered the workers to carry out passive resistance, which meant to go on strike. That way, there would be nothing for the French to take away. The French reacted harshly, killing over 100 workers and expelling over 100,000 protesters from the region. More importantly, the halt in industrial production in Germany's most important region caused the collapse of the German currency.

Think!

Is it possible to answer the question 'Could Germany afford the reparations payments?' with a simple yes or no? Explain your answer.

SOURCE 4

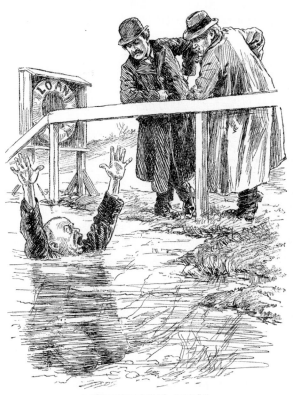

A TRANSPARENT DODGE.

Germany. "HELP! HELP! I DROWN! THROW ME THE LIFE-BELT!"
Mr. Lloyd George. } "TRY STANDING UP ON YOUR FEET."
M. Briand . . . }

A British cartoon from 1921. The two watchers are the leaders of France and Britain.

SOURCE 5

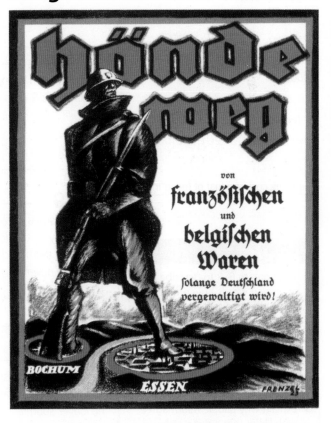

A 1923 German poster discouraging people from buying French and Belgian goods, as long as Germany is under occupation. The poster reads, 'Hands off French and Belgian goods as long as Germany is raped!'. Bochun and Essen are two industrial towns in the Ruhr.

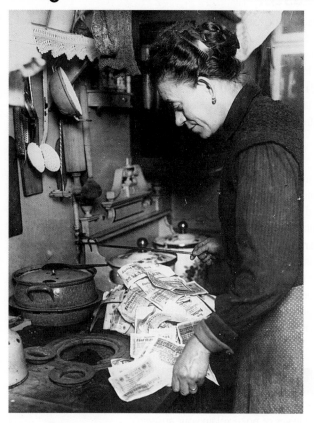

A photograph taken in 1923 showing a woman using banknotes to start her fire.

Hyperinflation

Because it had no goods to trade, the government simply printed money. For the government this seemed an attractive solution. It paid off its debts in worthless marks, including war loans of over £2,200 million. The great industrialists were able to pay off all their debts as well.

This set off a chain reaction. With so much money in circulation, but not enough goods to buy with it, prices and wages rocketed, but people soon realised that this money was worthless. Workers needed wheelbarrows to carry home their wages. Wages began to be paid daily instead of weekly. The price of goods could rise between joining the back of a queue in a shop and reaching the front!

Poor people suffered, but the greatest casualties were the richer Germans – those with savings. A prosperous middle-class family would find that their savings, which might have bought a house in 1921, by 1923 would not even buy a loaf of bread. Pensioners found that their monthly pension would not even buy one cup of coffee.

It was clear to all, both inside and outside Germany, that the situation needed urgent action. In August 1923 a new government under Gustav Stresemann took over.

- He called off the passive resistance in the Ruhr.
- He called in the worthless marks and burned them, replacing them with a new currency called the Rentenmark.
- He negotiated to receive American loans under the Dawes Plan.
- He even renegotiated the reparations payments.

The economic crisis was solved very quickly. Some historians suggest that this is evidence that Germany's problems were not as severe as its politicians had made out.

It was also increasingly clear, however, that the hyperinflation had done great political damage to the Weimar government. Their right-wing opponents had yet another problem to blame them for, and the government had lost the support of the middle classes.

	1918	0.63 marks
	1922	163 marks
January	1923	250 marks
July	1923	3465 marks
September	1923	1,512,000 marks
November	1923	201,000,000,000 marks

The rising cost of a loaf of bread in Berlin.

One afternoon I rang Aunt Louise's bell. The door was opened merely a crack. From the dark came a broken voice: 'I've used 60 billion marks' worth of gas. My milk bill is 1 million. But all I have left is 2000 marks. I don't understand any more.'

E Dobert, *Convert to Freedom*, 1941.

. . . the causes of hyperinflation were complex, but the Germans did not see it that way. They blamed reparations and the Weimar Republic which had accepted them and had presided over the chaos of 1923. Many middle-class Germans never forgave the republic for the blow they believed it had dealt to them.

British historian Finlay McKichan, writing in 1992.

Believe me, our misery will increase. The State itself has become the biggest swindler . . . Horrified people notice that they can starve on millions . . . we will no longer submit . . . we want a dictatorship!

Adolf Hitler attacks the Weimar government in a speech, 1924.

Think!

1 Use Sources 6–8 to describe in your own words how ordinary Germans were affected by the collapse of the mark.
2 Read Source 10. Choose two of Sources 6–10 to illustrate a leaflet containing a published version of Hitler's speech. Explain your choice.
3 Explain why people might agree with Hitler that a dictatorship would solve Germany's problems.

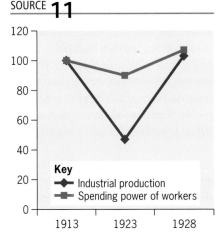

Comparison of aspects of the German economy in 1913, 1923 and 1928.

Think!

1 List the factors that helped Germany's economy to recover.
2 In what ways did economic recovery affect the lives of ordinary Germans?

Revision Tip

Hyperinflation

♦ Make sure you can describe two causes and two effects of the hyperinflation.
♦ Describe the actions of Stresemann to tackle the currency crisis.
♦ Ideally, see if you can explain at least one reason why Germans believed the Treaty caused the hyperinflation.
♦ Try explaining to someone else whether you think Stresemann's actions were effective.

The Dawes Plan

♦ Make sure you can describe how the Dawes Plan worked.
♦ Describe one way in which German politics was more settled in this period.
♦ Try explaining to someone else why the Nazis were unsuccessful in this period.

The Weimar Republic under Stresemann

Achievements

The economy

Although Chancellor for only a few months, Stresemann was a leading member of every government from 1923 to 1929. He was a more skilful politician than Ebert, and, as a right-winger, he had wider support. He was also helped by the fact that through the 1920s the rest of Europe was gradually coming out of its post-war depression. Slowly but surely, he built up Germany's prosperity again. Under the Dawes Plan (see page 37), reparations payments were spread over a longer period, and 800 million marks in loans from the USA poured into German industry. Some of the money went into German businesses, replacing old equipment with the latest technology. Some of the money went into public works like swimming pools, sports stadia and apartment blocks. As well as providing facilities, these projects created jobs.

By 1927 German industry seemed to have recovered very well. In 1928 Germany finally achieved the same levels of production as before the war and regained its place as the world's second greatest industrial power (behind the USA). Wages for industrial workers rose and for many Germans there was a higher standard of living. Reparations were being paid and exports were on the increase. The government was even able to increase welfare benefits and wages for state employees.

Politics

Even politics became more stable. To begin with, there were no more attempted revolutions after 1923 (see page 239). One politician who had been a leading opponent of Ebert in 1923 said that 'the Republic is beginning to settle and the German people are becoming reconciled to the way things are.' Source 12 shows that the parties that supported Weimar democracy did well in these years. By 1928 the moderate parties had 136 more seats in the Reichstag than the radical parties. Hitler's Nazis gained less than 3 per cent of the vote in the 1928 election. Just as importantly, some of the parties who had co-operated in the 'revolution' of 1918 began to co-operate again. The Socialists (SPD), Catholic Centre Party, German Democratic Party (DDP) and the German People's Party (DVP) generally worked well together in the years 1924–29.

SOURCE 12

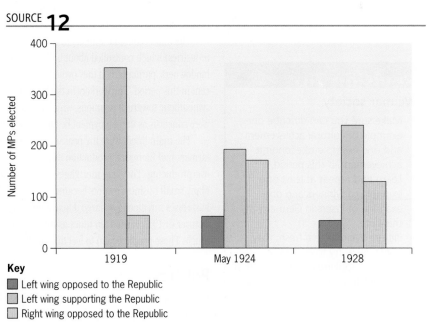

Support for the main political parties in Germany, 1919–28.

SOURCE 13

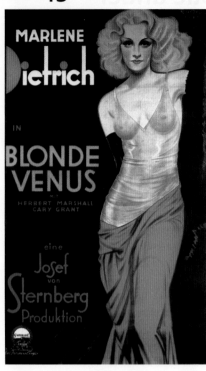

Poster for one of Marlene Dietrich's films.

SOURCE 14

What we have today is a coalition of ministers, not a coalition of parties. There are no government parties, only opposition parties. This state of things is a greater danger to the democratic system than ministers and parliamentarians realise.

Gustav Stolper, a Reichstag member for the DDP in 1929.

Revision Tip

Weimar society

♦ Make sure you can describe one example of cultural achievement and one example of economic achievement in this period.

♦ Learn and repeat at least one example of winners and one example of losers in Germany at this time.

♦ Picture Weimar as a fresh, rosy apple. Now try to explain to someone looking at the apple that it might have worms in. What are the worms?

Culture

There was also a cultural revival in Germany. In the Kaiser's time there had been strict censorship, but the Weimar constitution allowed free expression of ideas. Writers and poets flourished, especially in Berlin. Artists in Weimar Germany turned their back on old styles of painting and tried to represent the reality of everyday life, even when that reality was sometimes harsh and shocking. Artists like George Grosz produced powerful paintings such as *Pillars of Society*, which criticised the politicians and business, church and army leaders of the Weimar period, showing them as callous and mindless. Other paintings by Grosz highlighted how soldiers had been traumatised by their experiences in the war.

The famous Bauhaus style of design and architecture developed. Artists such as Walter Gropius, Paul Klee and Wassily Kandinsky taught at the Bauhaus design college in Dessau. The Bauhaus architects rejected traditional styles to create new and exciting buildings. They produced designs for anything from houses and shops to art galleries and factories. The first Bauhaus exhibition attracted 15,000 visitors.

The 1920s were a golden age for German cinema, producing one of its greatest ever international stars, Marlene Dietrich, and one of its most celebrated directors, Fritz Lang. Berlin was famous for its daring and liberated night life. Going to clubs was a major pastime. In 1927 there were 900 dance bands in Berlin alone. Cabaret artists performed songs criticising political leaders that would have been banned in the Kaiser's days. These included songs about sex that would have shocked an earlier generation of Germans.

Foreign policy

Stresemann's greatest triumphs were in foreign policy. In 1925 he signed the Locarno Treaties, guaranteeing not to try to change Germany's western borders with France and Belgium. As a result, in 1926 Germany was accepted into the League of Nations. Here Stresemann began to work, quietly but steadily, on reversing some of the terms of the Treaty of Versailles, particularly those concerning reparations and Germany's eastern frontiers. By the time he died in 1929, Stresemann had negotiated the Young Plan, which further lightened the reparations burden on Germany and led to the final removal of British, French and Belgian troops from the Rhineland.

Problems

The economy

The economic boom in Weimar Germany was precarious. The US loans could be called in at short notice, which would cause ruin in Germany.

The main economic winners in Germany were big businesses (such as the steel and chemicals industries) which controlled about half of Germany's industrial production. Other winners were big landowners, particularly if they owned land in towns – the value of land in Berlin rose by 700 per cent in this period. The workers in the big industries gained as well. Most Weimar governments were sympathetic towards the unions, which led to improved pay and conditions. However, even here there were concerns as unemployment began to rise – it was 6 per cent of the working population by 1928.

The main losers were the peasant farmers and sections of the middle classes. The peasant farmers had increased production during the war. In peacetime, they found themselves overproducing. They had mortgages to pay but not enough demand for the food they produced. Many small business owners became disillusioned during this period. Small shopkeepers saw their businesses threatened by large department stores (many of which were owned by Jews). A university lecturer in 1913 earned ten times as much as a coal miner. In the 1920s he only earned twice as much. These people began to feel that the Weimar government offered them little.

Politics

Despite the relative stability of Weimar politics in this period, both the Nazis and Communists were building up their party organisations. Even during these stable years there were four different chancellors and it was only the influence of party leaders which held the party coalitions together (see Source 14).

More worrying for the Republic was that around 30 per cent of the vote regularly went to parties opposed to the Republic. Most serious of all, the right-wing organisations which posed the greatest threat to the Republic were quiet rather than destroyed. The right-wing Nationalist Party (DNVP) and the Nazis began to collaborate closely and make themselves appear more respectable. Another event which would turn out to be very significant was that the German people elected Hindenburg as President in 1926. He was opposed to democracy and wrote to the Kaiser in exile for approval before he took up the post!

Culture

The Weimar culture was colourful and exciting to many. However, to many people living in Germany's villages and country towns, the culture of the cities seemed to represent a moral decline, made worse by American immigrants and Jewish artists and musicians. As you have read, the Bauhaus design college was in Dessau. What you were not told is that it was in Dessau because it was forced out of Weimar by hostile town officials.

Organisations such as the Wandervogel movement were a reaction to Weimar's culture. The Wandervogel called for a return to simple country values and wanted to see more help for the countryside and less decadence in the towns. It was a powerful feeling which the Nazis successfully harnessed in later years.

Foreign policy

There was also the question of international relations. Nationalists attacked Stresemann for joining the League of Nations and for signing the Locarno Pact because it meant Germany accepted the Treaty of Versailles. Communists also attacked Locarno, seeing it as part of a plot against the Communist government in the USSR. Germany was still a troubled place.

Focus Task

To what extent did the Weimar Republic recover after 1923?

Draw a diagram like this then complete it to summarise the strengths (+) and weaknesses (-) of the Weimar Republic in 1929.

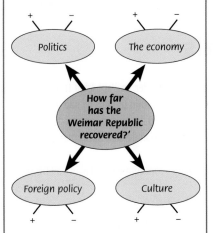

You could give each sector a mark out of ten. Finally, you need to decide on an overall judgement: in your opinion, how far had the Weimar Republic recovered? In your answer, do remember that, in the view of many historians, it was probably a major achievement for the Weimar Republic just to have survived.

Key Question Summary

Was the Weimar Republic doomed from the start?

1 Germany emerged from the First World War in a poor state, short of food and goods and in debt. It was an angry, bitter and divided society – politically (between left- and right-wing views) and socially (rich and poor).

2 The Weimar Republic was created in this turbulent time. Its constitution was very democratic but it had weaknesses. In particular, its system of proportional representation meant that it was difficult for any political party to get a clear majority and provide strong government.

3 It signed the armistice to end the war ('stab in the back') and the hated Treaty of Versailles. This gave Germans a poor view of democratic government and the Weimar Republic from the beginning.

4 It was beset by early crises, attacked from the left (Spartacists, 1919) and right (Kapp Putsch, 1920 and Munich Putsch, 1923), creating political instability.

5 The Treaty of Versailles had a devastating impact on Germany, economically (reparations, loss of territory and industry) and psychologically (war guilt, national pride). One consequence, the occupation of the Ruhr, led to the hyperinflation of 1923.

6 The economy recovered after 1924 as Germany was put on a sounder financial footing. However, prosperity depended on American loans, and unemployment remained a problem.

7 Germany was more stable politically and extremists parties, like the Nazis, did not do well in elections.

8 The Great Depression undermined the Weimar Republic. Its economic policies were unpopular and its weaknesses were revealed.

9.2 Why was Hitler able to dominate Germany by 1934?

Profile

Adolf Hitler – the early years, 1889–1919

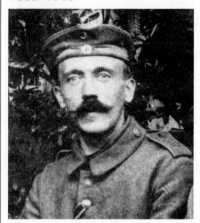

- Born in Austria in 1889.
- He got on badly with his father but was fond of his mother.
- At 16 he left school and went to Vienna to become a painter. However, he was not successful and between 1909 and 1914 he was virtually a 'down and out' on the streets of Vienna.
- During this period he developed his hatred of foreigners and Jews.
- When war broke out in 1914, Hitler joined the German army and served with distinction, winning the Iron Cross.
- Hitler found it very hard to accept the armistice and was completely unable to accept the Treaty of Versailles.
- He despised the Weimar democracy and like many Germans looked back to the 'glorious days' of the Kaiser.
- After the war, Hitler stayed in the army, working in Munich spying on extremist groups. It was in this job that he came across the German Workers' Party. He liked their ideas and joined in 1919.

Factfile

Twenty-Five Point Programme

The most important points were:
- the abolition of the Treaty of Versailles
- union of Germany and Austria
- only 'true' Germans to be allowed to live in Germany. Jews in particular were to be excluded
- large industries and businesses to be nationalised
- generous old age pension
- a strong central government.

Focus

Stresemann's government succeeded in stabilising Germany. However, as you have already seen, the extremist opponents of the Weimar government had not disappeared. Through the 1920s they were organising and regrouping, waiting for their chance to win power.

One of these extremist groups was the Nazi Party. You are now going to look back at what it had been doing since 1919 and examine its changing fortunes through the 1920s and early 1930s.

Your key question examines how the Nazis turned themselves from an obscure fringe party in the 1920s to the most popular party in Germany by 1933. You will see that there are a range of factors including Hitler's skills as a leader and the economic Depression that hit Germany in the 1930s.

You will also examine the ruthless way that once elected as Chancellor Hitler consolidated his power by removing all possible opposition.

Focus Points
- What did the Nazi Party stand for in the 1920s?
- Why did the Nazis have little success before 1930?
- Why was Hitler able to become Chancellor by 1933?
- How did Hitler consolidate his power in 1933–34?

Hitler and the Nazis

The Nazis began as the German Workers' Party, led by Anton Drexler. In 1919 Adolf Hitler joined the party. Drexler soon realised that Hitler had great talent and within months he had put him in charge of propaganda and the political ideas of the party. In 1920 the party announced its Twenty-Five Point Programme (see Factfile), and renamed itself the National Socialist German Workers' Party, or Nazis for short.

In 1921 Hitler removed Drexler as leader. Hitler's energy, commitment and above all his power as a speaker were soon attracting attention.

SOURCE 1

The most active political force in Bavaria at the present time is the National Socialist Party . . . It has recently acquired a political influence quite disproportionate to its actual numerical strength . . . Adolf Hitler from the very first has been the dominating force in the movement and the personality of this man has undoubtedly been one of the most important factors contributing to its success . . . His ability to influence a popular assembly is uncanny.

American intelligence report on political activities in Germany, 1922.

Revision Tip

- Make sure you can describe two aims of the Nazis (use pages 240–241 as well for this).
- Try to explain one way in which the Munich Putsch was a disaster for the Nazis and one way it was a success.

SOURCE 2

Hitler knew how to whip up those crowds jammed closely in a dense cloud of cigarette smoke – not by argument, but by his manner: the roaring and especially the power of his repetitions delivered in a certain infectious rhythm . . . He would draw up a list of existing evils and imaginary abuses and after listing them, in higher and higher crescendo, he screamed: 'And whose fault is it? It's all . . . the fault . . . of the Jews!'

A person who went to Nazi meetings describes the impact of Hitler's speeches. From *A Part of Myself: Portrait of an Epoch*, by C Zuckmayer.

SOURCE 3

'Power!' screamed Adolf. 'We must have power!' 'Before we gain it,' I replied firmly, 'let us decide what we propose to do with it.'

Hitler, who even then could hardly bear contradiction, thumped the table and barked: 'Power first – afterwards we can act as circumstances dictate.'

Leading Nazi Otto Strasser recalls a conversation with Hitler in the early 1920s.

Think!

A foreign intelligence service wants to keep an eye on Hitler and the Nazi Party. They want to know about this new man:
♦ his background
♦ abilities
♦ why his ideas are proving popular with some Germans
♦ why the Munich Putsch failed
♦ why Hitler got off so lightly.
Use the sources and information on these two pages to write a short report under each heading.

Source Analysis ▶

1 What impression does Source 4 give of the Putsch and Hitler's role in it?
2 Why would you have concerns about it as a source for finding out what happened?

Hitler had a clear and simple appeal. He stirred nationalist passions in his audiences. He gave them scapegoats to blame for Germany's problems: the Allies, the Versailles Treaty, the 'November Criminals' (the Socialist politicians who signed the Treaty), the Communists and the Jews.

His meetings were so successful that his opponents tried to disrupt them. To counter this, he set up the SA, also known as storm troopers or brownshirts, in 1921. These hired thugs protected Hitler's meetings but also disrupted those of other parties.

By 1923 the Nazis were still very much a minority party, but Hitler had given them a high profile.

The Munich Putsch, 1923

By November 1923 Hitler believed that the moment had come for him to topple the Weimar government. The government was preoccupied with the economic crisis. Stresemann had just called off Germany's passive resistance in the Ruhr (see pages 233–34). On 8 November, Hitler hijacked a local government meeting and announced he was taking over the government of Bavaria. He was joined by the old war hero Ludendorff.

Nazi storm troopers began taking over official buildings. The next day, however, the Weimar government forces hit back. Police rounded up the storm troopers and in a brief exchange of shots sixteen Nazis were killed by the police. The rebellion broke up in chaos. Hitler escaped in a car, while Ludendorff and others stayed to face the armed police.

Hitler had miscalculated the mood of the German people. In the short term, the Munich Putsch was a disaster for him. People did not rise up to support him. He and other leading Nazis were arrested and charged with treason. At the trial, however, Hitler gained enormous publicity for himself and his ideas, as his every word was reported in the newspapers.

In fact, Hitler so impressed the judges that he and his accomplices got off very lightly. Ludendorff was freed altogether and Hitler was given only five years in prison, even though the legal guidelines said that high treason should carry a life sentence. In the end, Hitler only served nine months of the sentence and did so in great comfort in Landsberg castle. This last point was very significant. It was clear that Hitler had some sympathy and support from important figures in the legal system. Because of his links with Ludendorff, Hitler probably gained the attention of important figures in the army. Time would show that Hitler was down, but not out.

SOURCE 4

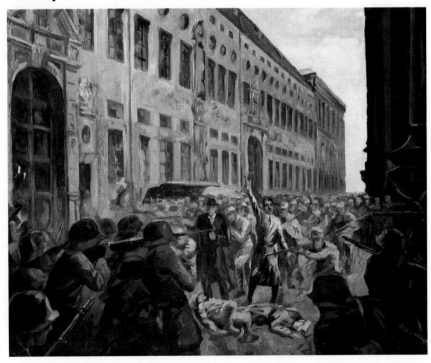

A painting of the Munich Putsch made by Arthur Wirth, one of the Nazis who took part in it. Hitler is in the centre and Ludendorff is in the black hat to Hitler's right.

SOURCE 5

When I resume active work, it will be necessary to pursue a new policy. Instead of working to achieve power by armed conspiracy we shall have to take hold of our noses and enter the Reichstag against the Catholic and Marxist deputies. If out-voting them takes longer than out-shooting them, at least the results will be guaranteed by their own constitution. Any lawful process is slow. Sooner or later we shall have a majority and after that we shall have Germany.

Hitler, writing while in prison in 1923.

Factfile

Hitler's views

In *Mein Kampf* and his later writings, Hitler set out the main Nazi beliefs:

➤ National Socialism: This stood for loyalty to Germany, racial purity, equality and state control of the economy.

➤ Racism: The Aryans (white Europeans) were the Master Race. All other races and especially the Jews were inferior.

➤ Armed force: Hitler believed that war and struggle were an essential part of the development of a healthy Aryan race.

➤ Living space ('Lebensraum'): Germany needed to expand as its people were hemmed in. This expansion would be mainly at the expense of Russia and Poland.

➤ The Führer: Debate and democratic discussion produced weakness. Strength lay in total loyalty to the leader (the Führer).

Source Analysis ▶

1 Read Source 6. List the demands made by Goebbels.

2 Would you say this source appeals more to the hearts of German people than to their minds? Support your answer with evidence from the source.

The Nazis in the wilderness, 1924–29

Hitler used his time in prison to write a book, *Mein Kampf* (My Struggle), which clarified and presented his ideas about Germany's future. It was also while in prison that he came to the conclusion that the Nazis would not be able to seize power by force. They would have to work within the democratic system to achieve power but, once in power, they could destroy that system.

As soon as he was released from prison, Hitler set about rebuilding the Nazi Party so that it could take power through democratic means. He saw the Communists building up their strength through youth organisations and recruitment drives. Soon the Nazis were doing the same.

They fought the Reichstag elections for the first time in May 1924 and won 32 seats. Encouraged by this, Hitler created a network of local Nazi parties which in turn set up the Hitler Youth, the Nazi Students' League and similar organisations.

SOURCE 6

The German people is an enslaved people. We have had all our sovereign rights taken from us. We are just good enough that international capital allows us to fill its money sacks with interest payments. That and only that is the result of a centuries-long history of heroism. Have we deserved it? No, and no again!

Therefore we demand that a struggle against this condition of shame and misery begin . . .

Three million people lack work and sustenance . . . The illusion of freedom, peace and prosperity that we were promised . . . is vanishing . . .

Thus we demand the right of work and a decent living for every working German.

While the front soldier was fighting in the trenches to defend his Fatherland, some Eastern Jewish profiteer robbed him of hearth and home. The Jew lives in palaces and the proletarian, the front soldier, lives in holes that do not deserve to be called 'homes'. That is . . . rather an injustice that cries out to the heavens. A government that does nothing is useless and must vanish, the sooner the better.

Therefore we demand homes for German soldiers and workers. If there is not enough money to build them, drive the foreigners out so that Germans can live on German soil.

Our people is growing, others diminishing. It will mean the end of our history if a cowardly and lazy policy takes from us the posterity that will one day be called upon to fulfil our historical mission.

Therefore we demand land on which to grow the grain that will feed our children.

We, however, demand a government of national labour, statesmen who are men and whose aim is the creation of a German state.

These days anyone has the right to speak in Germany – the Jew, the Frenchman, the Englishman, the League of Nations, the conscience of the world and the Devil knows who else. Everyone but the German worker. He has to shut up and work. Every four years he elects a new set of torturers, and everything stays the same. That is unjust and treasonous. We need tolerate it no longer. We have the right to demand that only Germans who build this state may speak, those whose fate is bound to the fate of their Fatherland.

Therefore we demand the annihilation of the system of exploitation! Up with the German worker's state! Germany for the Germans!

A pamphlet called 'We demand', written in 1927 by Nazi propaganda expert Joseph Goebbels.

Focus Task A

What did the Nazis stand for in the 1920s?

1 Using the information and sources from pages 238–41, draw up a diagram or chart to represent the Nazis' ideas. You can use this for revision so make the headings big and bold. You can use the ones below and/or add others of your own:
   ◆ The Treaty of Versailles
   ◆ Greater Germany
   ◆ The German people
   ◆ Lebensraum
   ◆ Race and the Jews
   ◆ Government/Weimar Republic
   ◆ Economic policies
   ◆ Social policies.
2 What was the biggest change in Nazi policy after 1923?

As you can see from Source 7, by 1927 the Nazis were still trying to appeal to German workers, as they had when the party was first founded. The results of the 1928 elections convinced the Nazis that they had to look elsewhere for support. The Nazis gained only twelve Reichstag seats and only a quarter of the Communist vote. Although their anti-semitic policies gained them some support, they had failed to win over the workers. Workers with radical political views were more likely to support the Communists. The great majority of workers supported the socialist Social Democratic Party (SPD), as they had done in every election since 1919. Indeed, despite the Nazis' arguments that workers were exploited, urban industrial workers actually felt that they were doing rather well in Weimar Germany in the years up to 1929.

Other groups in society were doing less well. The Nazis found that they gained more support from groups such as the peasant farmers in northern Germany and middle-class shopkeepers and small business people in country towns. Unlike Britain, Germany still had a large rural population who lived and worked on the land – probably about 35 per cent of the entire population. They were not sharing in Weimar Germany's economic prosperity. The Nazis highlighted the importance of the peasants in their plans for Germany, promising to help agriculture if they came to power. They praised the peasants as racially pure Germans. Nazi propaganda also contrasted the supposedly clean and simple life of the peasants with that of the allegedly corrupt, immoral, crime-ridden cities (for which they blamed the Jews). The fact that the Nazis despised Weimar culture also gained them support among some conservative people in the towns, who saw Weimar's flourishing art, literature and film achievements as immoral.

SOURCE 8

At one of the early congresses I was sitting surrounded by thousands of SA men. As Hitler spoke I was most interested at the shouts and more often the muttered exclamations of the men around me, who were mainly workmen or lower-middle-class types. 'He speaks for me . . . Ach, Gott, he knows how I feel' . . . One man in particular struck me as he leant forward with his head in his hands, and with a sort of convulsive sob said: 'Gott sei Dank [God be thanked], he understands.'

E Amy Buller, *Darkness over Germany*, published in 1943. Buller was an anti-Nazi German teacher.

In 1925 Hitler enlarged the SA. About 55 per cent of the SA came from the ranks of the unemployed. Many were ex-servicemen from the war. He also set up a new group called the SS. The SS were similar to the SA but were fanatically loyal to Hitler personally. Membership of the party rose to over 100,000 by 1928.

Hitler appointed Joseph Goebbels to take charge of Nazi propaganda. Goebbels was highly efficient at spreading the Nazi message. He and Hitler believed that the best way to reach what they called 'the masses' was by appealing to their feelings rather than by rational argument. Goebbels produced posters, leaflets, films and radio broadcasts; he organised rallies; he set up 'photo opportunities'.

Despite these shifting policies and priorities, there was no electoral breakthrough for the Nazis. Even after all their hard work, in 1928 they were still a fringe minority party who had the support of less than 3 per cent of the population. They were the smallest party with fewer seats than the Communists. The prosperity of the Stresemann years and Stresemann's success in foreign policy made Germans uninterested in extreme politics.

SOURCE 7

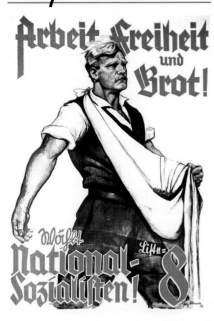

A Nazi election poster from 1928, saying 'Work, freedom and bread! Vote for the National Socialists.'

Focus Task B

Why did the Nazis have little success before 1930?

On the right are some factors which explain the Nazis' lack of success.

At the moment these factors are organised in alphabetical order. Work in groups to rearrange these factors into what you think is their order of importance.

◆ disastrous Putsch of 1923
◆ disruption of meetings by political enemies
◆ lack of support in the police and army
◆ most industrial workers supported left-wing parties
◆ Nazi aims were irrelevant to most Germans
◆ successes of Weimar government (for example in the economy, foreign policy)

The Depression and the rise of the Nazis

In 1929 the American stock market crashed and sent the USA into a disastrous economic depression. In a very short time, countries around the world began to feel the effects of this depression. Germany was particularly badly affected. American bankers and businessmen lost huge amounts of money in the crash. To pay off their debts they asked German banks to repay the money they had borrowed. The result was economic collapse in Germany. Businesses went bankrupt, workers were laid off and unemployment rocketed.

SOURCE 9

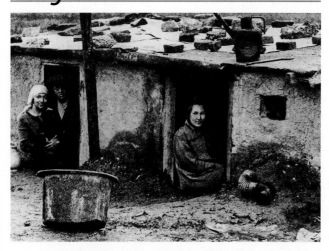

The German mining region of Upper Silesia in 1932: unemployed miners and their families moved into shacks in a shanty town because they had no money to pay their rent.

SOURCE 10

No one knew how many there were of them. They completely filled the streets. They stood or lay about in the streets as if they had taken root there. They sat or lay on the pavements or in the roadway and gravely shared out scraps of newspapers among themselves.

An eyewitness describes the unemployed vagrants in Germany in 1932.

The Depression was a worldwide problem. It was not just Germany that suffered. Nor was the Weimar government the only government having difficulties in solving the problem of unemployment. However, because Germany had been so dependent on American loans, and because it still had to pay reparations to the Allies, the problems were most acute in Germany.

In addition, it seemed that the Weimar Constitution, with its careful balance of power, made firm and decisive action by the government very difficult indeed (see Factfile, page 230).

Think!

Draw a diagram to show how the Wall Street Crash in New York could lead to miners losing their jobs in Silesia (Source 9). You could refer to Chapter 2 or Chapter 10.

SOURCE 11

Key
— Unemployed
▮ Communist vote
▯ Nazi vote

Number of seats in the Reichstag / Unemployed (millions)

1928　1930　July 1932　Nov 1932

Support for the Nazis and Communists, and unemployment, 1928–32.

Enter the Nazis!

Hitler's ideas now had a special relevance:

- Is the Weimar government indecisive? Then Germany needs a strong leader!
- Are reparations adding to Germany's problems? Then kick out the Treaty of Versailles!
- Is unemployment a problem? Let the unemployed join the army, build Germany's armaments and be used for public works like road building!

The Nazis' Twenty-Five Points (see page 238) were very attractive to those most vulnerable to the Depression: the unemployed, the elderly and the middle classes. Hitler offered them culprits to blame for Germany's troubles – the Allies, the 'November Criminals' and the Jews. None of these messages was new and they had not won support for the Nazis in the Stresemann years. The difference now was that the democratic parties simply could not get Germany back to work.

In the 1930 elections the Nazis got 107 seats. In November 1932 they got nearly 200. They did not yet have an overall majority, but they were the biggest single party.

Why did the Nazis succeed in elections?

When the Nazis were well established in power in Germany in the 1930s, their propaganda chief, Goebbels, created his own version of the events of 1929–33 that brought Hitler to power. In this version, it was Hitler's destiny to become Germany's leader, and the German people finally came to recognise this. How valid was this view? On pages 243–44 you are going to investigate

Nazi campaigning

Nazi campaign methods were modern and effective. The Nazis' greatest campaigning asset was Hitler. He was a powerful speaker. Hitler ran for president in 1932. Despite his defeat, the campaign raised his profile hugely. He was years ahead of his time as a communicator. Using films, radio and records he brought his message to millions. He travelled by plane on a hectic tour of rallies all over

SOURCE 12

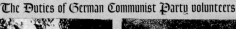
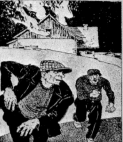
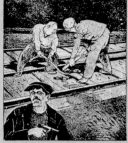
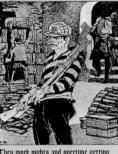
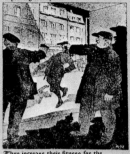

The Duties of German Communist Party volunteers

Unselfishly they help the farmers to dry the harvest.

Particular detachments are responsible for improving transport.

They work nights and overtime getting together useful equipment.

They increase their fitness for the fatherland with target practice.

An English translation of a 1931 Nazi election poster.

SOURCE 13

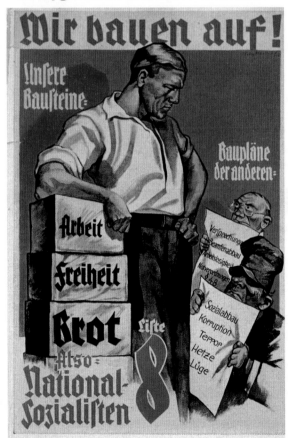

A Nazi election poster from July 1932. The Nazis proclaim 'We build!' and promise to provide work, freedom and bread. They accuse the opposing parties of planning to use terror, corruption, lies and other strategies as the basis for their government.

Germany. He appeared as a dynamic man of the moment, the leader of a modern party with modern ideas. At the same time, he was able to appear to be a man of the people, someone who knew and understood the people and their problems.

Nazi posters and pamphlets such as Sources 12 and 13 could be found everywhere. Their rallies impressed people with their energy, enthusiasm and sheer size. Nazis relied on generalised slogans rather than detailed policies – 'uniting the people of Germany behind one leader'; 'going back to traditional values' – though they were never very clear about what this meant in terms of policies. This made it hard to criticise them. When they *were* criticised for a specific policy, they were quite likely to drop it. (For example, when industrialists expressed concern about Nazi plans to nationalise industry, they simply dropped the policy.) The Nazis repeated at every opportunity that they believed Jews, Communists, Weimar politicians and the Treaty of Versailles were the causes of Germany's problems. They expressed contempt for Weimar's democratic system and said that it was unable to solve Germany's economic problems.

At this time, there were frequent street battles between Communist gangs and the police. Large unruly groups of unemployed workers gathered on street corners. In contrast, the SA and SS gave an impression of discipline and order. Many people felt the country needed this kind of order. The Nazis also organised soup kitchens and provided shelter in hostels for the unemployed.

SOURCE 14

My mother saw a storm trooper parade in the streets of Heidelberg. The sight of discipline in a time of chaos, the impression of energy in an atmosphere of universal hopelessness seems to have won her over.

Albert Speer, writing in 1931. Later, he was to become an important and powerful Nazi leader.

Nazi support rocketed. For example, in Neidenburg in East Prussia Nazi support rose from 2.3 per cent in 1928 to over 25 per cent in 1931, even though the town had no local Nazi Party and Hitler never went there.

SOURCE 15

He began to speak and I immediately disliked him. I didn't know then what he would later become. I found him rather comical, with his funny moustache. He had a scratchy voice and a rather strange appearance, and he shouted so much. He was shouting in this small room, and what he was saying was very simplistic. I thought he wasn't quite normal. I found him spooky.

An eyewitness account of one of Hitler's meetings.

Revision Tip

- ◆ Give two examples of places where Nazi support rose.
- ◆ Could you explain negative cohesion to someone who has never heard the phrase?

SOURCE **16**

Our opponents accuse us National Socialists, and me in particular, of being intolerant and quarrelsome. They say that we don't want to work with other parties. They say the National Socialists are not German at all, because they refuse to work with other political parties. So is it typically German to have thirty political parties? I have to admit one thing – these gentlemen are quite right. We are intolerant. I have given myself this one goal – to sweep these thirty political parties out of Germany.

Hitler speaking at an election rally, July 1932.

SOURCE **17**

The so-called race of poets and thinkers is hurrying with flags flying towards dictatorship . . . the radicalism of the Right [Nazis] has unleashed a strong radicalism on the Left [Communists]. The Communists have made gains almost everywhere. The situation is such that half the German people have declared themselves against the present state.

The Reich Interior Minister commenting on the rise of the Nazis and the Communists in 1932.

'Negative cohesion'

As Source 15 on page 243 shows, not everyone was taken in by Hitler's magnetism. But even some of the sceptics supported the Nazis. The historian Gordon Craig believed that this was because of 'negative cohesion'. People supported the Nazis not because they shared Nazi views (that would be positive cohesion) but because they shared Nazi fears: if you hate what I hate, then I'll support you!

Disillusionment with democracy

Perhaps the biggest negative was a dissatisfaction with democracy in Weimar Germany. Politicians seemed unable to tackle the problems of the Depression. When the Depression began to bite, Chancellor Brüning actually cut government spending and welfare benefits. He urged Germans to make sacrifices. Some historians think that he was deliberately making the situation worse in order to get the international community to cancel reparations payments. Other historians think that he was afraid of hyperinflation as in 1923.

Brüning called new elections in 1930. This was a disastrous decision, as it gave the Nazis the opportunity to exploit the discontent in Germany. The new elections resulted in yet another divided Reichstag. The impression was that democracy involved politicians squabbling over which job they would get. Meanwhile, they did nothing about the real world, where unemployment was heading towards 6 million and the average German's income had fallen by 40 per cent since 1929. The Reichstag seemed irrelevant. It met for only five days in 1932. Brüning relied on President Hindenburg's emergency powers, bypassing the democratic process altogether.

The Communist threat

As the crisis deepened, Communist support was rising too. The Nazis turned this to their advantage. 'Fear of Communism' was another shared negative.

Business leaders feared the Communists because of their plans to introduce state control of businesses. They were also concerned about the growing strength of Germany's trade unions. They felt the Nazis would combat these threats and some began to put money into Nazi campaign funds.

Farmers were also alarmed by the Communists. In the USSR, the Communist government had taken over all of the land. Millions of peasants had been killed or imprisoned in the process. In contrast, the Nazis promised to help Germany's desperately struggling small farmers.

Decadence

As for modern decadent Weimar culture – the Nazis could count on all those who felt traditional German values were under threat. The Nazis talked about restoring these old-fashioned values.

The Social Democratic Party made a grave mistake in thinking that German people would not fall for these vague promises and accusations. They underestimated the fear and anger that German people felt towards the Weimar Republic.

Revision Tip

Take the three headings on this page (Disillusionment, Communism, Decadence). Prepare a PowerPoint slide explaining each one. Limit yourself to three bullet points and five words per bullet point.

Focus Task

How did the Depression help the Nazis?

Did people rally to support Hitler for positive reasons – or do you think Gordon Craig was right that it was for negative reasons – out of fear and disillusionment? Work through questions 1–4 to help you make up your mind.

1 Look carefully at Sources 11–14. For each source, write two sentences explaining whether you think it is evidence that:
   ♦ supports the view of Goebbels
   ♦ supports the view of Craig
   ♦ could be used to support either interpretation.
2 Now work through the text and other sources on pages 242–44. Make a list of examples and evidence that seem to support either viewpoint.
3 Decide how far you agree with each of the following statements and give them a score on a scale of 1–5.
   ♦ Very few people fully supported the Nazis.
   ♦ The key factor was the economic depression. Without it, the Nazis would have remained a minority fringe party.
   ♦ The politicians of the Weimar Republic were mainly responsible for the rise of the Nazis.
4 Write a short paragraph explaining your score for each statement.

How did Hitler become Chancellor?

July 1932

November 1932

December 1932

January 1933

After the Reichstag elections of July 1932 the Nazis were the largest single party (with 230 seats) but not a majority party. Hitler demanded the post of Chancellor from the President. However, Hindenburg was suspicious of Hitler and refused. He allowed the current Chancellor Franz von Papen to carry on. He then used his emergency powers to pass the measures that von Papen hoped would solve the unemployment problem. However, von Papen was soon in trouble. He had virtually no support at all in the Reichstag and so called yet another election.

In November 1932 the Nazis again came out as the largest party, although their share of the vote fell. Hitler regarded the election as a disaster. He had lost more than 2 million votes along with 38 seats in the Reichstag. The signs were that the Hitler tide had finally turned. The Nazis started to run out of funds. Hitler is said to have threatened suicide.

Hindenburg again refused to appoint Hitler as Chancellor. In December 1932 he chose Kurt von Schleicher, one of his own advisers and a bitter rival of von Papen. But within a month, however, von Schleicher too was forced to resign.

By this time it was clear that the Weimar system of government was not working. The system of balances and proportional representation meant that no political group was able to provide strong rule. This had left the 84-year-old President Hindenburg to more or less run the country using his emergency powers, supported by army leaders and rich industrialists. In one sense, Hindenburg had already overthrown the principles of democracy by running Germany with emergency powers. If he was to rescue the democratic system, he needed a Chancellor who actually had support in the Reichstag.

Through January 1933 Hindenburg and von Papen met secretly with industrialists, army leaders and politicians. On 30 January, to everyone's surprise, they offered Hitler the post of Chancellor. With only a few Nazis in the Cabinet and von Papen as Vice Chancellor, they were confident that they could limit Hitler's influence and resist his extremist demands. The idea was that the policies would be made by the Cabinet, which was filled with conservatives like von Papen. Hitler would be there to get support in the Reichstag for those policies and to control the Communists.

So Hitler ended up as Chancellor through a behind-the-scenes deal by some German aristocrats. Both Hindenburg and von Papen were sure that they could control Hitler. They were very wrong.

SOURCE 18

The majority of Germans never voted for the Nazis.

The Nazis made it clear they would destroy democracy and all who stood in their way. Why then didn't their enemies join together to stop Hitler? . . . Had the Communists and Socialists joined forces they would probably have been strong enough both in the Reichstag and on the streets to have blocked the Nazis. The fact was that by 1932–3 there were simply not enough Germans who believed in democracy and individual freedom to save the Weimar Republic.

S Williams, in *The Rise and Fall of Hitler's Germany*, published in 1986, assesses the reasons for Hitler's success.

Revision Tip

- Make sure you can describe three of the events (in date order) that brought Hitler to power in 1933.
- 'Hindenburg offered Hitler the post of Chancellor because every other alternative had failed.' Could you explain one point for and one point against this argument?

Focus Task

How did Hitler become Chancellor in 1933?

Here is a list of factors that helped Hitler come to power.

Nazi strengths

- Hitler's speaking skills
- Propaganda campaigns
- Their criticisms of the Weimar system of government
- Nazi policies
- Support from big business
- Violent treatment of their opponents

Opponents' weaknesses

- Failure to deal with the Depression
- Failure to co-operate with one another
- Attitudes of Germans to the democratic parties

Other factors

- Weaknesses of the Weimar Republic
- Scheming of Hindenburg and von Papen
- The impact of the Depression
- The Treaty of Versailles
- Memories of the problems of 1923

1 For each factor, write down one example of how it helped Hitler.
2 Give each factor a mark out of 10 for its importance in bringing Hitler to power.
3 Choose what you think are the five most important factors and write a short paragraph on each, explaining why you have chosen it.
4 If you took away any of those factors, would Hitler still have become Chancellor?
5 Were any of those five factors also present in the 1920s?
6 If so, explain why the Nazis were not successful in the 1920s.

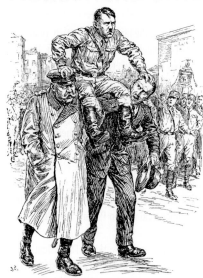

THE TEMPORARY TRIANGLE.

A British cartoon from early 1933. Hitler, as Chancellor, is being supported by Hindenburg and Von Papen. He needed their support and, although they were not happy with the idea, they needed his popularity with the masses

Think!

1 Some people suggest that the Nazis burnt down the Reichstag themselves. Explain why the Nazis might have wanted to do this.
2 Explain why the Enabling Act was so important to Hitler.
   a) Why might Hitler have executed people such as von Schleicher who were nothing to do with the SA?
   b) Why do you think Hitler chose the support of the army over the support of the SA?

Revision Tip

♦ Make sure you can describe how the Nazis reacted to the Reichstag Fire.
♦ Can you explain how the Enabling Act helped Hitler secure his power?

Hitler consolidates his position

It is easy to forget, but when Hitler became Chancellor in January 1933 he was in a very precarious position (see Source 19). Few people thought he would hold on to power for long. Even fewer thought that by the summer of 1934 he would be the supreme dictator of Germany. He achieved this through a clever combination of methods – some legal, others dubious. He also managed to defeat or reach agreements with those who could have stopped him.

The Reichstag Fire

Once he was Chancellor, Hitler took steps to complete a Nazi takeover of Germany. He called another election for March 1933 to try to get an overall Nazi majority in the Reichstag. Germany's cities again witnessed speeches, rallies, processions and street fighting. Hitler was using the same tactics as in previous elections, but now he had the resources of state media and control of the streets. Even so, success was in the balance. Then on 27 February there was a dramatic development: the Reichstag building burnt down. Hitler blamed the Communists and declared that the fire was the beginning of a Communist uprising. He demanded special emergency powers to deal with the situation and was given them by President Hindenburg. The Nazis used these powers to arrest Communists, break up meetings and frighten voters.

There have been many theories about what caused the fire, including that it was an accident, the work of a madman, or a Communist plot. Many Germans at the time thought that the Nazis might have started the fire themselves.

The defeat in 1918 did not depress me as greatly as the present state of affairs. It is shocking how day after day naked acts of violence, breaches of the law, barbaric opinions appear quite undisguised as official decree. The Socialist papers are permanently banned. The 'Liberals' tremble. The Berliner Tageblatt *was recently banned for two days; that can't happen to the* Dresdener Neueste Nachrichten, *it is completely devoted to the government . . . I can no longer get rid of the feeling of disgust and shame. And no one stirs; everyone trembles, keeps out of sight.*

An extract for 17 March 1933 from the diary of Victor Klemperer, a Jew who lived in Dresden and recorded his experiences from 1933 to 1941.

In the election, the Nazis won their largest-ever share of the votes and, with the support of the smaller Nationalist Party, Hitler had an overall majority. Using the SA and SS, he then intimidated the Reichstag into passing the Enabling Act which allowed him to make laws without consulting the Reichstag. Only the SPD voted against him. Following the election, the Communists had been banned. The Catholic Centre Party decided to co-operate with the Nazis rather than be treated like the Communists. In return, they retained control of Catholic schools. The Enabling Act made Hitler a virtual dictator. For the next four years if he wanted a new law he could just pass it. There was nothing President Hindenburg or anyone else could do.

Even now, Hitler was not secure. He had seen how the Civil Service, the judiciary, the army and other important groups had undermined the Weimar Republic. He was not yet strong enough to remove his opponents, so he set about a clever policy that mixed force, concessions and compromise (see Factfile on page 247).

Focus Task

How did Hitler consolidate his power in 1933–34?

Work in groups of three or four. Take one of these topics each. Report back your answers to the others then try to summarise in just a headline each how the following helped Hitler consolidate power:
♦ the Reichstag Fire
♦ the Enabling Act
♦ the Night of the Long Knives.

Nazi consolidation of power

- **30 January 1933** Hitler appointed Chancellor; Goering Minister of Interior.
- **17 February** Goering ordered local police forces to co-operate with the SA and SS.
- **27 February** Reichstag fire. Arrest of 4,000 Communists and other Nazi opponents on the same night.
- **28 February** Emergency Decree issued by Hindenburg:
  - police to arrest suspects and hold them without trial, search houses, ban meetings, close newspapers and radio stations
  - Hitler took over regional governments.
- **5 March** Reichstag elections: government used control of radio and police to intimidate opponents. Nazi election slogan was 'The battle against Marxism'. Won 43.9 per cent of vote.
- **13 March** Goebbels appointed head of Ministry for Propaganda. Took control of all media.
- **24 March** The Enabling Act allowed Hitler to pass decrees without the President's involvement. This made Hitler a legal dictator.
- **7 April** Civil Service administration, court, and education purged of 'alien elements', i.e. Jews and other opponents of the Nazis.
- **1 May** Workers granted May Day holiday.
- **2 May** Trade unions banned; all workers to belong to new German Labour Front (DAF).
- **9 June** Employment Law: major programme of public works (e.g. road building) to create jobs.
- **14 July** Law against the Formation of New Parties: Germany became a one-party state.
- **20 July** Concordat (agreement) with the Roman Catholic Church: government protected religious freedom; Church banned from political activity.
- **January 1934** All state governments taken over.
- **30 June** Night of the Long Knives.
- **August** On death of Hindenburg, Hitler became Führer. German armed forces swore oath of loyalty to him.

Revision Tip

- Choose three events from the Factfile above and make sure you can describe them accurately.
- Give the Enabling Act and the Night of The Long Knives marks out of 10 for their importance. Now prepare two points that justify your marks.

The Night of the Long Knives

Within a year any opponents (or potential opponents) of the Nazis had either left Germany or been taken to special concentration camps run by the SS. Other political parties were banned.

Hitler was still not entirely secure, however. The leading officers in the army were not impressed by him and were particularly suspicious of Hitler's SA and its leader Ernst Röhm. The SA was a badly disciplined force and, what's more, Röhm talked of making the SA into a second German army. Hitler himself was also suspicious of Röhm. Hitler feared that Röhm's control over the 4 million SA men made him a potentially dangerous rival.

Hitler had to choose between the army and the SA. He made his choice and acted ruthlessly. On the weekend of 29–30 June squads of SS men broke into the homes of Röhm and other leading figures in the SA and arrested them. Hitler accused Röhm of plotting to overthrow and murder him. Over the weekend Röhm and possibly as many as 400 others were executed. These included the former Chancellor von Schleicher, a fierce critic of Hitler, and others who actually had no connection with Röhm. This purge came to be known as the Night of the Long Knives.

Hindenburg thanked Hitler for his 'determined action which has nipped treason in the bud'. The army said it was well satisfied with the events of the weekend.

The SA was not disbanded. It remained as a Nazi paramilitary organisation, but was very much subordinate to the SS. Many of its members were absorbed by the army and the SS.

The Army oath

Soon after the Night of the Long Knives, Hindenburg died and Hitler took over as Supreme Leader (Führer) of Germany. On 2 August 1934 the entire army swore an oath of personal loyalty to Adolf Hitler as Führer of Germany. The army agreed to stay out of politics and to serve Hitler. In return, Hitler spent vast sums on rearmament, brought back conscription and made plans to make Germany a great military power again.

Key Question Summary

Why was Hitler able to dominate Germany by 1934?

1. The Nazi Party was formed in 1919 and Hitler soon became its leader.
2. Its 25-point programme appealed to ex-soldiers and those on the right but it did not enjoy wider support.
3. While in prison after the Munich Putsch of 1923, Hitler wrote *Mein Kampf*, setting out his ideas.
4. The Nazi Party reorganised itself in the 1920s but was still a fringe party in the 1928 elections.
5. The Great Depression led to unemployment and economic hardship, circumstances in which the Nazis could flourish.
6. Nazi criticisms of the Weimar government and the Treaty of Versailles were popular along with their ideas on rebuilding Germany.
7. They used innovative techniques – rallies, slogans, films, radio, posters and pamphlets – to put across their ideas.
8. Hitler was a great asset as a highly effective speaker who appeared to understand the people's problems and express their hopes.
9. Disillusionment with the Weimar Republic pushed Germans towards extremist parties, both the Nazis and the Communists.
10. There was violence and lawlessness and groups like businessmen and farmers, who feared Communism, liked the Nazis' anti-Communist message.
11. The Nazis became the biggest single party in the 1932 elections.
12. The leaders of the Weimar Republic thought they could use Hitler to their advantage by making him Chancellor. But he used emergency powers and the Enabling Act to establish himself as dictator.

9.3 How effectively did the Nazis control Germany, 1933–45?

Focus

There was supposed to be no room for opposition of any kind in Nazi Germany. The aim was to create a totalitarian state. In a totalitarian state there can be no rival parties, no political debate. Ordinary citizens must divert their whole energy into serving the state and to doing what its leaders want.

In this section you will examine how the Nazis combined the strategies of terror and propaganda to control Germany.

Focus Points

- How much opposition was there to the Nazi regime?
- How effectively did the Nazis deal with their political opponents?
- How did the Nazis use culture and the mass media to control the people?
- Why did the Nazis persecute many groups in German society?
- Was Nazi Germany a totalitarian state?

Focus Task

Summarise the information on these two pages in a table like this:

Method of control	Controlled by	Duties	How it helped Hitler to make his position secure

The police state

The Nazis had a powerful range of organisations and weapons that they used to control Germany and terrorise Germans into submission.

The Gestapo

The Gestapo (secret state police) was the force which was perhaps most feared by the ordinary German citizen. Under the command of Reinhard Heydrich, Gestapo agents had sweeping powers. They could arrest citizens on suspicion and send them to concentration camps without trial or even explanation.

Modern research has shown that Germans thought the Gestapo were much more powerful than they actually were. As a result, many ordinary Germans informed on each other because they thought the Gestapo would find out anyway.

The police and the courts

The police and courts also helped to prop up the Nazi dictatorship. Top jobs in local police forces were given to high-ranking Nazis reporting to Himmler. As a result, the police added political 'snooping' to their normal law and order role. They were, of course, under strict instructions to ignore crimes committed by Nazi agents. Similarly, the Nazis controlled magistrates, judges and the courts, which meant that opponents of Nazism rarely received a fair trial.

The SS

SOURCE 1

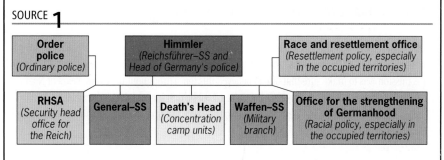

Order police (Ordinary police)		Himmler (Reichsführer–SS and Head of Germany's police)		Race and resettlement office (Resettlement policy, especially in the occupied territories)	

RHSA (Security head office for the Reich)	General–SS	Death's Head (Concentration camp units)	Waffen–SS (Military branch)	Office for the strengthening of Germanhood (Racial policy, especially in the occupied territories)

The elements of the SS during wartime.

The SS was formed in 1925 from fanatics loyal to Hitler. After virtually destroying the SA in 1934, it grew into a huge organisation with many different responsibilities. It was led by Heinrich Himmler. SS men were of course Aryans, very highly trained and totally loyal to Hitler. Under Himmler, the SS had primary responsibility for destroying opposition to Nazism and carrying out the racial policies of the Nazis.

Two important sub-divisions of the SS were the Death's Head units and the Waffen-SS. The Death's Head units were responsible for the concentration camps and the slaughter of the Jews. The Waffen-SS were special SS armoured regiments which fought alongside the regular army.

Revision Tip

♦ Make sure you can describe at least two methods of control the Nazis used.
♦ Choose one method and make sure you can explain how it was effective.

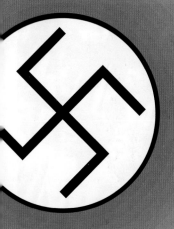

Concentration camps

Concentration camps were the Nazis' ultimate sanction against their own people. They were set up almost as soon as Hitler took power. The first concentration camps in 1933 were simply makeshift prisons in disused factories and warehouses. Soon these were purpose-built. These camps were usually in isolated rural areas, and run by SS Death's Head units. Prisoners were forced to do hard labour. Food was very limited and prisoners suffered harsh discipline, beatings and random executions. By the late 1930s, deaths in the camps became increasingly common and very few people emerged alive from them. Jews, Socialists, Communists, trade unionists, churchmen and anyone else brave enough to criticise the Nazis ended up there.

SOURCE 2

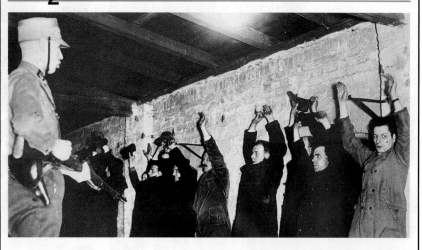

Nazi storm troopers arrest suspected Communists, 1933.

SOURCE 3

The Nazis gained 52 per cent of the vote in the March 1933 elections. This government will not be content with 52 per cent behind it and with terrorising the remaining 48 per cent, but will see its most immediate task as winning over that remaining 48 per cent . . . It is not enough for people to be more or less reconciled to the regime.

Goebbels at his first press conference on becoming Minister for Propaganda, March 1933.

Source Analysis ▼

Look at Source 4. How does the rally:
a) make it clear who the leader is
b) give people a sense of belonging
c) provide colour and excitement
d) show the power of the state
e) show the Nazis' ability to create order out of chaos?

Propaganda, culture and mass media in Nazi Germany

One reason why opposition to Hitler was so limited was the work of Dr Joseph Goebbels, Minister for Enlightenment and Propaganda. Goebbels passionately believed in Hitler as the saviour of Germany. His mission was to make sure that others believed this too. Throughout the twelve years of Nazi rule Goebbels constantly kept his finger on the pulse of public opinion and decided what the German public should and should not hear. He aimed to use every resource available to him to make people loyal to Hitler and the Nazis.

The Nuremberg rallies

Goebbels organised huge rallies, marches, torchlit processions and meetings. Probably the best example was the Nuremberg rally which took place in the summer each year. There were bands, marches, flying displays and Hitler's brilliant speeches. The rallies brought some colour and excitement into people's lives. They gave them a sense of belonging to a great movement. The rallies also showed the German people the power of the state and convinced them that 'every other German' fully supported the Nazis. Goebbels also recognised that one of the Nazis' main attractions was that they created order out of chaos and so the whole rally was organised to emphasise order.

SOURCE 4

A Hitler speaks to the assembled Germans.

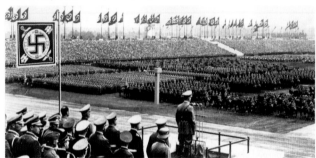

B A parade through the streets.

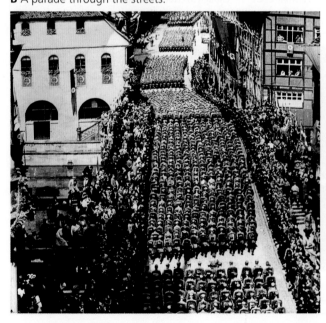

C German youth marching with spades.

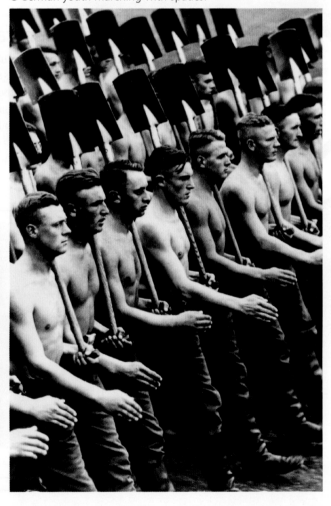

The annual rally at Nuremberg. The whole town was taken over and the rally dominated radio broadcasts and newsreels.

SOURCE 5

Hitler's dictatorship differed in one fundamental point from all its predecessors in history. It was the first dictatorship in the present period of modern technical development which made complete use of all technical means for the domination of its own country.

Through technical devices like the radio and loud-speaker, eighty million people were deprived of independent thought. It was thereby possible to subject them to the will of one man … The nightmare of many a man that one day nations could be ruled by technical means was realised in Hitler's totalitarian system.

Albert Speer, a leading Nazi, speaking at the Nuremberg war trials.

SOURCE 6

There are cinema evenings to be caught up with, very enjoyable ones – if only there were not each time the bitterness of the Third Reich's self-adulation and triumphalism. The renewal of German art – recent German history as reflected in postage stamps, youth camp, enthusiastic welcome for the Führer in X or Y. Goebbels' speech on culture to the Germanised theatre people, the biggest lecture theatre in the world, the biggest autobahn in the world, etc. etc. – the biggest lie in the world, the biggest disgrace in the world. It can't be helped . . .

From the diary of Victor Klemperer for 8 August 1937.

The media and culture

Less spectacular than the rallies but possibly more important was Goebbels' control of the media. In contrast with the free expression of Weimar Germany, the Nazis controlled the media and all aspects of culture strictly.

● No **books** could be published without Goebbels' permission (not surprisingly the best seller in Nazi Germany was *Mein Kampf*). In 1933 he organised a high-profile 'book-burning'. Nazi students came together publicly to burn any books that included ideas unacceptable to the Nazis.

● **Artists** suffered the same kinds of restriction as writers. Only Nazi-approved painters could show their works. These were usually paintings or sculptures of heroic-looking Aryans, military figures or images of the ideal Aryan family.

● Goebbels also controlled the **newspapers** closely. They were not allowed to print anti-Nazi ideas. Within months of the Nazi takeover, Jewish editors and journalists found themselves out of work and anti-Nazi newspapers were closed down. The German newspapers became very dull reading and Germans bought fewer newspapers as a result – circulation fell by about 10 per cent.

● The **cinema** was also closely controlled. All films – factual or fictional, thrillers or comedies – had to carry a pro-Nazi message. The newsreels which preceded feature films were full of the greatness of Hitler and the massive achievements of Nazi Germany. There is evidence that Germans avoided these productions by arriving late! Goebbels censored all foreign films coming into Germany.

● He banned **jazz music**, which had been popular in Germany as elsewhere around Europe. He banned it because it was 'Black' music and black people were considered an inferior race. Goebbels plastered Germany with posters proclaiming the successes of Hitler and the Nazis and attacking their opponents.

● Goebbels also loved new technology and quickly saw the potential of **radio broadcasting** for spreading the Nazi message. He made cheap radios available so all Germans could buy one (see Source 7) and he controlled all the radio stations. Listening to broadcasts from the BBC was punishable by death. Just in case people did not have a radio Goebbels placed loudspeakers in the streets and public bars. Hitler's speeches and those of other Nazi leaders were repeated on the radio over and over again until the ideas expressed in them – German expansion into eastern Europe, the inferiority of the Jews – came to be believed by the German people.

Throughout this period Goebbels was supported in his work by the SS and the Gestapo. When he wanted to close down an anti-Nazi newspaper, silence an anti-Nazi writer, or catch someone listening to a foreign radio station, they were there to do that work for him.

SOURCE 7

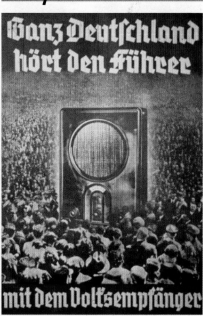

Poster advertising cheap Nazi-produced radios. The text reads 'All Germany hears the Führer on the People's Radio.' The radios had only a short range and were unable to pick up foreign stations.

Case study: The 1936 Olympics

Think!

1 In what ways was the Berlin Olympics a propaganda success for Goebbels?
2 In what ways was it a failure?
3 Why do you think Nazi propaganda was more successful within Germany than outside it?
4 You have already come across many examples of Nazi propaganda. Choose one example which you think is the clearest piece of propaganda. Explain your choice.

Revision Tip

♦ Describe how the Nazis exploited the 1936 Olympics.
♦ Can you explain one way in which the Olympics were a propaganda success and one way they were a failure?

One of Goebbels' greatest challenges came with the 1936 Olympic Games in Berlin. Other Nazis were opposed to holding the Games in Berlin, but Goebbels convinced Hitler that this was a great propaganda opportunity both within Germany and internationally.

Goebbels and Hitler also thought that the Olympics could be a showcase for their doctrine that the Aryan race was superior to all other races. However, there was international pressure for nations such as the USA to boycott the Games in protest against the Nazis' repressive regime and anti-Jewish politics. In response the Nazis included one token Jew in their team!

Goebbels built a brand new stadium to hold 100,000 people. It was lit by the most modern electric lighting. He brought in television cameras for the first time. The most sophisticated German photo-electronic timing device was installed. The stadium had the largest stop clock ever built. With guests and competitors from 49 countries coming into the heart of Nazi Germany, it was going to take all Goebbels' talents to show that Germany was a modern, civilised and successful nation. No expense was spared. When the Games opened, the visitors were duly amazed at the scale of the stadium, the wonderful facilities, and the efficiency of the organisation. However, they were also struck, and in some cases appalled, by the almost fanatical devotion of the people to Hitler and by the overt presence of army and SS soldiers who were patrolling or standing guard everywhere.

To the delight of Hitler and Goebbels, Germany came top of the medal table, way ahead of all other countries. However, to their great dismay, a black athlete, Jesse Owens, became the star of the Games. He won four gold medals and broke eleven world records in the process. The ten black members of the American team won thirteen medals between them. So much for Aryan superiority!

To the majority of German people, who had grown used to the Nazi propaganda machine, the Games appeared to present all the qualities they valued in the Nazis – a grand vision, efficiency, power, strength and achievement. However, to many foreign visitors who were not used to such blatant propaganda it backfired on the Nazi regime.

SOURCE 8

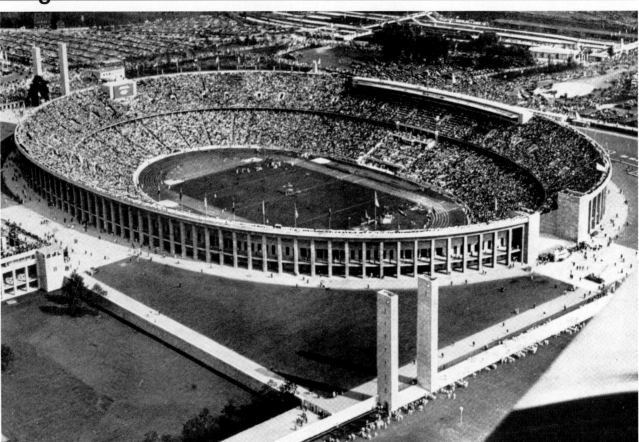

The stadium built for the 1936 Olympics.

How did the Nazis deal with the Churches?

The relationship between the Churches and the Nazis was complicated. In the early stages of the Nazi regime, there was some co-operation between the Nazis and the Churches. Hitler signed a Concordat with the Catholic Church in 1933. This meant that Hitler agreed to leave the Catholic Church alone and allowed it to keep control of its schools. In return, the Church agreed to stay out of politics.

Hitler tried to get all of the Protestant Churches to come together in one official Reich Church. The Reich Church was headed by the Protestant Bishop Ludwig Müller. However, many Germans still felt that their true loyalties lay with their original Churches in their local areas rather than with this state-approved Church.

Hitler even encouraged an alternative religion to the Churches, the pagan German Faith Movement (see Source 10).

Many churchgoers either supported the Nazis or did little to oppose them. However, there were some very important exceptions. The Catholic Bishop Galen criticised the Nazis throughout the 1930s. In 1941 he led a popular protest against the Nazi policies of killing mentally ill and physically disabled people, forcing the Nazis temporarily to stop. He had such strong support among his followers that the Nazis decided it was too risky to try to silence him because they did not want trouble while Germany was at war.

Protestant ministers also resisted the Nazis. Pastor Martin Niemöller was one of the most high-profile critics of the regime in the 1930s. Along with Dietrich Bonhoeffer, he formed an alternative Protestant Church to the official Reich Church. These church leaders suffered a similar fate to Hitler's political opponents. Niemöller spent the years 1938–45 in a concentration camp for resisting the Nazis. Dietrich Bonhoeffer preached against the Nazis until the Gestapo stopped him in 1937. He then became involved with members of the army's intelligence services who were secretly opposed to Hitler. He helped Jews to escape from Germany. Gradually he increased his activity. In 1942 he contacted the Allied commanders and asked what peace terms they would offer Germany if Hitler were overthrown. He was arrested in October 1942 and hanged shortly before the end of the war in April 1945.

SOURCE 9

Most postwar accounts have concentrated on the few German clerics who did behave bravely . . . But these were few. Most German church leaders were shamefully silent. As late as January 1945, the Catholic bishop of Würzburg was urging his flock to fight on for the Fatherland, saying that 'salvation lies in sacrifice'.

British historian and journalist Charles Wheeler, writing in 1996.

SOURCE 10

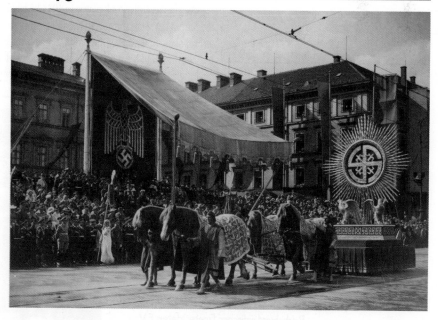

A parade organised by the German Faith Movement. This movement was a non-Christian movement based on worship of the sun.

The persecution of minorities

The Nazis believed in the superiority of the Aryan race. Through their twelve years in power they persecuted members of other races, and many minority groups such as gypsies, homosexuals and mentally handicapped people. They persecuted any group that they thought challenged Nazi ideas. Homosexuals were a threat to Nazi ideas about family life; the mentally handicapped were a threat to Nazi ideas about Germans being a perfect master race; gypsies were thought to be an inferior people.

The persecution of such minorities varied. In families where there were hereditary illnesses, sterilisation was enforced. Over 300,000 men and women were compulsorily sterilised between 1934 and 1945. A so-called 'euthanasia programme' was begun in 1939. At least 5,000 severely mentally handicapped babies and children were killed between 1939 and 1945 either by injection or by starvation. Between 1939 and 1941, 72,000 mentally ill patients were gassed before a public outcry in Germany itself ended the extermination. The extermination of the gypsies, on the other hand, did not cause an outcry. Five out of six gypsies living in Germany in 1939 were killed by the Nazis. Similarly, there was little or no complaint about the treatment of so-called 'asocials' – homosexuals, alcoholics, the homeless, prostitutes, habitual criminals and beggars – who were rounded up off the streets and sent to concentration camps.

You are going to investigate this most disturbing aspect of Nazi Germany by tracing the story of Nazi treatment of the Jewish population in which anti-semitism culminated in the dreadful slaughter of the 'Final Solution'.

Hitler and the Jews

Anti-semitism means hatred of Jews. Throughout Europe, Jews had experienced discrimination for hundreds of years. They were often treated unjustly in courts or forced to live in ghettos. One reason for this persecution was religious, in that Jews were blamed for the death of Jesus Christ! Another reason was that they tended to be well educated and therefore held well-paid professional jobs or ran successful stores and businesses.

Hitler hated Jews insanely. In his years of poverty in Vienna, he became obsessed by the fact that Jews ran many of the most successful businesses, particularly the large department stores. This offended his idea of the superiority of Aryans. Hitler also blamed Jewish businessmen and bankers for Germany's defeat in the First World War. He thought they had forced the surrender of the German army.

As soon as Hitler took power in 1933 he began to mobilise the full powers of the state against the Jews. They were immediately banned from the Civil Service and a variety of public services such as broadcasting and teaching. At the same time, SA and later SS troopers organised boycotts of Jewish shops and businesses, which were marked with a star of David.

Focus Task

Why did the Nazis persecute so many groups in Germany?

You have seen how the Nazis persecuted people who opposed them politically, e.g. the Communists, socialists and trade unionists. But why did they persecute so many other groups?
Complete a table as follows. In the first column, list the groups mentioned in this section. In the second column explain why these groups were targeted, and in the third column note Nazi actions towards them and what happened to them.

Revision Tip

Make sure you can describe how the Nazis persecuted the Jews and one other group. It is important to be able to explain Nazi theories on race and how these led to persecution.

SOURCE 11

To read the pages [of Hitler's Mein Kampf*] is to enter a world of the insane, a world peopled by hideous and distorted shadows. The Jew is no longer a human being, he has become a mythical figure, a grimacing leering devil invested with infernal powers, the incarnation of evil.*

A Bullock, Hitler: *A Study in Tyranny*, published in 1990.

SOURCE 12

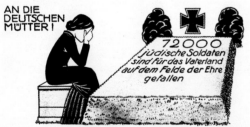

A poster published in 1920, directed at 'All German mothers'. It explains that over 12,000 German Jews were killed fighting for their country in the First World War.

SOURCE 13

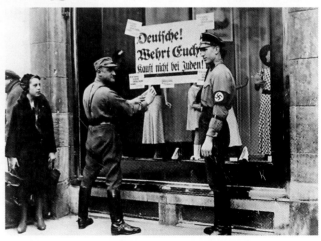

SA and SS men enforcing the boycott of Jewish shops, April 1933.

SOURCE **14**

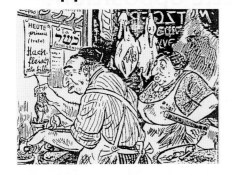

A cartoon from the Nazi newspaper *Der Stürmer*, 1935. Jews owned many shops and businesses. These were a constant target for Nazi attacks.

In 1935 the Nuremberg Laws took away German citizenship from Jews. Jews were also forbidden to marry or have sex with pure-blooded Germans. Goebbels' propaganda experts bombarded German children and families with anti-Jewish messages. Jews were often refused jobs, and people in shops refused to serve them. In schools, Jewish children were humiliated and then segregated.

Kristallnacht

In November 1938 a young Jew killed a German diplomat in Paris. The Nazis used this as an excuse to launch a violent revenge on Jews. Plain-clothes SS troopers were issued with pickaxes and hammers and the addresses of Jewish businesses. They ran riot, smashing up Jewish shops and workplaces. Ninety-one Jews were murdered. Hundreds of synagogues were burned. Twenty thousand Jews were taken to concentration camps. Thousands more left the country. This event became known as *Kristallnacht* or 'The Night of Broken Glass'. Many Germans watched the events of *Kristallnacht* with alarm and concern. The Nazi-controlled press presented *Kristallnacht* as the spontaneous reaction of ordinary Germans against the Jews. Most Germans did not believe this. However, hardly anyone protested. The few who did were brutally murdered.

SOURCE **15**

[The day after Kristallnacht] the teachers told us: don't worry about what you see, even if you see some nasty things which you may not understand. Hitler wants a better Germany, a clean Germany. Don't worry, everything will work out fine in the end.

Henrik Metelmann, member of the Hitler Youth, in 1938.

SOURCE **16**

I hate the treatment of the Jews. I think it is a bad side of the movement and I will have nothing to do with it. I did not join the party to do that sort of thing. I joined the party because I thought and still think that Hitler did the greatest Christian work for twenty-five years. I saw seven million men rotting in the streets, often I was there too, and no one . . . seemed to care . . . Then Hitler came and he took all those men off the streets and gave them health and security and work . . .

H Schmidt, Labour Corps leader, in an interview in 1938.

SOURCE **17**

I feel the urge to present to you a true report of the recent riots, plundering and destruction of Jewish property. Despite what the official Nazi account says, the German people have nothing whatever to do with these riots and burnings. The police supplied SS men with axes, house-breaking tools and ladders. A list of the addresses of all Jewish shops and flats was provided and the mob worked under the leadership of the SS men. The police had strict orders to remain neutral.

Anonymous letter from a German civil servant to the British consul, 1938.

SOURCE **18**

Until Kristallnacht, many Germans believed Hitler was not engaged in mass murder. [The treatment of the Jews] seemed to be a minor form of harassment of a disliked minority. But after Kristallnacht no German could any longer be under any illusion. I believe it was the day that we lost our innocence. But it would be fair to point out that I myself never met even the most fanatic Nazi who wanted the extermination [mass murder] of the Jews. Certainly we wanted the Jews out of Germany, but we did not want them to be killed.

Alfons Heck, member of the Hitler Youth in 1938, interviewed for a television programme in 1989.

Source Analysis

1 Read Sources 15–18. How useful is each source to a historian looking at the German reaction to *Kristallnacht*?
2 Taken together, do they provide a clear picture of how Germans felt about *Kristallnacht*?

Revision Tip

It is important that you can describe how actions against the Jews increased in the 1930s. Make sure you can:
♦ describe the 1933 boycott; the Nuremberg Laws and Kristallnacht.
♦ explain how each was more severe than the one before it.

Think!

Could Germans have protested effectively about *Kristallnacht*? Explain your answer with reference to pages 248–56.

SOURCE 19

The average worker is primarily interested in work and not in democracy. People who previously enthusiastically supported democracy showed no interest at all in politics. One must be clear about the fact that in the first instance men are fathers of families and have jobs, and that for them politics takes second place and even then only when they expect to get something out of it.

A report by a Socialist activist in Germany, February 1936.

SOURCE 20

November 1933

Millions of Germans are indeed won over by Hitler and the power and the glory are really his. I hear of some actions by the Communists . . . But what good do such pinpricks do? Less than none, because all Germany prefers Hitler to the Communists.

April 1935

Frau Wilbrandt told us that people complain in Munich when Hitler or Goebbels appear on film but even she (an economist close to the Social Democrats) says: 'Will there not be something even worse, if Hitler is overthrown, Bolshevism?' (That fear keeps Hitler where he is again and again.)

Extracts from the diaries of Victor Klemperer, a Jewish university lecturer in Germany.

Revision Tip

♦ There are three important factors on this page which explain lack of opposition to the Nazis (Nazi successes; economic fears; propaganda). Make sure you can give an example of each one.

♦ Give each a mark out of ten (but no two marks the same) and prepare an explanation that supports your mark. Be especially clear why you gave one factor a higher mark than another.

Why was there little opposition?

The Nazis faced relatively little open opposition during their twelve years in power. In private, Germans complained about the regime and its actions. Some might refuse to give the Nazi salute. They might pass on anti-Nazi jokes and rude stories about senior Nazis. However, serious criticism was always in private, never in public. Historians have debated why this was so. The main answer they have come up with may seem obvious to you if you've read pages 248–49. It was terror! All the Nazis' main opponents had been killed, exiled or put in prison. The rest had been scared into submission. However, it won't surprise you to learn that historians think the answer is not quite as simple as that. It takes more than just terror to explain why there was so little opposition to the Nazis.

'It's all for the good of Germany' – Nazi successes

Many Germans admired and trusted Hitler. They were prepared to tolerate rule by terror and to trade their political freedom in return for work, foreign policy success and what they thought was strong government.

● Economic recovery was deeply appreciated.
● Many felt that the Nazis were bringing some much needed discipline back to Germany by restoring traditional values and clamping down on rowdy Communists.
● Between 1933 and 1938 Hitler's success in foreign affairs made Germans feel that Germany was a great power again after the humiliations of the First World War.

'I don't want to lose my job' – economic fears

German workers feared losing their jobs if they did express opposition. Germany had been hit so hard by the Depression that many were terrified by the prospect of being out of work again. It was a similar situation for the bosses. Businesses that did not contribute to Nazi Party funds risked losing Nazi business and going bankrupt, and so in self-defence they conformed as well. If you asked no questions and kept your head down, life in Nazi Germany could be comfortable. 'Keeping your head down' became a national obsession.

'Have you heard the good news?' – propaganda

Underlying the whole regime was the propaganda machine. This ensured that many Germans found out very little about the bad things that were happening, or if they did they only heard them with a positive, pro-Nazi slant. Propaganda was particularly important in maintaining the image of Hitler. The evidence suggests that personal support for Hitler remained high throughout the 1930s and he was still widely respected even as Germany was losing the war in 1944.

Key Question Summary

How effectively did the Nazis control Germany, 1933–45?

1 The Nazis had a powerful range of organisations to control Germany: the SS, the Gestapo, the police and the courts, and concentration camps.
2 There was little opposition because of the terror they inspired, economic progress and success in foreign affairs, overturning the Treaty of Versailles and making Germany a strong military power.
3 The Nazis built a highly successful propaganda machine and used mass media to control what people knew.
4 They sought to control culture, banning books which contained ideas they did not like. Paintings, plays and films had to put across a pro-Nazi message and show idealised images of the Aryan family.
5 The Nazis persecuted many groups that did not fit in with their notions of racial purity, such as disabled people, homosexuals and gypsies.
6 They particularly persecuted the Jews, depriving them of their jobs, businesses and homes and forcing them into ghettos.
7 In 1942 they introduced a programme of mass extermination called the Final Solution.

9.4 What was it like to live in Nazi Germany?

Focus

It was Hitler's aim to control every aspect of life in Germany, including the daily lives of ordinary people. In the *Volksgemeinschaft* almost everyone had a role in making Germany great again.

Central to the Nazi vision was the role of young people: young men who would be turned into loyal soldiers and young women who would be turned into strong mothers. The workers were no longer working just for pay but they were working to provide the goods that the Fatherland needed.

However if you did not fit into the Nazi plan for Germany then you had a desperate time. From the very earliest stages of the regime minority groups who did not fit with the Nazi ideal of what a German person should be like were persecuted mercilessly. Measures against Jews, the homeless, the mentally ill, gypsies and homosexuals became more and more extreme, ending in the mass murder of the Holocaust.

In this section you will examine the experiences of these different groups.

Focus Points

♦ How did young people react to the Nazi regime?
♦ How successful were Nazi policies towards women and the family?
♦ Did most people in Germany benefit from Nazi rule?
♦ How did the coming of war change life in Nazi Germany?

Young people in Nazi Germany

It was Hitler's aim to control every aspect of life in Germany, including the daily life of ordinary people. If you had been a sixteen-year-old Aryan living in Nazi Germany you would probably have been a strong supporter of Adolf Hitler.

At school

The Nazis had reorganised every aspect of the school curriculum to make children loyal to them. At school you would have learned about the history of Germany. You would have been outraged to find out how the German army was 'stabbed in the back' by the weak politicians who had made peace. You might well remember the hardships of the 1920s for yourself, but at school you would have been told how these were caused by Jews squeezing profits out of honest Germans. By the time you were a senior pupil, your studies in history would have made you confident that loyalty to the Führer was right and good. Your biology lessons would have informed you that you were special, as one of the Aryan race which was so superior in intelligence and strength to the *Untermenschen* or sub-human Jews and Slavs of eastern Europe. In maths you would have been set questions like the one in Source 3 on page 258.

SOURCE 1

Our state is an educational state . . . It does not let a man go free from the cradle to the grave. We begin with the child when he is three years old. As soon as he begins to think, he is made to carry a little flag. Then follows school, the Hitler Youth, the storm troopers and military training. We don't let him go; and when all that is done, comes the Labour Front, which takes possession of him again, and does not let him go till he dies, even if he does not like it.

Dr Robert Ley, who was Chief of the Labour Front and in charge of making 'good citizens' out of the German people.

Source Analysis ▲

1 Read Source 1. Do you think that the speaker is proud of what he is saying?

SOURCE 2

It is my great educative work I am beginning with the young. We older ones are used up . . . We are bearing the burden of a humiliating past . . . But my magnificent youngsters! Are there finer ones in the world? Look at these young men and boys! What material! With them I can make a new world.

Hitler, speaking in 1939.

SOURCE 3

The Jews are aliens in Germany. In 1933 there were 66,060,000 inhabitants of the German Reich of whom 499,862 were Jews. What is the percentage of aliens in Germany?

A question from a Nazi maths textbook, 1933.

Think

1 Do you think the real aim of the question in Source 3 is to improve mathematical skills?
2 Read Source 5. Eugenics is the study of how to produce perfect offspring by choosing parents with ideal qualities. How would this help the Nazis?

SOURCE 6

It was a great feeling. You felt you belonged to a great nation again. Germany was in safe hands and I was going to help to build a strong Germany. But my father of course felt differently about it. [He warned] 'Now Henrik, don't say to them what I am saying to you.' I always argued with my father as I was very much in favour of the Hitler regime which was against his background as a working man.

Henrik Metelmann describes what it was like being a member of the Hitler Youth in the 1930s.

SOURCE 7

Hitler looked over the stand, and I know he looked into my eyes, and he said: 'You my boys are the standard bearers, you will inherit what we have created.' From that moment there was not any doubt I was bound to Adolf Hitler until long after our defeat. Afterwards I told my friends how Hitler had looked into my eyes, but they all said: 'No! It was my eyes he was looking into.'

A young German describes his feelings after a Hitler Youth rally.

SOURCE 4

All subjects – German language, History, Geography, Chemistry and Mathematics – must concentrate on military subjects, the glorification of military service and of German heroes and leaders and the strength of a rebuilt Germany. Chemistry will develop a knowledge of chemical warfare, explosives, etc, while Mathematics will help the young to understand artillery, calculations, ballistics.

A German newspaper, heavily controlled by the Nazis, approves of the curriculum in 1939.

SOURCE 5

8.00	German (every day)
8.50	Geography, History or Singing (alternate days)
9.40	Race Studies and Ideology (every day)
10.25	Recess, Sports and Special Announcements (every day)
11.00	Domestic Science or Maths (alternate days)
12.10	Eugenics or Health Biology (alternate days)
1.00–6.00	Sport
Evenings	Sex education, Ideology or Domestic Science (one evening each)

The daily timetable for a girls' school in Nazi Germany

In the Hitler Youth

As a member of the Hitler Youth or League of German Maidens, you would have marched in exciting parades with loud bands. You would probably be physically fit. Your leisure time would also be devoted to Hitler and the Nazis. You would be a strong cross-country runner, and confident at reading maps. After years of summer camps, you would be comfortable camping out of doors and if you were a boy you would know how to clean a rifle and keep it in good condition.

SOURCE 8

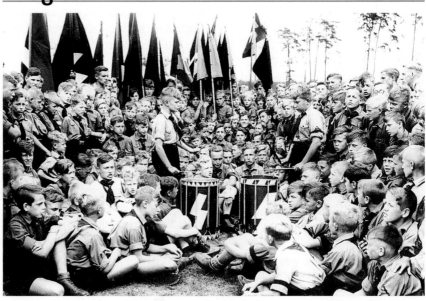

Members of the Hitler Youth in the 1930s. From a very early age children were encouraged to join the Nazi youth organisations. It was not compulsory, but most young people did join.

SOURCE 9

Children have been deliberately taken away from parents who refused to acknowledge their belief in National Socialism . . . The refusal of parents to allow their young children to join the youth organisation is regarded as an adequate reason for taking the children away.

A German teacher writing in 1938.

Think!

1 Make a list of the main differences between your life and the life of a sixteen-year-old in Nazi Germany.
2 Totalitarian regimes through history have used children as a way of influencing parents. Why do you think they do this?
3 Read Source 6. Why do you think Henrik's father asks Henrik not to repeat what he says to him?

SOURCE 11

We didn't know much about Nazi ideals. Nevertheless, we were politically programmed: to obey orders, to cultivate the soldierly virtue of standing to attention and saying 'Yes, Sir' and to stop thinking when the word Fatherland was uttered and Germany's honour and greatness were mentioned.

A former member of the Hitler Youth looks back after the war.

Revision Tip

♦ Make sure you can describe:
  – at least one way the Nazis tried to control young people.
  – at least two ways the Nazis tried to control or win over young people.
♦ What points can you find to support the view that the Nazis' attempts to win over or control young people succeeded?
♦ What points suggest that the Nazis failed?

At home

As a child in Nazi Germany, you might well feel slightly alienated (estranged) from your parents because they are not as keen on the Nazis as you are. They expect your first loyalty to be to your family, whereas your Hitler Youth leader makes it clear that your first loyalty is to Adolf Hitler. You find it hard to understand why your father grumbles about Nazi regulation of his working practices – surely the Führer (Hitler) is protecting him? Your parents find the idea of Nazi inspectors checking up on the teachers rather strange. For you it is normal.

SOURCE 10

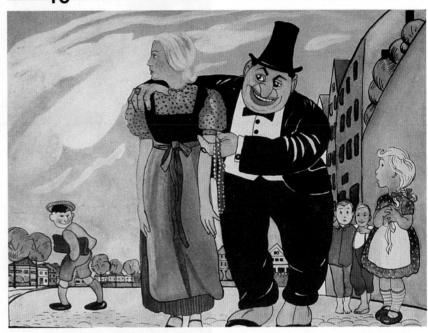

Illustration from a Nazi children's book. The children are being taught to distrust Jews.

Many young people were attracted to the Nazi youth movements by the leisure opportunities they offered. There were really no alternatives. All other youth organisations had been absorbed or made illegal. Even so, only half of all German boys were members in 1933 and only 15 per cent of girls. You can read what happened to young people in wartime on page 267.

Focus Task

How did young people react to the Nazi regime?

1 Young people were among the most fanatical supporters of the Nazi regime. Use pages 257–59 to write three paragraphs to explain why the Nazis were successful in winning them over. Include the following points:
  ♦ why the Nazis wanted to control young people
  ♦ how they set about doing it
  ♦ what the attractions of the youth movements were.
2 The Nazi regime was not successful in keeping the loyalty of all young people. Add a fourth paragraph to your essay to explain why some young people rejected the Nazi youth movements.

Women in Nazi Germany

Source Analysis ▶

What does Source 12 show about the Nazis' view of women?

SOURCE **12**

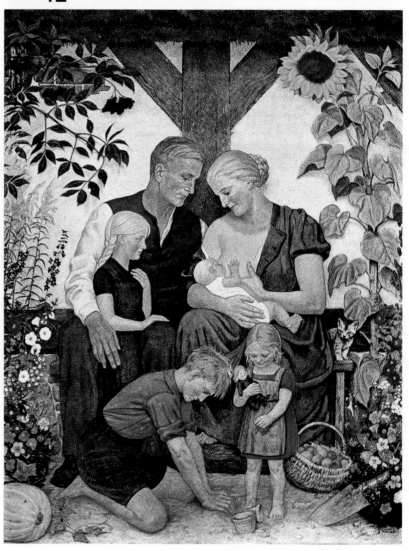

A painting showing the Nazis' view of an ideal German family.

All the Nazi leaders were men. The Nazis were a very male-dominated organisation. Hitler had a very traditional view of the role of the German woman as wife and mother. It is worth remembering that many *women* agreed with him. In the traditional rural areas and small towns, many women felt that the proper role of a woman was to support her husband. There was also resentment towards working women in the early 1930s, since they were seen as keeping men out of jobs. It all created a lot of pressure on women to conform to what the Nazis called 'the traditional balance' between men and women. 'No true German woman wears trousers' said a Nazi newspaper headline when the film star Marlene Dietrich appeared wearing trousers in public.

Alarmed at the falling birth rate, Hitler offered tempting financial incentives for married couples to have at least four children. You got a 'Gold Cross' for having eight children, and were given a privileged seat at Nazi meetings. Posters, radio broadcasts and newsreels all celebrated the ideas of motherhood and homebuilding. The German Maidens' League reinforced these ideas, focusing on a combination of good physical health and housekeeping skills. This was reinforced at school (see Source 5 on page 258).

With all these encouragements the birth rate did increase from fifteen per thousand in 1933 to twenty per thousand in 1939. There was also an increase in pregnancies outside marriage. These girls were looked after in state maternity hostels.

SOURCE **13**

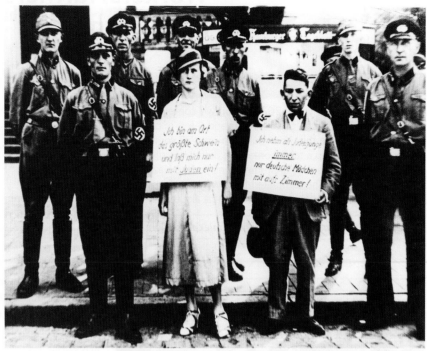

A German woman and her Jewish boyfriend being publicly humiliated by the SA in 1933. The notices say: (woman) 'I'm the biggest pig in town and only get involved with Jews'; (man) 'As a Jewish boy I always take only German girls up to my room'.

SOURCE **14**

I went to Sauckel [the Nazi minister in charge of labour] with the proposition that we should recruit our labour from the ranks of German women. He replied brusquely that where to obtain which workers was his business. Moreover, he said, as Gauleiter [a regional governor] he was Hitler's subordinate and responsible to the Führer alone . . . Sauckel offered to put the question to Goering as Commissioner of the Four-Year Plan . . . but I was scarcely allowed to advance my arguments. Sauckel and Goering continually interrupted me. Sauckel laid great weight on the danger that factory work might inflict moral harm on German womanhood; not only might their 'psychic and emotional life' be affected but also their ability to bear children.

Goering totally concurred. But just to be absolutely sure, Sauckel went immediately to Hitler and had him confirm the decision. All my good arguments were therefore blown to the winds.

Albert Speer, *Inside The Third Reich*, 1970. Speer was Minister of Armaments and War Production.

There were some prominent women in Nazi Germany. Leni Riefenstahl was a high-profile film producer. Gertrude Scholz-Klink was head of the Nazi Women's Bureau, although she was excluded from any important discussions (such as the one to conscript female labour in 1942). Many working-class girls and women gained the chance to travel and meet new people through the Nazi women's organisation. Overall, however, opportunities for women were limited. Married professional women were forced to give up their jobs and stay at home with their families, which many resented as a restriction on their freedom. Discrimination against women applicants for jobs was encouraged.

The impact of war

In the late 1930s the Nazis had to do an about-turn as they suddenly needed more women workers because the supply of unemployed men was drying up. Many women had to struggle with both family and work responsibilities. However, even during the crisis years of 1942–45 when German industry was struggling to cope with the demand for war supplies, Nazi policy on women was still torn between their traditional stereotype of the mother, and the actual needs of the workplace. For example, there was no chance for German women to serve in the armed forces, as there was in Allied countries.

Focus Task

How successful were the Nazi policies for women?

Read these two statements:

> 'Nazi policy for women was confused.'

> 'Nazi policy for women was a failure.'

For each statement explain whether you agree or disagree with it and use examples from the text to support your explanation.

Workers, farmers and businesses in Nazi Germany

SOURCE **15**

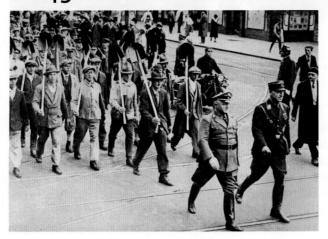

Previously unemployed men assemble for the building of the first autobahn, September 1933.

Economic recovery and rearmament

Hitler and the Nazis came to power because they promised to use radical methods to solve the country's two main problems – desperate unemployment and a crisis in German farming. In return for work and other benefits, the majority of the German people gave up their political freedom. Was it worth it?

At first, many Germans felt it was, particularly the 5 million who were unemployed in 1933. Hitler was fortunate in that by 1933 the worst of the Depression was over. Even so, there is no doubt that the Nazis acted with energy and commitment to solve some of the main problems. The brilliant economist **Dr Hjalmar Schacht** organised Germany's finances to fund a huge programme of work creation. The National Labour Service sent men on **public works projects** and conservation programmes, in particular to build a network of motorways or **autobahns**. Railways were extended or built from scratch. There were major house-building programmes and grandiose new public building projects such as the Reich Chancellery in Berlin.

Other measures brought increasing prosperity. One of Hitler's most cherished plans was **rearmament**. In 1935 he reintroduced **conscription** for the German army. In 1936 he announced a **Four-Year Plan** under the control of **Goering** to get the German economy ready for war (it was one of the very few clear policy documents that Hitler ever wrote).

Conscription reduced unemployment. The need for weapons, equipment and uniforms created jobs in the coal mines, steel and textile mills. Engineers and designers gained new opportunities, particularly when Hitler decreed that Germany would have a world-class air force (the Luftwaffe). As well as bringing economic recovery, these measures boosted Hitler's popularity because they boosted **national pride**. Germans began to feel that their country was finally emerging from the humiliation of the Great War and the Treaty of Versailles, and putting itself on an equal footing with the other great powers.

SOURCE **16**

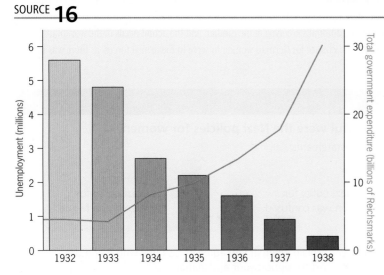

Unemployment and government expenditure in Germany, 1932–38. Economic recovery was almost entirely funded by the state rather than from Germans investing their own savings. Despite this, unemployment fell steadily and Germany was actually running short of workers by 1939.

SOURCE 17

Early one morning, a neighbour of ours, a trade-union secretary, was taken away in a car by the SS and police. His wife had great difficulty finding out what had happened to him. My mother was too scared to be seen talking to her and Father became very quiet and alarmed and begged me not to repeat what he had said within our four walls about the whole Nazi set-up . . .

I loved it when we went on our frequent marches, feeling important when the police had to stop the traffic to give us right of way and passing pedestrians had to raise their arm in the Nazi salute. Whenever we were led out on a march, it was always into the working-class quarters. We were told that this was to remind the workers, but I sometimes wondered what we wanted to remind them of, after all most of our fathers were workers . . .

From *Through Hell for Hitler*, the memoirs of Henrik Metelmann, published in 1970. Metelmann came from a working-class family in Hamburg but was an enthusiastic member of the Hitler Youth and served in the German army in the Second World War.

The Nazis and the workers

Hitler promised (and delivered) lower unemployment which helped to ensure popularity among **industrial workers**. These workers were important to the Nazis: Hitler needed good workers to create the industries that would help to make Germany great and establish a new German empire in eastern Europe. He won the loyalty of industrial workers by a variety of initiatives.

- Propaganda praised the workers and tried to associate them with Hitler.
- Schemes such as **Strength Through Joy (KDF)** gave them cheap theatre and cinema tickets, organised courses, trips and sports events, and even cut-price cruises on luxury liners.
- Many thousands of workers saved five marks a week in the state scheme to buy the **Volkswagen Beetle**, the 'people's car'. It was designed by Ferdinand Porsche and became a symbol of the prosperous new Germany, even though no workers ever received a car because all car production was halted by the war in 1939.
- Another important scheme was the **Beauty of Labour** movement. This improved working conditions in factories. It introduced features not seen in many workplaces before, such as washing facilities and low-cost canteens.

What was the price of these advances? Workers lost their main political party, the SDP. They lost their trade unions and for many workers this remained a source of bitter resentment. All workers had to join the **DAF (General Labour Front)** run by **Dr Robert Ley**. This organisation kept strict control of workers. They could not strike for better pay and conditions. In some areas, they were prevented from moving to better-paid jobs. Wages remained comparatively low, although prices were also strictly controlled. Even so, by the late 1930s, many workers were grumbling that their standard of living was still lower than it had been before the Depression (see Source 16).

The Nazis and the farming communities

The **farmers** had been an important factor in the Nazis' rise to power. Hitler did not forget this and introduced a series of measures to help them. In September 1933 he introduced the **Reich Food Estate** under **Richard Darre**. This set up central boards to buy agricultural produce from the farmers and distribute it to markets across Germany. It gave the peasant farmers a guaranteed market for their goods at guaranteed prices. The second main measure was the **Reich Entailed Farm Law**. It gave peasants state protection for their farms: banks could not seize their land if they could not pay loans or mortgages. This ensured that peasants' farms stayed in their hands.

The Reich Entailed Farm Law also had a racial aim. Part of the Nazi philosophy was **'Blood and Soil'**, the belief that the peasant farmers were the basis of Germany's master race. They would be the backbone of the new German empire in the east. As a result, their way of life had to be protected. As Source 19 shows, the measures were widely appreciated.

However, rather like the industrial workers, some peasants were not thrilled with the regime's measures. The Reich Food Estate meant that efficient, go-ahead farmers were held back by having to work through the same processes as less efficient farmers. Because of the Reich Entailed Farm Law, banks were unwilling to lend money to farmers. It also meant that only the eldest child inherited the farm. As a result, many children of farmers left the land to work for better pay in Germany's industries. **Rural depopulation** ran at about 3 per cent per year in the 1930s – the exact opposite of the Nazis' aims!

SOURCE 18

Annual food consumption in working class families, 1927–37 (% change).

SOURCE 19

Thousands of people came from all over Germany to the Harvest Festival celebrations . . . We all felt the same happiness and joy. Harvest festival was the thank you for us farmers having a future again. I believe no statesman has ever been as well loved as Adolf Hitler was at that time.

Lusse Essig's memories of the 1930s. Lusse was a farm worker who later worked for the Agriculture Ministry.

Big business and the middle classes

The record of the Nazis with the **middle classes** was also mixed. Certainly many middle-class business people were grateful to the Nazis for eliminating the Communist threat to their businesses and properties. They also liked the way in which the Nazis seemed to be bringing order to Germany. For the owners of small businesses it was a mixed picture. If you owned a small engineering firm, you were likely to do well from government orders as rearmament spending grew in the 1930s. However, if you produced consumer goods or ran a small shop, you might well struggle. Despite Hitler's promises, the large department stores which were taking business away from local shops were not closed.

It was **big business** that really benefited from Nazi rule. The big companies no longer had to worry about troublesome trade unions and strikes. Companies such as the chemicals giant IG Farben gained huge government contracts to make explosives, fertilisers and even artificial oil from coal. Other household names today, such as Mercedes and Volkswagen, prospered from Nazi policies.

'National community': *Volksgemeinschaft*

We have divided this section by social group, but the Nazis would not want Germans to see their society that way. Hitler wanted all Germans (or more exactly all 'racially pure' Germans) to think of themselves as part of a **national community**, or *Volksgemeinschaft*. Under Nazi rule, workers, farmers, and so on, would no longer see themselves primarily as workers or farmers; they would see themselves as Germans. Their first loyalty would not be to their own social group but to Germany and the Führer. They would be so proud to belong to a great nation that was racially and culturally superior to other nations that they would put the interests of Germany before their own. Hitler's policies towards each group were designed to help win this kind of loyalty to the Nazi state.

The evidence suggests that the Nazis never quite succeeded in this: Germans in the 1930s certainly did not lose their self-interest, nor did they embrace the national community wholeheartedly. However, the Nazis did not totally fail either! In the 1930s Germans did have a strong sense of national pride and loyalty towards Hitler. For the majority of Germans, the benefits of Nazi rule made them willing – on the surface at least – to accept some central control in the interests of making Germany great again.

Revision Tip

Look back at pages 262–264. There is a lot here and it might help you to get right down to basics, so make sure you can describe:

♦ two ways in which the Nazis helped tackle the problem of unemployment.
♦ two ways the Nazis tried to improve life for workers.
♦ one way the Nazis tried to improve life for farmers.
♦ one reason why middle classes and one reason why big business might have approved of the Nazis.

Focus Task

Did most people in Germany benefit from Nazi rule?

Here are some claims that the Nazi propaganda machine made about how life in Germany had been changed for the better during the 1930s:

♦ 'Germans now have economic security.'
♦ 'Germans no longer need to feel inferior to other states. They can be proud of their country.'
♦ 'The Nazi state looks after its workers very well indeed.'
♦ 'The Nazis have ensured that Germany is racially pure.'
♦ 'The Nazis are on the side of the farmers and have rescued Germany's farmers from disaster.'
♦ 'The Nazis have made Germany safe from Communism.'

You are now going to decide how truthful these claims actually are.

1 Look back over pages 248–64. Gather evidence that supports or opposes each claim. You could work in groups taking one claim each.
2 For each claim, decide whether, overall, it is totally untrue; a little bit true; mostly true; or totally true.
3 Discuss:
  a) Which of the groups you have studied do you think benefited most from Nazi rule?
  b) Who did not benefit from Nazi rule and why not?

Focus Task

How did the war change life in Germany?

1 Draw a timeline from 1939 to 1945 down the middle of a page.
2 On the left, make notes from pages 265–68 on how the war was going for Germany's army.
3 On the right, make notes to show how the war affected Germans at home in Germany.
4 Choose one change from the right-hand column that you think had the greatest impact on ordinary Germans and explain your choice.

Factfile

Germany's War Economy

➤ When war broke out it did not bring massive changes to the German economy because Germany had been preparing for it since the mid-1930s.
➤ In the early stages of the war, Germany was short of raw materials. This was made worse when the British navy blockaded sea routes into Germany.
➤ As the German forces conquered territories they took raw materials and goods from these territories. For example, Germany took around 20 per cent of Norway's entire production in 1940.
➤ From 1942 German production was shifted towards armaments to supply the army fighting against Russia.
➤ Huge corporations like IG Farben produced chemicals, explosives and the infamous gas used in the death camps.
➤ German factories used forced labour from occupied countries. Most factories had a significant number of prisoners in their workforce and estimates suggest that forced labourers made up around 25 per cent of the workforce.
◆ By 1944 there had been a vast increase in military production. Production of aircraft and tanks trebled compared to 1942.
◆ Production was hampered by Allied bombing and some factories were moved underground.
◆ There is an ongoing debate about the effectiveness of the Nazi war economy. The traditional view is that the economy was mismanaged until 1942 and then improved. However, this account is based on the writings of Albert Speer. Some historians believe he exaggerated his own importance and that the war economy became more efficient after 1942 simply because Germany focused production away from civilian goods and into military equipment.

The impact of the Second World War on Germany

Through the 1930s, Hitler fulfilled his promises to the German people that he would:

- reverse the Treaty of Versailles
- rebuild Germany's armed forces
- unite Germany and Austria
- extend German territory into eastern Europe.

He fulfilled each of these aims, but started the Second World War in the process.

Germans had no great enthusiasm for war. People still had memories of the First World War. But in war, as in peace time, the Nazis used all methods available to make the German people support the regime.

Food rationing was introduced soon after war began in September 1939. Clothes rationing followed in November 1939. Even so, from 1939 to 1941 it was not difficult to keep up civilian morale because the war went spectacularly well for Germany. Hitler was in control of much of western and eastern Europe and supplies of luxury goods flowed into Germany from captured territories.

However, in 1941 Hitler took the massive gamble of invading the Soviet Union, and for the next three years his troops were engaged in an increasingly expensive war with Russian forces who 'tore the heart out of the German army', as the British war leader, Winston Churchill, put it. As the tide turned against the German armies, civilians found their lives increasingly disrupted. They had to cut back on heating, work longer hours and recycle their rubbish. Goebbels redoubled his censorship efforts. He tried to maintain people's support for the war by involving them in it through asking them to make sacrifices. They donated an estimated 1.5 million fur coats to help to clothe the German army in Russia.

At this stage in the war, the German people began to see and hear less of Hitler. His old speeches were broadcast by Goebbels, but Hitler was increasingly preoccupied with the detail of the war. In 1942 the 'Final Solution' began (see pages 268–69), which was to kill millions of Jewish civilians in German-occupied countries.

From 1942, Albert Speer began to direct Germany's war economy (see Factfile). All effort focused on the armament industries. Postal services were suspended and letter boxes were closed. All places of entertainment were closed, except cinemas – Goebbels needed these to show propaganda films. Women were drafted into the labour force in increasing numbers. Country areas had to take evacuees from the cities and refugees from eastern Europe.

These measures were increasingly carried out by the SS. In fact, the SS became virtually a state within the German state. This SS empire had its own armed forces, armaments industries and labour camps. It developed a business empire that was worth a fortune. However, even the SS could not win the war, or even keep up German morale.

With defeat looming, support for the Nazis weakened. Germans stopped declaring food they had. They stayed away from Nazi rallies. They refused to give the 'Heil Hitler' salute when asked to do so. Himmler even contacted the Allies to ask about possible peace terms.

The July bomb plot

In July 1944, some army officers came close to removing Hitler. By this stage of the war, many army officers were sure that the war was lost and that Hitler was leading Germany into ruin. One of these was a colonel in the army, Count von Stauffenberg. On 20 July he left a bomb in Hitler's conference room. The plan was to kill Hitler, close down the radio stations, round up the other leading Nazis and take over Germany. It failed on all counts, for the revolt was poorly planned and organised. Hitler survived and the Nazis took a terrible revenge, killing 5,000 in reprisal.

SOURCE 20

Goebbels does not always tell you the truth. When he tells you that England is powerless do you believe that? Have you forgotten that our bombers fly over Germany at will? The bombs that fell with these leaflets tell you . . . The war lasts as long as Hitler's regime.

Translation of a leaflet dropped by the Allies on Berlin.

SOURCE 21

The greatest effect on [civilian] morale will be produced if a new blow of catastrophic force can be struck at a time when the situation already appears desperate.

From a secret report to the British government, 1944.

Think!

What do Sources 20–23 tell you about
a) the aims of the bombing
b) the success of the bombing?

Revision Tip

Make sure you can:
♦ describe three changes which the war caused for Germans.
♦ explain how at least one change affected Germans for the worse.

The bombing of Dresden

It was the bombing of Germany which had the most dramatic effect on the lives of German civilians. In 1942 the Allies decided on a new policy towards the bombing of Germany. Under Arthur 'Bomber' Harris the British began an all-out assault on both industrial and residential areas of all the major German cities. One of the objectives was to cripple German industry, the other was to lower the morale of civilians and to terrorise them into submission.

The bombing escalated through the next three years, culminating in the bombing of Dresden in February 1945 which killed between 35,000 and 150,000 people in two days. Sources 21–23 tell you more about that bombing.

SOURCE 22

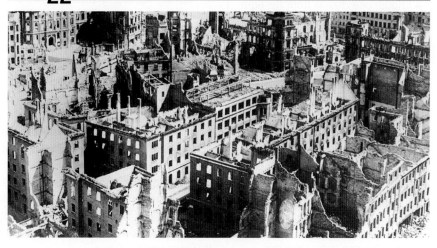

The centre of Dresden after the bombing in February 1945.

SOURCE 23

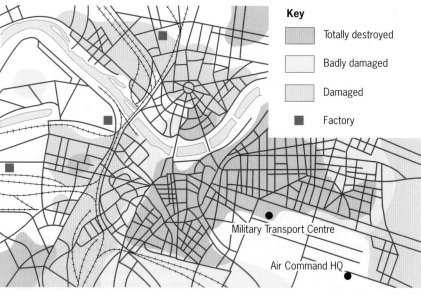

Key

■ Totally destroyed
□ Badly damaged
▨ Damaged
■ Factory

Military Transport Centre

Air Command HQ

A map showing the destruction of Dresden. Dresden was an industrial city, but the major damage was to civilian areas.

By 1945 the German people were in a desperate state. Food supplies were dwindling. Already 3.5 million German civilians had died. Refugees were fleeing the advancing Russian armies in the east.

Three months after the massive destruction of Dresden, Germany's war was over. Hitler, Goebbels and other Nazi war leaders committed suicide or were captured. Germany surrendered. It was now a shattered country. The Nazi promises lay in tatters and the country was divided up into zones of occupation run by the British, French, US and Soviet forces (see page 88).

SOURCE 24

The formation of cliques, i.e. groupings of young people outside the Hitler Youth, has been on the increase before and particularly during the war to such a degree that one must speak of a serious risk of political, moral and criminal subversion of our youth.

From a report by the Nazi youth leadership, 1942.

Revision Tip

♦ The Edelweiss Pirates and Swing movements are important examples of resistance. Make sure you can describe each movement.
♦ Prepare two points to argue that the Pirates were a more serious threat to the Nazis than the Swing Movement.

How did war affect young people?

In 1939 membership of a Nazi youth movement was made compulsory. But by this time the youth movements were going through a crisis. Many of the experienced leaders had been drafted into the German army. Others – particularly those who had been leaders in the pre-Nazi days – had been replaced by keener Nazis. Many of the movements were now run by older teenagers who rigidly enforced Nazi rules. They even forbade other teenagers to meet informally with their friends.

As the war progressed, the activities of the youth movements focused increasingly on the war effort and military drill. The popularity of the movements decreased and indeed an anti-Hitler Youth movement appeared. The Nazis identified two distinct groups of young people who they were worried about: the Swing movement and the Edelweiss Pirates.

The 'Swing' movement

This was made up mainly of middle-class teenagers. They went to parties where they listened to English and American music and sang English songs. They danced American dances such as the 'jitterbug' to banned jazz music. They accepted Jews at their clubs. They talked about and enjoyed sex. They were deliberately 'slovenly'. The Nazis issued a handbook helping the authorities to identify these degenerate types. Some were shown with unkempt, long hair; others with exaggeratedly English clothes.

The Edelweiss Pirates

The Edelweiss Pirates were working-class teenagers. They were not an organised movement, and groups in various cities took different names: 'The Roving Dudes' (Essen); the 'Kittelbach Pirates' (Düsseldorf); the 'Navajos' (Cologne). The Nazis, however, classified all the groups under the single name 'Edelweiss Pirates' and the groups did have a lot in common.

The Pirates were mainly aged between fourteen and seventeen (Germans could leave school at fourteen, but they did not have to sign on for military service until they were seventeen). At the weekends, the Pirates went camping. They sang songs, just like the Hitler Youth, but they changed the lyrics of songs to mock Germany and when they spotted bands of Hitler Youth they taunted and sometimes attacked them. In contrast with the Hitler Youth, the Pirates included boys and girls. The Pirates were also much freer in their attitude towards sex, which was officially frowned upon by the Hitler Youth.

The Pirates' activities caused serious worries to the Nazi authorities in some cities. In December 1942 the Gestapo broke up 28 groups containing 739 adolescents. The Nazi approach to the Pirates was different from their approach to other minorities. As long as they needed future workers for industry and future soldiers they could not simply exterminate all these teenagers or put them in concentration camps (although Himmler did suggest that). They therefore responded uncertainly – sometimes arresting the Pirates, sometimes ignoring them.

In 1944 in Cologne, Pirate activities escalated. They helped to shelter army deserters and escaped prisoners. They stole armaments and took part in an attack on the Gestapo during which its chief was killed. The Nazi response was to round up the so called 'ringleaders'. Twelve were publicly hanged in November 1944.

Neither of the groups described above had strong political views. They were not political opponents of the Nazis. But they resented and resisted Nazi control of their lives.

SOURCE 25

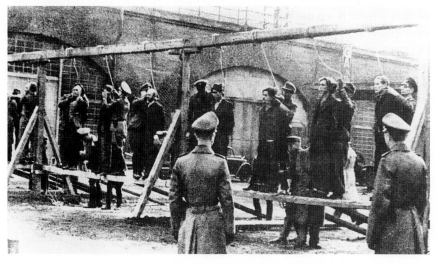

The public hanging of twelve Edelweiss Pirates in Cologne in 1944.

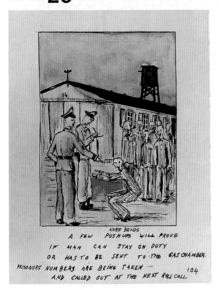

A drawing by a prisoner in Auschwitz concentration camp. The prisoners are being made to do knee bends to see if they are fit enough to work. If not they will be killed in the gas chambers.

The extermination of the Jews is the most dreadful chapter in German history, doubly so because the men who did it closed their senses to the reality of what they were doing by taking pride in the technical efficiency of their actions and, at moments when their conscience threatened to break in, telling themselves that they were doing their duty . . . others took refuge in the enormity of the operation, which lent it a convenient depersonalisation. When they ordered a hundred Jews to get on a train in Paris or Amsterdam, they considered their job accomplished and carefully closed their minds to the thought that eventually those passengers would arrive in front of the ovens of Treblinka.

American historian Gordon Craig, 1978.

Think!

The systematic killing of the Jews by the Nazis is generally known today as the Holocaust, which means 'sacrifice'. Many people prefer the Jewish term Sho'ah, which means 'destruction'. Why do you think this is?

How did war affect the Jews?

The ghettos

Persecution of the Jews developed in intensity after the outbreak of war in 1939. After defeating Poland in 1939, the Nazis set about 'Germanising' western Poland. This meant transporting Poles from their homes and replacing them with German settlers. Almost one in five Poles died in the fighting and as a result of racial policies of 1939–45. Polish Jews were rounded up and transported to the major cities. Here they were herded into sealed areas, called ghettos. The able-bodied Jews were used for slave labour but the young, the old and the sick were simply left to die from hunger and disease.

Mass murder

In 1941 Germany invaded the USSR. The invasion was a great success at first. However, within weeks the Nazis found themselves in control of 3 million Russian Jews in addition to the Jews in all of the other countries they had invaded. German forces had orders to round up and shoot Communist Party activists and their Jewish supporters. The shooting was carried out by special SS units called *Einsatzgruppen*. By the autumn of 1941, mass shootings were taking place all over occupied eastern Europe. In Germany, all Jews were ordered to wear the star of David on their clothing to mark them out.

The 'Final solution'

In January 1942, senior Nazis met at Wannsee, a suburb of Berlin, for a conference to discuss what they called the 'Final Solution' to the 'Jewish Question'. At the Wannsee Conference, Himmler, head of the SS and Gestapo, was put in charge of the systematic killing of all Jews within Germany and German-occupied territory. Slave labour and death camps were built at Auschwitz, Treblinka, Chelmo and other places. The old, the sick and young children were killed immediately. The able-bodied were first used as slave labour. Some were used for appalling medical experiments. Six million Jews, 500,000 European gypsies and countless political prisoners, Jehovah's Witnesses, homosexuals and Russian and Polish prisoners of war were sent to these camps to be worked to death, gassed or shot.

Resistance

Many Jews escaped from Germany before the killing started. Other Jews managed to live under cover in Germany and the occupied territories. Gad Beck, for instance, led the Jewish resistance to the Nazis in Berlin. He was finally captured in April 1945. On the day he was due to be executed, he was rescued by a detachment of troops from the Jewish regiment of the Red Army who had heard of his capture and had been sent to rescue him. There were 28 known groups of Jewish fighters, and there may have been more. Many Jews fought in the resistance movements in the Nazi-occupied lands. In 1945 the Jews in the Warsaw ghetto rose up against the Nazis and held out against them for four weeks. Five concentration camps saw armed uprisings and Greek Jews managed to blow up the gas ovens at Auschwitz.

We know that many Germans and other non-Jews helped Jews by hiding them and smuggling them out of German-held territory. The industrialist Oskar Schindler protected and saved many by getting them on to his 'list' of workers. The Swedish diplomat Raoul Wallenberg worked with other resisters to provide Jews with Swedish and US passports to get them out of the reach of the Nazis in Hungary. He disappeared in mysterious circumstances in 1945. Of course, high-profile individuals such as these were rare. Most of the successful resisters were successful because they kept an extremely low profile and were discovered neither by the Nazis then, nor by historians today.

Make sure you know what these terms mean and are able to define them confidently.
♦ Autobahn
♦ Bauhaus
♦ Beauty of Labour
♦ Communist (Bolshevik)
♦ Concentration camps
♦ Consolidation
♦ Democracy
♦ Diktat
♦ Edelweiss Pirates
♦ Final Solution
♦ Freikorps
♦ Gestapo
♦ Hitler Youth
♦ Holocaust
♦ Inflation
♦ League of German Maidens
♦ National Community
♦ Nazism
♦ Negative cohesion
♦ Nuremburg Laws
♦ Propaganda
♦ Putsch
♦ Rearmament
♦ Reparations
♦ Spartacists
♦ SA
♦ SS
♦ Strength Through Joy

Revision Tip

♦ Make sure you can describe the ghettos and the Final Solution.
♦ Identify three examples that show how Nazi actions against Jews and other groups became more violent as the war went on.

Exam Practice

See pages 168–175 and pages 316–319 for advice on the different types of questions you might face.
1 (a) What was the Munich Putsch? **[4]**
  (b) Explain why the Nazis launched the Munich Putsch in 1923. **[6]**
  (c) 'The Munich Putsch was a total failure for Adolf Hitler.' How far do you agree with this statement? Explain your answer. **[10]**
Component 3 or 4 questions
2 How important was the Depression in bringing about the end of the Weimar Republic?
3 How significant was the work of Himmler in maintaining Nazi control of Germany after 1933?

Focus Task

Was Germany a totalitarian state?

A totalitarian state is one where:
♦ **no opposition** is allowed;
♦ people are expected to show **total loyalty and obedience** to the state;
♦ every aspect of life is **controlled** by the state for its own benefit.
You are going to prepare for a debate on the question: Was Nazi Germany a totalitarian state? Clearly Hitler wanted Germany to be like this, but did the Nazis achieve it?

Stage A: Research

Read through this chapter gathering as much evidence as you can on either side. Use the text and the sources and your own research. Here are a few references to get you started.

p.247	p.249	p.250	p.267	p.251
Factfile	Source 2	Source 3	Source 25	Source 6
p.255	p.258	p.261	p.268	p.253
Source 16	Source 7	Source 14	Source 27	Source 9

Summarise your evidence in a table (be sure to note where you found this evidence).

Stage B: Reach your judgement

Share your evidence with others. Discuss it. Do you think that the Nazis managed to turn Germany into a totalitarian state?

Stage C: Write your speech

Aim for just one minute (200–250 words). State your view. Use evidence to support your arguments.

What was it like to live in Nazi Germany?

1 Young people were expected to join the Hitler Youth. There were separate organisations for boys and girls.
2 The boys focused on activities to teach them to be soldiers. The girls focused on healthy living and preparing for motherhood.
3 The school curriculum was also used to indoctrinate young people. Teachers were among the keenest supporters of the Nazis.
4 Not all young people liked the Nazis and once the war started opposition to the Hitler Youth among young people increased and groups like the Edelweiss Pirates actively resisted.
5 The Nazis rewarded German women for having children – the more the better. They discouraged women from working and encouraged them to stay at home and look after children.
6 However later on they also needed women to become workers so they had to change their policies to encourage women to do both.
7 The Nazis promised to end unemployment, which they did but only by drafting hundreds of thousands of people into the army or putting political opponents to forced labour.
8 The economy recovered in the 1930s but business was geared to getting ready for war, making weapons or becoming self-sufficient in raw materials.
9 For those who did not fit Nazi ideas life was terrible. The Jews suffered in particular, facing restrictions, then persecution or exile, and in the end forced labour and genocide.
10 The war went well for Germany to start with. However after Germany invaded Russia in 1941 the tide turned. German resources were directed into a fighting an unwinnable war against the USSR. The German economy and the Nazi regime collapsed.

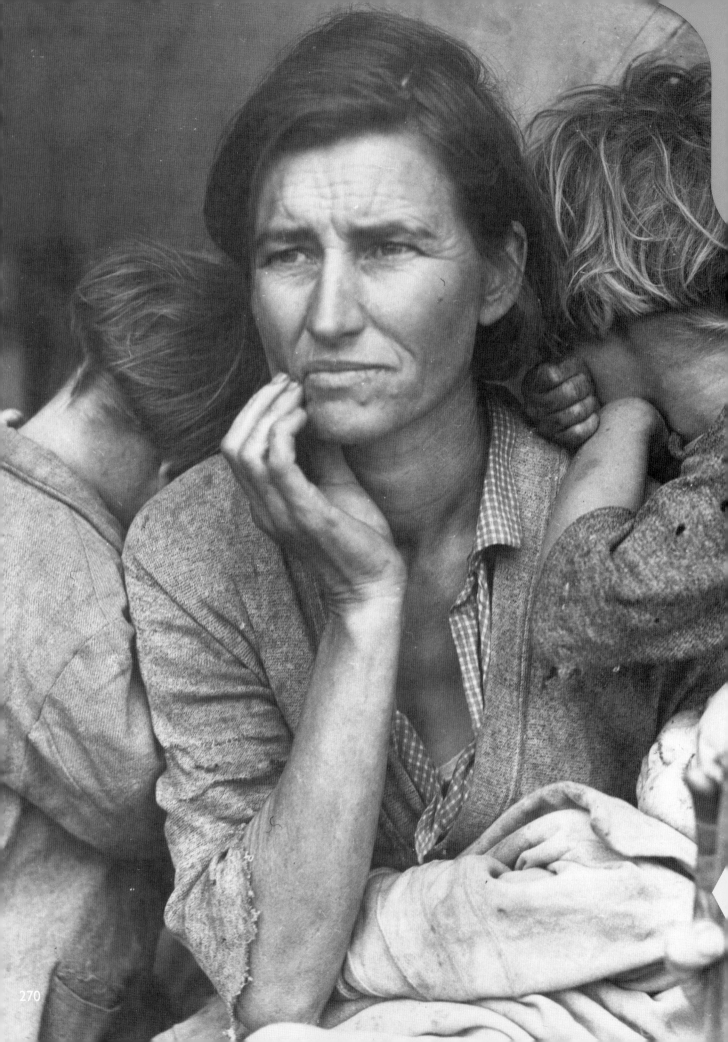

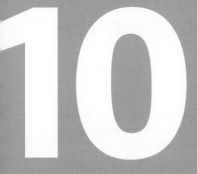

10

The USA 1919–41

KEY QUESTIONS

10.1 How far did the US economy boom in the 1920s?

10.2 How far did US society change in the 1920s?

10.3 What were the causes and consequences of the Wall Street Crash?

10.4 How successful was the New Deal?

At the end of the First World War the USA was the richest and most powerful country in the world. The next two decades were a turbulent time: a boom then a bust; a time of opportunity for some but a time of trauma for others.

In 10.1 you will look at the booming US economy in the 1920s. You will look at the causes of this economic boom and also its consequences. Most important of all, you will investigate which Americans shared in the new prosperity and what happened to those who did not.

In 10.2 you will examine the changes that took place in the 1920s, particularly for women, immigrants and African Americans.

In 10.3 you will examine the economic disaster that plunged the USA into crisis – the Wall Street Crash of 1929 – and how the Crash led to a deep economic depression.

In 10.4 you will look at the New Deal: the measures President Roosevelt used to help the USA recover. You will examine the range of measures taken, the thinking behind those measures and how people reacted to them. Most of all you will think hard about whether or not the New Deal should be seen as a success or not.

Timeline

This timeline shows the period you will be covering in this chapter. Some of the key dates are filled in already. To help you get a complete picture of the period make your own much larger version and add other details to it as you work through the chapter.

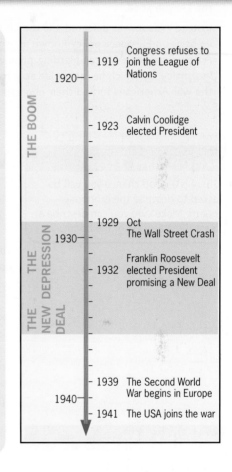

THE BOOM	1919	Congress refuses to join the League of Nations
	1920	
	1923	Calvin Coolidge elected President
THE NEW DEAL / THE DEPRESSION	1929	Oct The Wall Street Crash
	1930	
	1932	Franklin Roosevelt elected President promising a New Deal
	1939	The Second World War begins in Europe
	1940	
	1941	The USA joins the war

◄ This photo was taken in California by Dorothea Lange during the Great Depression of the early 1930s. It was taken in a temporary camp for workers who had come to California to find a job. It is called 'Migrant Mother' and is one of the most famous and widely used photographs about this period.

1 What impression does this photo give you of the woman?

2 This was a carefully constructed photo – what does the photographer want you to feel and think and how has she achieved that?

10.1 How far did the US economy boom in the 1920s?

As you saw in Chapter 1, after the First World War President Wilson determined that from then on the USA should take a lead in world affairs. He proposed an international League of Nations that would be like a world parliament that prevented aggression between countries. As you saw in Chapter 2, Wilson failed in this attempt. He even failed to get the USA to agree to join the League at all.

Instead Wilson was defeated and the USA turned its back on Europe, a policy known as 'isolationism'. A new President, Warren Harding, promised a return to 'normalcy' by which he meant life as it had been before the war. Americans turned their energies to what they did best – making money! Over the next ten years the USA, already the richest country in the world, became richer still as its economy boomed.

In 10.1 you will examine the reasons for this boom and also the extent. You will also see that while some people in America benefited greatly from the boom there were significant proportions – possibly even the majority – who did not share in the boom at all.

Focus Points

♦ On what factors was the economic boom based?
♦ Why did some industries prosper while others did not?
♦ Why did agriculture not share in the prosperity?
♦ Did all Americans benefit from the boom?

Revision Tip

There is a good chance you will be asked to describe the economic boom. Make sure you can describe at least three aspects of the boom.

What was the boom?

The 'boom' is the name given to the dynamic growth of the American economy in the decade after the First World War.

In the 1920s American businesses grew more quickly than ever before. They found faster and cheaper ways of making goods than ever before. As production went up prices came down so ordinary people bought more household goods than ever before: millions of fridges and cars were sold; hundreds of millions of nylon stockings.

Many families bought new houses in the suburbs of America's rapidly growing cities. And with money to spare they spent more on leisure – so the music, radio, cinema industries and even sport were booming.

Company profits were booming and confidence was booming too. Business leaders were prepared to take risks and ordinary people were too. Banks had money to spare so they invested it in the stock market or lent it to ordinary Americans to do so. The value of stocks and shares went up and up.

The government built more roads than ever before. More homes were supplied with electricity and phone lines than ever before. There was more building being done in the boom years of the 1920s than ever before. And, as if to symbolise the massive confidence of the time, cities built higher skyscrapers than ever before.

It seemed that everything was going up, up, up!

This may all sound too good to be true – and it was! The whole system came crashing down with a bang in 1929 but that is another story which you will investigate on page 298. For now you will focus on the boom years and why exactly American industry was so successful in the 1920s.

Think!

What was the boom?

Automobiles	Entertainment
Advertising	Cities
Electricity	Transport
Credit	Mass consumption
Mass production	

1 These cards show nine key features of the 1920s economic boom. Make your own set of cards – large enough to write some information on the back.
2 As you read this chapter write notes on each card to summarise how this was changing in the 1920s and how it contributed to the boom.
3 Working on a larger piece of paper make notes about how these different features are linked.
NB Keep your cards. They will be useful for the Focus Task on page 277. They will also be useful when it comes to revision.

Factors behind the economic boom

Industrial strength

The USA was a vast country, rich in natural resources. It had a growing population (123 million by 1923). Most of this population was living in towns and cities. They were working in industry and commerce, usually earning higher wages than in farming. So these new town dwellers became an important market for the USA's new industries. Most US companies had no need to export outside the USA, and most US companies had access to the raw materials they needed in the USA.

SOURCE

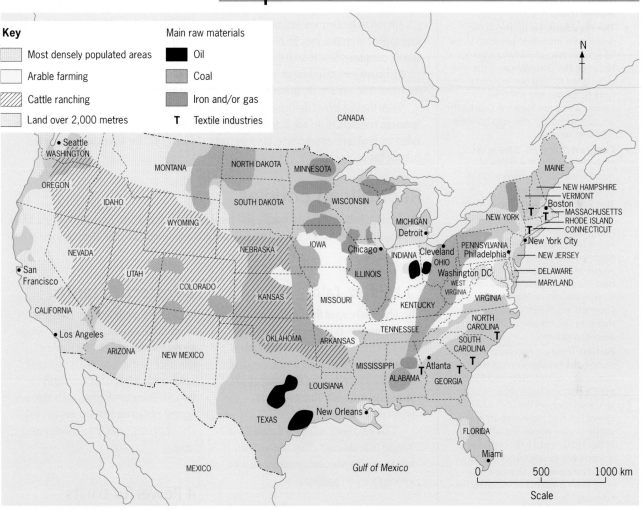

Key

	Most densely populated areas
	Arable farming
	Cattle ranching
	Land over 2,000 metres

Main raw materials

	Oil
	Coal
	Iron and/or gas
T	Textile industries

The USA's main centres of population and main natural resources around 1920.

Think!

Why did it benefit American industry to have raw materials, especially coal, oil and cotton, so easily available within the USA?

Revision Tip

On this page and the next four there are quite a few factors explaining the boom. Focus on two per page. Make sure you can explain how the factor contributed to the boom.

Ever since the 1860s and 1870s, American industry had been growing vigorously. By the time of the First World War, the USA led the world in most areas of industry. It had massive steel, coal and textile industries. It was the leading oil producer. It was foremost in developing new technology such as motor cars, telephones and electric lighting. In fact, electricity and electrical goods were a key factor in the USA's economic boom. Other new industries such as chemicals were also growing fast. The USA's new film industry already led the world.

The managers of these industries were increasingly skilled and professional, and they were selling more and more of their products not just in the USA but in Europe, Latin America and the Far East.

American agriculture had become the most efficient and productive in the world. In fact, farmers had become so successful that they were producing more than they could sell, which was a very serious problem (see page 278). In 1914, however, most Americans would have confidently stated that American agriculture and industry were going from strength to strength.

US system of government

- **The federal system:** The USA's federal system means that all the individual states look after their own internal affairs (such as education). Questions that concern all of the states (such as making treaties with other countries) are dealt with by Congress.
- **The Constitution:** The Constitution lays out how the government is supposed to operate and what it is allowed to do.
- **The President:** He (or she) is the single most important politician in the USA. He is elected every four years. However, the Constitution of the USA is designed to stop one individual from becoming too powerful. Congress and the Supreme Court both act as 'watchdogs' checking how the President behaves.
- **Congress:** Congress is made up of the Senate and the House of Representatives. Congress and the President run the country.
- **The Supreme Court:** This is made up of judges, who are usually very experienced lawyers. Their main task is to make sure that American governments do not misuse their power or pass unfair laws. They have the power to say that a law is unconstitutional (against the Constitution), which usually means that they feel the law would harm American citizens.
- **Parties:** There are two main political parties, the Republicans and the Democrats. In the 1920s and 1930s, the Republicans were stronger in the industrial north of the USA while the Democrats had more support in the south. On the whole, Republicans in the 1920s and 1930s preferred government to stay out of people's lives if possible. The Democrats were more prepared to intervene in everyday life.

The First World War

The Americans tried hard to stay out of the fighting in the First World War. But throughout the war they lent money to the Allies, and sold arms and munitions to Britain and France. They sold massive amounts of foodstuffs as well. This one-way trade gave American industry a real boost. In addition, while the European powers slugged it out in France, the Americans were able to take over Europe's trade around the world. American exports to the areas controlled by European colonial powers increased during the war.

There were other benefits as well. Before the war Germany had one of the world's most successful chemicals industries. The war stopped it in its tracks. By the end of the war the USA had far outstripped Germany in the supply of chemical products. Explosives manufacture during the war also stimulated a range of by-products which became new American industries in their own right. Plastics and other new materials were produced.

Aircraft technology was improved during the First World War. From 1918 these developments were applied to civilian uses. In 1918 there were virtually no civilian airlines. By 1930 the new aircraft companies flew 162,000 flights a year.

Historians have called the growth and change at this time the USA's second industrial revolution. The war actually helped rather than hindered the 'revolution'.

When the USA joined the fighting it was not in the war long enough for the war to drain American resources in the way it drained Europe's. There was a downturn in the USA when war industries readjusted to peacetime, but it was only a blip. By 1922 the American economy was growing fast once again.

Republican policies

A third factor behind the boom was the policies of the Republican Party. From 1920 to 1932 all the US presidents were Republican, and Republicans also dominated Congress. Here are some of their beliefs.

1 Laissez-faire

Republicans believed that government should interfere as little as possible in the everyday lives of the people. This attitude is called 'laissez-faire'. In their view, the job of the President was to leave the businessman alone – to do his job. That was where prosperity came from.

This was closely related to their belief in 'rugged individualism'. They admired the way Americans were strong and got on with solving their own problems.

2 Protective tariffs

The Republicans believed in import tariffs which made it expensive to import foreign goods. For example, in 1922 Harding introduce the Fordney–McCumber tariff which made imported food expensive in the USA. These tariffs protected businesses against foreign competition and allowed American companies to grow even more rapidly.

3 Low taxation

The Republicans kept taxation as low as possible. This brought some benefits to ordinary working people, but it brought even more to the very wealthy. The Republican thinking was that if people kept their own money, they would spend it on American goods and wealthy people would reinvest their money in industries.

4 Powerful trusts

Trusts were huge super-corporations, which dominated industry. Woodrow Wilson and the Democrats had fought against trusts because they believed it was unhealthy for men such as Carnegie (steel) and Rockefeller (oil) to have almost complete control of one vital sector of industry. The Republicans allowed the trusts to do what they wanted, believing that the 'captains of industry' knew better than politicians did what was good for the USA.

SOURCE **2**

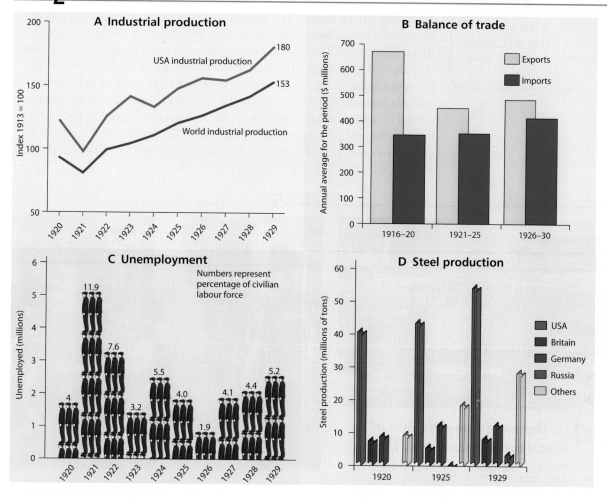

The growth of the US economy in the 1920s.

1 How could the Republicans use Source 2 to justify their policies?
2 How could critics of Republican policies use Source 2 to attack the Republicans?

Which factors have you chosen from pages 274 and 275? Practise explaining how they caused the boom rather than just describing them.

New industries, new methods

Through the 1920s new industries and new methods of production were developed in the USA. The country was able to exploit its vast resources of raw materials to produce steel, chemicals, glass and machinery. Electricity was changing America too. Before the First World War industry was still largely powered by coal. By the 1920s electricity had taken over. In 1918 only a few homes were supplied; by 1929 almost all urban homes had it. These new industries in turn became the foundation of an enormous boom in consumer goods. Telephones, radios, vacuum cleaners and washing machines were mass-produced on a vast scale. These new techniques, together with mass production methods, meant that huge amounts of goods could be produced much more cheaply and so more people could afford them.

Things that used to be luxuries were now made cheaper by new inventions and mass production. For example, silk stockings had once been a luxury item reserved for the rich. In 1900 only 12,000 pairs had been sold. In the 1920s rayon was invented, which was a cheaper substitute for silk. In 1930, 300 million pairs of stockings were sold to a female population of around 100 million.

SOURCE **3**

We are quick to adopt the latest time and labour saving devices in business. The modern woman has an equal right to employ in her home the most popular electric cleaner: The Frantz Premier. Over 250,000 are in use. We have branches and dealers everywhere. Our price is modest – time payments if desired.

Advertisement for the Frantz Premier vacuum cleaner.

The car

The most important of these new booming industries was the motor-car or automobile industry. The motor car had only been developed in the 1890s. The first cars were built by blacksmiths and other skilled craftsmen. They took a long time to make and were very expensive. In 1900 only 4,000 cars were made. Car production was revolutionised by Henry Ford. In 1913 he set up the world's first moving production line, in a giant shed in Detroit. Each worker on the line had one or two small jobs to do as the skeleton of the car moved past him. At the beginning of the line, a skeleton car went in; at the end of the line was a new car. The most famous of these was the Model T. More than 15 million were produced between 1908 and 1925. In 1927 they came off the production line at a rate of one every ten seconds. In 1929, 4.8 million cars were made. In 1925 they cost $290. This was only three months' wages for an American factory worker.

SOURCE **4**

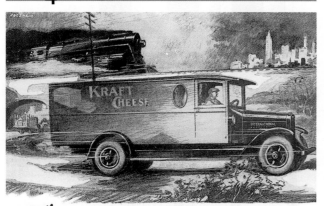

For 1927 the most complete line of 4 and 6-cylinder Speed Trucks

INTERNATIONAL HARVESTER COMPANY

INTERNATIONAL TRUCKS

The new roads gave rise to a new truck industry. In 1919 there were 1 million trucks in the USA. By 1929 there were 3.5 million.

SOURCE **6**

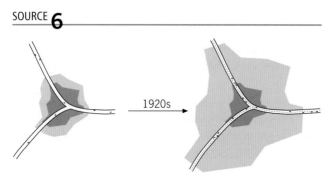

1920s

The car made it possible for more Americans to live in their own houses in the suburbs on the edge of towns. For example, Queens outside New York doubled in size in the 1920s. Grosse Point Park outside Detroit grew by 700 per cent.

SOURCE **5**

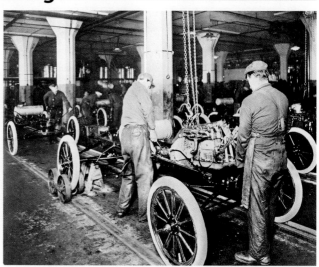

Ford's production line in 1913.

By the end of the 1920s the motor industry was the USA's biggest industry. As well as employing hundreds of thousands of workers directly, it also kept workers in other industries in employment. Glass, leather, steel and rubber were all required to build the new vehicles. Automobiles used up 75 per cent of US glass production in the 1920s! Petrol was needed to run them. And a massive army of labourers was busily building roads throughout the country for these cars to drive on. In fact, road construction was the biggest single employer in the 1920s.

Owning a car was not just a rich person's privilege, as it was in Europe. There was one car to five people in the USA compared with one to 43 in Britain, and one to 7,000 in Russia. The car made it possible for people to buy a house in the suburbs, which further boosted house building. It also stimulated the growth of hundreds of other smaller businesses, ranging from hot dog stands and advertising bill boards to petrol stations and holiday resorts.

SOURCE **7**

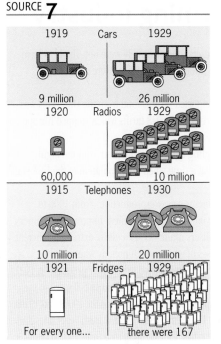

1919	Cars	1929	

9 million — 26 million

1920 Radios 1929
60,000 — 10 million

1915 Telephones 1930
10 million — 20 million

1921 Fridges 1929
For every one... — there were 167

Sales of consumer goods, 1915–30. Overall, the output of American industry doubled in the 1920s.

Mass consumption

It is no good producing lots of goods if people don't buy them. Mass production requires mass consumption.

So, the big industries used sophisticated sales and marketing techniques to get people to buy their goods. New electrical companies such as Hoover became household names. They used the latest, most efficient techniques proposed by the 'Industrial Efficiency Movement'.

- Mass nationwide advertising had been used for the first time in the USA during the war to get Americans to support the war effort. Many of the advertisers who had learned their skills in wartime propaganda now set up agencies to sell cars, cigarettes, clothing and other consumer items. Poster advertisements, radio advertisements and travelling salesmen encouraged Americans to spend.
- There was a huge growth in the number of mail-order companies. People across America, especially in remote areas, could buy the new consumer goods from catalogues. In 1928 nearly one-third of Americans bought goods from Sears, Roebuck and Company catalogue. This greatly expanded the market for products.
- Even if they did not have the money, people could borrow it easily. Or they could take advantage of the new 'Buy now, pay later' hire purchase schemes. Eight out of ten radios and six out of ten cars were bought on credit. Before the war, people expected to save up until they could afford something. Now they could buy on credit.
- A brand-new kind of shop emerged – the chain store – the same shop selling the same products all across the USA.

This all worked very well as you can see from Source 7.

A state of mind

One thing that runs through all the factors you have looked at so far is an attitude or a state of mind. Most Americans believed that they had a right to 'prosperity'. For many it was a main aim in life to have a nice house, a good job and plenty to eat, and for their home to be filled with the latest consumer goods. Consuming more and more was seen as part of being American.

In earlier decades, thrift (being careful with money and saving 'for a rainy day') had been seen as a good quality. In the 1920s this was replaced by a belief that spending money was a better quality.

There was confidence in the USA in the 1920s. Business people had the confidence to invest in the new industries, to experiment with new ideas and to set up businesses and employ people. Ordinary Americans had confidence to buy goods, sometimes on credit, because they were sure they could pay for them, or to invest in industry itself by buying shares. Confidence is vital to any economic boom.

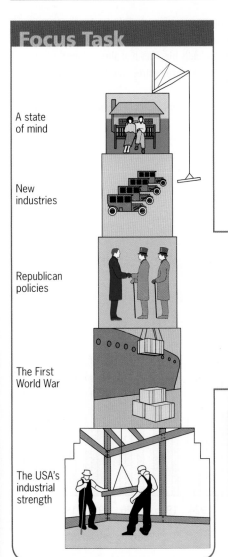

Focus Task

A state of mind

New industries

Republican policies

The First World War

The USA's industrial strength

What factors caused the economic boom?

1 The diagram on the left shows you the main factors on which the economic boom in the 1920s was based. Put a copy of the diagram in the centre of a large piece of paper. Write notes to summarise how each factor contributed to the boom using pages 273–77.

2 One historian has said: 'Without the new automobile industry, the prosperity of the 1920s would scarcely have been possible.' Explain whether you agree or disagree with this statement. Support your explanation by referring to the sources and information on pages 273–77.

Revision Tip

So have you got five or more factors which explain the boom? If so:
- Choose two factors you think were connected and practise explaining how they were connected.
- Decide which one you think is the most important (or if you think the boom cannot be explained that way, say why).

SOURCE **8**

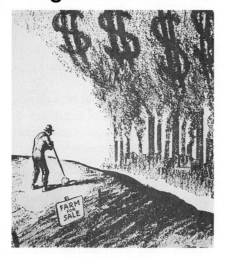

A cartoon showing the situation faced by American farmers in the 1920s.

Problems in the farming industry

While many Americans were enjoying the boom, farmers most definitely were not. Total US farm income dropped from $22 billion in 1919 to just $13 billion in 1928. There were a number of reasons why farming had such problems.

Declining exports   After the war, Europe imported far less food from the USA. This was partly because Europe was poor, and it was partly a response to US tariffs which stopped Europe from exporting to the USA (see page 274).

New competitors   Farmers were also struggling against competition from the highly efficient Canadian wheat producers. All of this came at a time when the population of the USA was actually falling and there were fewer mouths to feed.

Over-production   Underlying all these problems was overproduction. From 1900 to 1920, while farming was doing well, more and more land was being farmed. Improved machinery, especially the combine harvester, and improved fertilisers made US agriculture extremely efficient. The result was that by 1920 it was producing surpluses of wheat which nobody wanted.

Falling prices   Prices plummeted as desperate farmers tried to sell their produce. In 1921 alone, most farm prices fell by 50 per cent (see Source 9). Hundreds of rural banks collapsed in the 1920s and there were five times as many farm bankruptcies as there had been in the 1900s and 1910s.

Not all farmers were affected by these problems. Rich Americans wanted fresh vegetables and fruit throughout the year. Shipments of lettuce to the cities, for example, rose from 14,000 crates in 1920 to 52,000 in 1928. But for most farmers the 1920s were a time of hardship.

This was a serious issue. About half of all Americans lived in rural areas, mostly working on farms or in businesses that sold goods to farmers. Problems in farming therefore directly affected more than 60 million Americans.

Six million rural Americans, mainly farm labourers, were forced off the land in the 1920s. Many of these were unskilled workers who migrated to the cities, where there was little demand for their labour. The African Americans were particularly badly hit. They had always done the least skilled jobs in the rural areas. As they lost their jobs on the farms, three-quarters of a million of them became unemployed.

It is no surprise that farming communities were the fiercest critics of the 'laissez-faire' policies of the Republican party.

SOURCE **9**

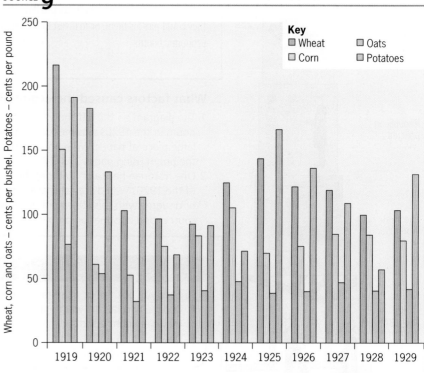

Farming prices in the 1920s.

Focus Task

Why did agriculture not share in the prosperity?

Write a 200-word caption explaining the message of Source 8. Refer to details in the source but also use the information in the text to explain the details, for example, explaining the reasons why the farmer might be looking enviously (or angrily) at the factories, or the events that might have led to his farm being for sale.

Problems in traditional industries

SOURCE 10

A graph showing % increase 1920–29 on the vertical axis (100 to 170) and years 1920 to 1929 on the horizontal axis. Lines show: Dividends to shareholders, Company profits, and Average earnings.

A comparison of the growth of profits and the growth of average earnings.

SOURCE 11

goes to the richest 5%

32%

10%

goes to the poorest 42%

The distribution of income in 1925.

Revision Tip

Find an industry where the following issues called problems: electrification; oil; lack of growth markets; declining profits. Your friends might come up with different ideas – that is fine, several industries suffered many similar problems.

You have already seen how the farmers – a very large group in American society – did not share in the prosperity of the 1920s. But they were not alone. Workers in many older industries did not benefit much either.

The coal industry was a big employer but it began to struggle. Firstly, like farming it was producing too much coal and this reduced the price of coal and therefore profits. At the same time coal was losing out to new power sources like electricity and oil. Although electricity producers used coal to generate electricity, the new generating technology was highly efficient so it did not need much coal to produce a lot of energy. Manufacturers were either switching to electricity or oil, or if they were using coal they had more efficient machinery which used less coal. The same pattern could be seen in areas like domestic heating boilers where users could get the same amount of heat with less coal.

Other industries such as leather, textiles and shoe-making also struggled. They were protected from competition from foreign imports by tariffs. However, they were not growth markets like the markets for electrical goods. They also suffered from competition from industries which used new man-made materials and were often mechanised. In the traditional industries generally growth was slow and profits were gradually declining. Workers in these industries suffered as they became increasingly mechanised. Skilled workers struggled to compete against both machinery and cheap labour in the southern states. Even if workers in these industries did get a pay rise, their wages did not increase on the same scale as company profits or dividends paid to shareholders.

In 1928 there was a strike in the coal industry in North Carolina, where the male workers were paid only $18 and women $9 for a 70-hour week, at a time when $48 per week was considered to be the minimum required for a decent life. In fact, for the majority of Americans wages remained well below that figure. It has been estimated that 42 per cent of Americans lived below the poverty line – they did not have the money needed to pay for essentials such as food, clothing, housing and heating for their families.

SOURCE 12

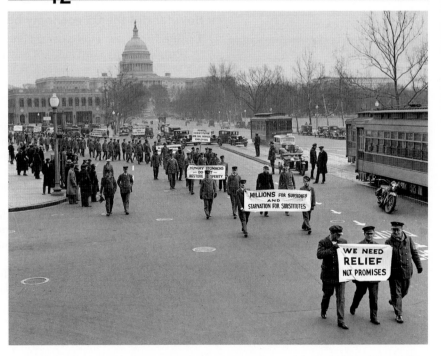

A hunger march in Washington during the brief recession which hit some industries in 1921–22.

Did all Americans share in the boom?

In 1928 a new Republican President, Herbert Hoover, was elected. He said:

SOURCE **13**

One of the oldest and perhaps the noblest of human activities [aims] has been the abolition of poverty . . . we in America today are nearer to the final triumph over poverty than ever before in the history of any land.

Herbert Hoover.

Gather evidence from pages 278–80 to contest Hoover's claim. Write a paper setting out in detail:

♦ how badly off some farmers have become since the war
♦ why farmers are poor and how Republican policies have contributed to this
♦ why workers in older industries are suffering and what has happened to their wages (give an example)
♦ why immigrant workers and African-Americans are not well off.

Try to use specific examples such as Chicago in the 1920s.

♦ Choose two points about Chicago which you think you could use in a question about whether all Americans shared in the boom.
♦ Explain to someone else how you would use those points.

Unemployment

What's more, throughout this period unemployment remained a problem. The growth in industry in the 1920s did not create many new jobs. Industries were growing by electrifying or mechanising production. The same number of people (around 5 per cent) were unemployed at the peak of the boom in 1929 as in 1920. Yet the amount of goods produced had doubled. These millions of unemployed Americans were not sharing in the boom. They included many poor whites, but an even greater proportion of African American and Hispanic people and other members of the USA's large immigrant communities.

The plight of the poor was desperate for the individuals concerned. But it was also damaging to American industry. The boom of the 1920s was a consumer-led boom, which means that it was led by ordinary families buying things for their home. But with so many families too poor to buy such goods, the demand for them was likely to begin to tail off. However, Republican policy remained not to interfere, and this included doing nothing about unemployment or poverty.

Case Study: Chicago in the 1920s

Chicago was one of America's biggest cities. It was the centre of the steel, meat and clothing industries, which employed many unskilled workers. Such industries had busy and slack periods. In slack periods the workers would be 'seasonally unemployed'. Many of these workers were Polish or Italian immigrants, or African American migrants from the southern United States. How far did they share in the prosperity of the 1920s?

- Only 3 per cent of semi-skilled workers owned a car. Compare that with richer areas where 29 per cent owned a car.
- Workers in Chicago didn't like to buy large items on credit. They preferred to save for when they might not have a job. Many bought smaller items on credit, such as radios.
- The poor whites did not use the new chain stores which had revolutionised shopping in the 1920s. Nearly all of them were in middle-class districts. Poorer white industrial workers preferred to shop at the local grocer's where the owner was more flexible and gave them credit.

How far did the US economy boom in the 1920s?

1 The 1920s saw unprecedented growth in mass consumption in the USA. People bought a vast range of new products which changed the way people lived their lives.
2 The period saw dynamic business growth and prosperity with the creation of vast new cities, characterised by skyscrapers, and new systems of transport to link towns and cities.
3 The boom was encouraged by the policies of the Republican party which believed in laissez-faire, low taxes and protective tariffs.
4 It was also underpinned by the development of new industries using new materials and innovative production techniques, especially mass production.
5 The motor car was particularly important, changing the American way of life and stimulating other industries.
6 Large sections of American society did not benefit to the same degree from prosperity including farmers and farm labourers – farming in the 1920s was very depressed through a combination of overproduction and environmental problems.
7 Older industries such as coal or leather suffered because of competition from new materials such as oil or plastics and because their methods and machinery became outdated.

10.2 How far did US society change in the 1920s?

Focus

The 1920s are often called the Roaring Twenties. The name suggests a time of riotous fun, loud music and wild enjoyment when everyone was having a good time.

You have already found out enough about the USA in the period to know that this is probably not how everyone saw this decade. For example, how do you think the poor farmers described on page 278 would react to the suggestion that the 1920s were one long party?

What is in no doubt is that this was a time of turmoil for many Americans. For those who joined in 'the party', it was a time of liberation and rebellion against traditional values. For those who did not, it was a time of anxiety and worry. For them, the changes taking place were proof that the USA was going down the drain and needed rescuing.

All this combined to make the 1920s a decade of contrasts. In this section you will examine these contrasts and the conflicts that resulted from them.

Focus Points

- What were the 'Roaring Twenties'?
- How widespread was intolerance in US society?
- Why was prohibition introduced, and then later repealed?
- How far did the roles of women change during the 1920s?

The USA in the Roaring Twenties

Town v. country

In 1920, for the first time in American history, more Americans lived in towns and cities than in the country. People flocked to them from all over the USA. The growing city with its imposing skyline of skyscrapers was one of the most powerful symbols of 1920s USA. In New York, the skyscrapers were built because there was no more land available. But even small cities, where land was not in short supply, wanted skyscrapers to announce to the country that they were sharing in the boom. As you can see from Source 2, throughout the 1920s cities were growing fast.

Throughout the 1920s there was tension between rural USA and urban USA. Many people in the country thought that their traditional values, which emphasised religion and family life, were under threat from the growing cities, which they thought were full of atheists, drunks and criminals. Certain rural states, particularly in the south, fought a rearguard action against the 'evil' effects of the city throughout the 1920s, as you will see on page 292.

Think!

Write an advertising slogan to go with Source 1, inviting workers to come to New York City.

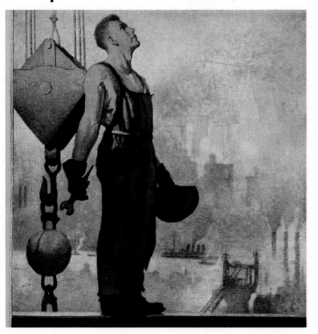

The Builder, painted by Gerrit A Beneker in the 1920s.

SOURCE 2

The change in the USA's urban and rural populations, 1900–40.

Entertainment

The term 'Roaring Twenties' is particularly associated with entertainment and changing morality. During the 1920s the entertainment industry blossomed. The average working week dropped from 47.4 to 44.2 hours so people had more leisure time. Average wages rose by 11 per cent (in real terms) so workers also had more disposable income. A lot of this spare time and money was channelled into entertainment.

Radio

Almost everyone in the USA listened to the radio. Most households had their own set. It was a communal activity – most families listened to the radio together. People who could not afford to buy one outright could purchase one in instalments. In poorer districts where people could not all afford a radio, they shared. By 1930 there was one radio for every two to three households in the poorer districts of Chicago. Those who didn't own a radio set went to shops or to neighbours to listen. The choice of programmes grew quickly. In August 1921 there was only one licensed radio station in America. By the end of 1922 there were 508 of them. By 1929 the new network NBC was making $150 million a year.

SOURCE 3

(i) Jazz employs primitive rhythms which excite the baser human instincts.

(ii) Jazz music causes drunkenness. Reason and reflection are lost and the actions of the persons are directed by the stronger animal passions.

Comments on jazz music in articles in the 1920s.

Jazz

The radio gave much greater access to new music. Jazz music became an obsession among young people. African Americans who moved from the country to the cities had brought jazz and blues music with them. Blues music was particularly popular among the African Americans, while jazz captured the imagination of both young white and African Americans.

Such was the power of jazz music that the 1920s became known as the Jazz Age. Along with jazz went new dances such as the Charleston, and new styles of behaviour which were summed up in the image of the flapper, a woman who wore short dresses and make-up and who smoked in public. One writer said that the ideal flapper was 'expensive and about nineteen'.

The older generation saw jazz and everything associated with it as a corrupting influence on the young people of the USA. The newspapers and magazines printed articles analysing the influence of jazz (see Source 3).

Sport

Sport was another boom area. Baseball became a big money sport with legendary teams like the New York Yankees and Boston Red Sox. Baseball stars like Babe Ruth became national figures. Boxing was also a very popular sport, with heroes like world heavyweight champion Jack Dempsey. Millions of Americans listened to sporting events on the radio.

SOURCE 4

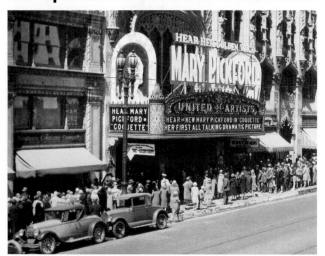

Crowds queuing for cinema tickets in New York. In 1920, 40 million tickets were sold per week and in 1929, 100 million.

Cinema

In a small suburb outside Los Angeles, called Hollywood, a major film industry was developing. All-year-round sunshine meant that the studios could produce large numbers of films or 'movies'. New stars like Charlie Chaplin and Buster Keaton made audiences roar with laughter, while Douglas Fairbanks thrilled them in daring adventure films. Until 1927 all movies were silent. In 1927 the first 'talkie' was made.

During the 1920s movies became a multi-billion dollar business and it was estimated that, by the end of the decade, a hundred million cinema tickets were being sold each week.

Even the poor joined the movie craze. For example, there were hundreds of cinemas in Chicago with four performances a day. Working people in Chicago spent more than half of their leisure budget on movies. Even those who were so poor that they were getting Mothers' Aid Assistance went often. It only cost ten or twenty cents to see a movie.

Morals

SOURCE 5

There was never a time in American history when youth had such a special sense of importance as in the years after the First World War. There was a gulf between the generations like a geological fault. Young men who had fought in the trenches felt that they knew a reality their elders could not even imagine. Young girls no longer consciously modelled themselves on their mothers, whose experience seemed unusable in the 1920s.

William E Leuchtenberg, *The Perils of Prosperity*, 1958.

Source 5 is one historian's description of this period. He refers to new attitudes among young women (see pages 284–85). The gulf he mentions was most obvious in sexual morals. In the generation before the war, sex had still been a taboo subject. After the war it became a major concern of tabloid newspapers, Hollywood films, and everyday conversation. Scott Fitzgerald, one of a celebrated new group of young American writers who had served in the First World War, said: 'None of the mothers had any idea how casually their daughters were accustomed to be kissed.'

The cinema quickly discovered the selling power of sex. The first cinema star to be sold on sex appeal was Theda Bara who, without any acting talent, made a string of wildly successful films with titles like *Forbidden Path* and *When a Woman Sins*. Clara Bow was sold as the 'It' girl. Everybody knew that 'It' meant 'sex'. Hollywood turned out dozens of films a month about 'It', such as *Up in Mabel's Room*, *Her Purchase Price* and *A Shocking Night*. Male stars too, such as Rudolph Valentino, were presented as sex symbols. Women were said to faint at the very sight of him as a half-naked Arab prince in *The Sheik* (1921).

Today these films would be considered very tame indeed, but at the time they were considered very daring. The more conservative rural states were worried by the deluge of sex-obsessed films, and 36 states threatened to introduce censorship legislation. Hollywood responded with its own censorship code which ensured that, while films might still be full of sex, at least the sinful characters were not allowed to get away with it!

Meanwhile, in the real world, contraceptive advice was openly available for the first time. Sex outside marriage was much more common than in the past, although probably more people talked about it and went to films about it than actually did it!

The car

The motor car was one factor that tended to make all the other features of the 1920s mentioned above more possible. Cars helped the cities to grow by opening up the suburbs. They carried their owners to and from their entertainments. Cars carried boyfriends and girlfriends beyond the moral gaze of their parents and they took Americans to an increasing range of sporting events, beach holidays, shopping trips, picnics in the country, or simply on visits to their family and friends.

Focus Task

What were the Roaring Twenties?

1 Draw a mind map to summarise the features of the Roaring Twenties. You can get lots of ideas from the text on pages 281–83, but remember that other factors may also be relevant; for example, material on the economy (pages 272–80). You can also add to your mind map as you find out about the period, particularly women (pages 284–85) and prohibition (pages 293–96).
2 Think about the way these new developments in the 1920s affected people's lives. Choose three aspects of the Roaring Twenties that you think would have had the greatest impact and explain why. Compare your choices with others in your class.

Women in 1920s USA

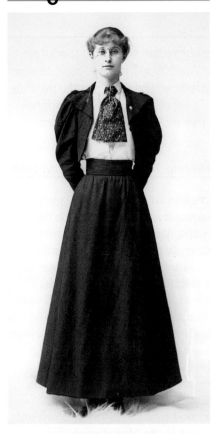

A school teacher in 1905.

Women formed half of the population of the USA and their lives were as varied as those of men. It is therefore difficult to generalise. However, before the First World War middle-class women in the USA, like those in Britain, were expected to lead restricted lives. They had to wear very restrictive clothes and behave politely. They were expected not to wear make-up. Their relationships with men were strictly controlled. They had to have a chaperone with them when they went out with a boyfriend. They were expected not to take part in sport or to smoke in public. In most states they could not vote. Most women were expected to be housewives. Very few paid jobs were open to women. Most working women were in lower-paid jobs such as cleaning, dressmaking and secretarial work.

In rural USA there were particularly tight restrictions owing to the Churches' traditional attitude to the role of women.

In the 1920s, many of these things began to change, especially for urban and middle-class women, for a range of reasons.

- **Impact of war** When the USA joined the war in 1917, some women were taken into the war industries, giving them experience of skilled factory work for the first time.
- **The vote** In 1920 they got the vote in all states.
- **The car** Through the 1920s, they shared the liberating effects of the car.
- **Housework** Their domestic work was made easier (in theory) by new electrical goods such as vacuum cleaners and washing machines.
- **Behaviour** For younger urban women many of the traditional roles of behaviour were eased as well. Women wore more daring clothes. They smoked in public and drank with men, in public. They went out with men, in cars, without a chaperone. They kissed in public.

Employment

In urban areas more women took on jobs – particularly middle-class women. They typically took on jobs created by the new industries. There were 10 million women in jobs in 1929, 24 per cent more than in 1920. With money of their own, working women became the particular target of advertising. Even women who did not earn their own money were increasingly seen as the ones who took decisions about whether to buy new items for the home. There is evidence that women's role in choosing cars triggered Ford, in 1925, to make them available in colours other than black.

Revision Tip

Select two changes for women in this period. Make sure you can describe both of them fully.

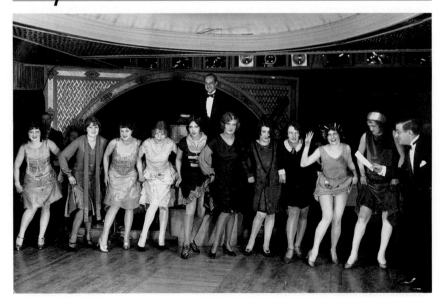

Flappers, identified by short skirts, bobbed hair, bright clothes, and lots of make-up, were the extreme example of liberated urban women

Choices

Films and novels also exposed women to a much wider range of role models. Millions of women a week saw films with sexy or daring heroines as well as other films that showed women in a more traditional role. The newspaper, magazine and film industries found that sex sold much better than anything else.

Women were less likely to stay in unhappy marriages. In 1914 there were 100,000 divorces; in 1929 there were twice as many.

Think!

1 Compare the clothes of the women in Sources 6 and 7. Write a detailed description of the differences between them.
2 Flappers were controversial figures in the 1920s. List as many reasons as possible for this.

SOURCE 8

It is wholly confusing to read the advertisements in the magazines that feature the enticing qualities of vacuum cleaners, mechanical refrigerators and ... other devices which should lighten the chores of women in the home. On the whole these large middle classes do their own housework ...

Women who live on farms ... do a great deal of work besides the labour of caring for their children, washing the clothes, caring for the home and cooking ... labour in the fields ... help milk the cows ...

The other largest group of American women comprises the families of the labourers ... the vast army of unskilled, semi-skilled and skilled workers. The wages of these men are on the whole so small [that] wives must do double duty – that is, caring for the children and the home and toil on the outside as wage earners.

Doris E Fleischman, *America as Americans See It*, FJ Ringel (ed.), 1932.

Source Analysis

How does Source 9 contrast with the image of women given by Source 7?

Profile

Eleanor Roosevelt

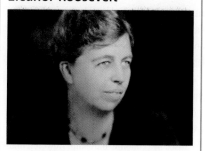

➤ Born 1884 into a wealthy family.
➤ Married Franklin D Roosevelt in 1905.
➤ Heavily involved in:
  – League of Women Voters
  – Women's Trade Union League
  – Women's City Club (New York)
  – New York State Democratic Party (Women's Division).
➤ Work concentrated on:
  – uniting New York Democrats
  – public housing for low-income workers
  – birth control information
  – better conditions for women workers.

Limitations

It might seem to you as if everything was changing, and for young, middle-class women living in cities a lot was changing in the 1920s. However, this is only part of the story.

Take work, for example. Women were still paid less than men, even when they did the same job. One of the reasons women's employment increased when men's did not was that women were cheaper employees.

In politics as well, women in no way achieved equality with men. They may have been given the vote but it did not give them access to political power. Political parties wanted women's votes, but they didn't particularly want women as political candidates as they considered them 'unelectable'. Although many women, such as Eleanor Roosevelt (see Profile), had a high public standing, only a handful of women had been elected by 1929.

How did women respond?

From films of the 1920s such as *Forbidden Path* (see page 283) you would think that all American women were living passionate lives full of steamy romance. However, novels and films of the period can be misleading.

Women certainly did watch such films, in great numbers. But there is no evidence that the majority of women began to copy what they saw in the 1920s. In fact the evidence suggests that the reaction of many women was one of opposition and outrage. There was a strong conservative element in American society. A combination of traditional religion and old country values kept most American women in a much more restricted role than young urban women enjoyed. For most, raising a family and maintaining a good home for their husbands were their main priorities.

SOURCE 9

Though a few young upper middle-class women in the cities talked about throwing off the older conventions – they were the flappers – most women stuck to more traditional attitudes concerning 'their place' ... most middle-class women concentrated on managing the home ... Their daughters, far from taking to the streets against sexual discrimination, were more likely to prepare for careers as mothers and housewives. Millions of immigrant women and their daughters ... also clung to traditions that placed men firmly in control of the family ... Most American women concentrated on making ends meet or setting aside money to purchase the new gadgets that offered some release from household drudgery.

JT Patterson, *America in the Twentieth Century*, 1999.

Focus Task

Did the roles of women change during the 1920s?

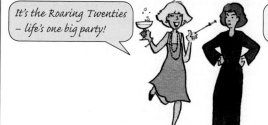

It's the Roaring Twenties – life's one big party!

It might be roaring for you, but life's more of a miaow for me!

You are going to write a script to continue this conversation.
Aim for 6 more scenes: 3 for each woman.
To get you started, draw up a table with two columns headed:
◆ Roaring Twenties
◆ Not so Roaring Twenties.
In each column summarise the points each speaker might make to support their view of the 1920s.

Revision Tip

Now select two ways in which life did not change for women and describe those.

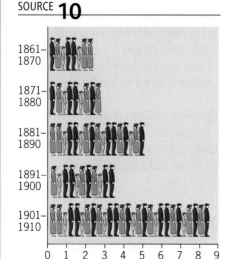

Immigration to the USA, 1861–1910.

Intolerance

At the same time as some young Americans were experiencing liberation, others were facing intolerance and racism.

The vast majority of Americans were either immigrants or descendants of recent immigrants. Source 11 shows you the ethnic background of the main groups.

As you can see from Source 10, immigration to the USA was at an all-time high from 1901 to 1910. Immigrants were flooding in, particularly Jews from eastern Europe and Russia who were fleeing persecution, and people from Italy who were fleeing poverty. Many Italian immigrants did not intend to settle in the USA, but hoped to make money to take back to their families in Italy.

The United States had always prided itself on being a 'melting pot'. In theory, individual groups lost their ethnic identity and blended together with other groups to become just 'Americans'. In practice, however, this wasn't always the case. In the USA's big cities the more established immigrant groups – Irish Americans, French Canadians and German Americans – competed for the best jobs and the best available housing. These groups tended to look down on the more recent eastern European and Italian immigrants. These in turn had nothing but contempt for African Americans and Mexicans, who were almost at the bottom of the scale.

SOURCE **11**

1,200,000	Canada & Newfoundland
700,000	Norway
1,000,000	Sweden
2,700,000	Russia
4,400,000	Germany
5,000,000	Great Britain
2,000,000	Ireland
3,300,000	Austria–Hungary
3,200,000	Italy
400,000	Balkans
600,000	France
200,000	West Indies
50,000	Mexico
250,000	China
175,000	Japan

USA

The ethnic background of Americans in the early 20th century.

The blaze of revolution is eating its way into the homes of the American workman, licking at the altars of the churches, leaping into the belfry of the school house, crawling into the sacred corners of American homes, seeking to replace the marriage vows with libertine laws, burning up the foundations of society.

Mitchell Palmer, US Attorney General, speaking in 1920.

The Red Scare

In the 1920s these racist attitudes towards immigrants were made worse by an increased fear of Bolshevism or Communism. The USA watched with alarm as Russia became Communist after the Russian Revolution of 1917. It feared that many of the more recent immigrants from eastern Europe and Russia were bringing similar radical ideas with them to the USA. This reaction was called the Red Scare.

In 1919 Americans saw evidence all around them to confirm their fears. There was a wave of disturbances. Some 400,000 American workers went on strike. Even the police in Boston went on strike and looters and thieves roamed the city. There were race riots in 25 towns.

Today, most historians argue that the strikes were caused by economic hardship. However, many prominent Americans in the 1920s saw the strikes as the dangerous signs of Communist interference. Fear of Communism combined with prejudice against immigrants was a powerful mix.

The fears were not totally unjustified. Many immigrants in the USA did hold radical political beliefs. Anarchists published pamphlets and distributed them widely in American cities, calling for the overthrow of the government. In April 1919 a bomb planted in a church in Milwaukee killed ten people. In May, bombs were posted to 36 prominent Americans. In June more bombs went off in seven US cities, and one almost succeeded in killing Mitchell Palmer, the US Attorney General. All those known to have radical political beliefs were rounded up. They were generally immigrants and the evidence against them was often flimsy. J. Edgar Hoover, a clerk appointed by Palmers, built up files on 60,000 suspects and in 1919–20 around 10,000 individuals were informed that they were to be deported from the USA.

SOURCE 13

The steamship companies haul them over to America and as soon as they step off the ships the problem of the steamship companies is settled, but our problem has only begun – Bolshevism, red anarchy, black-handers and kidnappers, challenging the authority and integrity of our flag . . . Thousands come here who will never take the oath to support our constitution and become citizens of the USA. They pay allegiance to some other country while they live upon the substance of our own. They fill places that belong to the wage earning citizens of America . . . They are of no service whatever to our people . . . They constitute a menace and a danger to us every day.

Republican Senator Heflin speaking in 1921 in a debate over whether to limit immigration.

SOURCE 14

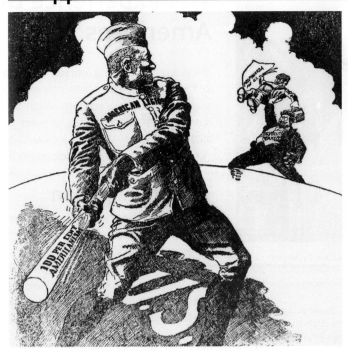

A 1919 cartoon entitled 'Come On!' showing attitudes to Communism in the USA. The character in the black suit looks like Trotsky and has 'Revolution maker' written on his chest. The piece of paper says 'Propaganda for US'.

Source Analysis

Look at Sources 12–14. Do they tell historians more about Communists or the enemies of Communism? Explain your answer.

Think!

Work in pairs.
1 One of you collect evidence to show that the Red Scare was the result of fear of Communism.
2 The other collect evidence to show that the Red Scare was the result of prejudice and intolerance.
3 Now try to come up with a definition of the Red Scare that combines both of your views.

Revision Tip

♦ Make sure you can describe two attacks that sparked off the Red Scare 1919–20.
♦ Make sure you can explain at least one reason for Palmer's downfall.
♦ Practise explaining to someone else why the Sacco and Vanzetti case received so much publicity.

Palmer discovered that these purges were popular, so he tried to use the fear of revolution to build up his own political support and run for president. Trade unionists, African Americans, Jews, Catholics and almost all minority groups found themselves accused of being Communists. In the end, however, Palmer caused his own downfall. He predicted that a Red Revolution would begin in May 1920. When nothing happened, the papers began to make fun of him and officials in the Justice Department who were sickened by Palmer's actions undermined him. Secretary of Labor Louis Post examined Palmer's case files and found that only 556 out of the thousands of cases brought had any basis in fact.

Sacco and Vanzetti

Two high-profile victims of the Red Scare were Italian Americans Nicola Sacco and Bartolomeo Vanzetti. They were arrested in 1920 on suspicion of armed robbery and murder. It quickly emerged that they were self-confessed anarchists. Anarchists hated the American system of government and believed in destroying it by creating social disorder. Their trial became less a trial for murder, more a trial of their radical ideas. The prosecution relied heavily on racist slurs about their Italian origins, and on stirring up fears about their radical beliefs. The judge at the trial said that although Vanzetti 'may not actually have committed the crime attributed to him he is nevertheless morally culpable [to blame] because he is the enemy of our existing institutions'.

Sacco and Vanzetti were convicted on flimsy evidence. A leading lawyer of the time said: 'Judge Thayer is . . . full of prejudice. He has been carried away by fear of Reds which has captured about 90 per cent of the American people.' After six years of legal appeals, Sacco and Vanzetti were executed in 1927, to a storm of protest around the world from both radicals and moderates who saw how unjustly the trial had been conducted. Fifty years later, they were pardoned.

Immigration quotas

In 1924 the government introduced a quota system that ensured that the largest proportion of immigrants was from north-west Europe (mainly British, Irish and German). From a high point of more than a million immigrants a year between 1901 and 1910, by 1929 the number arriving in the USA had fallen to 150,000 per year. No Asians were allowed in at all.

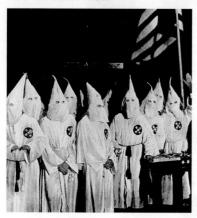
Source Analysis

1 What does Source 15 tell you about the motives of Klan violence?
2 Describe the scene you can see in Source 17 as though you were reporting it on the radio.
3 What does Source 17 reveal about attitudes towards racial violence at this time in the USA?

The experience of African Americans

African Americans had long been part of America's history. The first Africans had been brought to the USA as slaves by white settlers in the seventeenth century. By the time slavery was ended in the nineteenth century, there were more African Americans than white people in the southern United States. White governments, fearing the power of African Americans, introduced many laws to control their freedom. They could not vote. They were denied access to good jobs and to worthwhile education, and well into the twentieth century they suffered great poverty.

The Ku Klux Klan

The Ku Klux Klan was a white supremacy movement. It used violence to intimidate African Americans. It had been in decline, but was revived after the release of the film *The Birth of a Nation* in 1915. The film was set in the 1860s, just after the Civil War. It glorified the Klan as defenders of decent American values against renegade African Americans and corrupt white businessmen. President Wilson had it shown in the White House. He said: 'It is like writing history with lightning. And my only regret is that it is all so terribly true.' With such support from prominent figures, the Klan became a powerful political force in the early 1920s.

SOURCE 15

A lad whipped with branches until his back was ribboned flesh . . . a white girl, divorcee, beaten into unconsciousness in her home; a naturalised foreigner flogged until his back was pulp because he married an American woman; a negro lashed until he sold his land to a white man for a fraction of its value.

RA Patton, writing in *Current History* in 1929, describes the victims of Klan violence in Alabama.

African Americans throughout the south faced fierce racism. For example, in 1930 James Cameron, aged sixteen, had been arrested, with two other African American men, on suspicion of the murder of a white man, and the rape of a white woman. They were in prison in Marion, Indiana. A mob arrived intending to lynch them (hang them without trial). The mob broke down the doors of the jail.

SOURCE 16

A huge and angry mob . . . had gathered from all over the state of Indiana. Ten to fifteen thousand of them at least, against three. Many in the crowd wore the headdress of the Ku Klux Klan.

The cruel hands that held me were vicelike. Fists, clubs, bricks and rocks found their marks on my body. The weaker ones had to be content with spitting. Little boys and little girls not yet in their teens, but being taught how to treat black people, somehow managed to work their way in close enough to bite and scratch me on the legs.

And over the thunderous din rose the shout of 'Nigger! Nigger! Nigger!'

James Cameron, *A Time of Terror*, 1982.

Cameron's two friends were killed. Miraculously Cameron was not. He still does not know what saved him. The crowd had the rope round his neck before they suddenly stopped and let him limp back to the door of the jail. He called it 'a miraculous intervention'.

Profile
Paul Robeson

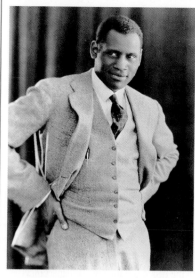

- Born 1898, son of a church minister who had been a former slave.
- Went to Columbia University and passed his law exams with honours in 1923.
- As a black lawyer, it was almost impossible for him to find work, so he became an actor – his big break was in the hit musical 'Showboat'.
- Visited Moscow in 1934 on a world tour and declared his approval of Communism saying 'Here, for the first time in my life, I walk in dignity.'
- As a Communist sympathiser, Robeson suffered in the USA – he was banned from performing, suffered death threats and had his passport confiscated.
- He left the USA in 1958 to live in Europe, but returned in 1963.

Revision Tip

Racial prejudice is a major part of the course. You need to be able to describe:
- two examples of intolerance which African Americans faced.
- at least two ways African Americans responded (look at page 290 as well).

Think!

Read the profile of Paul Robeson. Imagine you are interviewing him on the radio. Write three questions you'd like to ask him.

SOURCE 17

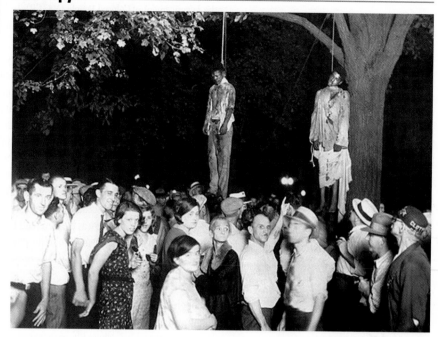

The scene outside the jail in Marion, Indiana. Abram Smith and Thomas Shipp have already been lynched.

Cameron's experience was not unusual. Thousands of African Americans were murdered by lynching in this period. Many reports describe appalling atrocities at which whole families, including young children, clapped and cheered. It is one of the most shameful aspects of the USA at this time.

Faced by such intimidation, discrimination and poverty, many African Americans left the rural south and moved to the cities of the northern USA. Through the 1920s the African American population of both Chicago and New York doubled: New York's from 150,000 to 330,000 and Chicago's from 110,000 to 230,000.

Improvements

In the north, African Americans had a better chance of getting good jobs and a good education. For example, Howard University was an exclusively African American institution for higher education.

In both Chicago and New York, there was a small but growing African American middle class. There was a successful 'black capitalist' movement, encouraging African Americans to set up businesses. In Chicago they ran a successful boycott of the city's chain stores, protesting that they would not shop there unless African American staff were employed. By 1930 almost all the shops in the South Side belt where African Americans lived had black employees.

There were internationally famous African Americans, such as the singer and actor Paul Robeson (see Profile). The popularity of jazz made many African American musicians into high-profile media figures. The African American neighbourhood of Harlem in New York became the centre of the Harlem Renaissance. Here musicians and singers made Harlem a centre of creativity and a magnet for white customers in the bars and clubs. African American artists flourished in this atmosphere, as did African American writers. The poet Langston Hughes wrote about the lives of ordinary working-class African Americans and the poverty and problems they suffered. Countee Cullen was another prominent poet who tried to tackle racism and poverty. In one famous poem ('For A Lady I Know') he tried to sum up attitudes of wealthy white employees to their African American servants:

> She even thinks that up in heaven
> Her class lies late and snores
> While poor black cherubs rise at seven
> To do celestial chores.

African Americans also entered politics. WEB DuBois founded the National Association for the Advancement of Colored People (NAACP). In 1919 it had 300 branches and around 90,000 members. It campaigned to end racial segregation laws and to get laws passed against lynching. It did not make much headway at the time, but the numbers of lynchings did fall.

Another important figure was Marcus Garvey. He founded the Universal Negro Improvement Association (UNIA). Garvey urged African Americans to be proud of their race and colour. He instituted an honours system for African Americans (like the British Empire's honours system of knighthoods). The UNIA helped African Americans to set up their own businesses. By the mid 1920s there were UNIA grocery stores, laundries, restaurants and even a printing workshop.

Garvey set up a shipping line to support both the UNIA businesses and also his scheme of helping African Americans to emigrate to Africa away from white racism. Eventually, his businesses collapsed, partly because he was prosecuted for exaggerating the value of his shares. He was one of very few businessmen to be charged for this offence, and some historians believe that J Edgar Hoover was behind the prosecution. Garvey's movement attracted over 1 million members at its height in 1921. One of these was the Reverend Earl Little. He was beaten to death by Klan thugs in the late 1920s, but his son went on to be the civil rights leader Malcolm X.

Problems

Although important, these movements failed to change the USA dramatically. Life expectancy for African Americans increased from 45 to 48 between 1900 and 1930, but they were still a long way behind the whites, whose life expectancy increased from 54 to 59 over the same period. Many African Americans in the northern cities lived in great poverty. In Harlem in New York they lived in poorer housing than whites, yet paid higher rents. They had poorer education and health services than whites. Large numbers of black women worked as low paid domestic servants. Factories making cars employed few blacks or operated a whites-only policy.

In Chicago African Americans suffered great prejudice from longer-established white residents. If they attempted to move out of the African American belt to adjacent neighbourhoods, they got a hostile reception (see Source 20).

SOURCE 18

If I die in Atlanta my work shall only then begin . . . Look for me in the whirlwind or the storm, look for me all around you, for, with God's grace, I shall come and bring with me countless millions of black slaves who have died in America and the West Indies and the millions in Africa to aid you in the fight for Liberty, Freedom and Life.

Marcus Garvey's last word's before going to jail in 1925.

SOURCE 19

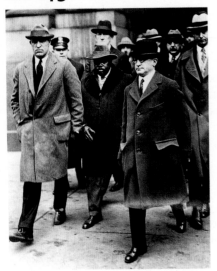

Marcus Garvey after his arrest.

SOURCE 20

There is nothing in the make up of a negro, physically or mentally, that should induce anyone to welcome him as a neighbour. The best of them are unsanitary . . . ruin follows in their path. They are as proud as peacocks, but have nothing of the peacock's beauty . . . Niggers are undesirable neighbours and entirely irresponsible and vicious.

From the *Chicago Property Owners' Journal*, 1920.

They got a similarly hostile reception from poor whites. In Chicago when African Americans attempted to use parks, playgrounds and beaches in the Irish and Polish districts, they were set upon by gangs of whites calling themselves 'athletic clubs'. The result was that African American communities in northern areas often became isolated ghettos.

Within the African American communities prejudice was also evident. Middle-class African Americans who were restless in the ghettos tended to blame newly arrived migrants from the south for intensifying white racism. In Harlem, the presence of some 50,000 West Indians was a source of inter-racial tension. Many of them were better educated, more militant and prouder of their colour than the newly arrived African Americans from the south.

Revision Tip

It is a good idea to prepare your ideas, ready for a question about whether life changed African Americans in the 1920s. Choose two points to help you explain how life improved, and two points to help explain how it did not change or got worse.

Think!

James Cameron, who wrote Source 16 on page 288 went on to found America's Black Holocaust Museum, which records the suffering of black African Americans through American history.

Write a 100-word summary for the museum handbook of the ways in which the 1920s were a time of change for African Americans.

'The vanishing Americans'

The native Americans were the original settlers of the North American continent. They almost disappeared as an ethnic group during the rapid expansion of the USA during the nineteenth century – declining from 1.5 million to around 250,000 in 1920. Those who survived or who chose not to leave their traditional way of life were forced to move to reservations in the mid-west.

SOURCE **21**

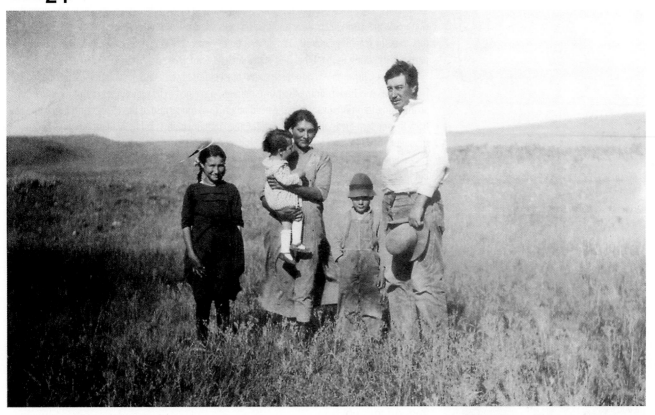

Photograph of a native American, Charlie Guardipee, and his family taken for a US government report of 1921. According to the report Charlie Guardipee had twenty horses, ten cattle, no chickens, no wheat, oats or garden, and no sickness in the family.

Think!

Make two lists:
a) evidence of prejudice and discrimination towards native Americans
b) evidence that the treatment of native Americans was improving in the 1920s.

Revision Tip

Make sure you can describe:
♦ at least two ways in which native Americans suffered in the 1920s.
♦ one improvement.

In the 1920s the government became concerned about the treatment of native Americans. Twelve thousand had served in the armed forces in the First World War, which helped to change white attitudes to them. The government did a census in the 1920s and a major survey in the late 1920s which revealed that most lived in extreme poverty, with much lower life expectancy than whites, that they were in worse health and had poorer education and poorly paid jobs (if they were able to get a job at all). They suffered extreme discrimination. They were quickly losing their land. Mining companies were legally able to seize large areas of native American land. Many native Americans who owned land were giving up the struggle to survive in their traditional way and selling up.

They were also losing their culture. Their children were sent to special boarding schools. The aim of the schools was to 'assimilate' them into white American culture. This involved trying to destroy the native Americans' beliefs, traditions, dances and languages. In the 1920s the native Americans were referred to as 'the vanishing Americans'.

However, the 1920s were in some ways a turning point. In 1924 native Americans were granted US citizenship and allowed to vote for the first time. In 1928 the Merriam Report proposed widespread improvement to the laws relating to native Americans, and these reforms were finally introduced under Roosevelt's New Deal in 1934.

The Monkey Trial

While the Sacco and Vanzetti trial became a public demonstration of anti-immigrant feelings, another trial in the 1920s – the Monkey Trial – became the focus of ill-feeling between rural and urban USA.

Most urban people in the 1920s would have believed in Charles Darwin's theory of evolution. This says that over millions of years human beings evolved from ape-like ancestors.

Many rural Americans, however, disagreed. They were very religious people. They were mostly Protestants. They went to church regularly and believed in the Bible. When the Bible told them that God made the world in six days, and that on the sixth day He created human beings to be like Him, they took the teachings literally. People with these views were known as Fundamentalists. They were particularly strong in the 'Bible Belt' states such as Tennessee.

At school, however, even in these states, most children were taught evolution. Fundamentalists felt that this was undermining their own religion. It seemed to be yet another example of the USA's abandoning traditional values in the headlong rush to modernise in the 1920s. They decided to roll back the modern ideas and so, in six states, the Fundamentalists led by William Jennings Bryan managed to pass a law banning the teaching of 'evolution'.

A biology teacher called John Scopes deliberately broke the law so that he could be arrested and put his case against Fundamentalism in the courts. The best lawyers were brought in for both sides and in July 1925, in the stifling heat of a Tennessee courtroom, the USA's traditionalists joined battle with its modernists.

The trial captured public imagination and the arguments on both sides were widely reported in the press. Scopes was convicted of breaking the law, but it was really American Fundamentalism itself which was on trial – and it lost! At the trial the anti-evolutionists were subjected to great mockery. Their arguments were publicly ridiculed and their spokesman Bryan, who claimed to be an expert on religion and science, was shown to be ignorant and confused. After the trial, the anti-evolution lobby was weakened.

Think!

1 Why do you think the trial became known as the Monkey Trial?
2 In what ways did the trial show American intolerance of other points of view?

Revision Tip

Try to summarise this page in three points:
♦ a reason for the Monkey Trial
♦ description of the trial
♦ results of the trial.

SOURCE 22

. . . for nearly two hours . . . Mr Darrow [lawyer for the defendant] goaded his opponent. [He] asked Mr Bryan if he really believed that the serpent had always crawled on its belly because it tempted Eve, and if he believed Eve was made from Adam's rib . . .

[Bryan's] face flushed under Mr Darrow's searching words, and . . . when one [question] stumped him he took refuge in his faith and either refused to answer directly or said in effect: 'The Bible states it; it must be so.'

From the report of the Monkey Trial in the *Baltimore Evening Sun*, July 1925.

Focus Task

How widespread was intolerance in the 1920s?

You have looked at various examples of intolerance and prejudice in the 1920s.
Draw up a chart like this, and fill it in to summarise the various examples.

Group	Pages	How did intolerance affect them?	How did they react? How did the situation change?
Immigrants	286–87		
Communists	286		
African Americans	288–90		
Native Americans	291		
Evolutionists	292		

Our nation can only be saved by turning the pure stream of country sentiment and township morals to flush out the cesspools of cities and so save civilisation from pollution.

A temperance campaigner speaking in 1917.

Source Analysis ▼

Sources 24 and 25 were published by supporters of prohibition.

Imagine that the examiner for your course is intending to use either source in your exam. Advise the examiner on:
♦ what questions to set on this source
♦ what to expect students to be able to write about the source.

Why was prohibition introduced?

In the nineteenth century, in rural areas of the USA there was a very strong 'temperance' movement. Members of temperance movements agreed not to drink alcohol and also campaigned to get others to give up alcohol. Most members of these movements were devout Christians who saw what damage alcohol did to family life. They wanted to stop that damage.

In the nineteenth century the two main movements were the Anti-Saloon League and the Women's Christian Temperance Union (see Sources 24 and 25).

The temperance movements were so strong in some of the rural areas that they persuaded their state governments to prohibit the sale of alcohol within the state. Through the early twentieth century the campaign gathered pace. It became a national campaign to prohibit (ban) alcohol throughout the country. It acquired some very powerful supporters. Leading industrialists backed the movement, believing that workers would be more reliable if they did not drink. Politicians backed it because it got them votes in rural areas. By 1916, 21 states had banned saloons.

SOURCE **24**

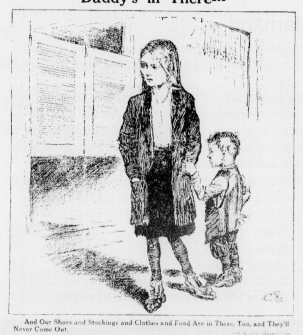

Daddy's in There---

And Our Shoes and Stockings and Clothes and Food Are in There, Too, and They'll Never Come Out.

A poster issued by the Anti-Saloon League in 1915.

SOURCE **25**

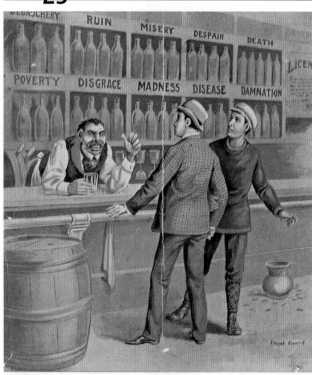

A poster issued by the Women's Christian Temperance Union.

Revision Tip

You should aim to be able to explain at least two reasons why Prohibition was brought in. Ideally, group your reasons under headings like Religion; Patriotism; Health, etc.

Supporters of prohibition became known as 'dries'. The dries brought some powerful arguments to their case. They claimed that '3000 infants are smothered yearly in bed, by drunken parents.' The USA's entry into the First World War in 1917 boosted the dries. Drinkers were accused of being unpatriotic cowards. Most of the big breweries were run by German immigrants who were portrayed as the enemy. Drink was linked to other evils as well. After the Russian Revolution, the dries claimed that Bolshevism thrived on drink and that alcohol led to lawlessness in the cities, particularly in immigrant communities. Saloons were seen as dens of vice that destroyed family life. The campaign became one of country values against city values.

In 1917 the movement had enough states on its side to propose the Eighteenth Amendment to the Constitution. This 'prohibited the manufacture, sale or transportation of intoxicating liquors'. It became law in January 1920 and is known as the Volstead Act.

Think!

1 Prohibition did not actually make it illegal to drink alcohol, only to make or supply it. Why not?
2 Is it possible to enforce any law when the population refuses to obey it? Try to think of laws that affect you today.

What was the impact of prohibition?

Prohibition lasted from 1920 until 1933. It is often said that prohibition was a total failure. This is not entirely correct. Levels of alcohol consumption fell by about 30 per cent in the early 1920s (see Source 26). Prohibition gained widespread approval in some states, particularly the rural areas in the mid-west, although in urban states it was not popular (Maryland never even introduced prohibition). The government ran information campaigns and prohibition agents arrested offenders (see Source 27). Two of the most famous agents were Isadore Einstein and his deputy Moe Smith. They made 4,392 arrests. Their raids were always low key. They would enter speakeasies (illegal bars) and simply order a drink. Einstein had a special flask hidden inside his waistcoat with a funnel attached. He preserved the evidence by pouring his drink down the funnel and the criminals were caught!

SOURCE 26

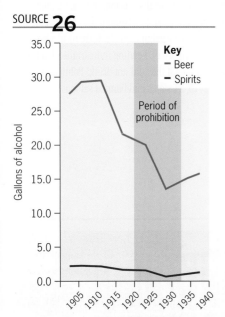

Average alcohol consumption of Americans (in US gallons) per year, 1905–40.

Key
— Beer
— Spirits

Period of prohibition

Gallons of alcohol: 35.0, 30.0, 25.0, 20.0, 15.0, 10.0, 5.0, 0.0

Years: 1905, 1910, 1915, 1920, 1925, 1930, 1935, 1940

SOURCE 27

	1921	1925	1929
Illegal distilleries seized	9,746	12,023	15,794
Gallons (US) of spirit seized	414,000	11,030,000	11,860,000
Arrests	34,175	62,747	66,878

Activities of federal prohibition agents.

Supply and demand

Despite the work of the agents, prohibition proved impossible to enforce effectively in the cities.

Enforcement was underfinanced. There were not enough agents – each agent was poorly paid and was responsible for a huge area.

By far the biggest problem was that millions of Americans, particularly in urban areas, were simply not prepared to obey this law. So bootleggers (suppliers of illegal alcohol) made vast fortunes. Al Capone (see page 296) made around $60 million a year from his speakeasies. His view was that 'Prohibition is a business. All I do is supply a public demand.' And the demand was huge. By 1925 there were more speakeasies in American cities than there had been saloons in 1919. Izzy Einstein filed a report to his superiors on how easy it was to find alcohol after arriving in a new city. Here are the results:

● Chicago: 21 minutes
● Atlanta: 17 minutes
● Pittsburg: 11 minutes
● New Orleans: 35 seconds (he was offered a bottle of whisky by his taxi driver when he asked where he could get a drink!)

SOURCE 28

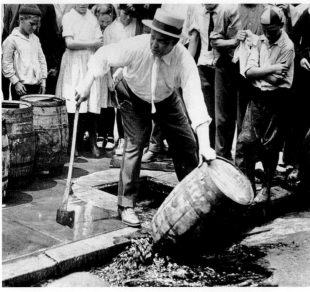

Alcohol being tipped down the drain. Vast quantities of bootleg (illegal) liquor were seized, but were only a fraction of the total.

Source Analysis

Which of Sources 26–28 is the most useful to the historian, or are they more useful when taken together? Explain your answer.

Revision Tip

The main debate about Prohibition is about why it failed. Even so it is worth selecting one or two examples of its success.

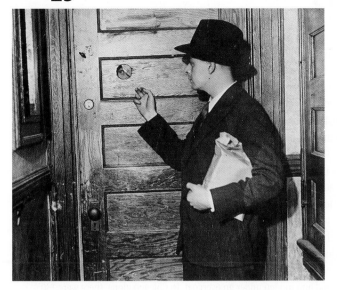

SOURCE **29**

A visit to a speakeasy.

SOURCE **30**

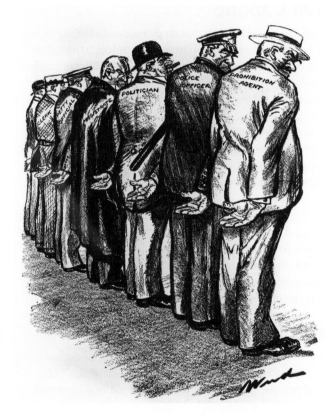

'The National Gesture': a cartoon from the prohibition era.

Illegal stills (short for distilleries) sprang up all over the USA as people made their own illegal whisky – moonshine. The stills were a major fire hazard and the alcohol they produced was frequently poisonous. Agents seized over 280,000 of these stills, but we have no clear way of knowing how many were not seized.

Most Americans had no need for their own still. They simply went to their favourite speakeasy. The speakeasies were well supplied by bootleggers. About two-thirds of the illegal alcohol came from Canada. The vast border between the USA and Canada was virtually impossible to patrol. Other bootleggers brought in alcohol by sea. They would simply wait in the waters outside US control until an opportunity to land their cargo presented itself. One of the most famous was Captain McCoy, who specialised in the finest Scotch whisky. This is where the phrase 'the real McCoy' comes from.

Corruption

Prohibition led to massive corruption. Many of the law enforcement officers were themselves involved with the liquor trade. Big breweries stayed in business throughout the prohibition era. This is not an easy business to hide! But the breweries stayed in operation by bribing local government officials, prohibition agents and the police to leave them alone.

In some cities, police officers were quite prepared to direct people to speakeasies. Even when arrests were made, it was difficult to get convictions because more senior officers or even judges were in the pay of the criminals. One in twelve prohibition agents was dismissed for corruption. The New York FBI boss, Don Chaplin, once ordered his 200 agents: 'Put your hands on the table, both of them. Every son of a bitch wearing a diamond is fired.'

SOURCE **31**

Statistics in the Detroit police court of 1924 show 7391 arrests for violations of the prohibition law, but only 458 convictions. Ten years ago a dishonest policeman was a rarity . . . Now the honest ones are pointed out as rarities . . . Their relationship with the bootleggers is perfectly friendly. They have to pinch two out of five once in a while, but they choose the ones who are least willing to pay bribes.

E Mandeville, in *Outlook* magazine, 1925.

Source Analysis

1 Explain the message of Source 30.
2 Read Source 31. How has prohibition affected the police in Detroit?
3 Which of Sources 30 and 31 do you most trust to give you accurate information about corruption during the Prohibition era?

Revision Tip

Make sure you can use the key terms in an answer about why Prohibition failed: bootlegger, speakeasy, demand, corruption.

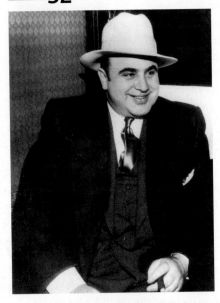

A portrait of Al Capone from 1930.

Gangsters

The most common image people have of the prohibition era is the gangster. Estimates suggest that organised gangs made about $2 billion out of the sale of illegal alcohol. The bootlegger George Remus certainly did well from the trade. He had a huge network of paid officials that allowed him to escape charge after charge against him. At one party he gave a car to each of the women guests, while all the men received diamond cuff links worth $25,000.

The rise of the gangsters tells us a lot about American society at this time. The gangsters generally came from immigrant backgrounds. In the early 1920s the main gangs were Jewish, Polish, Irish and Italian. Gangsters generally came from poorer backgrounds within these communities. They were often poorly educated, but they were also clever and ruthless. Dan O'Banion (Irish gang leader murdered by Capone), Pete and Vince Guizenberg (hired killers who worked for Bugsy Moran and died in the St Valentine's Day Massacre), and Lucky Luciano (Italian killer who spent ten years in prison) were some of the most powerful gangsters. The gangs fought viciously with each other to control the liquor trade and also the prostitution, gambling and protection rackets that were centred on the speakeasies. They made use of new technology, especially automobiles and the Thompson sub-machine gun, which was devastatingly powerful but could be carried around and hidden under an overcoat. In Chicago alone, there were 130 gangland murders in 1926 and 1927 and not one arrest. By the late 1920s fear and bribery made law enforcement ineffective.

Chicago and Al Capone

The gangsters operated all over the USA, but they were most closely associated with Chicago. Perhaps the best example of the power of the gangsters is Chicago gangster boss Al Capone. He arrived in Chicago in 1919, on the run from a murder investigation in New York. He ran a drinking club for his boss Johnny Torio. In 1925 Torio retired after an assassination attempt by one of his rivals, Bugsy Moran. Capone took over and proved to be a formidable gangland boss. He built up a huge network of corrupt officials among Chicago's police, local government workers, judges, lawyers and prohibition agents. He even controlled Chicago's mayor, William Hale Thompson. Surprisingly, he was a high-profile and even popular figure in the city. He was a regular at baseball and American football games and was cheered by the crowd when he took his seat. He was well known for giving generous tips (over $100) to waiters and shop girls and spent $30,000 on a soup kitchen for the unemployed.

Capone was supported by a ruthless gang, hand picked for their loyalty to him. He killed two of his own men whom he suspected of plotting against him by beating their brains out with a baseball bat. By 1929 he had destroyed the power of the other Chicago gangs, committing at least 300 murders in the process. The peak of his violent reign came with the St Valentine's Day Massacre in 1929. Capone's men murdered seven of his rival Bugsy Moran's gang, using a false police car and two gangsters in police uniform to put Moran's men off their guard.

The end of prohibition

The St Valentine's Day Massacre was a turning point. The papers screamed that the gangsters had graduated from murder to massacre. It seemed that prohibition, often called 'The Noble Experiment', had failed. It had made the USA lawless, the police corrupt and the gangsters rich and powerful. When the Wall Street Crash was followed by the Depression in the early 1930s, there were also sound economic arguments for getting rid of it. Legalising alcohol would create jobs, raise tax revenue and free up resources tied up in the impossible task of enforcing prohibition. The Democrat President Franklin D Roosevelt was elected in 1932 and prohibition was repealed in December 1933.

Think!

In other chapters of this book, you have seen profiles of important historical figures.

Use the information and sources to produce two different profiles of Al Capone.

♦ The first profile is the kind of profile that might appear in this book.
♦ The second profile is one that might have appeared inside a news magazine of the time in 1930 after the St Valentine's Day Massacre.

Make sure you can explain to your teacher why the two profiles are different.

These points might be useful to you:

♦ born in 1889 in New York
♦ arrived in Chicago in 1919
♦ took over from Johnny Torio in 1925
♦ jailed in 1931 for not paying taxes
♦ released in January 1939
♦ died in 1947 from syphilis.

Revision Tip

Add these terms to your list of terms you should know how to explain in relation to Prohibition: gangster, Chicago.

Focus Task A

Why did prohibition fail?

In the end prohibition failed. Here are four groups who could be blamed for the failure of prohibition.

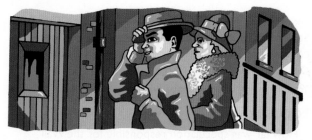

a) the American people who carried on going to illegal speakeasies making prohibition difficult to enforce

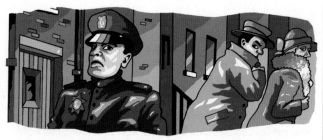

b) the law enforcers who were corrupt and ignored the law breakers

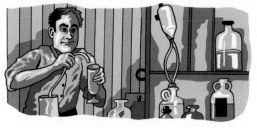

c) the bootleggers who continued supplying and selling alcohol

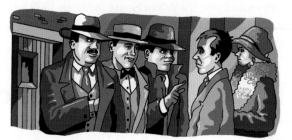

d) the gangsters who controlled the trade through violence and made huge profits

1 For each of the above groups find evidence on pages 293–96 to show that it contributed to the failure of prohibition.

2 Say which group you think played the most important role in the failure. Explain your choice.

3 Draw a diagram to show links between the groups.

Focus Task B

Why was prohibition introduced in 1920 and then abolished in 1933?

Many people who were convinced of the case for prohibition before 1920 were equally convinced that it should be abolished in 1933.
Write two letters.

The first should be from a supporter of prohibition to his or her Congressman in 1919 explaining why the Congressman should vote for prohibition. In your letter, explain how prohibition could help to solve problems in America.

The second should be from the same person to the Congressman in 1933 explaining why the Congressman should vote against prohibition. In your letter, explain why prohibition has failed.

Key Question Summary

How far did US society change in the 1920s?

1 The 'Roaring Twenties' is a name given to this period to get across the sense of vibrancy, excitement and change.

2 The 1920s saw enormous social and cultural change in the cities with new attitudes to behaviour, entertainment, dress styles and morals. This was not shared by many in traditional, conservative rural communities.

3 There was also a growth in prejudice and intolerance, particularly towards new immigrants. This was highlighted by the Sacco and Vanzetti case.

4 The divide between the urban and rural USA was evident in different attitudes to the role of women in society, views on morality and religious values (as shown in the Monkey Trial).

5 In 1920 the manufacture and sale of alcohol was prohibited. But prohibition was difficult to enforce and had disastrous effects, leading to the growth of organised crime, lawlessness and corruption in politics and business.

10.3 What were the causes and consequences of the Wall Street Crash?

Focus

In 1928 there was a presidential election. Nobody doubted that the Republicans would win. The US economy was still booming. After so much success, how could they lose?

They did win, by a landslide, and all seemed well. One of the earliest statements from the new President Herbert Hoover was: 'We in America today are nearer to the final triumph over poverty than ever before'. When Hoover formally moved into the White House in March 1929 he pointed out that Americans had more bathtubs, oil furnaces, silk stockings and bank accounts than any other country.

Six months later it was a very different picture. The Wall Street stock market crashed, the American economy collapsed, and the USA entered a long depression that destroyed much of the prosperity of the 1920s.

You are going to investigate what went wrong.

Focus Points

- How far was speculation responsible for the Wall Street Crash?
- What impact did the Crash have on the economy?
- What were the social consequences of the Crash?
- Why did Roosevelt win the election of 1932?

Factfile

Investment and the stock market

- To set up a company you need money to pay staff, rent premises, buy equipment, etc.
- Most companies raise this money from investors. In return, these investors own a share in the company. They become 'shareholders'.
- These shareholders can get a return on their money in two ways:
  a) by receiving a dividend – a share of the profits made by the company
  b) by selling their shares.
- If the company is successful, the value of the shares is usually higher than the price originally paid for them.
- Investors buy and sell their shares on the stock market. The American stock market was known as Wall Street.
- The price of shares varies from day to day. If more people are buying than selling, then the price goes up. If more are selling than buying, the price goes down.
- For much of the 1920s the price of shares on the Wall Street stock market went steadily upwards.

Revision Tip

Speculation sounds simple but it is not easy to explain.
- Make sure you can describe two examples which show how speculation worked.
- Practise explaining why speculation was attractive to Americans.
- Also practise explaining why it was risky to the US economy.

Causes of the Wall Street Crash

To understand the Wall Street Crash you first need to understand how the stock market is supposed to work (see Factfile).

Speculation

You can see that investment on the stock market would be quite attractive during an economic boom. The American economy was doing well throughout the 1920s. Because the economy kept doing well, there were more share buyers than sellers and the value of shares rose.

It seemed to many Americans that the stock market was an easy and quick way to get rich. Anyone could buy shares, watch their value rise and then sell the shares later at a higher price. Many Americans decided to join the stock market. In 1920 there had been only 4 million share owners in America. By 1929 there were 20 million, out of a population of 120 million (although only about 1.5 million were big investors).

Around 600,000 new investors were speculators. Speculation is a form of gambling. Speculators don't intend to keep their shares for long. They borrow money to buy some shares, then sell them again as soon as the price has risen. They pay off their loan and still have a quick profit to show for it. In the 1920s speculators didn't even have to pay the full value of the shares. They could buy 'on the margin', which meant they only had to put down 10 per cent of the cash needed to buy shares and could borrow the rest. Women became heavily involved in speculation. Women speculators owned over 50 per cent of the Pennsylvania Railroad, which became known as the 'petticoat line'. It was not only individuals who speculated. Banks themselves got involved in speculation. And certainly they did nothing to hold it back. American banks lent $9 billion for speculating in 1929.

Through most of the 1920s the rise in share prices was quite steady. There were even some downturns. But in 1928 speculation really took hold. Demand for shares was at an all-time high, and prices were rising at an unheard-of rate. In March, Union Carbide shares stood at $145. By September 1928 they had risen to $413.

One vital ingredient in all this is confidence. If people are confident that prices will keep rising, there will be more buyers than sellers. However, if they think prices might stop rising, all of a sudden there will be more sellers and . . . crash, the whole structure will come down. This is exactly what happened in 1929.

The stock market hysteria reached its apex that year [1929] . . . Everyone was playing the market . . . On my last day in New York, I went down to the barber. As he removed the sheet he said softly, 'Buy Standard Gas. I've doubled . . . It's good for another double.' As I walked upstairs, I reflected that if the hysteria had reached the barber level, something must soon happen.

Cecil Roberts, *The Bright Twenties*, 1938.

Weaknesses in the US economy

The construction industry (one of the leading signs of health in any economy) had actually started its downturn as far back as 1926. You have already seen how farming was in trouble in the 1920s. You have also seen the decline in coal, textile and other traditional trades. There were other concerns, such as the unequal distribution of wealth and the precarious state of some banks. In the decade before the Crash, over 500 banks had failed each year. These were mainly small banks who lent too much.

By 1929 other sectors of the economy were showing signs of strain after the boom years of the 1920s. The boom was based on the increased sale of consumer goods such as cars and electrical appliances. There were signs that American industries were producing more of these goods than they could sell. The market for these goods was largely the rich and the middle classes. By 1929 those who could afford consumer goods had already bought them. The majority of Americans who were poor could not afford to buy them, even on the generous hire purchase and credit schemes on offer.

Companies tried high-pressure advertising. In 1929 American industry spent a staggering $3 billion on magazine advertising. But with workers' wages not rising and prices not falling, demand decreased.

In the past, American industry would have tried to export its surplus goods. But people in Europe could not afford American goods either. In addition, after nine years of American tariffs, Europe had put up its own tariffs to protect its industries.

By the summer of 1929 these weaknesses were beginning to show. Even car sales were slowing, and in June 1929 the official figures for industrial output showed a fall for the first time for four years. Speculators on the American stock exchange became nervous about the value of their shares and began to sell.

As you can see from the Factfile, the slide in share values started slowly. But throughout September and October it gathered pace. Many investors had borrowed money to buy their shares and could not afford to be stuck with shares worth less than the value of their loan. Soon other investors sold their shares and within days panic set in. On Tuesday 29 October 1929 it became clear to the speculators that the banks were not going to intervene to support the price of shares, and so Wall Street had its busiest and its worst day in history as speculators desperately tried to dump 13 million shares at a fraction of the price they had paid for them.

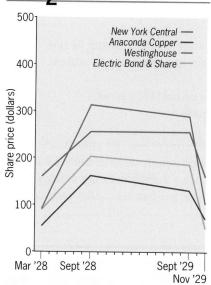

New York Central —
Anaconda Copper —
Westinghouse —
Electric Bond & Share —

Selected share prices, 1928–29.

Factfile

The Wall Street Crash, 1929

➤ **June** Factory output starts declining. Steel production starts declining.

➤ **3 Sept** The hottest day of the year. The last day of rising prices.

➤ **5 Sept** 'The Babson Break': Roger Babson, economic forecaster, says 'Sooner or later a crash is coming and it may be terrific.' The index of share prices drops ten points.

➤ **6 Sept** Market recovers.

➤ **Mon 21 Oct** Busy trading. Much selling. So much trading that the 'ticker' which tells people of changes in price falls behind by 1½ hours. Some people don't know they are ruined until after the exchange closes. By then it is too late to do anything about it.

➤ **Thu 24 Oct** Busiest trading yet. Big falls. Banks intervene to buy stock. Confidence returns. Prices stabilise.

➤ **Mon 28 Oct** Massive fall. Index loses 43 points. It is clear that the banks have stopped supporting share prices.

➤ **Tue 29 Oct** Massive fall. People sell for whatever they can get.

Revision Tip

Make sure you can describe:
♦ two weaknesses in the US economy in the late 1920s.
♦ two events leading up to the Crash.

Focus Task

How far was speculation responsible for the Wall Street Crash?

Work in groups.

1 Here are five factors that led to the Wall Street Crash. For each one explain how it helped to cause the Crash:
   ♦ poor distribution of income between rich and poor
   ♦ overproduction by American industries
   ♦ the actions of speculators
   ♦ no export market for US goods
   ♦ decision by the banks not to support share prices.

2 If you think other factors are also important, add them to your list and explain why they helped to cause the Crash.

3 Decide whether there is one factor that is more important than any of the others. Explain your choice.

The economic consequences of the Wall Street Crash

At first, it was not clear what the impact of the Crash would be. In the short term, the large speculators were ruined. The rich lost most because they had invested most. For example:

- The Vanderbilt family lost $40 million.
- Rockefeller lost 80 per cent of his wealth – but he still had $40 million left.
- The British politician Winston Churchill lost $500,000.
- The singer Fanny Brice lost $500,000.
- Groucho and Harpo Marx (two of the Marx Brothers comedy team) lost $240,000 each.

They had always been the main buyers of American goods, so there was an immediate downturn in spending. Many others had borrowed money in order to buy shares that were now worthless. They were unable to pay back their loans to the banks and insurance companies, so they went bankrupt. Some banks themselves also went bankrupt.

SOURCE 3

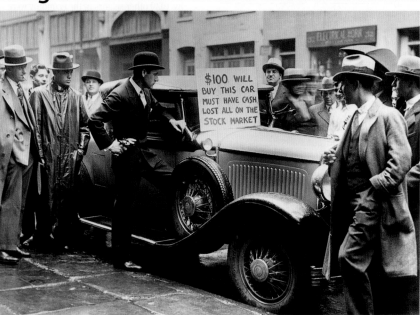

An attempt to make some cash after the Wall Street Crash, 1929.

At first, however, these seemed like tragic but isolated incidents. President Hoover reassured the nation that prosperity was 'just around the corner'. He cut taxes to encourage people to buy more goods and by mid 1931 production was rising again slightly and there was hope that the situation was more settled.

In fact, it was the worst of the Depression that was 'just around the corner', because the Crash had destroyed the one thing that was crucial to the prosperity of the 1920s: confidence.

This was most marked in the banking crisis. In 1929, 659 banks failed. As banks failed people stopped trusting them and many withdrew their savings. In 1930 another 1,352 went bankrupt. The biggest of these was the Bank of the United States in New York, which went bankrupt in December 1930. It had 400,000 depositors – many of them recent immigrants. Almost one-third of New Yorkers saved with it. This was the worst failure in American history. To make matters worse, 1931 saw escalating problems in European banks, which had a knock-on effect in the USA. Panic set in. Around the country a billion dollars was withdrawn from banks and put in safe deposit boxes, or stored at home. People felt that hard currency was the only security. Another 2,294 banks went under in 1931.

Revision Tip

The impact of the Crash is a big theme. There are so many examples to choose from it is helpful to narrow it down.

- Choose four examples and make sure you can describe those thoroughly.
- Make sure at least one of your examples is about the collapse of banks and one is about unemployment.

SOURCE 4

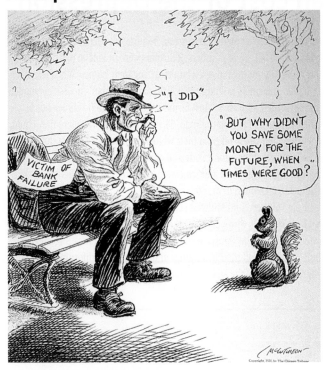

A cartoon by American cartoonist John McCutcheon, 1932. The man on the bench has lost all his savings because of a bank failure.

So while Hoover talked optimistically about the return of prosperity, Americans were showing their true feelings. They now kept their money instead of buying new goods or shares. Of course, this meant that banks had less money to give out in loans to businesses or to people as mortgages on homes. What is worse is that banks were calling in loans from businesses, which they needed to keep running, so even more businesses collapsed or cut back. The downward spiral was firmly established. Businesses cut production further and laid off more workers. They reduced the wages of those who still worked for them. Between 1928 and 1933 both industrial and farm production fell by 40 per cent, and average wages by 60 per cent.

As workers were laid off or were paid less, they bought even less. This reduction in spending was devastating. The American economy had been geared up for mass consumption and relied on continued high spending. Now this was collapsing and fewer goods bought equated to fewer jobs. By 1932 the USA was in the grip of the most serious economic depression the world had ever seen. By 1933 there were 14 million unemployed, and 5,000 banks had gone bankrupt. The collapse in the urban areas soon had an impact on the countryside. Farm prices were already low before the Crash for the reasons we saw on page 278. Now people in the towns could not afford to buy so much food and the prices went into freefall. Soon they were so low that the cost of transporting animals to market was higher than the price of the animals themselves. Total farm income had slipped to just $5 billion. The USA could have sold more products to other countries but they were also affected by the Crash. Also, because the US government had put tariffs on imported goods, these countries could not sell their goods in America and earn the dollars to buy American goods. The USA's international trade was drastically reduced from $10 billion in 1929 to $3 billion in 1932 – another blow to the US economy.

Source Analysis

Look at Source 4. Do you think the cartoonist is sympathetic or critical of the man on the bench? Explain your opinion.

Focus Task

What impact did the Crash have on the American economy?

You can see how a downward spiral was started by the Crash. Draw a diagram with notes to explain how the following were connected to each other. Show how the effect they had on one another continued to make the economic situation worse over time.

♦ Wall Street Crash
♦ the banking crisis
♦ business failure or contraction
♦ wage cuts and unemployment
♦ reduced spending.

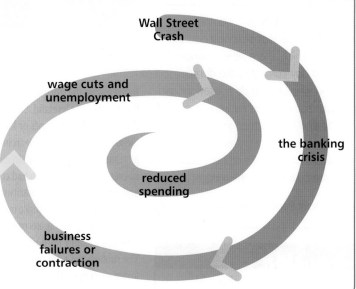

SOURCE 5

During the last three months I have visited . . . some 20 states of this wonderfully rich and beautiful country. A number of Montana citizens told me of thousands of bushels of wheat left in the fields uncut on account of its low price that hardly paid for the harvesting. In Oregon I saw thousands of bushels of apples rotting in the orchards. At the same time there are millions of children who, on account of the poverty of their parents, will not eat one apple this winter.

. . . I saw men picking for meat scraps in the garbage cans of the cities of New York and Chicago. One man said that he had killed 3,000 sheep this fall and thrown them down the canyon because it cost $1.10 to ship a sheep and then he would get less than a dollar for it.

The farmers are being pauperised [made poor] by the poverty of industrial populations and the industrial populations are being pauperised by the poverty of the farmers. Neither has the money to buy the product of the other; hence we have overproduction and under-consumption at the same time.

Evidence of Oscar Ameringer to a US government committee in 1932.

SOURCE 7

Last summer, in the hot weather, when the smell was sickening and the flies were thick, there were a hundred people a day coming to the dumps . . . a widow who used to do housework and laundry, but now had no work at all, fed herself and her fourteen-year-old son on garbage. Before she picked up the meat she would always take off her glasses so that she couldn't see the maggots.

From *New Republic* magazine, February 1933.

Revision Tip

As with the economic effects of the Crash, the key here is to focus. Choose three examples of hardships and make sure you can describe those thoroughly. Make sure at least one of your examples is about Hoovervilles.

The human cost of the Depression

People in agricultural areas were hardest hit by the Depression, because the 1920s had not been kind to them anyway. As farm income fell, huge numbers of farmers were unable to pay their mortgages. Some farmers organised themselves to resist banks seizing their homes. When sheriffs came to seize their property, bands of farmers holding pitch forks and hangman's nooses persuaded the sheriffs to retreat. Others barricaded highways. Most farmers, however, had no choice but to pack their belongings into their trucks and live on the road. They picked up work where they could. Black farmers and labourers were often worse off than their white neighbours. They lost their land and their farms first. Hunger stalked the countryside and children fell ill and died from malnutrition. Yet this was happening while wheat and fruit were left to rot and animals killed because farmers could not afford to take them to market.

But worse was to come in the Southern and Midwest states where over-farming and drought caused the topsoil to turn to dust. This was whipped up by the wind to create an area known as the dustbowl. The dust covered everything, as Source 6 shows; it got into every crack and crevice making life unbearable. Many packed up all their belongings and headed for California to look for work. The plight of these migrants is one of the enduring impressions of the Depression.

SOURCE 6

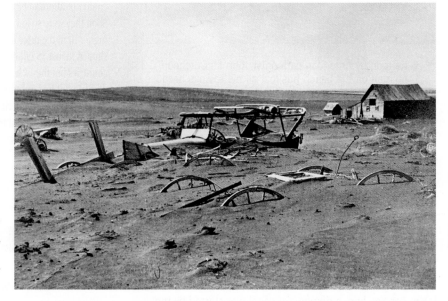

A dustbowl farm. Overfarming, drought and poor conservation turned farmland into desert.

In the towns, the story was not much better. Unemployment rose rapidly. For example, in 1932 in the steel city of Cleveland, 50 per cent of workers were now unemployed and in Toledo 80 per cent. Forced to sell their homes or kicked out because they could not pay the rent, city workers joined the army of unemployed searching for work of any kind. Thousands were taken in by relatives but many ended up on the streets. At night the parks were full of the homeless and unemployed. In every city, workers who had contributed to the prosperity of the 1920s now queued for bread and soup dished out by charity workers. A large number of men (estimated at 2 million in 1932) travelled from place to place on railway freight wagons seeking work. Thousands of children could be found living in wagons or on tents next to the tracks. Every town had a so-called Hooverville. This was a shanty town of ramshackle huts where the migrants lived, while they searched for work. The rubbish tips were crowded with families hoping to scrape a meal from the leftovers of more fortunate people. Through 1931, 238 people were admitted to hospital in New York suffering from malnutrition or starvation. Forty-five of them died.

SOURCE 8

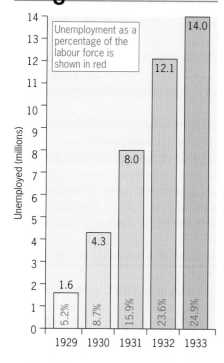

Unemployment in the USA, 1929–33.

Chart showing unemployment (millions) with unemployment as a percentage of the labour force shown in red:

Year	Unemployed (millions)	Percentage
1929	1.6	5.2%
1930	4.3	8.7%
1931	8.0	15.9%
1932	12.1	23.6%
1933	14.0	24.9%

SOURCE 9

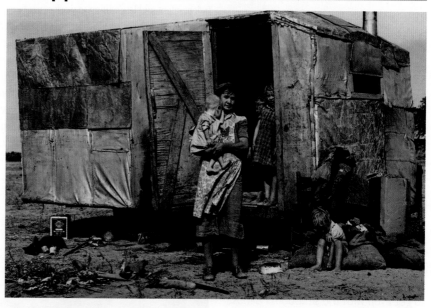

A Hooverville shanty town on wasteland in Seattle, Washington.

SOURCE 10

There is not an unemployed man in the country that hasn't contributed to the wealth of every millionaire in America. The working classes didn't bring this on, it was the big boys . . . We've got more wheat, more corn, more food, more cotton, more money in the banks, more everything in the world than any nation that ever lived ever had, yet we are starving to death. We are the first nation in the history of the world to go to the poorhouse in an automobile.

Will Rogers, an American writer, 1931. Rogers had a regular humorous column in an American magazine which was popular with ordinary people.

SOURCE 11

A migrant family.

Source Analysis

1 Read Source 10. What do you think Will Rogers means by 'the big boys?'
2 Explain how a writer such as Rogers can be useful to a historian studying the impact of the Depression in the 1930s.

Focus Task

What were the social consequences of the Crash?

1 You have been asked to prepare an exhibition of photos which compares the life of Americans during the boom times of the 1920s with the depressed years of the 1930s. Choose two pictures from the 1920s and two from the 1930s which you think present the greatest contrast. Explain your choice.
2 Do you think everyone suffered equally from the Depression? Explain your answer by referring to Sources 5–11. In particular, think about how the effects of the Depression in the countryside were different/similar to those in the towns and cities.

Source Analysis ▼

1 Source 12 had a very powerful effect on Americans. Explain why.
2 From Sources 13 and 14 make a list of criticisms of Hoover and his government.

The 1932 presidential election

In the 1932 election President Hoover paid the price for being unable to solve the problems of the Depression. It was partly his own fault. Until 1932 he refused to accept that there was a major problem. He insisted that 'prosperity is just around the corner'. This left him open to bitter criticisms such as Source 14. A famous banner carried in a demonstration of Iowa farmers said: 'In Hoover we trusted and now we are busted.'

Hoover was regarded as a 'do nothing' President. This was not entirely fair on Hoover. He tried to restart the economy in 1930 and 1931 by tax cuts. He tried to persuade business leaders not to cut wages. He set up the Reconstruction Finance Company, which propped up banks to stop them going bankrupt. He did put money into public works programmes, e.g. the Hoover Dam on the Colorado River, but too little to have a real impact on unemployment. He tried to protect US industries by introducing tariffs, but this simply strangled international trade and made the Depression worse.

To most observers these measures looked like mere tinkering. The measures the government was taking did not match up to the scale of the problems the country was facing. Hoover and most Republicans were very reluctant to change their basic policies. They believed that the main cause of the Depression had been economic problems in Europe, not weaknesses in the USA's economy. They said that business should be left alone to bring back prosperity. Government help was not needed. They argued that business went in cycles of boom and bust, and therefore prosperity would soon return. In 1932 Hoover blocked the Garner–Wagner Relief Bill, which would have allowed Congress to provide $2.1 billion to create jobs.

Even more damaging to Hoover's personal reputation, however, was how little he tried to help people who were suffering because of the Depression. He believed that social security was not the responsibility of the government. Relief should be provided by local government or charities. The Republicans were afraid that if the government helped individuals, they would become less independent and less willing to work.

Hoover's reputation was particularly damaged by an event in June 1932. Thousands of servicemen who had fought in the First World War marched on Washington asking for their war bonuses (a kind of pension) to be paid early. The marchers camped peacefully outside the White House and sang patriotic songs. Hoover refused to meet them. He appointed General Douglas MacArthur to handle the situation. MacArthur convinced himself (with little or no evidence) that they were Communist agitators. He ignored Hoover's instructions to treat the marchers with respect. Troops and police used tear gas and burned the marchers' camps. Hoover would not admit he had failed to control MacArthur. He publicly thanked God that the USA still knew how to deal with a mob.

SOURCE 12

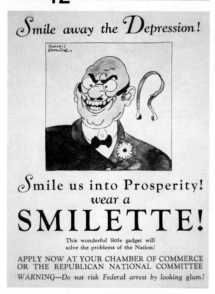

A 1932 Democrat election poster.

SOURCE 13

Never before in this country has a government fallen . . . so low . . . in popular estimation or been [such] an object of cynical contempt. Never before has [a President] given his name so freely to latrines and offal dumps, or had his face banished from the [cinema] screen to avoid the hoots and jeers of children.

Written by a political commentator.

SOURCE 14

Farmers are just ready to do anything to get even with the situation. I almost hate to express it, but I honestly believe that if some of them could buy airplanes they would come down here to Washington to blow you fellows up . . . The farmer is a naturally conservative individual, but you cannot find a conservative farmer today. Any economic system that has in its power to set me and my wife in the streets, at my age what can I see but red?

President of the Farmers' Union of Wisconsin, AN Young, speaking to a Senate committee in 1932.

SOURCE 15

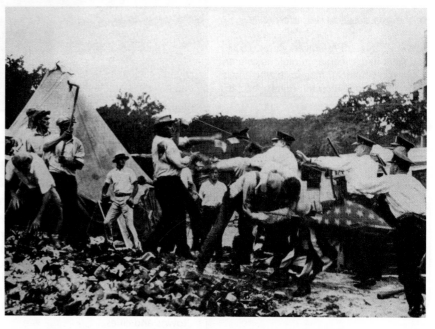

Police attacking the war bonus marchers.

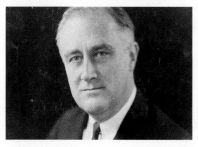
Franklin D Roosevelt

There could be no greater contrast to Hoover than his opponent in the 1932 election, the Democrat candidate, Franklin D Roosevelt. Roosevelt's main characteristics as a politician were:

- He was not a radical, but he believed in 'active government' to improve the lives of ordinary people although only as a last resort if self-help and charity had failed.
- He had plans to spend public money on getting people back to work. As Governor of New York, he had already started doing this in his own state.
- He was not afraid to ask for advice on important issues from a wide range of experts, such as factory owners, union leaders and economists.

The campaign

With such ill-feeling towards Hoover being expressed throughout the country, Roosevelt was confident of victory, but he took no chances. He went on a grand train tour of the USA in the weeks before the election and mercilessly attacked the attitude of Hoover and the Republicans.

Roosevelt's own plans were rather vague and general (see Source 16). But he realised people wanted action, whatever that action was. In a 20,800 km campaign trip he made sixteen major speeches and another 60 from the back of his train. He promised the American people a 'New Deal'. It was not only his policies that attracted support; it was also his personality. He radiated warmth and inspired confidence. He made personal contact with the American people and seemed to offer hope and a way out of the terrible situation they were in.

The election was a landslide victory for Roosevelt. He won by 7 million votes and the Democrats won a majority of seats in Congress. It was the worst defeat the Republicans had ever suffered.

Key Question Summary

What were the causes and consequences of the Wall Street Crash?

1. In October 1929 the Wall Street stock market crashed with a devastating impact on America and the rest of the world.
2. The Crash was partly to do with uncontrolled speculation but it was also the result of underlying weaknesses in the American economy; in particular, industry was overproducing goods which it could not sell.
3. The main consequences for the economy were huge losses for investors, bank failures, factories closing, mass unemployment, the collapse of farm prices and a drastic reduction in foreign trade.
4. The human cost was devastating: unemployment, homelessness, poverty and hunger. Families were split and 'Hoovervilles' appeared on the edges of cities.
5. Farmers lost their land and were dispossessed. Poverty was rampant in rural areas. Matters were made even worse by the dustbowl, which led to mass migration from central southern America to California.
6. President Hoover was unable to deal with the crisis. He believed that government should not interfere too much: the system would repair itself. The measures he undertook were too little too late and he did not do enough to provide relief to those who were suffering.
7. In 1932, Americans elected Franklin D Roosevelt as President. He promised a New Deal to help people and get America back to work.

SOURCE 16

Millions of our citizens cherish the hope that their old standards of living have not gone forever. Those millions shall not hope in vain. . . . I pledge myself, to a New Deal for the American people. This is more than a political campaign; it is a call to arms. Give me your help, not to win votes alone, but to win this crusade to restore America . . . I am waging a war against Destruction, Delay, Deceit and Despair . . .

Roosevelt's pre-election speech, 1932.

Revision Tip

Make sure you can describe:

♦ two actions taken by Hoover
♦ two factors which damaged Hoover
♦ two reasons why people supported Roosevelt.

Focus Task

Why did Roosevelt win the 1932 election?

In many ways Roosevelt's victory needs no explanation. Indeed, it would have been very surprising if any President could have been re-elected after the sufferings of 1929–32. But it is important to recognise the range of factors that helped Roosevelt and damaged Hoover.

Write your own account of Roosevelt's success under the following headings:

♦ The experiences of ordinary people, 1929–32
♦ The policies of the Republicans
♦ Actions taken by the Republicans
♦ Roosevelt's election campaign and personality.

10.4 How successful was the New Deal?

Focus

During his election campaign Roosevelt had promised the American people a New Deal. It was not entirely clear what measures that might include. What was clear was that Franklin D Roosevelt planned to use the full power of the government to get the US out of depression. He set out his priorities as follows:

♦ getting Americans back to work
♦ protecting their savings and property
♦ providing relief for the sick, old and unemployed

♦ getting American industry and agriculture back on their feet.

In 10.4 you will examine how far he succeeded.

Focus Points

♦ What was the New Deal as introduced in 1933?
♦ How far did the character of the New Deal change after 1933?
♦ Why did the New Deal encounter opposition?
♦ Why did unemployment persist despite the New Deal?
♦ Did the fact that the New Deal did not solve unemployment mean that it was a failure?

SOURCE 1

This is the time to speak the truth frankly and boldly . . . So let me assert my firm belief that the only thing we have to fear is fear itself – nameless, unreasoning, unjustified terror which paralyses efforts to convert retreat into advance . . . This nation calls for action and action now . . . Our greatest primary task is to put people to work . . . We must act and act quickly.

Roosevelt's inauguration speech, 4 March 1933.

SOURCE 2

The bank rescue of 1933 was probably the turning point of the Depression. When people were able to survive the shock of having all the banks closed, and then see the banks open up again, with their money protected, there began to be confidence. Good times were coming. It marked the revival of hope.

Raymond Moley, one of Roosevelt's advisers during the Hundred Days Congress session.

Revision Tip

The various agencies can be a bit confusing. Make sure you can describe the aims and the work of at least the National Industrial Recovery Act and the Tennessee Valley Authority.

The Hundred Days

In the first hundred days of his presidency, Roosevelt worked round the clock with his advisers (who became known as the 'Brains Trust') to produce an enormous range of sweeping measures.

One of the many problems affecting the USA was its loss of confidence in the banks.

The day after his inauguration Roosevelt ordered all of the banks to close and to remain closed until government officials had checked them over. A few days later 5,000 trustworthy banks were allowed to reopen. They were even supported by government money if necessary. At the same time, Roosevelt's advisers had come up with a set of rules and regulations which would prevent the reckless speculation that had contributed to the Wall Street Crash.

These two measures, the **Emergency Banking Act** and the **Securities Exchange Commission**, gave the American people a taste of what the New Deal was to look like, but there was a lot more to come. One of Roosevelt's advisers at this time said, 'During the whole Hundred Days Congress, people didn't know what was going on, but they knew something was happening, something good for them.' In the Hundred Days, Roosevelt sent fifteen proposals to Congress and all fifteen were adopted. Just as importantly, he took time to explain to the American people what he was doing and why he was doing it. Every Sunday he would broadcast on radio to the nation. An estimated 60 million Americans tuned in to these **'fireside chats'**. Nowadays, we are used to politicians doing this. At that time it was a new development.

The **Federal Emergency Relief Administration** tackled the urgent needs of the poor. $500 million was spent on soup kitchens, blankets, employment schemes and nursery schools.

The **Civilian Conservation Corps** (CCC) was aimed at unemployed young men. They could sign on for periods of six months, which could be renewed if they could still not find work. Most of the work done by the CCC was on environmental projects in national parks. The money earned generally went back to the men's families. Around 2.5 million were helped by this scheme.

The **Agricultural Adjustment Administration** (AAA) tried to take a long-term view of the problems facing farmers. It set quotas to reduce farm production in order to force prices gradually upwards. At the same time, the AAA helped farmers to modernise and to use farming methods that would conserve and protect the soil. In cases of extreme hardship, farmers could also receive help with their mortgages. The AAA certainly helped farmers, although modernisation had the unfortunate effect of putting more farm labourers out of work.

The final measure of the Hundred Days passed on 18 June was the **National Industrial Recovery Act** (NIRA). It set up two important organisations. The **Public Works Administration** (PWA) used government money to build schools, roads, dams, bridges and airports. These would be vital once the USA had recovered, and in the short term they created millions of jobs. The **National Recovery Administration** (NRA) improved working conditions in industry and outlawed child labour. It also set out fair wages and sensible levels of production. The idea was to stimulate the economy by giving workers money to spend, without overproducing and causing a slump. It was voluntary, but firms which joined used the blue eagle as a symbol of presidential approval. Over 2 million employers joined the scheme.

SOURCE 3

A

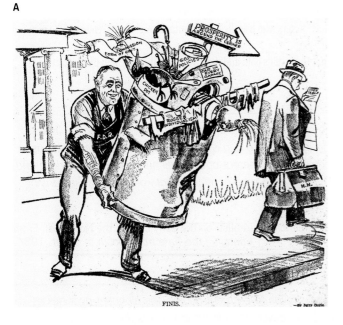

FINIS.

B

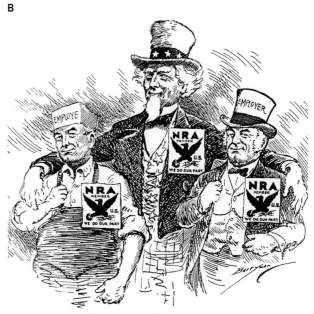

Two 1933 American cartoons.

Source Analysis

Look carefully at the two cartoons in Source 3A and 3B.

1 Use the text on pages 304–307 to help you to understand all the details. You could annotate your own copy.
2 Put the message of each cartoon into your own words.

The Tennessee Valley Authority

As you can see from Source 4, the Tennessee Valley was a huge area that cut across seven states. The area had great physical problems. In the wet season, the Tennessee river would flood. In the dry it would reduce to a trickle. The farming land around the river was a dust bowl. The soil was eroding and turning the land into desert. The area also had great social problems. Within the valley people lived in poverty. The majority of households had no electricity. The problems of the Tennessee Valley were far too large for one state to deal with and it was very difficult for states to co-operate.

Roosevelt therefore set up an independent organisation called the **Tennessee Valley Authority** (TVA), which cut across the powers of the local state governments. The main focus of the TVA's work was to build a series of dams on the Tennessee river (see Source 5). They transformed the region. The dams made it possible to irrigate the dried-out lands. They also provided electricity for this underdeveloped area. Above all, building the dams created thousands of jobs in an area badly hit by the Depression.

SOURCE 4

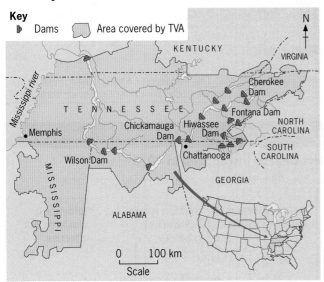

The Tennessee Valley and the work of the TVA.

SOURCE 5

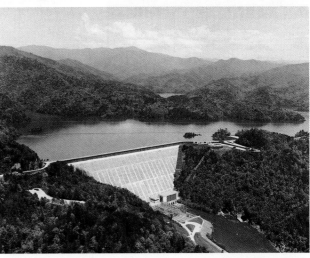

The Fontana Dam, one of the TVA's later projects. Dams such as these revitalised farmland, provided jobs and brought electric power to the area.

Source Analysis

1 What do Sources 6–8 agree about?
2 What do they disagree about?

Revision Tip

There was a lot of activity in the Hundred Days but you need to focus on effects. Make sure you can give examples of at least three ways the Hundred Days had an impact on Americans.

Impact

The measures introduced during the Hundred Days had an immediate effect. They restored confidence in government. Reporters who travelled the country brought back reports of the new spirit to be seen around the USA.

Historians too agree that Roosevelt's bold and decisive action did have a marked effect on the American people.

SOURCE 6

Wandering around the country with one of New York's baseball teams, I find that [what was] the national road to ruin is now a thriving thoroughfare. It has been redecorated. People have come out of the shell holes. They are working and playing and seem content to let a tribe of professional worriers do their worrying for them.

Rudd Rennie, an American journalist, on the early days of the New Deal. From *Changing the Tune from Gloom to Cheer*, 1934.

SOURCE 7

The CCC, the PWA, and similar government bodies (the alphabet agencies as Americans called them) made work for millions of people. The money they earned began to bring back life to the nation's trade and businesses. More customers appeared in the shops . . . As people started to buy again, shopkeepers, farmers and manufacturers began to benefit from the money the government was spending on work for the unemployed. This process was described by Roosevelt as 'priming the pump'. By this he meant that the money the Federal Government was spending was like a fuel, flowing into the nation's economic machinery and starting it moving again.

DB O'Callaghan, *Roosevelt and the USA*, published in 1966.

SOURCE 8

As Roosevelt described it, the 'New Deal' meant that the forgotten man, the little man, the man nobody knew much about, was going to be dealt better cards to play with . . . He understood that the suffering of the Depression had fallen with terrific impact upon the people least able to bear it. He knew that the rich had been hit hard too, but at least they had something left. But the little merchant, the small householder and home owner, the farmer, the man who worked for himself — these people were desperate. And Roosevelt saw them as principal citizens of the United States, numerically and in their importance to the maintenance of the ideals of American democracy.

Frances Perkins, *The Roosevelt I Knew*, 1947. Perkins was Labour Secretary under Roosevelt from 1933.

Focus Task

What was the New Deal as introduced in 1933?

Look back over pages 306–08 and complete your own copy of this table.

New Deal measure/agency	Issue/problem it aimed to tackle	Action taken/ powers of agency	Evidence it was/was not effective

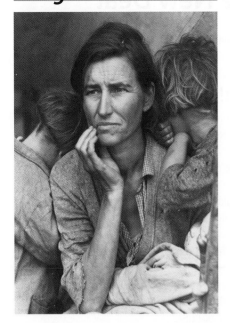

Migrant Mother (number 6) by Dorothea Lange, taken in Nipomo, California, March 1936. Many farmers migrated to California where farming had been less badly hit by the Depression.

The Second New Deal

Despite his achievements, by May 1935 Roosevelt was facing a barrage of criticism. Some critics (like Senator Huey Long, see page 310) complained that he was doing too little, others (mainly the wealthy business sector) too much. The USA was recovering less quickly than Europe. Business was losing its enthusiasm for the NRA (for example Henry Ford had cut wages). Roosevelt was unsure what to do. He had hoped to transform the USA, but it didn't seem to be working.

Tuesday, 14 May 1935 turned out to be a key date. Roosevelt met with a group of senators and close advisers who shared his views and aims. They persuaded him to take radical steps to achieve his vision and make the USA a fairer place for all Americans (see Source 8). One month later, he presented the leaders of Congress with a huge range of laws that he wanted passed. This became known as the Second New Deal and was aimed at areas that affected ordinary people – for example strengthening unions to fight for the members' rights, financial security in old age – as well as continuing to tackle unemployment. The most significant aspects were:

The **Wagner Act** forced employers to allow trade unions in their companies and to let them negotiate pay and conditions. It made it illegal to sack workers for being in a union.

The **Social Security Act** provided state pensions for the elderly and for widows. It also allowed state governments to work with the federal government to provide help for the sick and the disabled. Most importantly, the Act set up a scheme for unemployment insurance. Employers and workers made a small contribution to a special fund each week. If workers became unemployed, they would receive a small amount to help them out until they could find work.

The **Works Progress Administration (WPA)**, later renamed the Works Project Administration, brought together all the organisations whose aim was to create jobs. It also extended this work beyond building projects to create jobs for office workers and even unemployed actors, artists and photographers. The photograph in Source 9 was taken by a photographer working for the Farm Security Administration. This project took 80,000 photos of farming areas during the New Deal. Source 10 was produced by an artist working for the Federal Arts Project. The government paid artists to paint pictures to be displayed in the city or town they featured.

The **Resettlement Administration (RA)** helped smallholders and tenant farmers who had not been helped by the AAA. This organisation moved over 500,000 families to better-quality land and housing. The **Farm Security Administration (FSA)** replaced the RA in 1937. It gave special loans to small farmers to help them buy their land. It also built camps to provide decent living conditions and work for migrant workers.

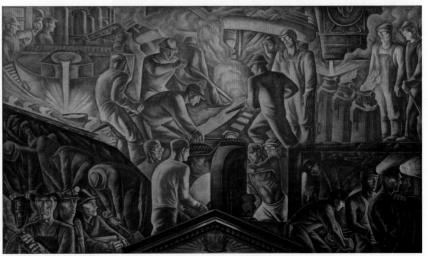

Steel Industry by Howard Cook, painted for the steel-making town of Pittsburgh, Pennsylvania.

Focus Task

How far did the character of the New Deal change after 1933?

Draw up two spider diagrams to compare the objectives and measures of the New Deal and the Second New Deal. Then explain how the measures of the Second New Deal were different from those in 1933.

Revision Tip

For the Second New Deal the key measures are the Wagner Act and the Social Security Act. Make sure you can describe them.

Source Analysis ▶

1 What impression of the New Deal does Source 10 attempt to convey?
2 Why do you think Roosevelt wanted artists and photographers to be employed under the New Deal?

Opposition to the New Deal

A programme such as Roosevelt's New Deal was unheard of in American history. It was bound to attract opposition and it did.

Not enough!

A number of high-profile figures raised the complaint that the New Deal was not doing enough to help the poor. Despite the New Deal measures, many Americans remained desperately poor. The hardest hit were African Americans and the poor in farming areas.

A key figure in arguing on behalf of these people was Huey Long. Long became Governor of Louisiana in 1928 and a senator in 1932. His methods of gaining power were unusual and sometimes illegal (they included intimidation and bribery). However, once he had power he used it to help the poor. He taxed big corporations and businesses in Louisiana and used the money to build roads, schools and hospitals. He employed African Americans on the same terms as whites and clashed with the Ku Klux Klan. He supported the New Deal at first, but by 1934 he was criticising it for being too complicated and not doing enough. He put forward a scheme called Share Our Wealth. All personal fortunes would be reduced to $3 million maximum, and maximum income would be $1 million a year. Government taxes would be shared between all Americans. He also proposed pensions for everyone over 60, and free washing machines and radios. Long was an aggressive and forceful character with many friends and many enemies. Roosevelt regarded him as one of the two most dangerous men in the USA. Long was assassinated in 1935.

Dr Francis Townsend founded a number of Townsend Clubs to campaign for a pension of $200 per month for people over 60, providing that they spent it that month, which would stimulate the economy in the process. A Catholic priest, Father Coughlin, used his own radio programme to attack Roosevelt. He set up the National Union for Social Justice and it had a large membership.

Too much!

The New Deal soon came under fire from sections of the business community and from Republicans for doing too much. There was a long list of criticisms:

- The New Deal was complicated and there were too many codes and regulations.
- Government should not support trade unions and it should not support calls for higher wages – the market should deal with these issues.
- Schemes such as the TVA created unfair competition for private companies.
- The New Deal schemes were like the economic plans being carried out in the Communist USSR and unsuitable for the democratic, free-market USA.
- Roosevelt was behaving like a dictator.
- High taxes discouraged people from working hard and gave money to people for doing nothing or doing unnecessary jobs (see Source 11).

Roosevelt was upset by the criticisms, but also by the tactics used against him by big business and the Republicans. They used a smear campaign against him and all connected to him. They said that he was disabled because of a sexually transmitted disease rather than polio. Employers put messages into their workers' pay packets saying that New Deal Schemes would never happen. Roosevelt turned on these enemies bitterly (see Source 14). And it seemed the American people were with him. In the 1936 election, he won 27 million votes – with the highest margin of victory ever achieved by a US president. He was then able to joke triumphantly, 'Everyone is against the New Deal except the voters.'

Source Analysis

Study Sources 11, 12 and 13. How would the author of Source 11 react to Source 12 and how would he react to Source 13? Make sure you can explain your answer.

SOURCE 11

The New Deal is nothing more or less than an effort to take away from the thrifty what the thrifty and their ancestors have accumulated, or may accumulate, and give it to others who have not earned it and never will earn it, and thus to destroy the incentive for future accumulation. Such a purpose is in defiance of all the ideas upon which our civilisation has been founded.

A Republican opponent of the New Deal speaking in 1935.

Think!

Look at the criticisms of the New Deal (above right). Roosevelt's opponents were often accused of being selfish. How far do the criticisms support or contradict that view?

SOURCE 12

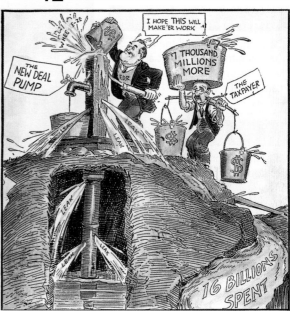

A cartoon published in an American newspaper in the mid 1930s.

SOURCE 13

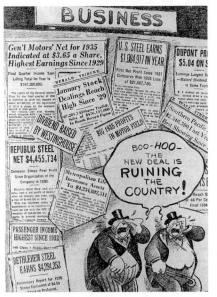

A 1930s cartoon attacking critics of the New Deal.

Source Analysis ▶

Look at Sources 15 and 16. One supports Roosevelt's actions and the other one doesn't. Explain which is which, and how you made your decision.

SOURCE 14

For twelve years this nation was afflicted with hear-nothing, see-nothing, do-nothing government. The nation looked to government but government looked away. Nine crazy years at the stock market and three long years in the bread-lines! Nine mad years of mirage and three long years of despair! Powerful influences strive today to restore that kind of government with its doctrine that government is best which is most indifferent . . . We know now that government by organised money is just as dangerous as government by organised mob. Never before in all our history have these forces been so united against one candidate – me – as they stand today. They are unanimous in their hate of me – and I welcome their hatred.

A speech by Roosevelt in the 1936 presidential election campaign.

Opposition from the Supreme Court

Roosevelt's problems were not over with the 1936 election. In fact, he now faced the most powerful opponent of the New Deal – the American Supreme Court. This Court was dominated by Republicans who were opposed to the New Deal. It could overturn laws if those laws were against the terms of the Constitution. In May 1935 a strange case had come before the US Supreme Court. The Schechter Poultry Corporation had been found guilty of breaking NRA regulations because it had: sold diseased chickens for human consumption; filed false sales claims (to make the company worth more); exploited workers; and threatened government inspectors.

It appealed to the Supreme Court. The Court ruled that the government had no right to prosecute the company. This was because the NRA was unconstitutional. It undermined too much of the power of the local states.

Roosevelt was angry that this group of old Republicans should deny democracy by throwing out laws that he had been elected to pass. He asked Congress to give him the power to appoint six more Supreme Court judges who were more sympathetic to the New Deal. But Roosevelt misjudged the mood of the American public. They were alarmed at what they saw as Roosevelt's attacking the American system of government. Roosevelt had to back down and his plan was rejected. Even so his actions were not completely pointless. The Supreme Court had been shaken by Roosevelt's actions and was less obstructive in the future. Most of the main measures in Roosevelt's Second New Deal were approved by the Court from 1937 onwards.

SOURCE 15

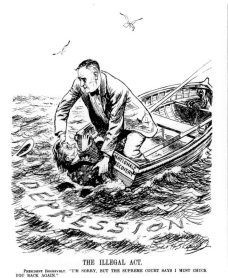

THE ILLEGAL ACT.
PRESIDENT ROOSEVELT. "I'M SORRY, BUT THE SUPREME COURT SAYS I MUST CHUCK YOU BACK AGAIN."

A *Punch* cartoon, June 1935.

SOURCE 16

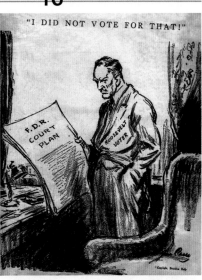

A cartoon from the *Brooklyn Daily Eagle*, February 1937.

Focus Task

Why did the New Deal encounter opposition?

The thought bubbles below show some of the reasons why people opposed the New Deal. Use the text and sources on these two pages to find examples of individuals who held each belief. Try to find two more reasons why people opposed the New Deal.

It won't work.

It'll harm me.

It'll harm the USA.

Focus Task A

How successful was the New Deal (1)?

-5 -4 -3 -2 -1 0 1 2 3 4 5

Failure is −5. Success is +5.

Pages 312–14 summarise the impact of the New Deal on various groups.

1 For each of the six aspects of the New Deal, decide where you would place it on the scale. Explain your score and support it with evidence from Chapter 10.4.

2 Compare your six 'marks' on the scale with those of someone else in your class.

3 Working together, try to come up with an agreed mark for the whole of the New Deal. You will have to think about the relative importance of different issues. For example, you might give more weight to a low mark in an important area than to a high mark in a less important area.

Verdicts on the New Deal

The events of 1936 took their toll on Roosevelt and he became more cautious after that. Early in 1937 prosperity seemed to be returning and Roosevelt did what all conservatives had wanted: he cut the New Deal budget. He laid off many workers who had been employed by the New Deal's own organisations and the cut in spending triggered other cuts throughout the economy. This meant that unemployment spiralled upwards once more.

The 1937 recession damaged Roosevelt badly. Middle-class voters lost some confidence in him. As a result, in 1938 the Republicans once again did well in the congressional elections. Now it was much harder for Roosevelt to push his reforms through Congress. However, he was still enormously popular with most ordinary Americans (he was elected again with a big majority in 1940). The problem was that the USA was no longer as united behind his New Deal as it had been in 1933. Indeed, by 1940 Roosevelt and most Americans were focusing more on the outbreak of war in Europe and on Japan's exploits in the Far East.

So was the New Deal a success? One of the reasons why this question is hard to answer is that you need to decide what Roosevelt was trying to achieve. We know that by 1940, unemployment was still high and the economy was certainly not booming. On the other hand, economic recovery was not Roosevelt's only aim. In fact it may not have been his main aim. Roosevelt and many of his advisers wanted to reform the USA's economy and society. So when you decide whether the New Deal was a success or not, you will have to decide what you think the aims of the New Deal were, as well as whether you think the aims were achieved.

Aspect 1: A new society?

SOURCE **17**

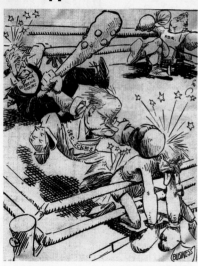

A 1937 cartoon from the *Portland Press Herald* showing Harold Ickes in conflict with big business.

- The New Deal restored the faith of the American people in their government.
- The New Deal was a huge social and economic programme. Government help on this scale would never have been possible before Roosevelt's time. It set the tone for future policies for government to help people.
- The New Deal handled billions of dollars of public money, but there were no corruption scandals. For example, the head of the Civil Works Administration, Harold Hopkins, distributed $10 billion in schemes and programmes, but never earned more than his salary of $15,000. The Secretary of the Interior, Harold Ickes, actually tapped the phones of his own employees to ensure there was no corruption. He also employed African Americans, campaigned against anti-semitism and supported the cause of native Americans.
- The New Deal divided the USA. Roosevelt and his officials were often accused of being Communists and of undermining American values. Ickes and Hopkins were both accused of being anti-business because they supported trade unions.
- The New Deal undermined local government.

Aspect 2: Industrial workers

- The NRA and Second New Deal strengthened the position of labour unions.
- Roosevelt's government generally tried to support unions and make large corporations negotiate with them.
- Some unions combined as the Committee for Industrial Organisation (CIO) in 1935 – large enough to bargain with big corporations.
- The Union of Automobile Workers (UAW) was recognised by the two most anti-union corporations: General Motors (after a major sit-in strike in 1936) and Ford (after a ballot in 1941).
- Big business remained immensely powerful in the USA despite being challenged by the government.
- Unions were still treated with suspicion by employers.
- Many strikes were broken up with brutal violence in the 1930s.
- Companies such as Ford, Republic Steel and Chrysler employed their own thugs or controlled local police forces.
- By the end of the 1930s there were over 7 million union members and unions became powerful after the war.

Aspect 3: Unemployment and the economy

SOURCE **18**

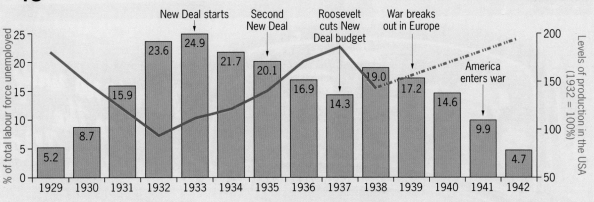

Unemployment, and the performance of the US economy during the 1930s.

- The New Deal created millions of jobs.
- It stabilised the American banking system.
- It cut the number of business failures.
- Projects such as the TVA brought work and an improved standard of living to deprived parts of the USA.
- New Deal projects provided the USA with valuable resources such as schools, roads and power stations.
- The New Deal never solved the underlying economic problems.

- The US economy took longer to recover than that of most European countries.
- Confidence remained low – throughout the 1930s Americans only spent and invested about 75 per cent of what they had before 1929.
- When Roosevelt cut the New Deal budget in 1937, the country went back into recession.
- There were six million unemployed in 1941.
- Only the USA's entry into the war brought an end to unemployment.

Aspect 4: African Americans

- Around 200,000 African Americans gained benefits from the Civilian Conservation Corps, other New Deal agencies, and relief programmes.
- Many African Americans benefited from New Deal slum clearance and housing projects.
- Some New Deal agencies discriminated against African Americans. There was racial segregation in the CCC. Mortgages were not given to black families in white neighbourhoods.
- More black workers were unemployed (35 per cent living on relief in 1935) but they were much less likely to be given jobs and the ones they did get were often menial.
- Domestic workers (the area in which many black women were employed) were not included in the Social Security Act.
- Roosevelt failed to put through any civil rights legislation, particularly laws against the lynching of African Americans. He feared that Democrat senators in the southern states would not support him.

Aspect 5: Women

- The New Deal saw some women achieve prominent positions. Eleanor Roosevelt became an important campaigner on social issues.
- Mary Macleod Bethune, an African American woman, headed the National Youth Administration.
- Frances Perkins was the Secretary of Labor. She removed 59 corrupt officials from the Labor Department and was a key figure in making the Second New Deal work in practice.
- Most of the New Deal programmes were aimed to help male manual workers rather than women (only about 8,000 women were involved in the CCC).
- Local governments tried to avoid paying out social security payments to women by introducing special qualifications and conditions.
- Frances Perkins was viciously attacked in the press as a Jew and a Soviet spy. Even her cabinet colleagues tended to ignore her at social gatherings.

Revision Tip

There is a lot happening on this page! When it comes to revision, choose two points from each aspect, one positive and one negative, and try to remember those.

Aspect 6: Native Americans

- The Indian Reorganisation Act 1934 provided money to help native Americans to buy and improve land and control their own tribal areas.
- The Indian Reservation Act 1934 helped native Americans to preserve and practise their traditions, laws and culture and develop their land as they chose.
- Native Americans remained a poor and excluded section of society.

SOURCE 20

African Americans queuing for government relief in 1937 in front of a famous government poster.

SOURCE 19

Many of Roosevelt's experiments were failures, but that is what experimentation entails. He would be satisfied he said if 75 per cent of them produced beneficial results. Experimentation depended on one of his distinctive characteristics: receptivity to new and untried methods and ideas.

Written by historian Samuel Rosemann.

Focus Task

How successful was the New Deal (2)?

This is a complicated question. You have already spent time thinking about it; now you are going to prepare to write an essay.

1 First recap some key points by answering these questions.

Roosevelt's aims	Unemployment and the economy
♦ What were Roosevelt's aims for the First New Deal? (see page 306) ♦ What new aims did the Second New Deal have? ♦ Which of these aims did Roosevelt succeed in? Which did he fail in?	♦ Why did unemployment remain high throughout the 1930s? ♦ Does this mean that Roosevelt's New Deal was not a success?
Opposition	*Criticisms and achievements*
♦ How far do you think opposition to the New Deal made it hard for the New Deal to work?	♦ Which criticism of the New Deal do you think is most serious? Why? ♦ Which achievement do you think is the most important? Why? ♦ Would Roosevelt have agreed with your choice? Why?

2 Now write your own balanced account of the successes and failures of the New Deal, reaching your own conclusion as to whether it was a success or not. Include:
 ♦ the nature and scale of the problem facing Roosevelt
 ♦ the action he took through the 1930s
 ♦ the impact of the New Deal on Americans
 ♦ the reasons for opposition to the New Deal
 ♦ your own judgement on its success.
Include evidence to back up your judgements.

Keywords

Make sure you know what these terms mean and are able to define them confidently.

- Competition
- Crash
- Credit
- Democrat
- Depression
- Flappers
- Hire purchase
- Hollywood
- Hooverville
- Hundred Days
- Jazz
- Ku Klux Klan
- Mail order
- Mass production
- NAACP
- New Deal
- Overproduction
- Prohibition
- Red Scare
- Repeal
- Republican
- Roaring Twenties
- Shares
- Speculation
- Stock market
- Supreme Court
- Tariff
- Temperance
- Tennessee Valley Authority

Key Question Summary

How successful was the New Deal?

1 Roosevelt's New Deal promised action to get industry and agriculture working, get Americans back to work and provide relief for those suffering from the Depression.

2 The first Hundred Days was a whirlwind of activity, putting into place a number of New Deal agencies to achieve his aims. These involved huge public works programmes, schemes to boost employment and measures to put agriculture and industry on a more sustainable basis. Millions of dollars were set aside for relief.

3 Roosevelt restored confidence in the banks and put financial bodies in America on a more stable footing.

4 He explained his actions to Americans and gave hope and optimism through his radio talks, 'fireside chats', to the nation.

5 The Tennessee Valley Authority was a special example of government planning across several states.

6 In 1935 Roosevelt introduced a Second New Deal, which was focused more on reform and creating a better life for ordinary Americans.

7 There was a lot of opposition to his policies from those who thought he was not doing enough to help and those who thought he was doing too much. Many thought that the New Deal was a huge waste of money and resources and was wrong in principle – it involved too much government interference and undermined American individualism and self-reliance.

8 The Supreme Court ruled some parts of the New Deal to be unconstitutional.

9 The American people re-elected Roosevelt in 1936 in a landslide victory.

10 The New Deal did not solve the underlying problems of the American economy or conquer unemployment. It was the Second World War which got it going again. Some groups in society did not do as well out of it as they might have hoped.

11 It did save the banking system, create millions of jobs and relieve the suffering of millions of Americans. It left much of lasting value, for example in roads, public buildings and schools. It set the tone for future government action in the USA.

Exam Practice

See pages 168–175 and pages 316–319 for advice on the different types of questions you might face.

1 (a) What was the Tennessee Valley Authority? **[4]**
  (b) Explain why Roosevelt introduced the Second New Deal in 1935. **[6]**
  (c) The New Deal was a failure. How far do you agree with this statement? Explain your answer. **[10]**

Component 3 or 4 questions

2 How important were Republican policies in the US economic boom of the 1920s?

3 How significant was the Second New Deal in helping the USA to recover from the Depression?

Paper 1: Depth Studies – Introduction

In your Paper 1 exam you will usually tackle two questions on the Core Content and one on your chosen Depth Study. The Depth Study questions are structured in the same way as the Core Content questions. We have analysed the types of question on pages 168–75 but in a nutshell they look like this:

There is a **source** or a **simple statement** to read or look at – however there are no questions on this, it is just to help you to focus your thinking about the topic. Then three parts:

a) a **knowledge** question worth 4 marks. This will often begin 'describe' or 'what'.
b) an **explanation** question worth 6 marks. This will often begin with 'explain' or 'why'.
c) an **evaluation** question worth 10 marks. You need to make a judgement (for example, agreeing or disagreeing with a statement) and back up your judgement with evidence and argument.

These questions should be tackled the same way as the questions on the interwar period, as we showed on pages 169–71.

A typical part (a) question

> **(a)** What were the main features of the Weimar constitution?

In a question like this, you should describe four features, such as Article 48, or the position of Chancellor.

A typical part (b) question

> **(b)** Why did Hitler become Chancellor in 1933?

Don't make the mistake of just describing the events of 1933. A good answer is likely to include longer-term factors such as the Depression or Nazi campaigning tactics, but would also need to show how what happened in 1933 finally gave Hitler the Chancellorship.

A typical part (c) question

> **(c)** 'Nazi education and youth policies were not effective in controlling young people'. How far do you agree with this statement?

This question is often answered badly because students simply list Nazi policies and don't explain whether or not they had the effect they intended. In a good answer you would be expected to:

- set out two to three events or developments and use them as evidence to support the argument that the Nazis were able to control young people
- set out two to three events or developments and use them as evidence to support the argument that Nazi policies failed.

We have worked through some examples for you on the following two pages.

> None of the answers on pages 317–318 is a real student answer. We have written them to help show the features.

Germany worked examples

There is nothing wrong with this response but it is far too long! Remember that this question is only worth 4 marks, so you should aim to make four points only, or two to three points with supporting detail.

(a) What methods did the Nazis use to control the population? **[4]**

The SS under Himmler were used to intimidate and terrorise people into obedience. There was also the Gestapo who were the secret police. They tapped telephones and spied on people. Political opponents were taken to concentration camps. Propaganda was also used to prevent opposition. This was the job of Goebbels who controlled what people read and heard. Newspapers were taken over or their content strictly controlled. Cheap radio sets were sold so people could hear Hitler's speeches.

This part of the answer correctly identifies a group who opposed the Nazis, but it is a bit vague in addressing the question of 'why'. It would be better to give specific examples such as the Communists had been targeted after the Reichstag Fire.

(b) Explain why some people opposed Nazi rule. **[6]**

The Communists opposed Nazi rule because of their political beliefs. Some youth groups such as the Edelweiss Pirates were anti-Nazi. They liked to listen to music and many gangs went looking for the Hitler Youth to beat them up. They sang songs but changed the lyrics to mock Germany.

The second part of this answer is only **describing** the youth opposition, rather than saying **why** people opposed the Nazis. With this example, the answer would need to explain how the popularity of youth groups fell as the war progressed because the activities were more focused on military drill and the war effort.

(c) 'The success of Nazi economic policy was more important than the police state in controlling opposition to the Nazis.' How far do you agree with this statement? Explain your answer. **[10]**

The Nazis' economic policies did help. They promised employment and did this through the development of public works such as the building of autobahns. Schemes like 'Strength Through Joy' gave workers cheap theatre and cinema tickets.

This answer starts well by addressing the question. It states clearly **why** economic policy helped to control opposition.

So some workers were won over by popular policies and this stopped opposition arising in the first place.

From 1935 conscription was applied and rearmament meant thousands of jobs in armament factories. So some people were scared of losing their jobs if they spoke out. Germany had been hit hard by the Depression and many were terrified of being out of work again.

This is the clinching bit that makes all the above supporting detail into an excellent **explanation**.

However, the police state was also important. The Nazis were very successful at getting rid of opposition. The SS went round terrorising people into obedience. It could arrest people without trial and put them into concentration camps where people were tortured or indoctrinated. The Gestapo spied on people. It had informers and encouraged people to inform on their neighbours and children on their families. It also tapped phones. The Germans thought the Gestapo was much more powerful than it actually was, so lots of people informed on each other purely because they thought the Gestapo would find out anyway.

Another reason that economic policy helped to stifle opposition here – again with a clear link back to the question. The answer goes on to examine the police state.

This is a very good example of showing how the two factors given are actually **linked** together. This is a valid way of **evaluating** reasons in a conclusion. The answer distinguishes between two types of opposition and shows how a different method was more successful for each.

In conclusion, I would say that economic successes were vital in controlling opposition amongst ordinary citizens but that the police state was also vital for dealing with the opposition when it did arise; the two actually worked together. The Nazis' main political opponents had been dealt with swiftly with the help of the SS and Gestapo, which left smaller pockets of opposition. Ordinary people with weaker political motivation were more easily won over by the Nazis' successes and the fear of losing their jobs.

Russia worked examples

318

(a) Describe the problems facing the Provisional Government after March 1917. **[4]**

> This is a very succinct response which is accurate and to the point.

The war effort was failing and some soldiers were deserting. The peasants were demanding land and some were starting to take it. The Bolsheviks had also started rioting after Lenin returned from exile. Workers in the cities were starving.

(b) Explain how Lenin secured the Bolsheviks' hold on power after the November Revolution of 1917. **[6]**

> These are all precise things that Lenin did, but haven't been explained to show how they were helping the Bolsheviks hold on to their power.

Lenin banned non-Bolshevik papers and set up the 'Cheka' secret police. The banks were placed under Bolshevik control.

> This is better because it is a much fuller explanation of how Lenin's actions were leading to the Bolsheviks' retention of power.

Lenin had promised free elections and these were held in late 1917. However, under the first democratic elections to the new Constituent Assembly, the Socialist Revolutionaries beat the Bolsheviks. This could have been the end of the Bolsheviks' power. However, Lenin simply sent the Red Guards to close down the assembly and to put down the protests against him.

> Another sound explanation, showing how Lenin was attempting to secure power through popularity with the people.

Finally, Lenin had to negotiate a peace treaty to end the war because he had promised the people 'bread, peace and land'. He hoped that this would increase the popularity of the Bolsheviks and they would stay in power.

(c) 'The main reason that the Reds won the Civil War was because the Whites were not unified.' How far do you agree with this statement? Explain your answer. **[10]**

> This is a full explanation of how the reason given in the statement led to Red success.

The success of the Reds was definitely helped by the lack of unity in their opposition. The Whites were made up of lots of different elements such as the Czech Legion, moderate socialists and ex-Tsarists. This meant they had different leaders and different objectives and therefore were not able to work together effectively. This allowed Trotsky to defeat them one by one.

> Remember that in this kind of question you need to identify and explain another reason, which has not been given in the statement. This answer has explained how War Communism was also a factor in the Reds' victory.

However, other things helped the Reds win the Civil War as well. For example, Lenin introduced War Communism. This system allowed Reds total control over people's lives and possessions in order to win the war. Ruthless discipline was introduced into the factories. Food was taken from peasant farmers by force in order to feed the Red Army and the workers in the cities. Strict rationing was introduced and the Cheka was used to terrify opponents. This policy ensured the Red Army was kept supplied and could continue to fight.

> The answer includes an attempted conclusion, but this is more of a summary. What you need to do here is to actively **compare** the factors, or to draw them together to show how they are **linked**. For example, you might say that although it was always going to be difficult for the Whites to win because they were such a broad alliance, it was the ruthless and harsh policy of War Communism, which determined that they were defeated by 1920 and that the Bolsheviks held onto their power so firmly.

I think that overall the Reds won because the Whites were not unified, which helped the Reds pick them off, and also because of War Communism, which allowed the Red Army to keep fighting.

Components 3 (coursework) and 4 (written paper alternative to coursework)

As well as Paper 1 and Paper 2, you have to tackle one more component. This is either coursework or a written paper. Whichever component you tackle the focus is on the significance of a given event, person or group.

If you are taking the coursework option your teacher will set and mark your question so it is difficult for us to offer very specific advice. However it will still focus on the same issue as the written paper, significance, so the following advice about the written alternative may still be useful.

Written paper alternative to coursework

Focus

In this paper you will be focusing on whichever Depth Study you have followed. There will be two questions and you have to choose one of them. The questions will ask you to make a judgement on how important or significant a particular event, person, group or development was. So you need to practise thinking about questions such as:

- How important was the Depression in explaining the failure of the League of Nations in the 1930s?
- How important was propaganda in maintaining Nazi control of Germany 1933–39?
- How significant was corruption in causing Prohibition to fail in the USA?
- How significant was Lenin in keeping the Bolsheviks in power in Russia after the 1917 revolution?

Your aims

A good answer to these questions will need to do the following things:

- **Make a strong case** that X (your given event, person or group) was or was not significant. You should aim to make a strong argument that focuses mostly on X.
- **Support your argument** by selecting relevant events **and** developments and explain how these events support the argument you are making.
- **Show you are aware of other factors** that you think are more/less significant than X. You should:
  - Explain why you think they are more or less significant than X.
  - Explain how they might be connected to X – how X and the other factors are interrelated (e.g. it could be that other factors created problems that gave an advantage to X)
- **Produce a well-argued conclusion** that sets out your view on the significance of X. This does **not** mean summarising the essay you have just written. It means saying that overall you think X was/was not the most significant factor and the reasoning which brought you to that conclusion (e.g. none of the other factors could have happened without X, or all the leading historians seem to argue X was not significant).

A possible approach

The important thing is to make up your mind on your key argument and then to use the rest of your research to support it. To help you think through the issue and reach a conclusion you could use a table like this.

Question	
...X was significant because:	**This mattered because:**

Question		
Other significant factors that played a part included	**This mattered because**	**More/less important than X because**

Here is an example of how you could begin to fill it out to analyse the following question about Lenin.

How significant was Lenin in keeping the Bolsheviks in power in Russia after the 1917 revolution?	
He was very significant because:	**This mattered because:**
He was the driving force behind the Bolshevik Party.	The Bolsheviks could not have taken and held power if they were not united and disciplined. No other Bolshevik leader had Lenin's authority over the Party or his ruthlessness.
He passed a range of decrees in 1917 including giving the land to the peasants, limiting working hours and banning opposition newspapers.	The land decree gained support for the Bolsheviks from the peasants and the working hours decrees gained support from the workers. Shutting down newspapers weakened Lenin's opponents.
Other points ...	

Other significant factors that played a part included	**This mattered because**	**More/less important than Lenin because**
Actions of Trotsky	He organised the Red Army which eventually defeated the Whites in the Civil War which saved the Bolsheviks.	
Weaknesses of Whites		

And remember...

Significance or importance is difficult to assess. These ideas might help you as you plan your argument.

- Did X bring about change in the way people acted?
- Did X change people's ideas and or beliefs?
- Did X force authorities (governments, monarchs, police forces, etc.) to change?
- Was the impact of X long lasting or short term?
- Did X have a major impact on people's lives? How many lives? For how long?
- If you remove X how far to you think events would have been different?

Glossary

Abyssinian crisis International tensions resulting from invasion of Abyssinia (present day Ethiopia) by Italy in 1935.

Agent Orange Poisonous chemical used by US forces in Vietnam to defoliate (remove leaves) from forest areas to deprive enemy of cover.

Alliance Arrangement between two countries to help or defend each other, usually in trade or war.

Anschluss Joining of Austria and Germany as one state – forbidden by Treaty of Versailles 1919 but carried out by Hitler in 1938.

Anti-Comintern Pact Alliance between Germany, Italy and Japan in 1936 to combat spread of Communism.

Appeasement Policy of Britain and France in 1930s allowing Hitler to break terms of Treaty of Versailles.

Arab nationalism Movement of Arab peoples in the Middle East to join together to resist outside influence and to oppose Israel in particular.

Armistice End to fighting.

Arms race Competition to build stockpiles of weapons

Article 10 Article of League of Nations Covenant which promised security to League members from attack by other states.

Assembly Main forum of League of Nations for discussing important issues.

Atomic bomb/H bomb Nuclear weapons, only used in WW2 by USA against Japan but a constant threat in the Cold War.

Autobahn High speed motorways built by the Nazis in Germany in the 1930s to create jobs.

Ayatollah A senior Muslim cleric

Baath Party Sunni Muslim political movement, most prominent in Iraq from 1960s. Strongly opposed to external interference in Arab world.

Bauhaus German design movement incorporating sleek lines and modern materials.

Bay of Pigs Bay in Cuba, scene of disastrous attempt by Cuban exiles to overthrow Fidel Castro. Caused humiliation for USA which backed the attack.

Beauty of Labour Nazi movement to improve conditions for industrial workers and try to win their support.

Berlin airlift Operation in 1948–49 using aircraft to transport supplies to West Berlin which had been cut off by USSR.

Berlin Blockade Action by USSR to cut road, rail and canal links between West Berlin and the rest of Germany. Aim was to force USA and allies to withdraw from West Berlin.

Berlin Wall Barrier constructed by Communist East German government to block movement between East and West Berlin. As well as a Wall there were fences, dogs and armed guards.

Big Three (1) Three main leaders at Versailles Peace Conference 1919 – Lloyd George (Britain); Wilson (USA); Clemenceau (France). (2) Leaders at Yalta and Potsdam Conferences 1945 – Roosevelt/Truman (USA); Churchill/Atlee (Britain); Stalin (USSR)

Blockade Tactic involving cutting off supplies to a city or country. Usually by sea but can also be land or air blockade.

Bolshevik/Bolshevism Russian political movement led by Lenin and following Communist ideas developed by Karl Marx and further developed by Lenin.

Brezhnev Doctrine Policy of USSR from 1968 which effectively meant no Eastern European states would be allowed to have a non-Communist government.

Budget The spending plans of a government. Can refer to a particular policy or the whole government spending plan.

Capitalism/Capitalist Political, social and economic system centred on democracy and individual freedoms such as free speech, political beliefs and freedom to do business.

Censorship System of controlling information to the public, usually employed by governments. Can refer to paper, radio, TV or online information.

CENTO Central Treaty Organisation – alliance of countries including Britain, Turkey and Pakistan designed to resist spread of Communism.

Checkpoint Charlie Most famous point where travel between Communist East Berlin and US controlled West Berlin was possible.

Chemical weapons Usually refers to weapons which employ poisonous gas to kill enemies.

CIA The Central Intelligence Agency is a US government department, formed in 1947, that gathers information (intelligence) about threats to the USA but which also funds direct action (such as the Bay of Pigs invasion) to support American foreign policy.

Civil War War between two sides within the same nation or group. Examples in Russia 1919–21 and Spain 1936–37.

Co-existence Living side by side without threatening the other side. Most famously put forward by Soviet leader Khrushchev when he proposed East and West could live in peaceful co-existence.

co-operation Working together – could be political, economic or legal

Cold War Conflict which ran from c1946 to 1989 between the USA and the USSR and their various allies. They never fought each other but used propaganda, spying and similar methods against other. Also sponsored other countries in regional wars.

Collective security Key principle of the League of Nations, that all members could expect to be secure because the other members of the League would defend them from attack.

Collectivisation Policy to modernise agriculture in the USSR 1928–40. Succeeded in modernising farming to some extent but with terrible human cost.

Comecon Organisation to control economic planning in Communist countries of Eastern Europe.

Cominform Organisation to spread Communist ideas and also make sure Communist states followed ideas of Communism practiced in USSR.

Commissions Organisations set up by the League of Nations to tackle economic, social and health problems.

Communism/Communist Political, economic and social system involving state control of economy and less emphasis on individual rights than Capitalism.

Communist bloc Eastern European states controlled by Communist governments from end of WW2 to 1989.

Competition Pressure from rivals, usually in business and often rivals in other countries.

Concentration camps Camps used by Nazis to hold political opponents in Germany.

Conference of Ambassadors Organisation involving Britain, France, Italy and Japan which met to sort out international disputes. Worked alongside League of Nations.

Conscription Compulsory service in the armed forces.

320

Consolidation   Making a position more secure, usually when a political party has just taken power.

Containment   US policy in Cold War to stop spread of Communism.

Conventional weapons   Non-nuclear weapons. Can refer to ground, air or sea including missiles.

Cossack   Elite troops of the Russian Tsars.

Council   Influential body within the League of Nations which contained the most powerful members of the League.

Coup   Revolution.

Covenant   Agreement or set of rules.

Crash   Collapse in value of US economy in 1929 which led to economic depression in 1930s.

Credit   Borrowing money, usually from a bank.

De-Stalinisation   Policy of Soviet leader Khrushchev in 1950s moving away from policies of Stalin.

Demilitarised zone   Area of land where troops cannot be stationed, e.g. Rhineland area of Germany after WW1.

Democracy   Political system in which population votes for its government in elections held on a regular basis.

Democrat   Member of one of the main US political parties.

Depression   Period of economic hardship in which trade is poor and usually leading to problems such as unemployment and possibly political unrest.

Dictator   Leader of a state who has total control and does not have to listen to opponents or face elections.

Dictatorship   System in which one person runs a country.

Diktat   Term used in Germany to describe the Treaty of Versailles because Germany had no say in the terms of the Treaty.

Diplomatic relations   How countries discuss issues with each other. Breaking off diplomatic relations can sometimes be a first step towards war.

Disarmament   Process of scrapping land, sea or air weapons.

Domino theory   Policy in which USA believed it had to stop countries becoming Communist otherwise they would fall to Communism like dominoes.

Draft   US term for compulsory military service.

Duma   Russian Parliament established after 1905 revolution in Russia and a source of opposition to Tsar 1905–17.

Ebert   President of Germany 1919–25. He was the first democratically elected President.

Economic depression   Period of economic downturn where trade between countries and inside countries declines, often leading to unemployment.

Edelweiss Pirates   Youth groups in Germany who opposed Nazis, especially in war years.

Final Solution   Nazi plan to exterminate the Jews and other races in Europe. Generally thought to have begun in 1942.

Five-Year Plan   Programme of economic development in the USSR from 1928 onwards. Achieved considerable progress in industry but with heavy human cost.

Flappers   Young women in 1920s, especially USA, who had greater freedom than previously because of job opportunities and changing attitudes.

Fourteen Points   Key Points set out by US President Woodrow Wilson for negotiating peace at end of WW1.

Free trade   Policy of trading between countries with no tariffs or duties, aim was to increase trade.

Freedom of speech   Ability to publish or speak any religious or political view without being arrested.

Freikorps   Ex-soldiers in Germany after WW1.

General strike   Large scale, co-ordinated strike by workers designed to stop essential services like power, transport etc.

Gestapo   Secret police in Nazi Germany.

Glasnost   Openness and transparency – policy of Soviet leader Mikhail Gorbachev in 1980s designed to allow people to have their views heard and criticise the government.

Guerrilla warfare   Type of warfare which avoids large scale battles and relies on hit and run raids

Hindsight   Looking back on historical events with the ability to see what happened since.

Hire purchase   System of buying goods in instalments so they could be enjoyed straight away.

Hitler Youth   Youth organisation in Nazi Germany designed to prepare young people for war and make them loyal Nazis.

Ho Chi Minh Trail   Route in Cambodia used by North Vietnamese and Viet Cong forces to supply forces fighting South Vietnamese and US forces.

Hollywood   Suburb of Los Angeles, home of the US film industry.

Holocaust   The mass murder of Jews and other racial groups by the Nazis in WW2.

Hooverville   Shanty town made up of temporary shacks, common in the economic depression of the 1930s in the USA and named after President Hoover.

Hundred Days   The initial period of President FD Roosevelt in 1933 in which he passed a huge range of measures to help bring economic recovery.

Hyperinflation   Process of money becoming worthless, most notable instance was in Germany in 1923.

ICBM   Inter Continental Ballistic Missile – nuclear missiles capable of travelling through space and almost impossible to stop.

idealist   Person motivated by particular beliefs e.g. commitment to right of peoples to rule themselves.

Indochina   Former name for Vietnam.

Inflation   Rising prices .

Intelligence (as in CIA)   Secret services of states e.g. CIA in USA or KGB in USSR.

Iron curtain   Term used by Churchill in 1946 to describe separation of Eastern and Western Europe into Communist and non-Communist blocs.

Isolationism   Policy in the USA in the 1920s which argued USA should not get involved in international disputes.

Jazz   Type of music which became extremely popular from 1920s, generally associated with African American musicians.

Kapp Putsch   Attempt to overthrow democratically elected government in Germany in 1920.

Kerensky   Leader of the Provisional Government which governed Russia after first revolution in 1917.

Ku Klux Klan   Secret Society in USA which aimed to keep white supremacy in USA and terrorised African Americans and other groups.

Landlord/peasant   Key figures in farming, particularly in Russia c.1900. Landlords owned land but also maintained Tsar's authority. Peasants worked for the landlords.

League of German Maidens   Organisation in Nazi Germany for girls designed to get girls to embrace Nazi beliefs and values.

League of Nations   Organisation set up to manage international disputes and prevent wars after WW1. Brainchild of US President Woodrow Wilson.

Lebensraum   Living Space – became part of Hitler's plans to conquer and empire for Germany in the 1930s.

Left-wing   Groups or individuals whose political beliefs are rooted in Socialism or Communism.

Lenin   Leader of the Bolshevik/Communist Party in Russia and a key figure in bringing them to power in 1917 and keeping power until his death in 1924.

MAD   Mutually Assured Destruction – the idea that no state would ever use nuclear weapons because they would themselves be destroyed by retaliation.

Mail order   Popular type of shopping in USA in 1920s, customers ordered from catalogues.

Manchurian crisis   International crisis sparked off when Japan invaded the Chinese province of Manchuria in 1931. Despite investigating, League of Nations failed to stop Japanese aggression.

Mandates   System by which Britain and France took control of territories ruled by Germany and Turkey which had been on the losing side in WW1.

Marshall Aid   Programme of US economic aid to Western Europe from 1947–51. Aim was to aid economic recovery but also to prevent more states becoming Communist.

Marshall Plan   Plan behind Marshall Aid. Although it was an economic programme it was also political. Some commentators argued it was an economic form of imperialism designed to allow the USA to dominate Western Europe.

Martial law   Rule by the military rather than a civil police force.

Martyr   Person who dies for a cause he or she believes in.

Marxist   Person who follows ideas of Karl Marx, a political commentator who believed that societies would eventually become Communist as workers overthrew bosses and took control of wealth and power.

Mass production   System of producing goods in factories using production lines in which workers specialised in one task. Made production quick and efficient and relatively cheap.

Mein Kampf   'My Struggle': the autobiography of Adolf Hitler in which he set out his theories about power and racial superiority.

Mensheviks   Opposition party in Russia in early 1900s, part of the Social Democratic Party before it split into Bolsheviks and Mensheviks.

Military force   Use of armed force (e.g. troops, bombing by aircraft) as opposed to political or economic methods.

Missile gap   Term to describe the alleged advantage of the USSR over the USA in nuclear missiles. Historians doubt whether the missile gap was as real as was claimed.

Mobilised   Armed forces told to prepare for war.

Moral condemnation   Criticism of a state for actions against another state – prelude to stronger action such as economic sanctions or military force.

Mullah   A man or woman well educated in the Islamic religion, often a term used to describe Islamic clergy.

Multi-national force   Force made up of more than one state. Often a political devise to make it appear that a policy is not driven by one state e.g. UN intervention in the Korean War in 1950 or the Gulf Wars of the 1990s.

Munich Agreement   Agreement in October 1938 in which Britain and France agreed to Hitler's demands to control the Sudetenland area of Czechoslovakia. This is generally seen as the final stage of the policy of Appeasement.

NAACP   National Association for the Advancement of Coloured people – organisation whose aim was to promote and support the cause of African Americans in the USA in the 1920s and 1930s.

Napalm   Highly explosive chemical weapon which spread a fireball over a large area. Used extensively in Vietnam war.

National Community   Key idea of Nazis in Germany in the 1930s – they wanted people to become part of and promote a 'National Community'.

Nationalism   Strong sense of pride in your own country, sometimes directed aggressively towards other countries or minority groups.

Nationalities   Racial groups within larger states e.g. Poles in the Russian Empire or Hungarians in the Austrian Empire.

NATO   North Atlantic Treaty Organisation: Alliance formed by USA and other western states which promised to defend members against any attack, particularly from the USSR.

Nazism   National Socialism, the political belief of Adolf Hitler and the Nazi party based on aggressive expansion of German lands and the superiority of the Aryan race.

Nazi–Soviet Pact   Agreement in 1939 between Hitler and Stalin to not attack each other and to divide Poland between them.

Negative cohesion   Term coined by historian Gordon Craig to describe the way different groups in Germany supported the Nazis not because they supported the Nazis but because they feared the opponents of the Nazis (particularly the Communists) more.

New Deal   Policies introduced by US President Roosevelt from 1933 onwards to try to tackle US economic problems.

New Economic Policy   Policy introduced by Lenin in the USSR after the Russian Civil War. Basically allowed limited amounts of private enterprise which went against Communist theory but was an emergency measure to help economy recover from war.

NKVD   Secret Police in USSR, later became KGB.

Nobel Peace Prize   Prize awarded to politicians who have made major contribution to bringing end to a conflict.

Normalcy   Term used by US President Warren Harding in the 1920s to describe return to normal life after WW1.

November Criminals   The German politicians who signed the Treaty of Versailles. This was a term of abuse exploited by extreme parties in Germany, especially the Nazis, to undermine democracy.

Nuclear deterrent   Term which referred to the nuclear weapons owned by each side in the Cold War. The fact that each side had these weapons stopped the other side from using theirs.

Nuremberg Laws   Series of laws passed in Germany in 1935 discriminating against Jews and other racial groups in Germany.

Okhrana   Secret police force of the Russian Tsars.

One-party state   State where only one political party is permitted by law such as Nazi Germany or the USSR under Communism.

Operation Rolling Thunder   Huge scale bombing campaign by USA against North Vietnam during Vietnam War.

Overproduction   Usually in agriculture – growing too much food so that demand is filled and prices fall.

Paris Peace Conference   Conference which ran from 1919-23 to decide how to officially end WW1. Resulted in Treaty of Versailles with Germany and three other treaties.

Peasants   Poor farmers who worked their own small plots of land and usually had to work the lands of landlords as well.

People power   Term to describe the rise of popular action against Communist regimes in 1989 which contributed to fall of Communism.

Perestroika   Restructuring – the idea of Soviet leader Mikhail Gorbachev in the later 1980s that the USSR needed to reform.

Polish Corridor   Strip of land which under the Treaty of Versailles 1919 gave Poland access to the sea but separated East Prussia from the rest of Germany.

Politburo   Main decision making group of the Communist Party in USSR, similar to British Cabinet.

Potsdam Conference   Conference held in August 1945 between President Truman (USA), Stalin (USSR) and Churchill, then Atlee (Britain). Discussed major issues including the Atomic Bomb and Soviet takeover of Eastern Europe.

Prague Spring   Reform movement in Czechoslovakia to change Communist rule in Czechoslovakia, eventually crushed by Soviet forces.

Prohibition   Amendment to US constitution passed in 1919 to ban production of alcohol.

Propaganda   Method of winning over a population to a particular idea or set of beliefs. Also used in wartime to raise morale.

Provisional Government   Government headed by Alexander Kerensky which took control of Russia after the March 1917 revolution which overthrew the Tsar.

Public opinion   View of majority or large section of population on an issue, most important in democracies where politicians often have to win over public opinion.

Purges   Policy pursued by Stalin in USSR in 1930s to remove potential opponents. Involved arrests, torture, show trials, deportations to labour camps and executions.

Putsch   Revolt designed to overthrow the existing government, most commonly associated with Kapp Putsch in 1920 and Nazis' attempted Putsch in Munich in 1923.

Radical   Term used to describe extreme political views.

Realist   Politician who accepts a particular course of action even though it is not what they would prefer to do.

Rearmament   Building up arms and armed forces, used as a means to fight unemployment by many states in the 1930s, including Nazi Germany and Britain.

Red Army   Armed forces of the Communists in the Russian Civil War 1918–21 and then the official forces of the Soviet Union.

Red Scare   Wave of fear about Communist infiltration of American political and social life to undermine it. Seen in the 1920s and also the 1940s and 1950s.

Remilitarisation   Reintroduction of armed forces into the Rhineland area of Germany 1936 even though this was banned by the Treaty of Versailles

Reparations   Compensation to be paid by Germany to France, Belgium, Britain and other states as a result of the First World War.

Repeal   The overturning of a law.

Republican   One of the two main political parties in the USA.

Reunification   Bringing back together of Germany in 1990 after it had been divided in 1945.

Rhineland   Area of Germany which bordered France. Under Treaty of Versailles it was demilitarised – no German forces were allowed there.

Right-wing   Political groups or individuals with beliefs usually in national pride, authoritarian government and opposed to Communism.

Roaring Twenties   Refers to 1920s in USA, a period of major social and economic change for many Americans.

Ruhr   Main industrial area of Germany.

Saar   Region on the border between France and Germany. Run by League of Nations from 1920 to 1935 when its people voted to become part of Germany.

Sanctions   Actions taken against states which break international law, most commonly economic sanctions e.g. refusing to supply oil.

Satellite state   State which is controlled by a larger state e.g. Eastern European states controlled by USSR after WW2

Search and destroy   Type of tactic used by US military in Vietnam to locate Vietcong fighters and kill them.

SEATO   South East Asia Treaty Organisation – alliance formed in 1954 designed mainly to block the spread of Communism.

Secret police   Police force specialising in dealing with threats to the state e.g. political opponents rather than normal crimes.

secret treaties   Agreements between states which were not made public and therefore led to suspicions from other states. A contributing factor to outbreak of WW1.

Secretariat   The section of the League of Nations which carried out administrative tasks and also the agencies of the League.

Self-determination   The right of nations to rule themselves rather than be part of larger empires.

Shares   System which allows large or small investors to own part of a company and get a share of its profits.

Shia (Shiite)   One of the main branches of the Muslim faith.

Show trials   Trials of political opponents which were given great publicity – most prominent in the USSR under Stalin in the 1930s.

Social Democratic Party   Main left wing (and generally most popular) political party in Germany in the 1920s and 1930s. Eventually banned by the Nazis when they came to power in 1933.

Socialism   Political system in which government takes strong control of economic and social life. In theory socialist societies would eventually become Communist societies.

Socialist Revolutionaries   Opposition group in Tsarist Russia, the most well supported group as they had the support of the peasants.

Solidarity   Polish trade union which emerged in the 1980s and opposed the Communist government there.

Soviet republics   The various smaller states which made up the USSR.

Soviet sphere of influence   Terms agreed at Yalta Conference in 1945 – Western powers agreed that Poland and other parts of Eastern Europe would be under Soviet influence.

Soviet Union   The former Russian empire after it became a Communist state in the 1920s.

Soviets   Councils of workers.

Spanish Civil War   Conflict in Spain which was seen as a rehearsal for WW2 when German and Italian forces intervened to support General Franco.

Spartacists   Communists in Germany in 1919 who wanted a revolution in Germany similar to the 1917 revolution in Russia.

Speculation   Buying shares in the hope that their price will rise when they can be sold at a profit.

SA   The Brownshirts – stormtroopers of the Nazi party

SS   Organisation within the Nazi party which began as Hitler's bodyguard but expanded to become a state within a state

Stalin   Leader of the USSR from 1929 to his death in 1953.

Stock market   Trading arena where investors can buy and sell shares in companies

Stolypin   Minister of the Tsar in imperial Russia.

Strength Through Joy   Leisure programme run by the Nazis in Germany to improve lives of ordinary people.

Sudetenland   Area of Czechoslovakia which bordered Germany and contained many German speakers. Taken over by Hitler in 1938 as part of the Munich Agreement.

Summit meeting   Meeting of leaders to discuss key issues e.g. US President Reagan and Soviet leader Gorbachev meetings in the 1980s.

Sunni   One of the main branches of the Muslim faith.

Superpower   A country in a dominant international position that is able to influence events.

Supreme Court   Highest court in the US, whose job was to rule if laws passed by the government were challenged as being unconstitutional.

Surveillance   Watching, usually by intelligence agencies or secret police.

Tariff/Tariffs   Taxes on imported goods which made them more expensive – often designed to protect makers of home produced goods.

Temperance   Movement which opposed alcohol.

Tennessee Valley Authority   Organisation set up by President Roosevelt to help provide economic development in the Tennessee Valley. Most famous projects were giant hydroelectric dams.

Tet Offensive   Attack launched by Vietcong and North Vietnamese forces in 1968. Seen by many as turning point in Vietnam War as US public turned against the war.

Trade sanctions   Restricting sale of goods to a nation or sales from a nation.

Trade union   Organisation which represents workers.

Treaty of Brest-Litovsk   Treaty between Germany and Russia in 1918 which ended war between the two. Germany took massive amounts of land and reparations.

Treaty of Versailles   Treaty which officially ended war between Allies and Germany in 1919. Controversial because of the terms which Germany claimed to be excessively harsh.

Trotsky   Leading figure in the Bolshevik Party, especially in the Russian Civil War 1918–21.

Truman Doctrine   Policy of US President Truman from 1947 to promise to help any state threatened by Communism.

Tsar   Ruler of Russia up until revolution in 1917.

Tsarina   Wife of Tsar.

Unanimous   Agreed by all.

United Nations   Organisation which succeeded League of Nations in 1945 and whose aim was to solve international disputes as well as promoting humanitarian causes.

US sphere of influence   Areas seen as under the control or political or economic influence of the USA.

USSR   The former Russian empire after it became a Communist state in the 1920s.

Viet Cong / Viet Minh   Underground army fighting against French rule in the 1950s and then government of South Vietnam and its US allies in Vietnam War.

Vietnamisation   Policy of handing over Vietnam War to South Vietnam forces.

Wall Street Crash   Collapse in value of US companies in October 1929 which led to widespread economic collapse.

War Communism   Policy pursued by Communist leader Lenin 1918–21 to try to build Communist society in Russia and also fight against his opponents. Caused major hardships and had to be temporarily replaced with New Economic Policy.

War guilt   Clause in Treaty of Versailles which forces Germany to accept blame for WW1.

Warsaw Pact   Alliance of USSR and Eastern European states to defend against attack and preserve Communist control in Eastern Europe.

West/Western Powers   Term generally used to refer to USA and its allies in the Cold War.

WMD (Weapons of Mass Destruction)   Missiles, bombs or shells which were armed with chemical, biological or nuclear weapons.

Yalta Conference   Conference between USA, USSR and Britain in 1945 to decide the shape of the world after WW2 ended.

Young Plan   American economic plan in 1929 to reorganise reparations payments to make it easier for Germany to pay.

Zemstva   Local councils in Tsarist Russia.

Photo acknowledgements

p.iii *t* © Bettmann/Corbis, *b* © Popperfoto/Getty Images; **pp.1, 2** © Bettmann/Corbis; **p.4** © Punch Limited; **p.6** © Hulton Archive: Getty Images; **p.7** © Solo Syndication/Associated Newspapers Ltd. Photo: British Cartoon Archive; **p.8** © Hulton Archive/Getty Images; **p.9** © Hulton Archive/Getty Images; **p.10** © Illustrated London News Ltd/Mary Evans Picture Library; **p.15** © Mary Evans Picture Library; **p.16** Cartoon by Will Dyson published by Daily Herald on 13 May 1919, British Cartoon Archive, University of Kent; **p.17** © Punch Limited/TopFoto; **p.22** © United Nations Library Geneva; **p.24** © Express Newspapers, London; **p.25** *l* © Punch Limited/TopFoto; **p.26** © The British Library. All rights reserved. *Star* 11/06/1919; **p.27** © Punch Limited/TopFoto; **p.28** *l* © United Nations Library Geneva *r* © FORGET Patrick/SAGAPOTO.com/Alamy; **p.34** © Punch Limited; **p.36** © Punch Limited; **p.41** © Solo Syndication/Associated Newspapers Ltd.; **p.43** © Solo Syndication/Associated Newspapers Ltd.; **p.45** © Punch Limited/TopFoto; **p.46** © Bildarchiv Preussischer Kulturbesitz; **p.47** © Punch Limited/TopFoto; **p.50** © Solo Syndication/Associated Newspapers Ltd. Photo: John Frost Historical Newspapers; **p.55** *t* © AKG London, *b* Cartoon by David Low, the Evening Standard 18 January 1935 © Solo Syndication/Associated Newspapers Ltd. Photo: British Cartoon Archive; **p.56** *l* © Bruce Alexander Russell, *r* © The Art Archive; **p.57** © Punch Limited/TopFoto; **p.58** © Topham Picturepoint/TopFoto; **p.59** *l* © Punch Limited/TopFoto; **p.61** © Solo Syndication/Associated Newspapers Ltd.; **p.63** *r* © Topham Picturepoint/TopFoto; **p.63** *l* © Popperfoto/Getty Images; **p.64** © Punch Limited/TopFoto; **p.65** © 2006 Alinari/TopFoto; **p.66** © TopFoto; **p.74** © Bettmann/Corbis; **p.76** © Associated Press/Topham/TopFoto; **p.78** © Solo Syndication/Associated Newspapers Ltd.; **p.83** *l* © Solo Syndication/Associated Newspapers Ltd.; **p.87** *l* © Hulton Archive/Getty Images; **p.88** © dpa/Corbis; **p.89** © Solo Syndication/Associated Newspapers Ltd.; by permission of Llyfrgell Genedlaethol Cymru/The National Library of Wales; **p.91** © Solo Syndication/Associated Newspapers Ltd.; **p.97** © Solo Syndication/Associated Newspapers Ltd.; **p.98** © VintageCorner/Alamy; **p.99** © Picture Post/Getty Images; **p.106** © Cartoon by Victor Weisz, London Evening Standard, 24 October 1962, Solo Syndication/Associated Newspapers Ltd./British Cartoon Archive; **p.107** © Solo Syndication/Associated Newspapers Ltd.; **p.110** © Associated Press/Topham; **p.115** © Nguyen Kong (Nick) Ut/Associated Press; **p.116** © CBS Photo Archive/Getty images; **p.117** 1967 Herblock Cartoon © The Herb Block Foundation; **p.118** © Associated Press/Topham/TopFoto; **p.124** © Solo Syndication/Associated Newspapers Ltd.; **p.126** © Everett Collection/Rex Features; **p.129** © Hulton Archive/Getty Images; **p.131** *t* © Topham/AP/Topfoto, *b* © Josef Koudelka/Magnum Photos; **p.134** *tl* © Topham Picturepoint/Topfoto, *tr* © Popperfoto/Getty Images, *bl* © Rolls Press/Popperfoto/Getty Images; **p.136** © Getty Images; **p.138** © Paul Popper/Popperfoto/Getty; **p.141** © Pictorial Press Ltd/Alamy; **p.143** *t* Novosti/Topham/Topfoto, *b* © Atlantic Syndication; **p.146** © Punch Limited; **p.150** © Vienna Report Agency/Sygma/Corbis; **p.152** © 2005 Roger-Viollet/Topfoto; **p.153** © IRNA/AFP/Getty Images; **p.154** © Solo Syndication/Associated Newspapers Ltd.; by permission of Llyfrgell Genedlaethol Cymru/The National Library of Wales; **p.156** © Michel Setboun/Corbis; **p.157** © ullsteinbild/TopFoto; **p.159** © Kaveh Kazemi/Getty Images; **p.163** © Cartoon by Nicholas Garland, Independent 10th August 1990/British Cartoon Archive, University of Kent; **p.164** © Cartoon by Nicholas Garland, Daily Telegraph 8th March 1991/British Cartoon Archive, University of Kent; **p.165** © Punch Limited; **p.176** © Topham Picturepoint/TopFoto; **p.177** © News of the World/NI Syndication; **p.178** © Nguyen Kong (Nick) Ut/Associated Press; **p.179** 1967 Herblock Cartoon © The Herb Block Foundation; **p.180** © The British Library. All rights reserved. *Star* 11/06/1919; **p.181** © Punch Limited; **p.182** © Bettmann/Corbis; **p.185** © Popperfoto/Getty Images; **p.186** © David King Collection; **p.189** *t* © Illustrated London News, *b* © David King Collection; **p.191** © RIA Novosti/TopFoto; **p.192** © RIA Novosti/TopFoto; **p.193** © David King Collection; **p.195** © Mary Evans Picture Library; **p.200** © RIA Novosti/TopFoto; **p.202** © Library of Congress Prints and Photographs Division, LC-DIG-ggbain-30798; **p.203** © Illustrated London News; **p.206** © The British Library. All rights reserved. BL063554; **p.207** © Bolshevik cartoon on the intervention of the USA, Britain and France in the Russian Civil War, 1919 (colour litho), Russian School, (20th century)/Private Collection/Peter Newark Military Pictures/The Bridgeman Art Library; **p.208** © Hulton Archive/Getty Images; **p.211** © David King Collection; **p.213** © Illustrated London News; **p.215** © David King Collection; **p.217** © Topham Picturepoint/TopFoto; **p.220** *l* © RIA Novosti/TopFoto; **p.221** *l* © David King Collection; **p.226** © war posters/Alamy; **p.232** © Graphik: Landesarchiv Berlin/N.N; **p.233** *l* © Punch Limited, *r* © Ullsteinbild/Topfoto; **p.234** © Bettman/Corbis; **p.236** © Paramount Pictures/Getty Images; **p.238** © Bettmann/Corbis; **p.239** © Scherl / Süddeutsche Zeitung Photo; **p.241** © David Crausby/Alamy; **p.242** © Scherl / Süddeutsche Zeitung Photo; **p.243** *b* © Hulton Archive/Getty Images; **p.246** © Punch Limited; **p.249** © Bundesarchiv Koblenz, Photo 102-02920A; **p.250** *tl & bl* © Hulton Archive/Getty Images, *r* © Scherl / Süddeutsche Zeitung Photo; **p.251** © war posters/Alamy; **p.252** © Topham Picturepoint/TopFoto; **p.253** © The Wiener Library/Rex Features; **p.254** *l* © Photo12/UIG/Getty Images, *r* © Ullstein Bild/TopFoto; **p.258** © Scherl / Süddeutsche Zeitung Photo; **p.259** © Ben Walsh; **p.260** © Weimar Archive/Mary Evans Picture Library; **p.261** © Ullstein Bild/TopFoto; **p.262** © Feltz/Topham Picturepoint/TopFoto; **p.266** © Popperfoto/ Getty Images; **p.267** © Rue des Archives/ Süddeutsche Zeitung Photo; **p.268** © Elek International Rights, NY (photo: Wiener Library); **p.270** © Library of Congress Prints and Photographs Division; LC-DIG-fsa-8b29516; **p.276** *r* © Bettman/Corbis; **p.278** © Cartoon of the 1920s depicting the difficult times of the American Farmers (colour litho) by Fitzpatrick, Daniel Robert (1891–1969) Private Collection/Peter Newark American Pictures/The Bridgeman Art Library; **p.279** © Bettman/Corbis; **p.281** © *The Builder* (colour litho) by Beneker, Gerrit Albertus (1882–1934), Private Collection/Peter Newark American Pictures/The Bridgeman Art Library; **p.282** © The Granger Collection, NYC/TopFoto; **p.284** *t & b* © Bettmann/Corbis; **p.285** © Underwood & Underwood/Corbis; **p.287** © San Francisco Examiner; **p.288** © Mary Evans Picture Library; **p.289** *l* © Hulton Archive/Getty Images, *r* © Bettmann/Corbis; **p.290** © Bettmann/Corbis; **p.291** © US National Archives, Rocky Mountains Division; **p.293** *l* © 'Wanted … a little boy's plea', c. 1915 (engraving), American School, (20th Century), Private Collection/Peter Newark American Pictures/The Bridgeman Art Library, *r* © Culver Pictures; **p.294** © Bettman/Corbis; **p.295** *t* © Bettman/Corbis, *b* © Clive Weed, *Judge*, June 12, 1926—American Social History Project; **p.296** © Underwood Archives/Getty Images; **p.300** © Popperfoto/Getty Images; **p.301** Charles Deering McCormick Library of Special Collections, Northwestern University Library, © John T. McCutcheon Jr.; **p.302** © Car and farm machinery buried by dust and sand, Dallas, South Dakota, 1936 (b/w photo) by American Photographer (20th Century), Private Collection/Peter Newark American Pictures/The Bridgeman Art Library; **p.303** *t* © Topham Picturepoint/Topfoto, *b* © The Art Archive/Alamy; **p.304** *t* © 'Smilette', Democrat Election Poster, 1932 (litho) by American School (20th Century), Private Collection/Peter Newark American Pictures/The Bridgeman Art Library, *b* © Gabriel Hackett/Getty Images; **p.305** © Library of Congress Prints and Photographs Division; LC-USZ62-117121; **p.307** *tl & tr* © The Granger Collection, NYC / TopFoto, *br* © Tennessee Valley Authority; **p.309** *t* © Library of Congress Prints and Photographs Division; LC-DIG-fsa-8b29516, *b* © Photographs in the Carol M. Highsmith Archive, Library of Congress, Prints and Photographs Division; **p.310** © The Granger Collection, NYC / TopFoto; **p.311** *tl* © Weidenfeld and Nicolson Archives, a division of the Orion Publishing Group, London, *c* © Punch Limited; **p.314** © 'World's Highest Standard of Living…', 1937, 1937 (litho), American School, (20th Century)/ Private Collection/Peter Newark American Pictures/The Bridgeman Art Library.

b = bottom, *c* = centre, *t* = top, *l* = left, *r* = right

Index